Biomaterials for Women's Health Engineering

Samantha G. Zambuto • Michelle L. Oyen
Editors

Biomaterials for Women's Health Engineering

Springer

Editors
Samantha G. Zambuto
University of Kentucky
Lexington, KY, USA

Michelle L. Oyen
Wayne State University
Detroit, MO, USA

ISBN 978-3-032-10744-2   ISBN 978-3-032-10745-9 (eBook)
https://doi.org/10.1007/978-3-032-10745-9

This Springer imprint is published by the registered company Springer Nature Switzerland AG
The registered company address is: Gewerbestrasse 11, 6330 Cham, Switzerland

Preface

Women make up nearly half of the global population yet remain underrepresented in science and medicine. Although rapid progress and interest in women's health over the past decade have provided an influx of research studies and rapid establishment of FemTech (technology solutions focused on females across the lifespan) companies, additional expertise, funding, and time are required to advance more aspects of women's health. This book aims to provide a guide to existing studies in biomaterials for women's health engineering and to highlight future opportunities for growth in this space.

In this book, we define "women" as all people for whom the selected topics are relevant. We define "women's health" as conditions that affect women differently from men or conditions that affect only women. The selected women's health topics expand beyond reproduction, fertility, obstetrics, and gynecology, and cover other relevant tissue and organ systems, such as orthopedic tissues, bones, and aortic valves. We define "women's health engineering" as applying the principles of core engineering disciplines to topics in women's health.

All sections and chapters revolve around biomaterials. We define "biomaterials" as materials used in biological and medical applications to support, enhance, or replace damaged tissue or to interact with cells for basic science, translational, or clinical purposes. Many biomaterials are described in this book, including synthetic and natural materials created in labs or from natural sources (e.g., animals, organs, plants, etc.). Biomaterials represent powerful engineering technology that can be used for in vitro, in vivo, and clinical studies and allow for precise control over the chemical composition, three-dimensional architecture, and mechanical properties of engineered systems.

The book is split into seven major parts encompassing organ and tissue systems or engineering technology and is authored by leaders and rising stars in the field of engineering for women's health. The first half of the book explores the female reproductive system, including the vagina and pelvic floor, uterus and cervix, and ovaries. Next, biomaterials for and biomaterials from the placenta, a temporary organ that grows alongside the fetus during pregnancy, are described. The subsequent section describes key sex differences between males and females and the role of hormones in orthopedic tissues and aortic valves. The penultimate section highlights important considerations for drug delivery to the placenta, uterus, breast, and ovaries as well as therapeutic applications of nanotechnology and exomes in the context of women's health. The final part of the book highlights engineering technology that has the potential to transform the field of women's health engineering, including on-a-chip technology, 3D bioprinting, and systems biology.

We wrote this book because this is what we wished we had when we were first learning about women's health engineering: a guide of what we know and what we don't know about women's health and a map directing us where to go next. We hope that this book will inspire multidisciplinary approaches by diverse research teams to solve problems in women's health.

We stand on the shoulders of giants: we thank all who came before us who made this work possible, all who contributed to this work as mentors of the next generation, and all the future pupils of these subjects. We in the past look forward to your innovations in the future.

Lexington, KY, USA Samantha G. Zambuto

Contents

Engineering Vaginal Health: Biomechanics, Diagnostics, and Devices . . 3
Ritika Singh, Monique Vaughan, and Raffaella De Vita

Composition and Dynamics of the Vaginal Extracellular Matrix 35
Fatemeh Vahidi Zaman, Mari J. E. Domingo, Matthew A. Salinas, Maria E. Florian Rodriguez, Isaac J. Pence, and Kristin S. Miller

Vaginal Tissue Engineering: Biomaterial Strategies and Opportunities 59
Samantha G. Zambuto

Biomaterials for Prolapse Repair 71
Sophya Breedlove, Amanda Artsen, and Katrina Knight

The Structure and Function of the Uterus and Cervix Across the Reproductive Lifespan: Considerations for Biomaterial Design 121
Daniella M. Fodera and Erin M. Louwagie

Biomechanics of the Uterus and Cervix Across Pregnancy and Disease: Considerations for Biomaterial Design 149
Erin M. Louwagie and Daniella M. Fodera

Mechanobiology of the Uterus and Maternal Fetal Interface During Pregnancy 181
Cecelia E. Curtis, Jessica Terray, and Adrienne K. Scott

Myometrial Contractility and Uterine Peristalsis: Translating Biological Complexity into Bioengineered Systems 205
Karla I. Ortega Sandoval, Astha Lamichhane, Ritu Dave, Antonina I. Frolova, and Shreya A. Raghavan

Biomaterial Tools for Modeling Endometriosis 231
Hannah S. Theriault and Brendan A. C. Harley

Engineering Applications for In Vitro Ovarian Follicle Culture 259
Taylor Schissel, Emily E. Thomas, and Ariella Shikanov

Biomaterials to Facilitate Revascularization and Improve Outcomes of Ovarian Tissue Transplantation 277
Despina I. Pavlidis and Ariella Shikanov

Biomaterials Related to the Placenta 305
Michelle L. Oyen

The Placenta as a Biomaterial 323
Renata Dos Reis Marques and Marley J. Dewey

Sex Differences in Bone: Considerations for Biomaterial Design 365
Aleczandria Tiffany and Vasiliki Kolliopoulos

Hormonal and Pregnancy-Related Changes on Bone Mechanical Properties: Considerations for Biomaterial Design 393
Laura C. Bowman, Heather C. M. Allaway, Patricia K. Thomas, and Anthony G. Lau

Biomaterial Design to Interrogate Sex-Biased Effects and Deliver Sex Hormones for Therapeutic Treatments in Orthopedic Tissues 409
Jennifer L. Robinson

Sex-Based Insights into Aortic Valve Disease and Scaffold Design 433
Joshita Suresh, Nafeesah Ibrahim, and Kristyn S. Masters

Engineering Biomaterial-Based Drug Delivery Technologies to Interface with the Placenta During Pregnancy 461
Kelsey L. Swingle

Uterine Drug-Delivery Systems 487
Lauren E. Mehanna, Claire E. Rowlands, and Brittany E. Givens

Nanotechnological Approaches for Targeted Drug Delivery to Combat Breast and Ovarian Cancer 513
Vinitha Rani, Abdulla Obadat, Kyle Boyes, and Needa Brown

Therapeutic Applications of Exosomes for Women's Reproductive Health 531
Alexandra M. Harrison, Yuanxin Xu, Adelyn A. Fisher, and Christina M. Bailey-Hytholt

Organ-on-Chip Technology for Women's Health Engineering 555
Cristina I. Bonilla Carrillo and Samantha G. Zambuto

Advancing Reproductive Tissue Engineering with Bioprinting 577
Pei Wen Xiao and Kayla J. Wolf

Other Engineering Technologies: Systems Biology Approaches for Understanding Maternal–Neonatal Immunology 597
Caitlin M. Sullivan and Sepideh Dolatshahi

Index 627

Vagina and Pelvic Floor

Engineering Vaginal Health: Biomechanics, Diagnostics, and Devices

Ritika Singh, Monique Vaughan, and Raffaella De Vita

Abstract Women's health has long been underrepresented in scientific research and medical innovation, leading to misdiagnosis, inadequate treatment, and reduced quality of care. Policies mandating the inclusion of women in clinical studies have spurred progress, but advancing women's health requires far greater investment in research and technology. The rapid expansion of the FemTech sector in recent years presents unprecedented opportunities to develop tools specifically designed to enhance female reproductive health. This chapter provides an overview of technologies designed to interact with the vagina, a reproductive organ that has often been overlooked in scientific and medical research. After a brief introduction to vaginal biomechanics, diagnostic methods are surveyed, ranging from vaginally inserted devices to advanced imaging technologies. Scoring systems for assessing vaginal health and dysfunction are also presented. Therapeutic and supportive devices, including pelvic floor strengthening tools, vaginal dilators and stents, and surgical implants, are reviewed. By consolidating these diverse technologies, the chapter highlights the numerous opportunities for innovation within FemTech in advancing vaginal and women's health while guiding investigators seeking to contribute to this rapidly expanding area.

Keywords FemTech · Vagina · Pelvic floor · Biomechanics · In vivo mechanical testing · Diagnostic devices · Therapeutic devices · Vaginal health

---

R. Singh · R. De Vita (✉)
Department of Mechanical Engineering, Virginia Tech, Blacksburg, VA, USA
e-mail: ritikas@vt.edu; devita@vt.edu

M. Vaughan
Department of Obstetrics and Gynecology, University of Virginia School of Medicine, Charlottesville, VA, USA
e-mail: mv4w@uvahealth.org

S. G. Zambuto, M. L. Oyen (eds.), *Biomaterials for Women's Health Engineering*,
https://doi.org/10.1007/978-3-032-10745-9_1

1 Introduction

In recent years, female-focused health technology, or FemTech, has experienced an unprecedented surge in innovation and investment. McKinsey, a global management consulting firm, estimates the current market size of FemTech to range from $500 million to $1 billion, with forecasts suggesting opportunities for double-digit revenue growth in the coming years [42]. Grand View Research [28] a market research and consulting firm, projects that the global FemTech market will reach $97.25 billion by 2030, as seen in Fig. 1. This rapid growth reflects recognition of the need to address long-standing gaps in women's health, particularly in areas such as reproductive care, maternal health, and pelvic floor disorders.

As shown in Fig. 2, pregnancy accounts for the largest share of the FemTech industry, whereas areas such as pelvic and uterine care, sexual health, and menopause receive comparatively less investment and attention [25]. Funding often focuses on pregnancy, reproductive, and menstrual health because of their strong clinical translation potential and relevance to the majority of women. Consequently, FemTech innovation is concentrated in these areas, while other aspects of women's health remain underrepresented.

Despite the recent surge of interest, fundamental biomedical research on many aspects of women's health, including reproductive, pelvic, and sexual health, menopause, maternal care, and chronic conditions that disproportionately affect women, remains limited. This underrepresentation stems from the historical treatment of the

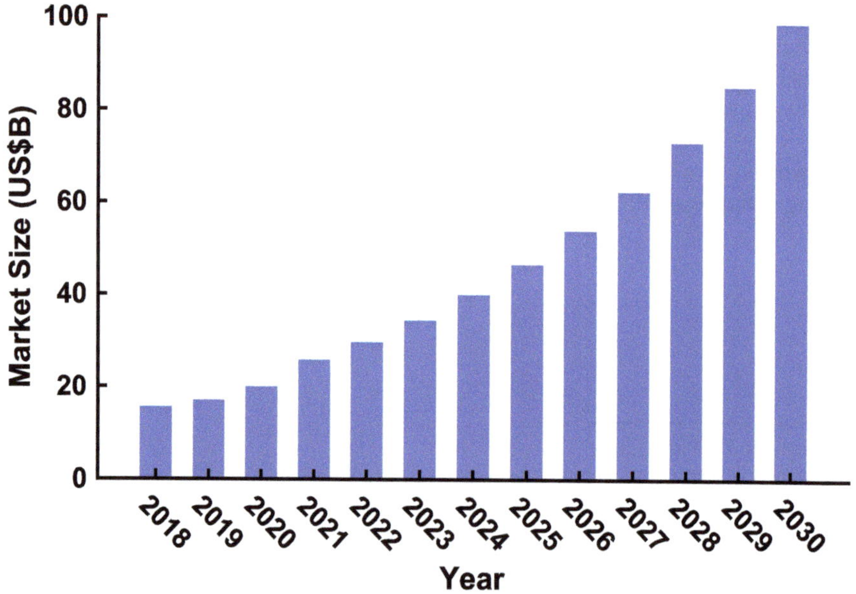

Fig. 1 Global FemTech market size (2018–2030) in billions of dollars, with projections based on an average compound annual growth rate (CAGR) of 16.37% (Adapted from [28])

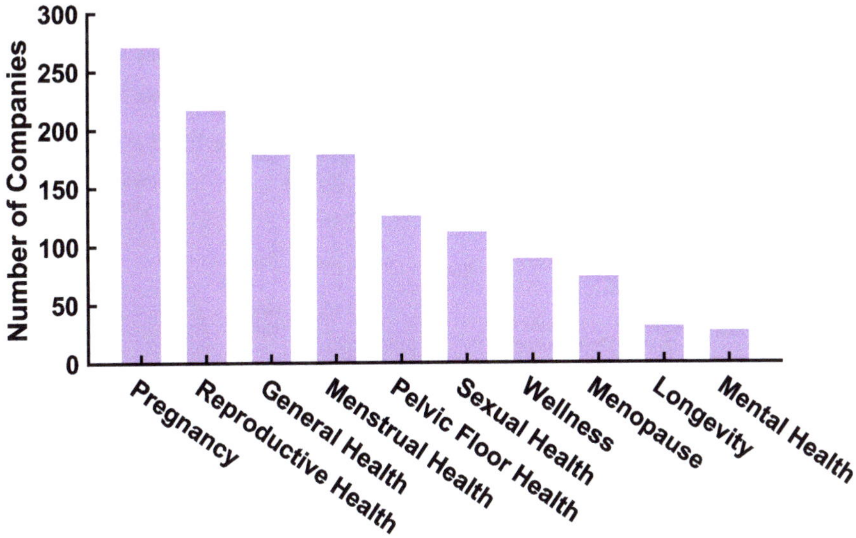

Fig. 2 Total number of FemTech companies worldwide by subsector prior to 2021 (Adapted from [25])

male body as the default model in medical science, which excluded female-specific physiology from both basic and translational research. As of 2015, the National Institutes of Health (NIH) mandates that sex be considered a biological variable in the design, analysis, and reporting of research involving vertebrate animals and humans [63]. This policy has driven a shift toward analyzing males and females separately, revealing substantial anatomical differences and sex-specific susceptibilities to various diseases, including, but not limited to, cardiovascular disorders and cancer [49, 51]. These developments have also underscored the critical need for targeted research investigating changes and injuries unique to the female body [12]. Notably, one domain experiencing a growing prioritization within the research community is the investigation of the structural, functional, and pathological characteristics of the vagina [7].

The vagina is a fibromuscular canal that connects the uterine cervix to the vulva, playing essential roles in sexual function, childbirth, and menstruation. It must accommodate significant physical stresses and biological changes, with anatomy that varies considerably among individuals, depending on age, hormonal status, and childbirth history [58]. The vagina consists of four layers: the epithelium, subepithelium (lamina propria), muscularis, and adventitia [44]. Each layer provides biomechanical properties, such as distensibility and strength, which arise from the interplay of collagen, elastin, and smooth muscle fibers. The whole anatomy of the vagina with surrounding pelvic floor organs and muscles can be visualized in Fig. 3. The bladder, rectum, and pelvic bones constitute adjacent structures, whereas the levator ani and coccygeus muscles provide support to pelvic organs from below by forming the pelvic diaphragm. This muscular support works together with passive

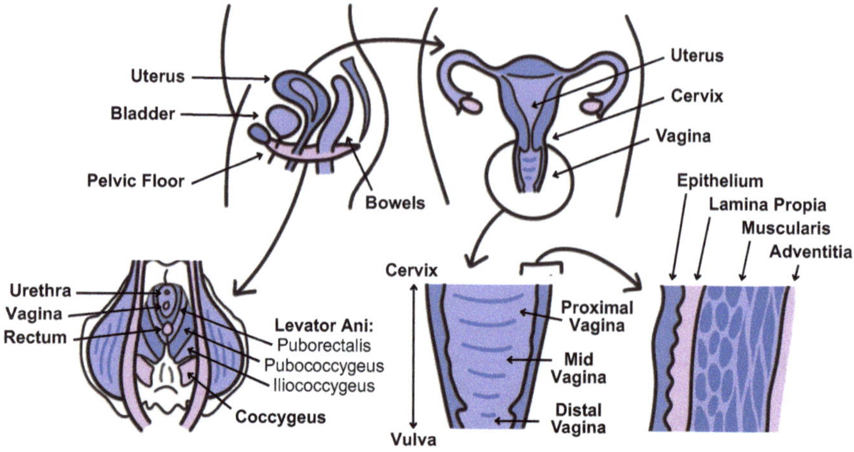

Fig. 3 The vagina lies between the urethra anteriorly and the rectum posteriorly, extending from the cervix to the vulva, and is closely integrated with surrounding pelvic structures. Adjacent organs include the bladder, uterus, and rectum, all of which are supported by the pelvic floor and a connective tissue framework. Structural support is provided not only by the pelvic bones and pelvic floor muscles, primarily the levator ani complex (puborectalis, pubococcygeus, iliococcygeus) and the coccygeus, but also by the endopelvic fascia and ligamentous supports such as the uterosacral and cardinal ligaments. The vaginal wall itself is composed of four layers: the epithelium, lamina propria, muscularis, and adventitia

suspensory structures, including the endopelvic fascia, uterosacral ligaments, and cardinal ligaments, which provide support from above and laterally [15]. Together, these systems maintain the position and function of the vagina and surrounding pelvic organs by balancing active muscular forces with connective tissue support across three levels of pelvic support: the upper level, where the vagina is anchored to the pelvic walls; the middle level, where it is supported by the pelvic sidewall and levator ani muscles; and the lower level, where it is fused with the pelvic floor and perineal body [13].

During puberty, gonadal hormones, primarily estrogens with contributions from adrenal androgens, drive the maturation of the vaginal epithelium, stroma, and musculature. In the reproductive years, cyclic ovarian hormones regulate vaginal structure and function, while pregnancy induces extensive remodeling, including increased vascularization, connective tissue turnover, and enhanced elasticity and distensibility to accommodate childbirth. With the onset of menopause, declining estrogen levels drive changes in the vagina, including reduced vascular perfusion and alterations in the vaginal microbiome. These hormonal changes result in epithelial thinning, decreased distensibility, loss of tissue elasticity, and overall compromise of vaginal structural and functional integrity [27]. Although part of normal remodeling, the changes that occur during pregnancy and menopause can increase susceptibility to injury, underscoring the need for research to mitigate dysfunction and disease [24].

Despite pregnancy-induced adaptations of the vaginal canal, the mechanical stresses of childbirth can still result in trauma [59]. Investigating structural and functional changes of the vaginal canal during pregnancy and childbirth may inform strategies to minimize perineal and vaginal lacerations. Importantly, large vaginal tears can serve as markers of underlying levator ani trauma, thus impacting the third level of pelvic support. This common but often undetected injury may contribute to later pelvic floor dysfunction, including pelvic organ prolapse. Additionally, research has investigated the effects of age and how menopause affects the vagina, primarily through estrogen deficiency that alters vaginal tissue structure and function. Declining sex hormone levels during menopause induce significant reproductive changes, notably thinning, drying, and reduced elasticity in the tissue [27].

The vagina is particularly vulnerable to dysfunction when the surrounding pelvic support structures, including muscles, ligaments, and fascia, are compromised. Such weakening can result in pelvic organ prolapse, defined as the descent of the bladder, uterus, rectum, or vaginal apex into or beyond the vaginal canal [39]. Broader pelvic floor dysfunction can manifest in different ways. When the muscles are weak or underactive, women may experience stress urinary incontinence, overactive bladder, pelvic organ prolapse, anal incontinence, and complications during and after childbirth [77]. Conversely, when the muscles are hypertonic and painful, symptoms may include myofascial pain, dyspareunia, vaginismus, vulvodynia, chronic pelvic pain, constipation, and painful intercourse [77]. Both presentations require targeted interventions to improve function and restore quality of life.

The vagina can be affected by invasive or high-risk interventions in the pelvic region, including surgical procedures and radiation therapy. For example, surgeries involving or adjacent to the vaginal canal, such as vaginal reconstruction surgery or cancer surgeries in the pelvic region, may cause tissue tearing and inflammation, which can compromise elasticity during the wound-healing process. In patients with cervical cancer, pelvic radiotherapy frequently induces vaginal stenosis, where radiation promotes scar tissue formation that shortens and narrows the canal, leading to discomfort and obstruction during pelvic examinations or sexual activity. Radiation-induced vaginal stenosis can also be accompanied by atrophic changes, including thinning, dryness, and inflammation of the vaginal walls [75].

Detailed characterization of the biomechanical properties of vaginal tissue provides the foundation for integrating mechanics into the design of next-generation FemTech solutions. These technologies, informed by biomechanics, can then be translated into evidence-based clinical interventions for treating vaginal conditions in humans, like prolapse, menopausal changes, stenosis, etc. Quantifying elastic and viscoelastic properties under both physiological and pathological conditions would enable more precise diagnosis and targeted treatment strategies. For example, the ability to measure and classify the mechanical severity of specific dysfunctions could allow clinicians to select or design specific biomaterials or mesh for pelvic organ prolapse, regenerative scaffolds for vaginal or perineal tears, or therapeutic devices for vaginal stenosis that match a patient's tissue properties, thereby promoting optimal healing. A data-driven, mechanics-informed approach would improve computational models of injury, disease, and disorder progression while guiding prevention and minimally invasive repair for safer, more personalized FemTech interventions.

2 Vaginal Tissue Biomechanics

Physiological remodeling of vaginal tissue occurs during puberty, pregnancy, and aging, whereas pathological alterations are observed in conditions including pelvic organ prolapse, genitourinary syndrome of menopause, and cancer-related treatments. Quantifying these mechanical changes is essential for both understanding normal adaptation and developing effective medical devices and therapeutic interventions. Ex vivo studies in animal models such as rodents, rabbits, sheep, and nonhuman primates have primarily employed uniaxial, biaxial, and inflation—extension testing techniques [18, 37]. Tissues are often subjected to quasi-static testing to determine their extensibility and ultimate tensile strength, along with complementary protocols such as stress–relaxation, creep, and cyclic loading, to capture their viscoelastic and fatigue behavior. To date, most investigations have relied on uniaxial tensile and inflation testing, with few applying planar biaxial methods (e.g., [17, 36, 38, 54–56, 64]). The overall number of publications investigating vaginal mechanical properties over the past 15 years remains limited (Fig. 4). Rather than revisiting the full breadth of prior literature, we direct readers to comprehensive reviews by Huntington et al. [37] and Dubik et al. [18], which synthesize ex vivo animal and human studies on vaginal mechanics.

The anatomy of the vagina varies across animal models and humans, as documented in a recent comparative study [53]. Figure 5 presents a schematic comparison of reproductive tract anatomy, including vaginal length. Rodent vaginas, for example, are much smaller than those of humans but share a distinct feature: a separate orifice connecting the vagina to the external introitus. As in humans, the vaginal canal in mice and rats extends from the uterine body to an external opening

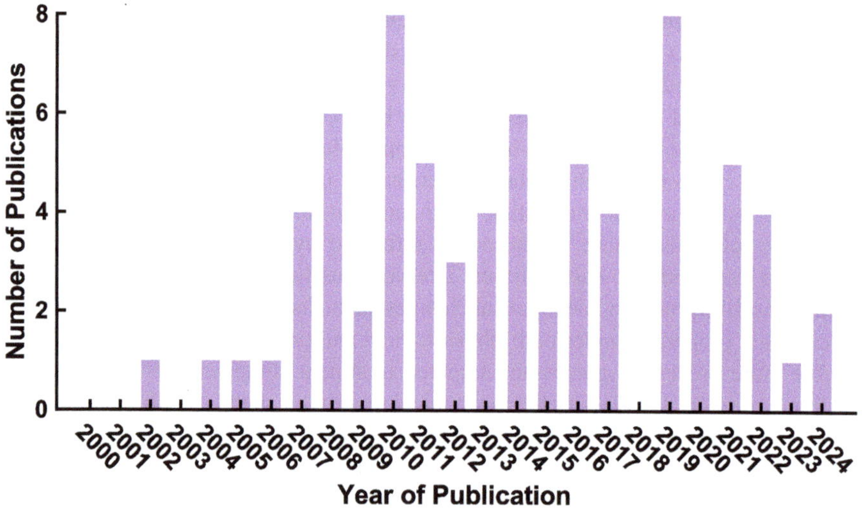

Fig. 4 Number of publications investigating vaginal mechanics in past 15 years (Adapted from [18])

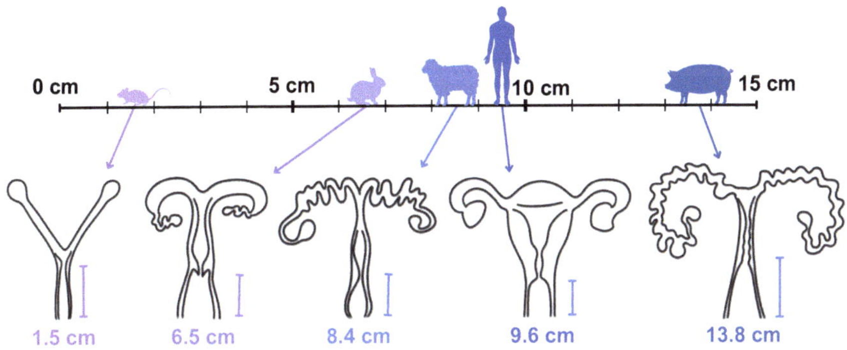

Fig. 5 Anatomical variations across animal models (human, pig, sheep, rabbit, and rodent), with the average vaginal length for each animal shown on a scale in cm

dorsal to the urethra. In contrast, rabbits, pigs, and sheep exhibit a different configuration in which the urethra merges with the vaginal tract to form a single urogenital sinus. Among these, pigs and sheep are the most comparable to humans in vaginal size. Despite these interspecies distinctions, animal models are indispensable because they provide a controlled experimental environment where confounding factors can be systematically managed, allowing for a more rigorous investigation of vaginal biomechanics and informing the design of standardized clinical studies. While human studies may be the most clinically relevant, they are inherently subject to ethical constraints and unavoidable confounding factors such as prior pelvic trauma, childbirth history, hormonal status, and age-related changes, as well as by individual anatomical and neuromuscular variation and differences in measurement conditions.

Ex vivo testing in animal models often fails to capture true in vivo behavior because it excludes essential physiological factors such as blood flow, hormonal signaling, and neuromuscular control. Methods that approximate in vivo mechanics more closely, rather than relying solely on ex vivo data, are therefore critical for advancing research-driven solutions that can be translated into effective clinical interventions and innovative FemTech applications for women's health. Using a custom-built testing system in female mice to compare in situ and ex vivo mechanical testing methods, our preliminary findings (Fig. 6) revealed marked differences in pressure–volume curves between in situ measurements, where the vagina remained in the body after sacrifice, and ex vivo testing conditions, where the tissue was completely isolated. These results suggest that ex vivo experiments may not faithfully represent the in vivo mechanical behavior of the vagina.

Currently, only a few studies have reported the in vivo mechanical behavior of vaginal tissue. In vivo testing revealed differences in vaginal distensibility across reproductive states in rats, measured with a balloon catheter coupled to a pressure transducer [1]. The results, illustrated in Fig. 7, show representative pressure–volume curves indicating that, for the same volume, virgin rats generated higher pressures than pregnant and postpartum rats. These results suggest that pregnancy

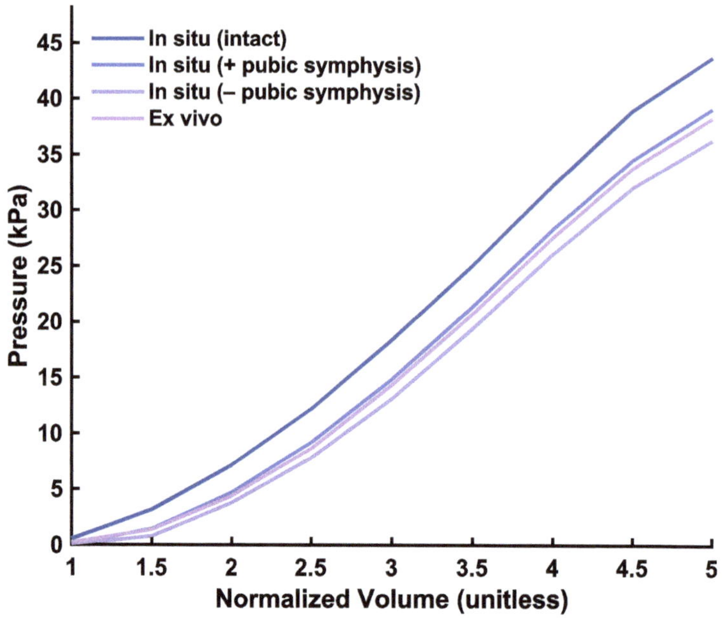

Fig. 6 Preliminary mean pressure–volume curves of the murine vagina during inflation measured in situ and ex vivo in 11 virgin mice post mortem. Inflation testing includes the following four methods, each performed on the same mouse: (1) in situ with only the outer skin removed to expose the peritoneum, (2) in situ with the bladder and fat tissue removed and the pubic symphysis intact, (3) in situ after removal of the pubic symphysis, and (4) ex vivo with the full reproductive tract fully isolated (Unpublished data from Singh and De Vita, 2025)

and vaginal delivery enhance vaginal compliance, with the tissue accommodating greater volumes before reaching comparable pressures. Although this approach applies in vivo testing to vaginal mechanics, its resolution is limited to overall pressure–volume relationships, without accounting for regional tissue contributions or intrinsic material properties.

In addition to animal studies, in vivo investigations in humans have examined how vaginal geometry relates to intraluminal pressure. Impedance planimetry (EndoFLIP^{TM}, Crospon Inc., Galway, Ireland) has been used during pregnancy to characterize cervical dimensions and to generate pressure-diameter data from the adjacent vaginal canal [30]. While the study primarily employed this tool to estimate cervical distensibility, it also provided pressure-diameter data, reported in Fig. 7 from the adjacent vaginal canal, thereby offering insight into its geometry and functional response.

Approaches such as pressure sensing and elastography have been used to probe vaginal physiology, though they capture functional rather than intrinsic mechanical behavior. Using high-definition manometry (ManoScan 360 HD^{TM}, Medtronic, Minnesota, USA), pressures were recorded in healthy participants both at rest and during pelvic floor contraction [68]. The data, illustrated in Fig. 8, shows

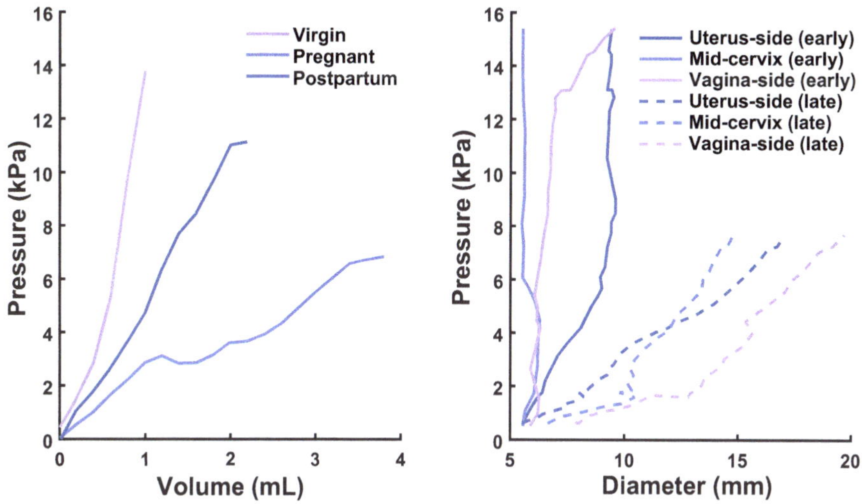

Fig. 7 Left: mean pressure–volume curves for seven virgin, ten pregnant, and ten postpartum rats during vaginal inflation testing (Adapted from [1]). Right: mean pressure-diameter curves for five early-pregnant and six late-pregnant women during cervical inflation (Adapted from [30])

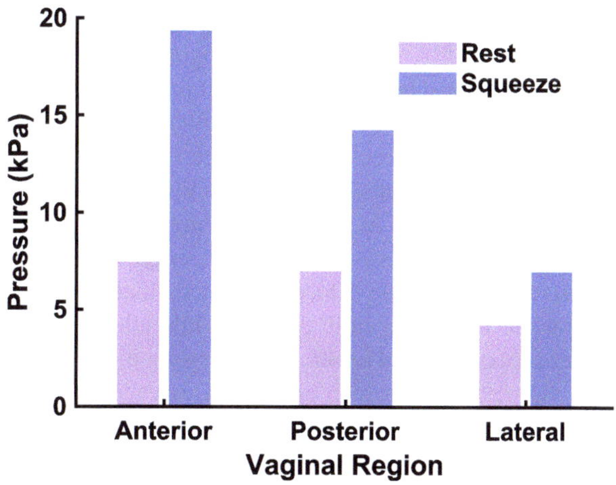

Fig. 8 A bar graph showing the maximum pressures recorded in the high-pressure vaginal zone, plotted separately for the anterior, posterior, and lateral (left and right) quadrants, both at rest and during voluntary contraction (Adapted from [68])

heterogeneous pressure distributions, with the anterior vagina bearing the highest loads and the lateral walls the lowest [68]. Although informative for understanding regional functional loading, pressure data alone is insufficient to quantify the material properties of the vaginal tissue without concurrent analysis of geometry or deformation.

Suction-based testing with a cutometer, widely used in dermatology to estimate viscoelastic tissue behavior, has also been adapted for gynecological applications. In one study, the device was applied to the vaginal walls during pelvic examination to

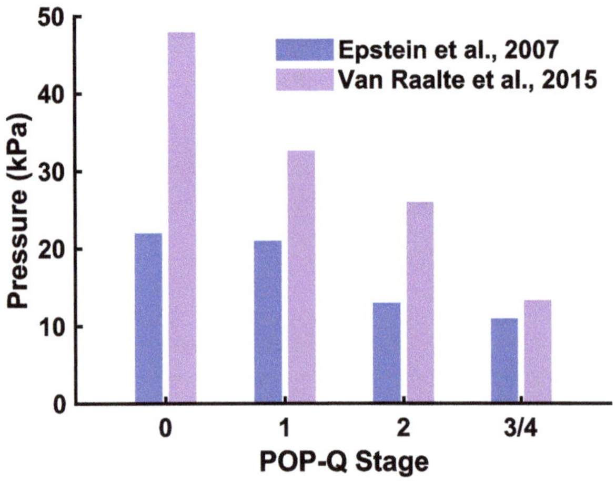

Fig. 9 Vaginal pressure vs POP-Q stage based on measurements from the DermaLab™ skin probe in 48 pelvic organ prolapse patients and based on measurements from the Vaginal Tactile Imager™ in 22 pelvic organ prolapse patients. These pressure values are averaged across all patients in each study (Adapted from [23] and [74])

compare recovery dynamics in women with and without pelvic organ prolapse (DermaLab™ skin probe, Cortex Technology, Denmark) [23]. Greater vaginal extensibility was found to correlate with more advanced Pelvic Organ Prolapse Quantification (POP-Q) stages, suggesting a role for altered tissue compliance in prolapse; the POP-Q system is defined and further discussed later. Similarly, another study applied tactile imaging (Vaginal Tactile Imager™, Advanced Tactile Imaging, New Jersey, USA), a form of elastography, to evaluate vaginal pressure profiles across different stages of pelvic organ prolapse [74]. This study shows that patients with more severe prolapse have "softer" tissue. Figure 9 compares the pressure values reported for each POP-Q stage in the two studies, highlighting differences between measurements obtained with the cutometer and the tactile imager.

Techniques such as manometry, impedance planimetry, and elastography are primarily research tools but are increasingly being adapted for clinical use through translational medicine. Once translated, these methods can complement existing diagnostic and therapeutic devices while allowing refinements and innovations to better support vaginal health. Incorporating biomechanical insights such as elasticity and viscoelasticity, which are linked to vaginal support and prolapse progression [18, 23, 74], may be helpful for improving diagnosis, guiding treatment, and fostering development of devices that ensure long-term functional outcomes.

3 Diagnostic Devices and Methods

The complete workflow for evaluating vaginal and pelvic floor health, together with related reproductive conditions, is summarized in Fig. 10. Within this workflow, diagnostic evaluation begins with a detailed clinical history and pelvic examination to assess for anatomical variations, visible tissue changes, structural abnormalities, or signs of trauma. This may be supplemented with laboratory tests, such as pH

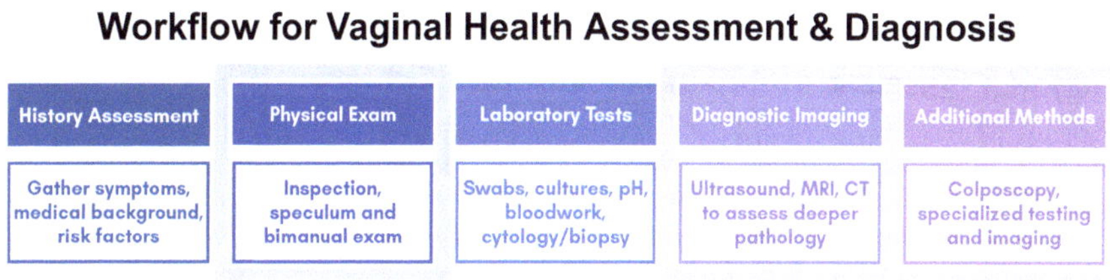

Fig. 10 Schematic of the diagnostic workflow for evaluating vaginal and pelvic floor health and diagnosing injuries, abnormalities, and disorders. Highlighted boxes indicate diagnostic steps requiring specialized engineering tools, underscoring their relevance to engineering applications

measurement, microscopy, and polymerase chain reaction tests, which analyze vaginal secretions for microbial imbalance, pH disturbances, and signs of infection. In some cases, tissue biopsy is performed to evaluate histopathological changes, including lesions, suspected malignancy, or inflammation, thereby aiding diagnosis and treatment decisions. Imaging modalities such as ultrasound, magnetic resonance imaging (MRI), and computed tomography (CT) extend the pelvic examination by visualizing soft tissue alterations, assessing vascular involvement, and identifying displacement or disruption of supporting structures. Diagnostic devices and advanced imaging modalities, including high-resolution manometry, elastography, and tactile imaging, discussed previously, can provide additional insights by characterizing vaginal tissue function and pelvic floor dynamics beyond conventional methods. This section focuses on pelvic examination, diagnostic imaging, and advanced instrumented techniques that rely directly on engineering design and technology (Fig. 10), in contrast to conventional laboratory-based tests. Many of these devices are introduced through the vaginal canal but are intended to assess not only the vagina but also adjacent structures such as the cervix, pelvic floor, uterus and surrounding reproductive organs.

3.1 Vaginally Inserted Diagnostic Devices

The first step in diagnosing vaginal disorders often involves tools that provide visualization during pelvic examination. Foremost among these is the vaginal speculum, introduced in the 1840s, which retracts the vaginal walls to permit inspection of the vagina and cervix and to facilitate sample collection [70] (Fig. 11). Despite numerous iterations, the bivalve configuration developed by J. Marion Sims remains the basis of current designs, with the Graves and Pederson "duckbill" specula from 1878 still the most widely used in practice. Traditional specula, however, present two important limitations: cervical visibility may be reduced by collapse of the lateral vaginal walls, and the vertical expansion mechanism often causes discomfort by stretching the vagina lengthwise rather than distributing pressure evenly around the circumference [5]. Several modern redesigns

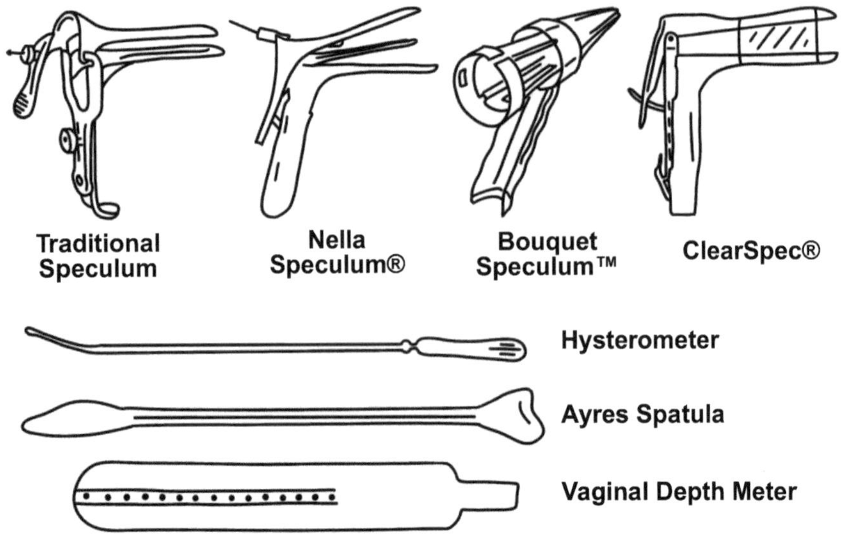

Fig. 11 Illustration of traditional and redesigned vaginal specula (traditional duckbill, Nella Speculum®, Bouquet Speculum™, and Clear Spec®) together with other diagnostic tools used during pelvic examination, including a hysterometer for uterine cavity assessment, sampling instruments such as the Ayre spatula, and a vaginal depth meter for canal measurement

intended to overcome the limitations of the traditional speculum, including the Nella Speculum® (Ceek Women's Health, Oregon, USA), Bouquet Speculum™ (Maternova inc., Rhode Island, USA), and ClearSpec® (ClearSpec Medical, Florida, USA) are shown in Fig. 11.

In addition to visualization, pelvic examinations also rely on tools designed for measurement, sampling, and imaging. For measurement, a vaginal depth meter is used to determine the length of the vaginal canal, one of the metrics used to assess the severity of pelvic organ prolapse (Fig. 11). By contrast, a hysterometer, also known as a uterine sound, is inserted through the cervix to measure the length of the uterine cavity, most often to guide intrauterine device insertion (Fig. 11). For sampling, the Ayre spatula, typically made of wood or plastic, is employed during Pap tests to gently scrape the cervical surface, providing cells for cytological screening that primarily targets cervical rather than vaginal abnormalities (Fig. 11). For imaging, the colposcope enables magnified visualization of the cervix, vagina, and vulva to detect abnormal cells or lesions, often in follow-up to an abnormal Pap test. More recently, a low-cost imaging probe (Callascope™, Calla Health Technologies, North Carolina, USA), currently under clinical evaluation, has been proposed as an alternative to the colposcope. Unlike conventional colposcopy, it does not require a speculum, making it well-suited for low-resource settings [16].

3.2 *From Manometry to MRI: Advanced Vaginal Diagnostic Technologies*

Clinicians commonly measure pelvic floor muscle function during a pelvic examination using the Oxford scale [45]. This involves instructing the patient to perform a voluntary pelvic floor contraction while the examiner evaluates the strength, endurance, and quality of the contraction through internal palpation. Muscle function is graded on a 0–4 scale, with 0 indicating no contraction and 4 representing a strong, sustained contraction. Although this digital palpation method remains the clinical standard due to its simplicity and accessibility, pressure-sensing devices and other instrumented methods have been developed, but are not yet widely adopted in routine practice (Fig. 12).

Vaginal pressure sensors are novel devices with diagnostic abilities that provide quantitative data on pelvic floor muscle strength and coordination. By producing pressure–time profiles during rest, voluntary contraction, and functional maneuvers, these sensors may be used in some cases to assist diagnosis and management of pelvic organ prolapse, urinary incontinence, and related disorders. Commercially available devices coexist with research prototypes that continue to expand their diagnostic scope. Vaginal manometry measures intravaginal pressure using a balloon-based manometer to record changes from rest to maximal voluntary

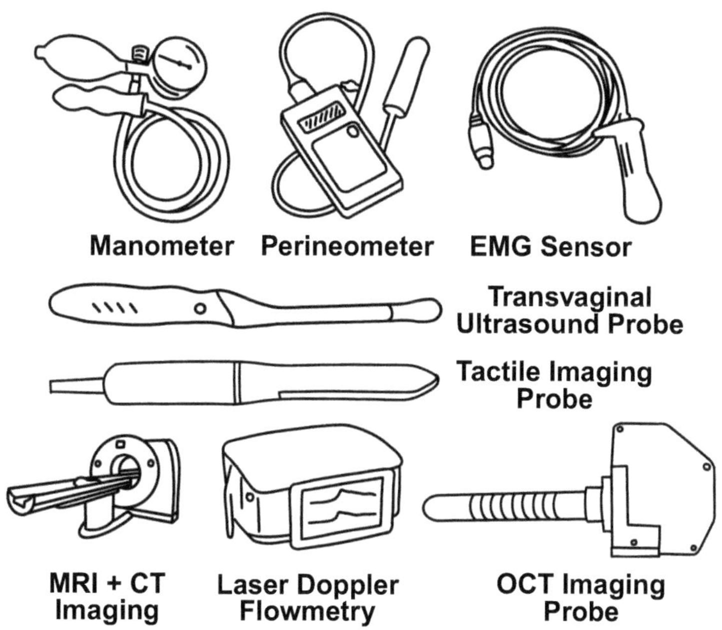

Fig. 12 Illustration of advanced vaginal diagnostic technologies, including devices for pressure and muscle activity measurement (manometer, perineometer, and EMG sensor), and other imaging modalities (transvaginal ultrasound, tactile imaging, MRI, CT, laser Doppler flowmetry, and OCT)

contraction [3] (Fig. 12). The perineometer, a related device, employs an inflatable probe connected to a pressure transducer to quantify contraction forces (Fig. 12). Pelvic floor muscle function can also be characterized using vaginal electromyography (EMG) sensors, which record electrical activity in the vaginal wall (Fig. 12). Available in various shapes (cylindrical, dumbbell, pear, or disk), these devices use small electrodes to capture neuromuscular signals and are applied in the diagnosis and management of pelvic floor dysfunction and urinary incontinence [40]. Although these devices can assist in the diagnosis of pelvic floor disorders, they are generally used as complements to therapeutic interventions such as biofeedback.

Imaging modalities provide diagnostic information by directly visualizing reproductive anatomy and function (Fig. 12). The most widely used technique is ultrasound, performed either transabdominally, across the abdomen during pregnancy to monitor fetal and maternal health, or transvaginally, which allows detailed evaluation of lesions such as ovarian masses and fibroids [62]. MRI has become the preferred modality in recent years, owing to its broader field of view and superior contrast resolution compared with ultrasound and CT. MRI enables accurate diagnosis of vaginal lesions, tumor staging, postoperative evaluation, and monitoring of treatment responses, including chemotherapy and radiotherapy [26]. It is also considered safe in pregnancy and is frequently employed to evaluate serious fetal or maternal complications, often with contrast gel to distend the canal and specialized coils to enhance spatial resolution. By contrast, CT is generally avoided during pregnancy because of fetal radiation risk, though it remains useful in selected nonpregnant cases. Beyond these standard modalities, advanced methods such as vaginal elastometry, laser Doppler flowmetry, and photoplethysmography are being explored to characterize biomechanical and vascular properties.

3.3 From Elastography to Optical Imaging: Emerging Vaginal Diagnostic Innovations

New technologies have been developed for vaginal health applications to quantify tissue elasticity, vascular physiology, and structural properties, extending diagnostic capabilities beyond conventional methods. While several devices have undergone clinical testing in humans, their adoption in routine practice continues to be limited. Representative examples are illustrated in Fig. 12.

Several approaches aim to characterize the mechanical behavior of vaginal tissue and, more specifically, vaginal tissue elasticity. Vaginal elastography measures the elastic properties of soft tissues to detect structural changes linked to prolapse or scarring. Originally developed to quantify skin viscoelasticity in dermatology, cutometers have been adapted to gynecological applications, using suction to measure vaginal tissue deformation and time-dependent recovery. Tactile imaging (Vaginal Tactile Imager™, Advanced Tactile Imaging, New Jersey, USA) replicates manual palpation by compressing tissue with a pressure-sensing probe to generate elasticity maps, capturing mechanical changes associated with prolapse and childbirth-related injury [2, 20] (Fig. 12). A more recent iteration combines tactile sensors with an ultrasound array in a single probe (Vaginal Tactile Ultrasound Imager™, Advanced Tactile Imaging, New Jersey, USA). It allows synchronized real-time visualization of tissue stiffness alongside anatomical detail [21]. This hybrid device helps overcome limitations of strain ultrasound imaging, which lacks stress information, and tactile imaging, which does not provide anatomical depth, though its complexity and cost continues to be obstacles to broader adoption. The vaginometer offers another mechanical approach by quantifying vaginal distension and flexibility, measuring maximum expansion up to the threshold of discomfort to define elasticity limits and the risk of trauma during sexual activity [52].

Other technologies focus on vascular and functional measurement. Laser Doppler imaging directly records genital blood flow, setting it apart from traditional vaginal photoplethysmography, which only provides indirect estimates of engorgement [4] (Fig. 12). Its clinical potential, however, is constrained by the lengthy scanning required to generate repeated measurements, making it less suitable for capturing rapid changes in sexual response.

More recently, high-resolution optical methods have been introduced. Intravaginal optical coherence tomography (OCT) and OCT angiography, delivered through a miniaturized probe modeled on standard laser treatment applicators, enable detailed visualization of vaginal tissue microstructure together with the vascular network [67] (Fig. 12). Initial evaluation in postmenopausal patients suggests potential for guiding laser treatments, but further validation is required before clinical adoption.

3.4 Scoring Systems for Vaginal Health and Dysfunction

Several scoring systems are used clinically to quantify the degree of injury, dysfunction, or pain in vaginal conditions. These range from clinician-reported scales based on physical examination to newer device-derived metrics.

One of the most widely adopted is the Pelvic Organ Prolapse Quantification system (POP-Q), which provides a standardized, site-specific framework for quantifying and staging pelvic support in women [9]. POP-Q measures six points (Aa, Ba, C, D, Ap, Bp) along with three landmarks, the genital hiatus (gh), total vaginal length (tvl), and perineal body (pb), each expressed in centimeters relative to the hymen, all of which are labeled in Fig. 13. Negative values for the six marked points indicate positions proximal to the hymen and positive values distal. Based on these measures, patients are assigned to a prolapse stage as indicated in Table 1. The system exhibits considerable reproducibility, is well-adapted for the monitoring of prolapse progression and evaluation of surgical outcomes, and provides enhanced precision in comparison to more rudimentary staging methods, such as the Baden-Walker system [65]. To facilitate communication with patients, the American Urogynecologic Society (AUGS) has also introduced an interactive POP-Q application for visualizing exam results.

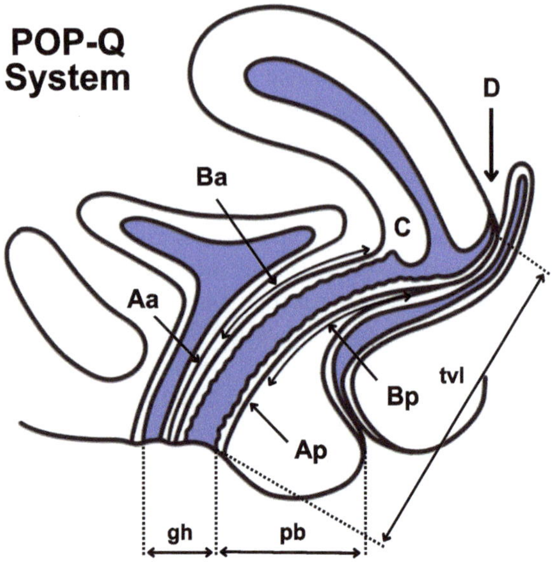

Fig. 13 Diagram of the pelvic organ prolapse quantification (POP-Q) system with the relevant POP-Q parameters labeled, including the anterior vaginal wall (points Aa and Ba), the apex/cervix/vaginal cuff (points C and D), and the posterior vaginal wall (points Ap and Bp). The genital hiatus (gh) and perineal body (pb) are also measured, along with the total vaginal length (tvl)

Table 1 Stages of pelvic organ prolapse based on the POP-Q system. Negative values indicate positions above the hymen (inside the vagina), and positive values indicate descent below the hymen

Stage	Extent of prolapse
Stage 0	No prolapse is observed. All anterior and posterior points (Aa, Ba, Ap, Bp) are at −3 cm, and the apex (C or D) is at total vaginal length (tvl)
Stage I	The most distal portion of the prolapse remains more than 1 cm above the hymenal plane. All points (Aa, Ba, Ap, Bp, C, D) are < -1 cm
Stage II	The most distal portion of the prolapse lies between 1 cm above and 1 cm below the hymen. That is, points Aa, Ba, Ap, Bp, C, and D range from −1 cm to +1 cm
Stage III	The most distal point of the prolapse lies beyond +1 cm relative to the hymen but does not exceed tvl − 2 cm. This corresponds to measurements for points Aa, Ba, Ap, Bp, C, and D in the range $\geq +2$ cm and $\leq$ tvl − 2 cm
Stage IV	Vaginal eversion has taken place, defined as descent of the most distal portion of the prolapse to within 2 cm of the total vaginal length, such that points Aa, Ba, Ap, Bp, C, and D are $\geq$ tvl − 2 cm

For conditions such as radiation-induced vaginal stenosis, expert consensus guidelines recommend using either the Common Terminology Criteria for Adverse Events (CTCAE) or the Late Effects of Normal Tissues—Subjective, Objective, Management, Analytic (LENT-SOMA) scale, as shown in Table 2 [75]. CTCAE, a general oncology grading system, classifies vaginal strictures on a five-point scale, ranging from 1 (asymptomatic with mild shortening or narrowing) to 5 (death). While widely applied in oncology, it is highly subjective and not specific to radiation-induced injuries. LENT-SOMA, developed by the European Organization for the Research and Treatment of Cancer (EORTC) and the Radiation Therapy

Table 2 Summary of late effects of normal tissues—subjective, objective, management, analytic (LENT-SOMA) scoring table for injury to the vagina, as defined by the Radiation Therapy Oncology Group and the European Organization for the Research and Treatment of Cancer (Adapted from [75])

	Grade 1	Grade 2	Grade 3	Grade 4
Subjective				
Dyspareunia	Occasional and minimal	Intermittent and tolerable	Persistent and intense	Refractory and excruciating
Dryness	Occasional	Intermittent	Persistent	Refractory
Bleeding	Occasional	Intermittent	Persistent	Refractory
Pain	Occasional and minimal	Intermittent and tolerable	Persistent and intense	Refractory and excruciating
Objective				
Stenosis, length	>2/3 normal length	1/3–2/3 normal length	<1/3 normal length	Obliteration
Dryness	Asymptomatic	Symptomatic	Secondary dysfunction	Complete atrophy
Ulceration, necrosis	Superficial, $\leq 1\ cm^2$	Superficial, $> 1\ cm^2$	Deep ulcer	Fistulae
Atrophy	Patchy	Confluent	Nonconfluent	Diffuse
Appearance	Telangiectasia without bleeding	Telangiectasia with gross bleeding	Extensive telangiectasia	Ulceration with bleeding or fistulae
Synechiae	Minimal adhesions	Partial	Complete	Obliteration
Bleeding	Occasional spotting	On contact	Intermittent	Persistent
Management				
Dyspareunia, pain	Occasional nonnarcotic	Regular nonnarcotic	Regular narcotic	Surgical intervention
Atrophy	Occasional hormone cream	Intermittent hormone cream	Regular hormone cream	Refractory to topical treatment
Bleeding	Iron therapy	Occasional transfusion	Frequent transfusions	Surgical intervention
Stenosis	Occasional dilation	Intermittent dilation	Persistent dilation	Surgical reconstruction
Dryness	Hormone replacement	Artificial lubrication	Refractory to treatment	Advanced intervention
Ulceration	Conservative	Debridement	Hyperbaric oxygen therapy (HBO_2)	Graft, surgical repair
Analytic				
MRI		Assessment of wall thickness, sinus, and fistula formation		
Ultrasound		Assessment of wall thickness, sinus, and fistula formation		
Examination under anesthesia		Assessment of wall diameter, length, and mucosal surface		

Oncology Group (RTOG), was designed specifically for radiation-related late tissue effects. It integrates multiple domains: subjective symptoms (e.g., dryness, pain), objective measures (e.g., vaginal length, ulceration), management strategies (e.g., dilation, lubrication), and analytic tests (MRI, ultrasound, biopsy). Scores range from 1 (mild) to 4 (severe), reflecting cumulative effects across these domains and providing a structured framework for grading late vaginal toxicity. While more comprehensive than CTCAE, its complexity limits routine clinical use.

Beyond clinician-reported scales, device-based approaches have recently been proposed. One example is the biomechanical integrity (BI) score, derived from vaginal tactile imaging, which translates biomechanical data into a composite index of pelvic floor function [72]. The score incorporates measures of tissue elasticity, pelvic support, muscle contraction, relaxation, and mobility, each contributing equally to the final value. Early studies in small patient cohorts suggest that the BI score may provide objective information on pelvic floor integrity, but its use is limited by the need for specialized equipment, recent regulatory approval, and lack of validation in larger, diverse populations [72, 74].

These systems highlight the trade-offs between clinical usability, comprehensiveness, and objectivity: the POP-Q and radiation scales are accessible and standardized but can be subjective or cumbersome, while emerging device-based metrics such as the BI score promise greater precision at the cost of complexity and limited availability.

4 Therapeutic Devices

Management of vaginal and pelvic floor disorders often involves a combination of hormonal, behavioral, pharmacologic, surgical, and device-based therapies, selected based on the nature and severity of anatomical and functional impairment. As illustrated in Fig. 14, treatment selection depends on the underlying diagnosis, symptom severity, tissue remodeling, and the mechanical or functional consequences of dysfunction. Hormonal therapies, including estrogen and dehydroepiandrosterone (DHEA), aim to restore mucosal integrity, microbes and pH balance, while behavioral interventions such as pelvic floor physical therapy target neuromuscular coordination and strength. Surgical approaches address persistent or severe anatomical disruption or prolapse through tissue repair or structural reinforcement. Within this broader context, therapeutic devices play an increasingly important role. They offer localized, minimally invasive solutions that act on tissue extensibility, luminal patency, or pelvic support.

This section focuses specifically on engineering-driven therapeutic devices interacting with the vaginal canal, designed to restore structure and function (Fig. 15). These include dilators, which mechanically preserve or expand the vaginal lumen; pessaries, which provide support for prolapsed organs; and implantable meshes or grafts, which reinforce compromised anatomical planes. As with

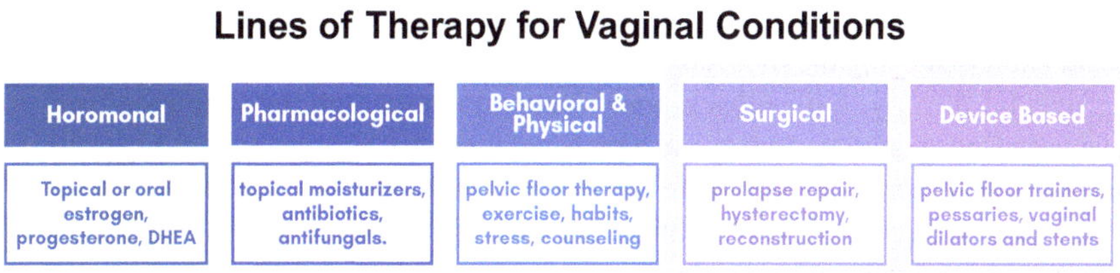

Fig. 14 Schematic of the therapeutic workflow for managing vaginal conditions, encompassing hormonal, behavioral/physical/psychosocial, surgical, device-based, and pharmacological interventions. Highlighted boxes indicate therapies where engineering innovations play a role, underscoring opportunities for engineering applications

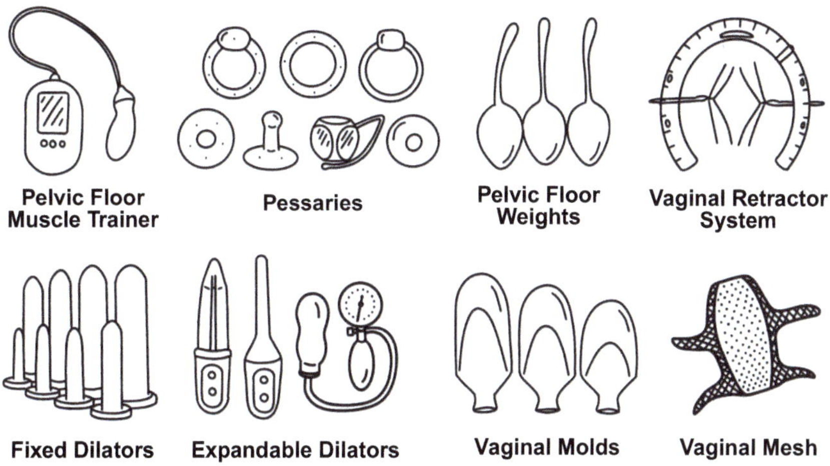

Fig. 15 Illustration of therapeutic vaginal devices, including conservative devices (muscle trainers, pessaries, and weights), rehabilitative devices (fixed dilators, expandable dilators, and vaginal molds), and surgical tools (vaginal retraction system and mesh), used in the conservative and surgical treatment of vaginal disorders

diagnostic tools, many of these therapeutic technologies rely on precise engineering of form, material properties, and deployment strategies and are informed by principles of biomechanics and tissue-device interaction.

4.1 From Pelvic Floor Therapy to Pessaries: Vaginal Support and Rehabilitation Strategies

Pelvic floor physical therapy, also referred to as pelvic floor muscle training, is a first-line conservative treatment for a wide range of pelvic floor disorders, including prolapse, and urinary and bowel incontinence. It primarily involves strengthening, relaxation, and coordination exercises, with home-based programs such as Kegel exercises being the most commonly recommended. Other approaches, including manual therapy, biofeedback, and electrical stimulation, may be employed in selected cases under the guidance of a physical therapist. Biofeedback devices utilize vaginal or rectal pressure sensors to provide real-time visual or auditory feedback on contraction strength and coordination, enabling patients to identify dysfunctional patterns and enhance muscle control [34]. Electrical stimulation devices deliver low-intensity current to elicit contractions and aid muscle isolation, while vaginal weights or cones provide a graded mechanical challenge for training [77] (Fig. 15). Pelvic floor physical therapy is supported by substantial evidence for both low-tone conditions (e.g., prolapse, incontinence) and high-tone conditions (e.g., pelvic pain, hypertonicity), although standardized guidelines for optimal modality, frequency, and duration are still lacking.

Complementing these exercise-based approaches, mechanical support devices provide another conservative option for managing pelvic floor dysfunction. Pessaries, long-established vaginal support devices, serve as a nonsurgical intervention for prolapse and incontinence and remain one of the most widely prescribed first-line treatments [29]. They are available in multiple designs, including rings, cubes, dishes, and donuts, to accommodate variations in pelvic floor anatomy and dysfunction [75] (Fig. 15). Each form serves different needs, from supporting prolapsed organs to reducing stress urinary incontinence, allowing individualized treatment that can be tailored to comfort and anatomy.

In recent years, novel pessary designs have been developed to improve usability and patient comfort (Fig. 15). For example, a recently Food and Drug Administration (FDA)-approved device (REIA™, Renovia Inc., New Hampshire, USA) incorporates a collapsible geometry and loop-assisted removal to reduce discomfort during insertion and removal [71]. Early studies report greater patient tolerance compared to traditional ring or Gellhorn pessaries, although a broader evaluation in larger cohorts is needed. Similarly, another recently FDA-approved design comprises a disposable, flexible vaginal ring pessary (ProVate™, ConTIPI Medical Ltd., Israel), which is inserted with an applicator and removed by pulling a string [79]. This pessary aims to provide support comparable to traditional pessaries and minimize adverse events and facilitate easier self-management of prolapse. The use of the device has been associated with significant improvements in prolapse symptoms, indicating high subjective efficacy; however, further studies are needed to compare outcomes with those of traditional pessaries directly. Most recently, another novel pessary design includes a patient-specific base design that can be adjusted to individual anatomy and was evaluated using finite element analysis [35]. By redirecting forces toward the lateral pelvic walls, it aims to reduce displacement and provide effective symptom relief, potentially delaying or avoiding surgical intervention. While this design has only been tested in a small cohort of eight patients with prolapse and requires further validation, it shows potential for engineering better data-driven pessaries.

4.2 From Vaginal Dilators to Supportive Stents: Management of Stenosis and Structural Dysfunction

Vaginal dilation therapy is widely prescribed for genito-pelvic pain and penetration disorders, as well as for managing vaginal narrowing following radiotherapy or surgery [48]. Conventional dilators are manufactured in graduated sets with fixed diameters and lengths, typically made of plastic, glass, or silicone (Fig. 15). Treatment involves regular insertion of progressively larger dilators in order to gently expand the vaginal and introital caliber over time. In postradiation or postsurgical contexts, vaginal dilation therapy is often applied over a period of several months. Many patients find conventional dilators uncomfortable or too rigid.

Newer devices have introduced circumferential expansion mechanisms in place of fixed sizes (Fig. 15). For example, an electronically controlled dilator (Milli™ Dilator, Materna Medical, California, USA) permits incremental expansion in 1 mm steps [48]. These devices aim to improve precision and user comfort. However, adherence to dilation therapy remains a challenge due to pain and insufficient clinical guidance).

Vaginal dilation therapy has also been explored as a preventive intervention in obstetric contexts with the goal of mitigating perineal lacerations at the time of vaginal delivery. A manually expandable balloon device (EPI-NO® Birth Trainer, TECSANA GmbH, Germany) has been marketed to pre-stretch the vagina prior to labor in an effort to reduce perineal trauma [41]. While occasionally recommended by midwives and physiotherapists, antenatal vaginal dilation not routinely prescribed in clinical practice since two recent systematic reviews showed no benefit in reducing perineal lacerations [6, 78]. A more recent example is the electromechanical Ellora™ Dilator (Materna Medical, California, USA), which is currently undergoing clinical testing as an intrapartum device designed to gradually stretch vaginal and pelvic tissues during labor, thereby reducing levator ani injury and cesarean section rates [32].

In contrast to vaginal dilators, vaginal stents are used in the immediate postoperative period to support grafts, preserve neovaginal architecture, and promote healing. They are integral to recovery after vaginoplasty, including in cases of vaginal agenesis or gender-affirming procedures, where stents help maintain patency and prevent contracture, often in conjunction with ongoing dilation [14]. While traditional stents, such as rigid acrylic or semi-rigid silicone dilators, are still commonly used, complications such as graft rejection, fibrosis, perforation, and discomfort may occur—some of which may also result from individual variation in surgical healing or graft integration rather than from the device itself. Recent innovations include hollow acrylic stents that permit drainage [61], tissue-conditioner-reinforced stents customized to patient dimensions [69], and 3D-printed molds based on MRI data (Fig. 15), incorporating features such as drainage channels and ergonomic handles [43].

Although these innovations demonstrate growing engineering sophistication, clinical validation is still limited. Most studies to date are case-based or descriptive, and robust trials are needed to establish efficacy, safety, and long-term outcomes.

4.3 From Mesh Implants to Surgical Scaffolds: Tools for Vaginal Reconstruction and Repair

Surgical treatment is often indicated for pelvic organ prolapse and related disorders when symptoms significantly impair quality of life and conservative therapies are insufficient. Reinforcement of weakened tissues commonly involves the use of grafts, most often fabricated from polypropylene mesh, a durable and biocompatible polymer (Fig. 15). This is most commonly used in a procedure called sacrocolpopexy, where mesh is used to attach the anterior, posterior, and apical vagina to the anterior longitudinal ligament of the sacrum, thereby elevating the vagina cephalad and restoring normal vaginal support. While polypropylene mesh is widely used in this procedure and considered the gold standard treatment for vaginal vault prolapse, it is associated with rare complications such as erosion, chronic pain, dyspareunia, and infection [47]. These outcomes reflect the complex mechanical and physiological environment of the vagina, which is characterized by dynamic loading, hormonal fluctuations, and constant microbial exposure. This environment presents unique challenges for implant integration and long-term performance. Indeed, Cochrane reviews report that transvaginal polypropylene mesh repairs for pelvic organ prolapse are associated with higher rates of mesh erosion and reoperation compared to native tissue repair, although comprehensive long-term outcomes are still limited [50]. As a result, FDA has banned transvaginal mesh use for pelvic organ prolapse repair in 2019 due to safety and effectiveness concerns [73]. Abdominal mesh, such as through sacrocolpopexy, is generally considered to have lower long-term recurrence rates and lower mesh complication rates and continues to be used.

Recent research has sought to develop alternative grafts for augmentation of prolapse repairs with improved safety and durability. Innovations include lightweight monofilament polypropylene, partially absorbable synthetic meshes (e.g., polypropylene, polylactic acid), biologic grafts derived from porcine dermis or cadaveric fascia, and polymer meshes coated with collagen or other biosynthetics to reduce erosion risk [47].

While an ideal mesh has yet to be realized, ongoing innovations and the introduction of advanced materials are laying the groundwork for its development. Tissue-engineered scaffolds, electrospun nanofiber constructs, and hydrogels represent emerging experimental strategies intended to better mimic the compliance and remodeling capacity of native vaginal tissue, though these remain largely at the preclinical stage [31]. For instance, one study explores an injectable hyaluronic acid–based fibrous hydrogel composite to augment uterosacral ligament suspension, demonstrating improved biomechanical strength and tissue integration compared to standard repair in a preclinical rat model [60]. Rather than summarizing all previous work, we refer readers to a recent review by Heidari et al. [31], which highlights advances in biomaterials, surface modification, drug-eluting designs, and technologies for bioresorbable meshes.

In addition to implants, vaginal surgery relies on specialized tools for tissue access and exposure. While the Sims speculum remains a standard instrument, newer systems offer circumferential retraction using elastic hooks or interchangeable blades, minimizing the need for additional instruments or assistants (Lone Star® Retractor System, Cooper Surgical, California, USA; Vaginal Multi-Trac Retractor Set, Marina Medical, Florida, USA) [33] (Fig. 15). Beyond conventional retraction devices, transvaginal robotic platforms are being developed to support minimally invasive approaches and increase surgical precision. One such system (Da Vinci™, Intuitive, California, USA) has been widely used in the operation room for the past 20 years since receiving FDA approval for many minimally invasive procedures, including vaginal surgeries such as prolapse repair and hysterectomies. Another system (Anovo™ Surgical System, Momentis Surgical Ltd., Israel), which was designed specifically for transvaginal surgeries, has also received FDA approval and is currently in clinical use.

5 Challenges and Limitations

Historically, women have been underrepresented in biomedical research, leaving critical gaps in the understanding of female-specific anatomy and physiology. This lack of foundational knowledge has hindered the design and validation of diagnostic and therapeutic devices for vaginal health. As a result, many existing tools rely on incomplete or non-translational datasets, leading to devices that are poorly tailored to women's needs. Even when promising technologies are developed, they often encounter substantial barriers to clinical adoption, including regulatory challenges, limited commercial investment, and sociocultural stigma surrounding vaginal health. These factors have collectively slowed the translation of innovative concepts into widely accessible clinical tools, contributing to persistent limitations in the care of vaginal disorders.

At the systemic level, recent analyses such as those from McKinsey report a rapid surge of interest in the FemTech industry, reflected in the growing number of publications, startups, and investments [42]. While FemTech is expanding quickly and showing promise in areas such as pregnancy and maternal health, significant gaps persist in other sectors, including oncology and menopause (Fig. 16). In 2020, only 5% of global research and development funding was dedicated to women's health, with 4% targeting women's cancers and just 1% addressing other women-specific conditions, a quarter of which was restricted to fertility research [10]. Funding continues to prioritize pregnancy and fertility, given their immediate clinical implications and large patient populations. By contrast, many conditions that

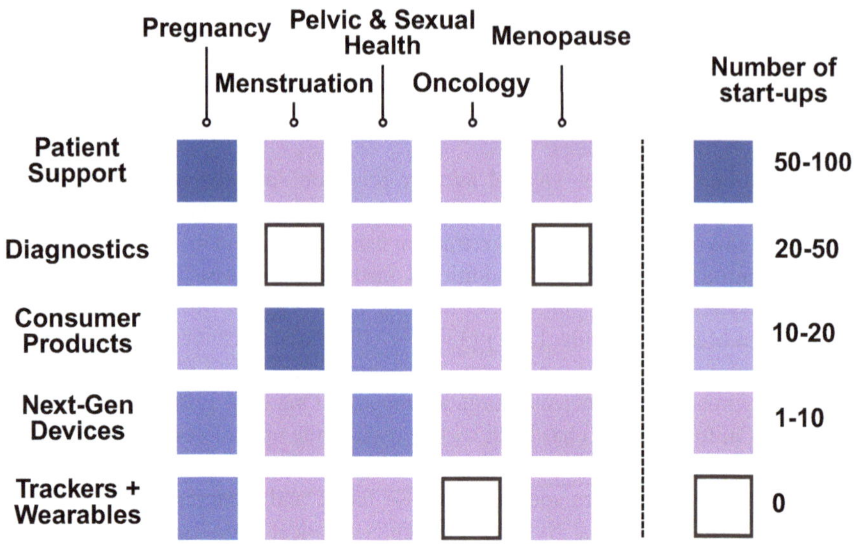

Fig. 16 Analysis of total number of FemTech start-ups worldwide over the past 20 years, based on the research by Kemble et al. [42] and data sourced from Pitchbook

are not life-threatening but still cause disability and reduced quality of life receive comparatively little attention, in part due to their clinical complexity, high costs, and the specialized expertise required to study them.

Company distribution patterns underscore the same imbalance. Figure 17 illustrates the distribution of FemTech companies in 2021 by product type, showing that some sectors attract disproportionately greater investment. For example, 228 companies focus on devices such as wearables and other hardware, whereas only 149 are dedicated to diagnostics [25]. Within this landscape, vaginal health technologies face particularly steep barriers, competing with more established FemTech sectors while also contending with persistent stigma around vaginal research and innovation. Figure 18 further highlights structural constraints in FemTech: despite rapid innovation, growth is limited by strict regulatory frameworks (e.g., FDA in the United States, Medicines and Healthcare products Regulatory Agency (MHRA) in the United Kingdom), usability concerns, and barriers to long-term adoption [28].

Clinician decision-making plays a key role in the adoption of new vaginal devices. Modernized speculum designs have been introduced to improve patient comfort, yet uptake in clinical practice has been gradual. Physicians are careful to balance innovation with evidence, cost, and practicality, particularly when alternatives involve higher expenses or have limited validation through rigorous trials [70]. This approach similarly affects advanced multifunctional imaging devices, such as tactile imaging and pressure sensing, which are currently considered nonessential for routine clinical practice [74]. Adoption can also be slowed by the need for specialized training, additional time, and resource investment. From a clinician's

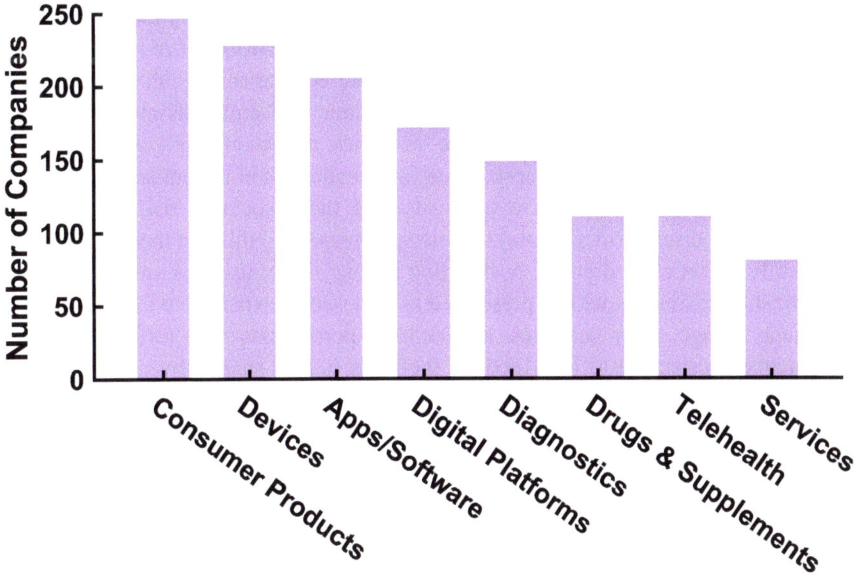

Fig. 17 Total number of FemTech companies by product type in 2021 (Adapted from [25])

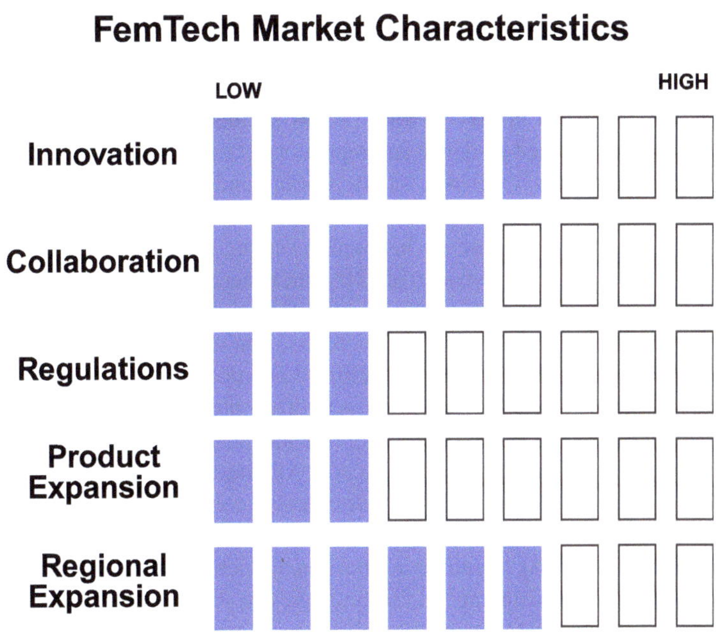

Fig. 18 Market characteristics across all FemTech companies, as indicated by a scoring out of 9, where a high score means high level of the characteristic (Adapted from Grand View Research [28])

standpoint, the decision to incorporate new technology is guided by robust evidence demonstrating safety, effectiveness, and meaningful improvement in patient care.

Equally important are the challenges patients encounter. Health interventions involving the vagina can evoke feelings of shame and embarrassment, reducing willingness to pursue them. For example, pessaries, though effective and accessible for managing pelvic organ prolapse, often face challenges in patient acceptance due to the need for frequent follow-up visits and the associated risk of infection [29]. Physical discomfort also plays a role with respect to dilation therapy: patients frequently report pain, dryness, or bleeding during dilator use, yet rigid plastic and silicone dilators remain widely prescribed as opposed to expandable ones [46]. Factors such as age, prior surgeries, and cultural perceptions may further influence acceptance. Resistance to new medical therapies is also shaped by external information sources, including social media, news reports, and high-profile class action lawsuits, such as those associated with vaginal mesh for prolapse [11]. Current clinical practices do not fully capture patients' lived experiences or the insights from available evidence, and incomplete or misleading media coverage can further reinforce patient reluctance.

Persistent research gaps continue to limit innovation in pelvic floor care, spanning both diagnostic and therapeutic technologies. The need for safer and more effective treatments remains pressing; however, advancements have been slowed by fragmented clinical data, inconsistent trial design, and a lack of coordinated research infrastructure. The vaginal mesh controversy has further underscored the importance of rigorous evaluation, as complications such as erosion and chronic pain have led to litigation across multiple continents and raised concerns about device safety and long-term outcomes [11]. While promising new strategies, including advanced biomaterials, and minimally invasive devices are in development, their clinical adoption is often delayed by limited evidence and regulatory classification as high risk (Class III), which necessitates extensive safety testing and slows approval timelines [47]. Significant gaps in education and implementation compound these barriers. Many patients receive little or no instruction on the correct use of pessaries or dilators, reducing the effectiveness of self-administered therapies and increasing the risk of discontinuation or noncompliance [57]. Similarly, in pelvic floor physical therapy, the lack of robust evidence and consensus on treatment modalities, session frequency, or duration complicates both clinical practice and the ability to compare outcomes across studies [8]. Without standardized protocols and evidence-based training, clinicians have limited tools to guide patients, and patients are often left without clear, actionable pathways for care. All these challenges illustrate how scientific, regulatory, and educational shortcomings collectively hinder progress in developing effective and accessible pelvic floor therapies.

Cost and accessibility continue to pose major challenges for implementing advanced diagnostic and therapeutic technologies in vaginal health. For example, while pelvic floor physical therapy is supported by evidence of clinical benefit, many patients face financial barriers due to high out-of-pocket expenses and inconsistent insurance coverage [77]. Similarly, high-resolution imaging modalities, such as MRI, offer superior diagnostic accuracy for identifying lesions, staging tumors, and guiding treatment decisions; yet, their use is often confined to specialized centers due to cost and infrastructure demands [26]. By contrast, ultrasound remains the most common imaging tool in clinical practice, suitable for general assessment but inadequate for detecting subtle or complex pathologies. In underserved regions, continued reliance on outdated equipment undermines efforts to improve cancer screening and gynecologic care. These disparities emphasize the need for affordable, scalable technologies specifically designed to strengthen vaginal and pelvic health across diverse care settings.

Even the most promising patient-specific innovations remain far from routine care. Studies on 3D-printed pessaries and custom vaginal molds demonstrate the potential of personalized solutions, yet the absence of standardized protocols and the scarcity of clinical trials continue to impede routine clinical adoption [35, 43]. These examples reflect broader systemic barriers: regulatory hurdles, clinician hesitancy, patient stigma and discomfort, insufficient evidence, and high development costs. Addressing these challenges will require a sustained commitment to translational research and infrastructure. In this context, the expanding FemTech sector presents a promising path forward. By supporting rigorous investigation, fostering multidisciplinary collaboration, and improving access to advanced diagnostic and therapeutic tools, FemTech can help bring emerging innovations into everyday clinical practice and improve care for individuals with vaginal and pelvic floor disorders.

6 Future Directions

Overcoming persistent barriers in women's health innovation will require systemic change, with expanded investment in research and technology as a first priority. Historically, funding has been narrowly concentrated on pregnancy and fertility, leaving conditions such as menopause, oncology, and pelvic disorders underrepresented. Expanding resources toward these neglected domains is essential to close research gaps and ensure that innovation addresses the full spectrum of women's health challenges [10, 42]. Achieving this will demand active participation from both public and private sectors, directing resources toward technologies that improve quality of life as well as survival [22, 66].

Progress also depends on stronger interdisciplinary collaboration. Engineers, scientists, clinicians, patients, and industry leaders must work together to design devices that are clinically relevant, effective, user-friendly, and accessible. Collaboration with providers ensures that design choices meet real clinical needs, while engagement with patients helps reduce stigma and improve usability. Sustained cooperation with regulators and governments will further accelerate translation from research concepts into deployable technologies [42]. Effective communication between stakeholders will be crucial to maintaining momentum and a shared purpose in advancing women's health technologies.

More accurate and representative experimental models are also needed. Traditional biomedical research often treats female physiology as a deviation from a male norm, leading to incomplete datasets. Emerging approaches, including animal studies, computational models, patient avatars, and humanized platforms, offer the potential to better capture the complexity of female biology [22]. The proposed "digital twin of the female pelvic floor" exemplifies this direction, enabling 3D visualization, disease prediction, and patient-specific treatment planning with machine learning [19]. While early in development, such models highlight the potential of precision approaches in vaginal and pelvic health.

The promise of technological innovation in vaginal health will only be realized if accompanied by rigorous clinical validation. New diagnostic and therapeutic devices should be tested through well-designed trials that establish safety, efficacy, and reliability. Emerging biomechanical imaging approaches (e.g., tactile imaging, scoring systems) illustrate the potential of quantitative assessments compared with traditional subjective measures such as pain scores or visual inspection [72]. For widespread adoption to occur, robust evidence must be accompanied by standardized protocols and regulatory frameworks specifically designed for vaginal health technologies.

Expanded investment, stronger collaboration, improved research models, and rigorous clinical validation can guide women's health research toward more effective and truly patient-centered solutions (Fig. 19). Through the integration of engineering and clinical knowledge, the future of vaginal health lies in technologies that are precise, accessible, and designed around the lived realities of patients, advancing both clinical outcomes and quality of life.

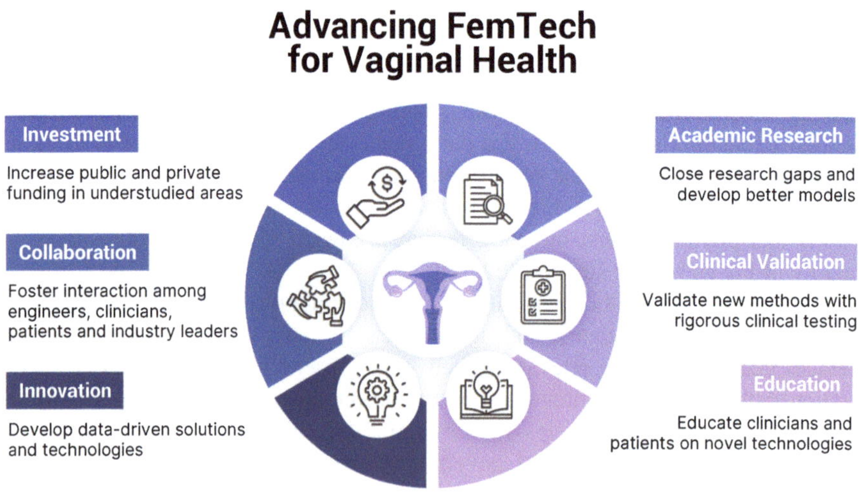

Fig. 19 Summary graphic illustrating strategies to advance FemTech and vaginal health such as investment, collaboration, innovation, clinical validation, and education

7 Conclusions

Women's health research is at an exciting turning point, and it is crucial to direct efforts where they will have the greatest impact. Vaginal health, in particular, has long been neglected due to stigma surrounding genital health, pervasive misogyny, and widespread ignorance of its vital role in women's overall well-being. The vagina is an extraordinarily powerful organ, capable of immense change and adaptation, and it deserves careful, specialized attention in both research and clinical care. Closing gaps in female-specific research, data, access, and investment can enable precise diagnostics, patient-specific treatments, and improved quality of life for women who have historically been underserved. Advancing vaginal health benefits not only individual patients but also society as a whole by supporting women's full participation in daily life, reducing long-term healthcare costs, and strengthening reproductive and public health. Only through coordinated research, inclusive collaboration, and continued investment can we eliminate disparities in women's health and ensure that innovation translates into meaningful care.

References

1. Alperin M, Feola A, Duerr R, Moalli P, Abramowitch S. Pregnancy-and delivery-induced biomechanical changes in rat vagina persist postpartum. Int Urogynecol J. 2010;21:1169–74.
2. Anumba DO, Gillespie S, Jha S, Abdi S, Kruger J, Taberner A, Nielsen PM, Li X. Postnatal pelvic floor muscle stiffness measured by vaginal elastometry in women with obstetric anal sphincter injury: A pilot study. Int Urogynecol J. 2020;31:567–75.
3. Barbosa-Silva J, de Oliveira Sato T, Jorge CH, Armijo-Olivo S, Driusso P. What are the cut-off points for vaginal manometry to differentiate women with a weak from those with a strong pelvic floor muscle contraction?: Vaginal manometry to classify a pelvic floor muscle contraction. Braz J Phys Ther. 2023;27(6):100572.
4. Bouchard KN, Pukall CF. Validation of laser Doppler flowmetry for the continuous measurement of women's genital response. Psychophysiol. 2023;60(5):e14230.
5. Bouquet JM, Naji R, Armas CA, Roldan V, Selkhi S, Bentley CZ, Zapata I, Fisher J. An innovative design for the vaginal speculum. Med Devices: Evi Res. 2023;16:211–218.
6. Brito LGO, Ferreira CHJ, Duarte G, Nogueira AA, Marcolin AC. Antepartum use of Epi-No birth trainer for preventing perineal trauma: systematic review. Int Urogynecol J. 2015;26(10): 1429–36.
7. Buchanan LM, Domingo MJ, White SE, Vanoven TN, Karbasion N, Bersi MR, Pence IJ, Florian-Rodriguez M, Miller KS. Advances in vaginal bioengineering: applications, techniques, and needs. Curr Res Physiol. 2023;6:100111.
8. Bugge C, Adams EJ, Gopinath D, Stewart F, Dembinsky M, Sobiesuo P, Kearney R. Pessaries (mechanical devices) for managing pelvic organ prolapse in women. Cochrane Database Systematic Rev. 2020;(11):1–55. https://www.cochranelibrary.com/cdsr/doi/10.1002/14651858.CD004010.pub4/pdf/full.
9. Bump RC, Mattiasson A, Bø K, Brubaker LP, DeLancey JO, Klarskov P, Shull JO, Smith AR. The standardization of terminology of female pelvic organ prolapse and pelvic floor dysfunction. Am Journal Obstet Gynecol. 1996;175(1):10–7.
10. Cheng R-fJ, Barone MA. Funding research on women's health. Nat Rev Bioeng. 2024;2:797–8.
11. Davey M. What does pelvic mesh do and why are women suing over it? 2017.

12. De Vita R, Munson J. Special issue on the advances in engineering for women's health. Ann Biomed Eng. 2021;49(8):1785–1787. https://doi.org/10.1007/s10439-021-02837-5
13. Delancey JO. Anatomic aspects of vaginal eversion after hysterectomy. Am J Obstet Gynecol. 1992;166:1717–24.
14. Deshmukh S, Priya M, Pisulkar SG, Dubey SA, Beri A, Bansod A, Jain R. Troubleshooting vaginal stents: a critical review of common problems and solutions. Cureus. 2024;16(8): e66388.
15. Donaldson K, Huntington A, De Vita R. Mechanics of uterosacral ligaments: current knowledge, existing gaps, and future directions. Ann Biomed Eng. 2021;49(8):1788–804.
16. Dotson ME, Cuenca E, Krieger M, Ramanujam N, Garcia P. Acceptability and feasibility of Callascope self-imaging of the cervix among women in Ventanilla, Peru: A mixed methods pilot study. J Womens Health Reproduct Med. 2021;5(3):12.
17. Dubik J, Tartaglione A, Miller DA, Dillard R, De Vita R. History-dependent deformations of rat vaginas under inflation. Integr Comp Biol. 2022;62(3):625–640. https://doi.org/10.1093/icb/icac110
18. Dubik J, Alperin M, De Vita R. The biomechanics of the vagina: a complete review of incomplete data. npj Women's Health. 2025;3(1):4.
19. Egorov V. Digital twin of the female pelvic floor. Open J Obstet Gynecol. 2024;14(11):1687.
20. Egorov V, Van Raalte H, Sarvazyan AP. Vaginal tactile imaging. IEEE Trans Biomed Eng. 2010;57(7):1736–44.
21. Egorov V, van Raalte H, Shobeiri SA. Tactile and ultrasound image fusion for functional assessment of the female pelvic floor. Open J Obstet Gynecol. 2021;11(6):674.
22. Ellingrud K, Pérez L, Petersen A, Sartori V. Closing the women's health gap: A $1 trillion opportunity to improve lives and economies, January 17 2024. Insight report.
23. Epstein LB, Graham CA, Heit MH. Systemic and vaginal biomechanical properties of women with normal vaginal support and pelvic organ prolapse. Am J Obstet Gynecol. 2007;197(2): 165–e1.
24. Farage M, Maibach H. Lifetime changes in the vulva and vagina. Arch Gynecol Obstet. 2006;273(4):195–202.
25. FemTech Analytics. FemTech market overview. 2021.
26. Ferreira DM, Bezerra ROF, Ortega CD, Blasbalg R, Viana PCC, Menezes MRd, Rocha MdS. Magnetic resonance imaging of the vagina: an overview for radiologists with emphasis on clinical decision making. Radiol Brasileira. 2015;48:249–59.
27. Gimenez C, Alperin M, De Vita R. The effect of menopause on vaginal tissue mechanics: a brief review. J Biomech Eng. 2024;146(6):060903.
28. Grand View Research. FemTech market size, share, & trends analysis report by type (devices, software, services), by application (pregnancy and nursing care), by end-use (direct to consumer), by region, and segment forecasts, 2025–2030. 2024.
29. Hagen S, Kearney R, Goodman K, Best C, Elders A, Melone L, Dwyer L, Dembinsky M, Graham M, Agur W, et al. Clinical effectiveness of vaginal pessary self-management vs clinic-based care for pelvic organ prolapse (TOPSY): a randomised controlled superiority trial. EClinicalMedicine. 2023;66:1–14.
30. Hee L, Liao D, Sandager P, Gregersen H, Uldbjerg N. Cervical stiffness evaluated in vivo by endoflip in pregnant women. PLoS One. 2014;9(3):e91121.
31. Heidari BS, Dodda JM, El-Khordagui LK, Focarete ML, Maroti P, Toth L, Pacilio S, El-Habashy SE, Boateng J, Catanzano O, et al. Emerging materials and technologies for advancing bioresorbable surgical meshes. Acta Biomaterialia. 2024;184:1–21.
32. Hesham H, Orejuela F, Rood KM, Turrentine M, Casey B, Khandelwal M, Dajao R, Azad S, Rosen T, Hoffman MK, et al. Effect of an intrapartum pelvic dilator device on levator ani muscle avulsion during primiparous vaginal delivery: a pilot randomized controlled trial. Int Urogynecol J. 2024;35(9):1839–49.
33. Hilton P, Monaghan JM. Operations on the vagina. Bonney's Gynaecological Surgery, p. 71. 2018.

34. Hite M, Curran T. Biofeedback for pelvic floor disorders. Clin Colon Rectal Surgery. 2021;34 (01):056–61.
35. Hong CX, Zhang S, Eltahawi A, Borazjani A, Kalami H, San AN, Sham D, Ameri G, McDermott CD. Patient-specific pessaries for pelvic organ prolapse using three-dimensional printing: a pilot study. Urogynecology. 2023;29(9):732–9.
36. Huntington A, Rizzuto E, Abramowitch S, Del Prete Z, De Vita R. Anisotropy of the passive and active rat vagina under biaxial loading. Ann Biomed Eng. 2019;47(1):272–281. https://doi.org/10.1007/s10439-018-02117-9
37. Huntington K, Donaldson A, De Vita R. Contractile properties of vaginal tissue. J Biomech Eng. 2020;142(8).
38. Huntington AD, Abramowitch PA, Moalli R, De Vita R. Strains induced in the vagina by smooth muscle contractions. Acta Biomater. 2021;129:178–187. https://doi.org/10.1016/j.actbio.2021.05.015
39. Jelovsek JE, Maher C, Barber MD. Pelvic organ prolapse. Lancet. 2007;369(9566):1027–38.
40. Kalantar-Zadeh K, Susic D, Hyett J. Vaginal sensors. ACS Sens. 2024;9(8):3810–27.
41. Kavvadias T, Hoesli I. The epino® device: efficacy, tolerability, and impact on pelvic floor—implications for future research. Obstet Gynecol Int. 2016;2016(1):3818240.
42. Kemble E, Pérez L, Sartori V, Tolub G, Zheng A. The dawn of the FemTech revolution. 2022.
43. Kisby CK, Agosta PO, Alexander A, Erie E, Morris JM, Gebhart JB. Three-dimensional–printed vaginal molds for use after McIndoe neovagina creation. Obstet Gynecol. 2022;140(2): 311–5.
44. Krstic RV. Human microscopic anatomy: an atlas for students of medicine and biology. Berlin: Springer; 1991.
45. Laycock J. Clinical evaluation of pelvic floor. In: Schussler B, Laycock J, Norton P, Stanton S, editors. Pelvic floor re-education: principles and practice. London: Springer-Verlag; 1994. p. 42–48.
46. Lee Y. Patients' perception and adherence to vaginal dilator therapy: a systematic review and synthesis employing symbolic interactionism. In: Patient Preference and Adherence. 2018, p. 551–60.
47. Lee D, Zimmern PE. An update on research and outcomes in surgical management of vaginal mesh complications. Exp Rev Med Devices. 2019;16(7):569–80.
48. Liu M, Juravic M, Mazza G, Krychman ML. Vaginal dilators: issues and answers. Sexual Med Rev. 2021;9(2):212–220.
49. Lucas-Domínguez R, Rius C, Liu Y, Sixto-Costoya A, Valderrama-Zurián JC. Sex and gender differences in cancer research and its application to clinical oncology and therapeutics. Clinics. 2025;80:100670.
50. Maher C, Feiner B, Baessler K, Schmid C. Surgical management of pelvic organ prolapse in women. Cochrane Database Systematic Rev. 2013;22(4):229–235.
51. Mahowald MK, Esmail K, Ezzeddine FMM, Choi C, Mieszczanska H, Velarde G. Sex disparities in cardiovascular disease. Methodist DeBakey Cardiovas J. 2024;20(2):107.
52. Matthes A, Zucca-Matthes G. Measurement of vaginal flexibility and its involvement in the sexual health of women. J Women's Health Care. 2016;5(302):2167–420.
53. McCracken JM, Calderon GA, Robinson AJ, Sullivan CN, Cosgriff-Hernandez E, Hakim JC. Animal models and alternatives in vaginal research: a comparative review. Reproduct Sci. 2021;28(6):1759–73.
54. McGuire JA, Abramowitch SD, Maiti S, De Vita R. Swine vagina under planar biaxial loads: an investigation of large deformations and tears. J Biomech Eng. 2019;141(4). https://doi.org/10.1115/1.4042437
55. McGuire J, Monclova J, Coariti-Salazar A, Stine C, Toussaint K Jr, Munson J, Dillard D, De Vita R. Tear propagation in vaginal tissue under inflation. Acta Biomater. 2021;127:193–204. https://doi.org/10.1016/j.actbio.2021.03.065
56. McGuire JA, Crandall SD, Abramowitch PA, De Vita R. Inflation and rupture of vaginal tissue. Interface Focus. 2019;9(4):20190029. https://doi.org/10.1098/rsfs.2019.0029

57. Miles T, Johnson N. Vaginal dilator therapy for women receiving pelvic radiotherapy. Cochrane Database Systematic Rev. 2014;(9):1–26. https://www.cochranelibrary.com/cdsr/doi/10.1002/14651858.CD007291.pub3/pdf/full.
58. Miller KS, Myers K, Oyen M. Bioengineering in women's health: part I. 2019.
59. Miller KS, Myers K, Oyen M. Bioengineering in women's health, volume 2: pregnancy—from implantation to parturition. 2019.
60. Miller B, Wolfe W, Gentry JL, Grewal MG, Highley CB, De Vita R, Vaughan MH, Caliari SR. Supramolecular fibrous hydrogel augmentation of uterosacral ligament suspension for treatment of pelvic organ prolapse. Adv Healthcare Mater. 2023;12(22):2300086.
61. Mohamed K, Krishnamurthy P, Yogitha K, Hussain SA. Hollow prosthetic vaginal dilator–a novel technique. J Evol Med Dental Sci. 2021;10(11):841–5.
62. Nahlawi S, Gari N. Sonography transvaginal assessment, protocols, and interpretation. Tampa: StatPearls Publishing LLC; 2021.
63. National Institutes of Health. NOT-OD-15-102: Consideration of Sex as a Biological Variable in NIH-funded Research. NIH Guide for Grants and Contracts, June 2015.
64. Pack E, Dubik J, Snyder W, Simon S, Clark R, De Vita R. Biaxial stress relaxation of vaginal tissue in pubertal gilts. J Biomech Eng. 2020;142(3). https://doi.org/10.1115/1.4045707
65. Persu C, Chapple CR, Cauni V, Gutue S, Geavlete P. Pelvic organ prolapse quantification system (POP–Q)–a new era in pelvic prolapse staging. J Med Life. 2011;4(1):75.
66. PitchBook. Femtech startups appear on track for record VC funding. 2024.
67. Qiu S, Arthur A, Jiang Y, Miao Y, Li Y, Wang J, Tadir Y, Lane F, Chen Z. Oct angiography in the monitoring of vaginal health. APL Bioeng. 2023;7(4):046112-1-046112-9.
68. Raizada V, Bhargava V, Jung S-A, Karstens A, Pretorius D, Krysl P, Mittal RK. Dynamic assessment of the vaginal high-pressure zone using high-definition manometery, 3-dimensional ultrasound, and magnetic resonance imaging of the pelvic floor muscles. Am J of Obstet Gynecol. 2010;203(2):172–e1.
69. Rathee M, Singhal SR, Malik S, Gupta G. Resilient customized hollow vaginal stent for the treatment of vaginal agenesis in Mayer–Rokitansky–Kuster–Hauser syndrome. Nigerian J Surgery. 2020;26(1):88–91.
70. Rossmann JS. Built to spec?: The vaginal speculum as a case study of inadequate design. 2008.
71. Strohbehn K, Wadensweiler PM, Richter HE, Grimes CL, Rardin CR, Rosenblatt PL, Toglia MR, Siddiqui G, Hanissian P. Effectiveness and safety of a novel, collapsible pessary for management of pelvic organ prolapse. Am J Obstet Gynecol. 2024;231:271-e1.
72. Takacs P, Rátonyi D, Koroknai E, van Raalte H, Lucente V, Egorov V, Krasznai ZT, Kozma B. Biomechanical integrity score of the female pelvic floor for stress urinary incontinence. Int Urogynecol J. 2024;35(6):1245–53.
73. US Food and Drug Administration. Pelvic organ prolapse (POP): surgical mesh considerations and recommendations. FDA: Silver Spring, MD. 2021.
74. van Raalte H, Egorov V. Tactile imaging markers to characterize female pelvic floor conditions. Open J Obstet Gynecol. 2015;5(9):505.
75. Varytė G, Bartkevičienė D. Pelvic radiation therapy induced vaginal stenosis: a review of current modalities and recent treatment advances. Medicina. 2021;57(4):336.
76. Viera AJ, Larkins-Pettigrew M. Practical use of the pessary. Am Family Phys. 2000;61(9):2719–26.
77. Wallace SL, Miller LD, Mishra K. Pelvic floor physical therapy in the treatment of pelvic floor dysfunction in women. Curr Opin Obstet Gynecol. 2019;31(6):485–93.
78. Zambuto SG, Scott AK, Hardi A, Oyen ML, Sutcliffe S, Lowder JL. The effect of antenatal vaginal dilators on perineal trauma: a systematic review and meta-analysis. Int J Gynecol Obstet. 2025.
79. Ziv E, Erlich T. Novel, disposable, self-inserted, vaginal device for the nonsurgical management of pelvic organ prolapse: efficacy, safety, and quality of life. BMC Women's Health. 2022;22(1):459.

Composition and Dynamics of the Vaginal Extracellular Matrix

Fatemeh Vahidi Zaman, Mari J. E. Domingo, Matthew A. Salinas, Maria E. Florian Rodriguez, Isaac J. Pence, and Kristin S. Miller

Abstract The vagina is a highly adaptable organ whose extracellular matrix (ECM) provides essential structural support throughout life, enabling functions such as intercourse, menstrual flow, and childbirth. This chapter describes the key ECM components in the vagina—collagens, elastic fibers, proteoglycans, glycoproteins, and enzymes—that together determine tissue function. Collagen types I and III form

Authors Fatemeh Vahidi Zaman and Mari J.E. Domingo contributed equally to this work.

F. Vahidi Zaman · M. J. E. Domingo · M. A. Salinas
Department of Bioengineering, University of Texas at Dallas, Richardson, TX, USA
e-mail: Fatemeh.VahidiZaman@UTDallas.edu; Mari.Domingo@UTDallas.edu; Matthew.Salinas@UTDallas.edu

M. E. Florian Rodriguez
Department of Obstetrics and Gynecology, University of Texas Southwestern Medical Center, Dallas, TX, USA
e-mail: Maria.florian-rodriguez@utsouthwestern.edu

I. J. Pence
Department of Bioengineering, University of Texas at Dallas, Richardson, TX, USA

Department of Biomedical Engineering, University of Texas Southwestern Medical Center, Dallas, TX, USA

Charles and Jane Pak Center for Mineral Metabolism and Clinical Research, University of Texas Southwestern Medical Center, Dallas, TX, USA

Department of Internal Medicine, University of Texas Southwestern Medical Center, Dallas, TX, USA
e-mail: Isaac.Pence@UTSouthwestern.edu

K. S. Miller (✉)
Department of Bioengineering, University of Texas at Dallas, Richardson, TX, USA

Department of Obstetrics and Gynecology, University of Texas Southwestern Medical Center, Dallas, TX, USA

Department of Biomedical Engineering, University of Texas Southwestern Medical Center, Dallas, TX, USA

Department of Mechanical Engineering, University of Texas at Dallas, Richardson, TX, USA
e-mail: Kristin.Miller@UTDallas.edu

S. G. Zambuto, M. L. Oyen (eds.), *Biomaterials for Women's Health Engineering*,
https://doi.org/10.1007/978-3-032-10745-9_2

the main fibrillar framework and structural support, while elastic fibers enable tissue recoil and resilience needed during physiological events such as pregnancy, childbirth, and intercourse. Proteoglycans and glycosaminoglycans maintain tissue hydration and help the vagina resist compressive forces; also, matrix metalloproteinases and their inhibitors regulate ECM remodeling. The vaginal wall consists of four layers, including epithelium, subepithelium, muscularis, and adventitia, each contributing to structural integrity, flexibility, and function. ECM composition changes dynamically across developmental stages: menstruation, pregnancy, postpartum recovery, and menopause. Improper ECM remodeling correlates with pelvic organ prolapse and the genitourinary syndrome of menopause. Finally, the chapter discusses noninvasive imaging techniques for quantifying ECM composition, supporting the design of biomaterials that mimic native vaginal ECM and improve pelvic floor disorder outcomes.

Keywords Vagina · Vaginal extracellular matrix · ECM remodeling · Collagen · Elastic fibers · Vaginal wall structure · Pregnancy and parturition · Postpartum remodeling · Menopause · Pelvic organ prolapse · Genitourinary syndrome of menopause

1 Introduction

The vagina is a fibromuscular, multilayered, tubular organ located in the female pelvic region (Fig. 1). It is proximally connected to the cervix, while the distal end marks the vaginal opening, or introitus [85, 109]. The main functions of the vagina are to serve as a passage for menses, facilitate intercourse, permit fetal delivery during childbirth, and provide support to surrounding pelvic organs [38, 46, 64]. Furthermore, the vaginal extracellular matrix (ECM) is a dynamic, three-dimensional network that helps dictate vaginal function [3, 56, 124, 131, 134, 141]. In this

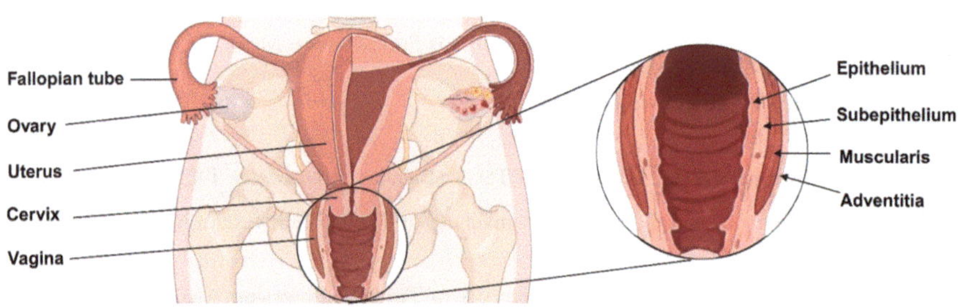

Fig. 1 Schematic of the female reproductive organs showing an intact external view on the left and a longitudinal cutaway view on the right to illustrate the vaginal lumen and wall layers. The magnified panel highlights the vaginal layers including epithelium, subepithelium, muscularis, and adventitia. Some figure components were created using BioRender.com

chapter, we introduce the structure of the vagina, key load-bearing components of the vaginal ECM, and their contributions to vaginal function. Additionally, we discuss how the ECM composition is dynamic, meaning it grows and remodels to accommodate biological changes such as pregnancy and aging. This constant adaptation of the ECM guides biomaterial design.

2 Vaginal Structure

The vaginal wall contains macroscopic transverse folds known as rugae, which are anatomical features that span multiple layers, including the epithelium and underlying connective tissue (Fig. 2) [135]. These folds increase surface area, enabling the ability to maintain moisture and support beneficial microbial colonization by keeping a highly acidic environmental pH of 3.8–4.2 [6, 114, 116]. Additionally, the rugae may contribute to tissue resilience during intercourse and childbirth, but their function is not fully understood [135]. Furthermore, these features contribute to the tissue's compliance during everyday activities and support overall reproductive health against infection.

The vaginal wall is composed of four distinct microscopic layers: the epithelium, subepithelium, muscularis, and adventitia, which work together through many cell types and ECM components (Fig. 2) [93]. Each layer has specialized functions and interacts with one another to support reproductive health, mechanical flexibility, and

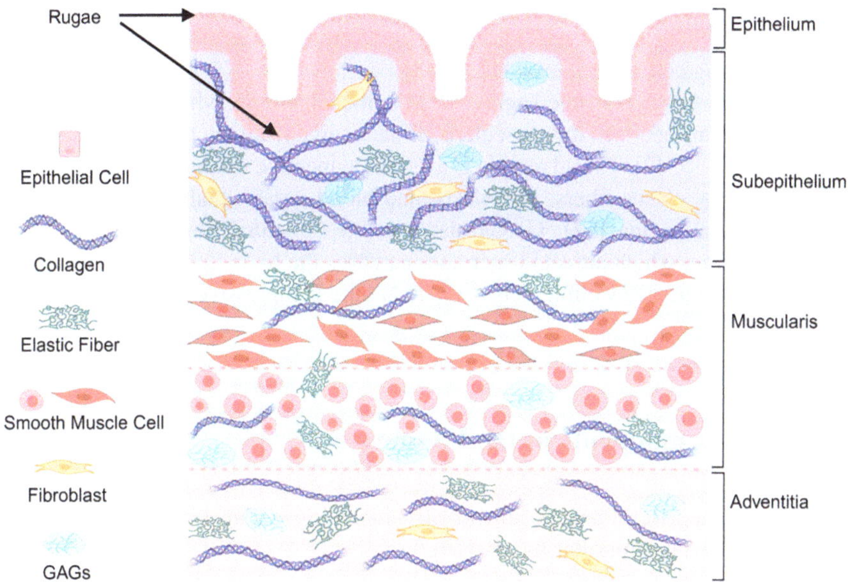

Fig. 2 Schematic of the vaginal layers and microstructural components. Some figure components were made in BioRender.com

the response to bacterial infections [17]. The following details each layer, starting from the epithelium to adventitia (Fig. 2). Notably, the muscularis and subepithelium layer are the thickest among the vaginal wall layers, whereas the thickness of the adventitia and epithelium vary substantially [148].

The vaginal epithelium serves as a protective barrier against pathogens [6]. Epithelium permits diffusion of small molecules, peptides, and steroid hormones, making it a viable route for drug delivery, which enables its bidirectional transport function of the tissue [144]. The vaginal epithelium undergoes continuous renewal through proliferation and differentiation of basal cells, which migrate toward the lumen and are eventually shed [90].

The subepithelium is a dense layer of connective tissue that contributes to passive mechanical properties such as the ability to stretch the tissue [47, 93]. Proper elastic fiber formation contributes to maintaining passive mechanical function [1, 29, 151, 152]. Within this layer, glycosaminoglycans (GAGs) play a key role in maintaining the structural organization of the ECM and regulating interactions between the subepithelium layer and the epithelial and muscularis layers [14]. GAGs also allow protein binding during the remodeling of the ECM [51].

The muscularis primarily comprises smooth muscle cells interspersed with connective tissue [86, 133]. The muscularis has a circular and longitudinal layer of smooth muscle cells [62]. It also contains elastin, collagen, and basement membrane components [80, 86]. These ECM components provide the structural support necessary for smooth muscle cells to generate and sustain contractile forces, which contributes to their functionality within the vagina [29, 152]. Contractility is an essential function of the vagina as it helps maintain its structural integrity. The contractile nature of the vagina also facilitates intercourse and childbirth [69]. Smooth muscle cells and ECM interact together by repairing collagen fibers and influencing cell morphology [123, 148].

The outermost layer of the vaginal ECM is the adventitia, which is a connective tissue layer that separates the muscularis of the vagina from the tissues surrounding the vagina [8, 36, 47]. The adventitia is a dense connective tissue layer composed of collagen fibers, elastic fibers, fibroblasts, and blood vessels that provide structural support to the vagina [57]. GAGs also provide structural support due to their negative charge, which attracts water and increases the hydration state of the layer. This hydration-based swelling helps counteract the compressive forces from neighboring organs [20].

3 ECM Components in the Vagina

The ECM comprises fibrillar components, including collagen and elastic fibers, surrounded by a non-fibrillar matrix [79].

3.1 Collagen

Collagen is the main component of vaginal ECM, accounting for about 35% of the total ECM content [10]. The average collagen fiber bundle diameter is between 50 and 350 micrometers [117]. Collagen fibers in the vaginal wall are thick, wavy (undulated) bundles that interweave to form a dense supportive network [10, 26, 137]. Collagen fibers in the vaginal wall also exhibit a complex orientation that supports its mechanical function [26, 28, 137]. Some collagen fibers are oriented along the circumferential and longitudinal axes, providing structural support along these two axes [28]. All collagens have a triple helix structure, and their structure classifies their respective subtype [52, 119]. Details on specific collagen structure and classification can be found in Gelse [52] and Ricard-Blum [120].

The fibrillar collagens type I and III are the main structural components of vaginal ECM, with the ratio of collagen type I/III being approximately one under normal physiological conditions [79, 89]. These collagen fibrils play an essential role in dictating the biomechanical properties of vaginal tissue [150]. For instance, collagen type I provides tensile strength, meaning it resists changes in shape while under loading conditions [98]. It can also bear most of the load during strenuous activities like childbirth, intercourse, or increases in intra-abdominal pressure [54]. Type III collagen enables tissue flexibility and compliance thereby contributing to vaginal mechanics [11, 79, 83, 98]. Both type I and III provide structural support during the wound repair process, promoting cell adhesion and migration, and replacing the provisional matrix with a stronger, more organized collagen network as the tissue matures [61, 79].

Collagen V exists in the vagina in smaller quantities, has shorter fibers, and has lower tensile strength than collagen I and III [79]. Collagen V also contributes to wound healing by regulating collagen fibril formation and increasing connective tissue strength; however, its specific role in the vagina remains unknown [15, 79]. Collagen type IV and VI are non-fibrillar and play roles in forming networks or supporting basement membranes and are minor components of the vagina [80, 89, 119]. Collagen types IV and VI establish a nonfibrous scaffold that increases the flexibility of the basement membrane [11]. However, the specific role in vaginal tissue remains unknown [79].

3.2 Elastic Fibers

Elastic fibers are the other fibrillar component of the ECM, comprising approximately 15% of the vaginal ECM [77]. The diameter of elastic fibers varies from 50 nanometers to 1 micrometer [140]. The structure of elastic fibers, characterized by a 90% elastin core surrounded by microfibrils, is well established in tissues such as the aorta and skin [115, 122, 147]. However, its structure is not well defined and presumed to be similar in vagina compared to established organ systems.

Elastogenesis is the multistep process that forms functional elastic fibers, primarily described in studies on arterial and dermal tissues [147]. First, smooth muscle cells and fibroblasts secrete microfibril components such as fibrillin-1 and fibrillin-2. Previous studies demonstrate this phenomenon in arteries, lungs, and skin; however, the specific cells responsible for producing elastic fiber components in the vagina remain unknown [115, 147]. These fibrillin proteins self-assemble extracellularly into microfibrillar scaffolds that support the deposition and alignment of tropoelastin, the soluble precursor of elastin and a subunit of elastic fibers. Tropoelastin is the highly extensible, springlike molecule that contributes to the recoil and resilience of elastic fibers [115, 147]. Smooth muscle cells and fibroblasts synthesize tropoelastin, which is then deposited onto the microfibrillar scaffold by proteins such as fibulin-5 [147, 157]. Finally, lysyl oxidase (LOX) enzymes catalyze oxidative cross-linking reactions, forming mature elastic fibers [115, 147, 154].

Elastic fibers provide resilience and recoil properties to the vagina to adapt to the high-volume changes in physiological conditions including intercourse, pregnancy, and childbirth [29, 42]. Additionally, elastic fibers maintain vaginal shape by preventing excessive deformation and maintaining the structural integrity of the vagina during these physiological events [1, 29, 42, 77]. Furthermore, they limit collagen fiber undulation, which increases the tissue's resistance to stretch under mechanical loads [48, 63]. This combination of resilience and stiffness ensures normal vaginal function while minimizing long-term tissue damage or pathological remodeling [23, 37].

3.3 Glycoproteins

In addition to collagenous proteins, the vaginal ECM also consists of glycoproteins, which are critical for cell-to-ECM interactions [89, 156]. Fibronectin, vitronectin, and laminin are non-collagenous ECM proteins that serve different specialized functions based on their binding domain [32]. Fibronectin contributes to cell adhesion, migration, and wound healing, while vitronectin supports cell adhesion and spreading [156]. Laminin is a basement membrane protein with essential roles in cellular migration, adhesion, and differentiation [82, 132, 138]. In the vaginal environment, this balance is essential for maintaining tissue elasticity, supporting wound healing, and adapting to mechanical stresses [32].

3.4 Proteoglycans

Part of the non-fibrillar ground matrix, proteoglycans are a subtype of glycoproteins that comprise a core protein covalently attached to a GAG chain. Small leucine-rich proteoglycans (SLRP) have a small molecular size of 36–42 kDa with 7–24 repeats of leucine amino acid sequences [158]. SLRPs assist with collagen fibril formation and cellular behavior [72, 76]. Specifically, decorin, lumican, and fibromodulin interact with fibrils of collagen and play a role in collagen fibril formation [87]. Decorin influences the spacing and size of collagen fibrils [127, 149]. Biglycan contributes to elastic fiber assembly and, in part, to collagen assembly [31, 101]. Syndecan binds to ECM components and growth factors [44, 71].

Information on GAGs in the vagina remain limited. As such, GAG structure and function will be generalized below. GAGs are the negatively charged complex carbohydrate components of proteoglycans [51]. GAGs consist of repeating disaccharide structures and enable proteoglycan function. The core disaccharide distinguishes different types of GAGs. For example, dermatan sulfate is the predominant GAG in the vagina and can contribute to wound healing and infection response [14, 78]. Chondroitin sulfate has diverse functions: it is responsible for tissue metabolism and maintaining ECM shape, cell adhesion, growth, receptor binding, and cell migration [103]. Heparan sulfate and heparin interact with cytokines and growth factors. They also contribute to ECM organization, modulating cellular growth and cellular signaling [20, 96]. Finally, the GAG with the simplest structure, hyaluronan, maintains the mechanical integrity of the tissue and sequesters water for tissue hydration [39]. Intra-abdominal pressure fluctuates throughout daily life due to coughing, laughing, sitting, exercising, and defecating contributing to repetitive compressive forces in the vagina [106, 111]. Because GAGs are highly negatively charged, proteoglycans have the capability of sequestering water for hydration, thus potentially contributing to the vagina's ability to withstand compressive forces [60, 158]. Furthermore, hydration is also critical for vaginal function to retain a physiological pH to preserve the vaginal microbiota [24].

3.5 *Matrix Metalloproteinases*

The vagina is a dynamic organ that constantly remodels its ECM to adapt to changes based on physical and biochemical cues. Matrix metalloproteinases (MMPs) are a group of enzymes that degrade the proteins in the ECM contributing to the remodeling process [2, 66]. MMPs are classified based on their primary amino acid sequence and specific substrates [66].

MMP-1 and MMP-8 initiate collagen degradation by cleaving a single peptide bond within each chain of the mature triple-helical collagen molecule, resulting in two distinct fragments [2, 67, 142, 155]. MMP-2 and MMP-9 play essential roles in weakening fibrous collagens, further degrading the cleavage fragments produced by MMP-1 [2]. Additionally, MMP-12, or macrophage metalloelastase, targets a broad range of ECM components, contributing to tissue breakdown and remodeling [91]. While specific MMPs found in the vagina are not well defined, MMP function during parturition and prolapse will be discussed in future sections. Overall, MMPs are essential for maintaining vaginal ECM homeostasis by turning over its components during physiological events [5, 153].

3.6 *Tissue Inhibitors*

Tissue inhibitors of metalloproteinases (TIMPs) are the primary regulators of MMP activity [2, 131]. Additionally, TIMPs bind to active MMPs' catalytic sites with a 1:1 molar ratio, controlling their regulation. TIMP subtypes (TIMP-1, 2, 3, 4) may inhibit different MMPs' activity [107, 153]. TIMP-1 and TIMP-3 bind to inactive site of MMP-9, while TIMP-2, TIMP-3, and TIMP-4 associate with MMP-2, influencing their activation and function [12]. Like MMPs, TIMP subtypes in the vagina have yet to be fully determined but will be expanded on with respect to postpartum recovery and prolapse.

4 ECM Remodeling

4.1 *Development and Menstruation*

During early embryonic development, Müllerian ducts facilitate formation of the female reproductive tract, including the upper two-thirds of the vagina. The urogenital sinus forms the lower third of the vagina [33]. This dual origin of the vagina explains the distal transition in vaginal epithelium [33]. Improper formation of the Müllerian ducts results in congenital anomalies affecting the reproductive tract such as Mayer–Rokitansky–Kuster–Hauser syndrome, absence of the vagina [121]. Following birth, the adolescent vagina does not change much until puberty. Once puberty begins, the 28-day menstrual cycle commences [46]. The menstrual cycle is a series of phases of hormonal and physical changes that allow for species reproduction and lasts for approximately 28 days [16].

Ovarian hormones, including estrogen and progesterone, regulate ECM protein metabolism in the reproductive tract throughout the menstrual cycle [131]. Additionally, changes in the expression of genes encoding MMPs, TIMPs, and LOX enzymes indicate that vaginal ECM components undergo dynamic alterations across different menstrual phases [131]. However, future research efforts still need to investigate collagen and elastin remodeling during menstruation.

4.2 *Pregnancy, Parturition, and Postpartum*

One critical function of the vagina is to permit delivery of the fetus from the uterus. During pregnancy, the vagina adapts from a stiff to compliant structure to expand enough in size to accommodate the extreme size of the fetus [30, 47, 139]. Humans are one of the few mammals in which the birth canal is smaller than the fetal head [104]. Contributing to the increase in tissue compliance, collagen area fraction decreases, and fibers become less densely packed compared to the non-pregnant state [35, 97, 125, 143]. At term, collagen fibers and fibrils decrease in diameter by about 20–25% compared to non-pregnant [97]. Components necessary for elastic fiber formation also vary throughout gestation. Fibulin-5, tropoelastin, and LOX1 decrease during pregnancy [41, 42], while elastin and elastic tissue-associated proteins significantly increase with pregnancy compared to the nonpregnant state [125, 143]. A decrease in MMP-2 and MMP-9 levels occurs during late pregnancy, which may help protect the elastic fibers from damage during delivery [153].

Immediately after delivery, collagen fibers are thin and dispersed, lacking orientation and organization due to both predelivery remodeling and deformation during parturition [35, 97]. Meanwhile, proteases that target elastic fibers, fibulin-5, tropoelastin, and LOX1 rapidly increase to counteract potential degradation [153]. This is, in part, regulated by an increase in TIMP-1 and decrease in TIMP-2. The upregulation of elastic fiber components increases elastogenesis, which may help with postpartum recovery [153]. In rodents, collagen, MMPs, and elastic fiber levels return to baseline non-pregnant levels 2–4 weeks after delivery [35, 40–42, 153].

In humans, MMP-9 levels significantly increase in postpartum compared to the first and third trimesters, possibly contributing to successful postpartum recovery [112]. With regard to multiple vaginal deliveries, remodeling has yet to be investigated in humans. However, in an ovine model, sheep with at least three vaginal deliveries have higher total collagen and lower elastin content compared to virgin, non-pregnant sheep tissues [143]. Elastic tissue-associated proteins also significantly decrease in parous tissue compared to non-pregnant and pregnant groups, suggesting that multiple deliveries may result in incomplete postpartum recovery [143]. Additional studies are needed to clarify the impact of parity and gravidity on the extent of postpartum tissue recovery.

4.3 Menopause

Menopause typically occurs between the ages of 40 and 60 and involves hormonal fluctuations that lead to irregular menstrual cycles and symptoms such as hot flashes in the body and vaginal dryness [68, 92]. Menopause represents the end of one's reproductive years and is clinically diagnosed after 12 consecutive months without menstruation [55].

Studies report contradictory results with regard to changes in collagen content with menopause. Babinski et al. [9] and Vodegel et al. [146] report decreased collagen and elasticity in the vaginal wall with menopause. However, others report increased collagen I and decreased collagen III after estrogen loss, suggesting collagen accumulation and tissue stiffening [98, 160]. Disorganized or fragmented collagen and reduced collagen I/III ratio has also been reported, pointing to structural weakening [88]. These differences likely arise from variations in species, tissue regions examined, and whether collagen turnover or static content was measured [70, 146].

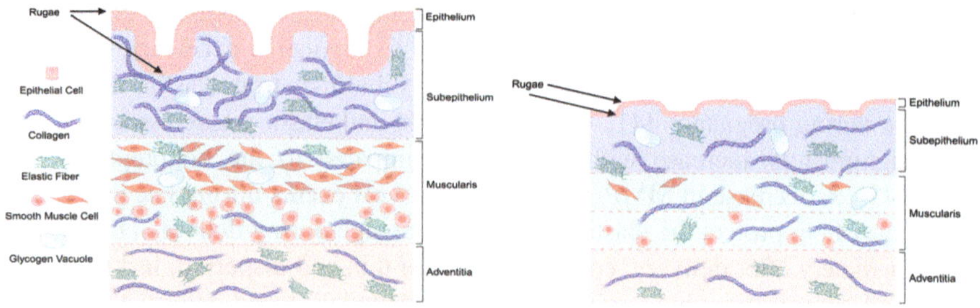

Fig. 3 The schematic illustrates major histological differences between premenopausal (left) and postmenopausal (right) vaginal tissue. In the premenopausal state, the epithelium is thick and rugae are well-defined, with abundant glycogen vacuoles, and dense elastic fibers [124]. Following menopause, the epithelium and muscularis become thinner with reduced rugal folds, fewer glycogen vacuoles, and a decrease in elastic fiber density [95, 152]

Elastin begins to form from the late fetal to the early postnatal period and gradually decreases through adulthood [100]. Specifically, during menopause, the significant drop in estrogen can cause an increase in elastin degradation, which may reduce the elasticity of the vaginal tissue [59, 113]. However, not all investigations detected a significant difference between the menopausal and control groups [53, 70, 74, 88, 146]. During menopause, declining estrogen levels cause the vaginal epithelium to become thinner, with fewer glycogen vacuoles and reduced epithelial cell layering, as shown in Fig. 3. In the underlying connective tissue, collagen fibers become sparse and disorganized, and this all contributes to the loss of elasticity and the flattening of vaginal rugae [19, 53]. Previous studies also confirm that the content, organization, and size of SMCs decrease with menopause [13, 21, 53, 81, 98, 128, 160]. However, one study showed no significant change in SMC content [70].

The menopausal transition plays a significant role in the development of chronic vaginal conditions such as vaginal atrophy (VA) [126, 130]. The genitourinary syndrome of menopause (GSM) is a chronic and progressive condition that affects the pelvic floor due to a decline in estrogen levels during menopause. GSM includes VA as a pelvic exam finding and symptoms such as vaginal dryness, discomfort, urinary problems, and sexual discomfort. GSM-related ECM changes in women closely resemble those observed in postmenopausal tissue, reflecting similar pathological alterations due to estrogen deficiency [7]. GSM encompasses both vaginal and urinary tract symptoms, whereas VA refers specifically to changes in vaginal tissue. VA is one of the primary manifestations of GSM, in which the vagina becomes thinner, drier, and inflamed [7, 50, 95]. It is common, especially in postmenopausal women, and studies show that between 50% and 85% of women experience some symptoms of VA and GSM [95].

The main reason for this syndrome is the reduction of estrogen hormone production, which results in epithelial layer thinning, and the loss of vaginal rugae becomes pronounced [50, 95]. VA exhibits similar ECM characteristics and changes to those observed during menopause, but at a more intensified level. A decline in collagen and elastin structure may lead to sexual discomfort and reduced physical well-being [65, 108]. With VA, collagen and elastin fibers in the subepithelial layer decrease [50, 95].

4.4 Pathology

Abnormal vaginal ECM remodeling can result in pathological conditions due to changes in composition and microstructure, leading to changes in mechanical and structural integrity [89]. Pelvic organ prolapse (POP), described as the descent of pelvic organs into the vaginal canal, is closely linked to ECM dysregulation and loss of structural integrity, which is influenced by factors such as aging, menopause, and childbirth [73, 145]. With POP, changes in the ECM content cause the vagina to lose its strength and functional structure [98].

Alteration in collagen content in POP is contradictory: some studies show decreased total collagen or reduced type III collagen, while others report elevated levels of immature collagen [4, 79, 161]. Shifts in collagen type ratios, particularly increased collagen I relative to III, are associated with POP and may result in reduced compliance and increased tissue stiffness [45, 98, 105]. In addition to compositional shifts, POP tissues show increased remodeling activity mediated by MMPs. MMP-2 and MMP-12 are upregulated early in prolapse onset, while MMP-9 activity rises with disease progression [2, 136]. These enzymatic changes correspond with a reduction in mature cross-linked collagen and an increase in immature collagen, ultimately weakening the mechanical strength of the vaginal wall [136].

POP is also associated with impaired elastogenesis, evidenced by decreased fibulin-5 levels, which play a critical role in elastic fiber assembly [18, 136]. Abnormal elastic fiber homeostasis is a common finding in prolapsed tissue, and changes in elastic fiber organization are strongly influenced by menopausal status, differing significantly between pre- and postmenopausal women [58]. LOXL1 expression varies between premenopausal and postmenopausal women with POP, indicating that different mechanisms may contribute to POP development across these groups [84]. Elastin content [34] and the width of elastic fibers [77] decrease with POP. Also, increased MMP activity and decreased TIMP expression are observed in prolapsed vaginal tissues suggesting an imbalance in ECM remodeling that further weakens connective tissue integrity [2]. These trends, along with condition-specific alterations in collagen and elastin content during pregnancy, postpartum, menopause, and GSM/VA, are summarized in Fig. 4.

Condition	Collagen	Elastin
Pregnancy	↓ (Rynkevic et al., 2017)	↑ (Ulrich et al., 2014)
Postpartum	↑ (Manabe et al., 1986)	↓ (Wieslander et al., 2008)
Menopause	↓ (Vodegel et al., 2023)	↓ (Jiang et al., 2014) = (Vodegel et al., 2023)
GSM + VA	↓ (Flores et al., 2022)	↓ (Flores et al., 2022)
POP	↓ (Jackson et al., 1996) ↑ (Kökçü et al., 2002)	↓ (Dahal et al., 2021)

Fig. 4 Summary of changes in collagen and elastin expression in the vagina across physiological and pathological conditions. Some figure components were made in BioRender.com

5 Future Directions

As a highly dynamic organ with a complex layered structure, the vaginal composition and structure pose challenges for comprehensive investigation. Specific tools provide a snapshot of these dynamics either for development or pathology; however, many of these approaches require the removal of tissue, which halts natural processes. Therefore, to better understand and study changes in the ECM in both animal models and directly in humans, researchers need noninvasive tools that can provide insights into compositional, structural, and functional aspects of vaginal tissue remodeling. In this context, imaging approaches offer the potential to study tissue and ECM level changes that are critical to tissue makeup, structural support, and functional performance of the vagina in both animals and directly in human subjects [17]. Given the range of size scales and the diversity of constituents critical to health maintenance and repair, various tools may provide valuable information to the field. For instance, structural changes in the support of the vagina related to ECM may be accessible using noninvasive imaging approaches such as magnetic resonance imaging (MRI) [162] or ultrasound (US) [94]. These tools are particularly well-suited to study human subjects as they are clinically accessible, do not require ionizing radiation, and primarily rely on intrinsic contrast. However, depending on the needed spatial resolution or source of contrast, US and MRI, respectively, may not provide a complete picture of the complex changes in specific layers of the vaginal ECM. In addition, other soft-tissue whole-body imaging tools, such as X-ray and computed tomography scans, are not ideal due to ionizing radiation exposure, spatial resolution, and specific soft tissue contrast [27]. Conversely, high spatial resolution tools like optical coherence tomography can image layer-specific changes in tissues using light scattering and have the potential to encode/measure mechanical properties using elastography methods [102]. Importantly, researchers can implement these tools in non−/minimally invasive approaches similar to endoscopy tools used for gynecology procedures. Unfortunately, this approach does not provide composition-specific measures that may be important for understanding development or disease processes.

To address this limitation, researchers have developed and proposed functional imaging tools to assess the mechanical properties of vaginal tissues. Some of these tools use tactile imaging to acquire a spatial map of tissue deformation [43]. Notably, recent implementations of this technique provide coarse spatial resolution compared to other imaging tools. However, the method can directly capture elastographic data from tissues. Despite the potential for direct measurement of vaginal functional/mechanical properties, this approach has not achieved broad utilization, perhaps due to the lack of structural or compositional information provided. As such, noninvasive tissue composition assessment poses challenges, especially for imaging. For example, magnetic resonance spectroscopic imaging methods may provide whole-body noninvasive imaging of specific biological constituents, but are prohibitively expensive, lack layer-specific spatial resolution, and can visualize only a limited range of biochemicals [25].

In parallel, researchers have implemented optical spectroscopy tools for other female reproductive tissues to study the composition of tissues and disease processes with non−/minimally invasive approaches. Specifically, researchers have used fluorescence, diffuse reflectance, and Raman spectroscopy to study cervical cancers [118, 129]. Furthermore, they have also applied Raman spectroscopy to mouse models and women to study compositional changes in the cervix during pregnancy and parturition [99, 110]. These tools are relatively low cost and may be translational compared with other imaging tools. Still, most approaches are based on point measurements instead of imaging, complicating data collection and limiting understanding of spatial heterogeneity. Prior work has combined structural and compositional optical methods into a single instrument for clinical investigations; however, these are currently incompatible for non−/minimally invasive imaging of vaginal anatomy [49]. Compositional tools generally lack structural or functional information that may be critical to understanding the complexity of development and disease in these dynamic, layered tissues.

Finally, a few preliminary investigations have applied high-resolution imaging techniques that can acquire both structural and compositional information [75, 163]. While investigated only for a subset of tissues and largely applicable to tissues removed from the body, these combined structural-compositional imaging tools may provide valuable information. If proven essential for understanding these dynamic processes, there may be potential to develop further combined imaging tools for clinical and investigational translation to study vaginal ECM in animal models or patient studies.

6 Conclusion

This chapter summarizes current knowledge on the vaginal ECM to date, emphasizing its role in supporting tissue structure, elasticity, and adaptation across physiological stages. It highlights the contributions of key ECM components, including collagens, elastin, proteoglycans, and enzymes, to vaginal function and remodeling.

Hormonal and mechanical influences shape ECM composition during life events such as pregnancy, postpartum recovery, and menopause, with imbalances linked to disorders like POP and GSM. Despite advances, challenges remain in capturing ECM changes in vivo. Continued development of integrated imaging and analytical approaches is essential for improving diagnosis, treatment, and biomaterial design.

In addition to understanding the structure and function of the vaginal ECM, researchers have started applying this knowledge to design biomaterials that can better mimic native tissue. Recent work has focused on both natural and synthetic scaffolds that aim to replicate the biocompatibility, biodegradability, and mechanical properties of healthy vaginal ECM [159]. Although tissue engineering has brought significant progress in implant material design, clinical outcomes for pelvic floor disorder treatments remain inconsistent. This inconsistency likely comes from limited understanding of how grafts interact with host tissues and mechanical loading, emphasizing the need for improved material models and carefully monitored clinical studies before introducing new implants into clinical use [22].

References

1. Akintunde AR, Robison KM, Capone DJ, Desrosiers L, Knoepp LR, Miller KS. Effects of elastase digestion on the murine vaginal wall biaxial mechanical response. J Biomech Eng. 2019;141:021011. https://doi.org/10.1115/1.4042014.
2. Alarab M, Kufaishi H, Lye S, Drutz H, Shynlova O. Expression of extracellular matrix-remodeling proteins is altered in vaginal tissue of premenopausal women with severe pelvic organ prolapse. Reprod Sci. 2014;21:704–15. https://doi.org/10.1177/1933719113512529.
3. Alberts B, Johnson A, Lewis J, Raff M, Roberts K, Walter P. The extracellular matrix of animals. In: Molecular biology of the cell. 4th ed. Garland Science; 2002.
4. Alperin M, Moalli PA. Remodeling of vaginal connective tissue in patients with prolapse. Curr Opin Obstet Gynecol. 2006;18:544–50. https://doi.org/10.1097/01.gco.0000242958.25244.ff.
5. Amabebe E, Ogidi H, Anumba DO. Matrix metalloproteinase-induced cervical extracellular matrix remodelling in pregnancy and cervical cancer. Reprod Fertil. 2022;3:R177–91. https://doi.org/10.1530/RAF-22-0015.
6. Anderson DJ, Marathe J, Pudney J. The structure of the human vaginal *stratum corneum* and its role in immune defense. Am J Rep Immunol. 2014;71:618–23. https://doi.org/10.1111/aji.12230.
7. Angelou K, Grigoriadis T, Diakosavvas M, Zacharakis D, Athanasiou S. The genitourinary syndrome of menopause: an overview of the recent data. Cureus. 2020;12:e7586. https://doi.org/10.7759/cureus.7586.
8. Aronson MP, Bates SM, Jacoby AF, Chelmow D, Sant GR. Periurethral and paravaginal anatomy: an endovaginal magnetic resonance imaging study. Am J Obstet Gynecol. 1995;173:1702–10. https://doi.org/10.1016/0002-9378(95)90413-1.
9. Babinski M d SD, Pires LAS, Fonseca Junior A, Manaia JHM, Babinski MA. Fibrous components of extracellular matrix and smooth muscle of the vaginal wall in young and postmenopausal women: stereological analysis. Tissue Cell. 2022;74:101682. https://doi.org/10.1016/j.tice.2021.101682.
10. Badiou W, Granier G, Bousquet P-J, Monrozies X, Mares P, de Tayrac R. Comparative histological analysis of anterior vaginal wall in women with pelvic organ prolapse or control subjects. A pilot study. Int Urogynecol J. 2008;19:723–9. https://doi.org/10.1007/s00192-007-0516-4.

11. Bailey A. Molecular mechanisms of ageing in connective tissues. Mech Ageing Dev. 2001;122:735–55. https://doi.org/10.1016/S0047-6374(01)00225-1.
12. Baker AH, Edwards DR, Murphy G. Metalloproteinase inhibitors: biological actions and therapeutic opportunities. J Cell Sci. 2002;115:3719–27. https://doi.org/10.1242/jcs.00063.
13. Basha ME, Chang S, Burrows LJ, Lassmann J, Wein AJ, Moreland RS, Chacko S. Effect of estrogen on molecular and functional characteristics of the rodent vaginal muscularis. J Sex Med. 2013;10:1219–30. https://doi.org/10.1111/jsm.12088.
14. Bezerra LRPS, Feldner PC, Kati LM, Girão MJBC, Sartori MG, Baracat EC, De Lima GR, Nader HB, Dietrich CP. Sulfated glycosaminoglycans of the vagina and perineal skin in pre- and postmenopausal women, according to genital prolapse stage. Int Urogynecol J. 2004;15: 266–71. https://doi.org/10.1007/s00192-004-1150-z.
15. Birk DE. Type V collagen: heterotypic type I/V collagen interactions in the regulation of fibril assembly. Micron. 2001;32:223–37. https://doi.org/10.1016/S0968-4328(00)00043-3.
16. Boland MR, Fieder M, John LH, Rijnbeek PR, Huber S. Female reproductive performance and maternal birth month: a comprehensive meta-analysis exploring multiple seasonal mechanisms. Sci Rep. 2020;10:555. https://doi.org/10.1038/s41598-019-57377-9.
17. Buchanan LM, Domingo MJE, White SE, Vanoven TN, Karbasion N, Bersi MR, Pence IJ, Florian-Rodriguez M, Miller KS. Advances in vaginal bioengineering: applications, techniques, and needs. Curr Res Physiol. 2023;6:100111. https://doi.org/10.1016/j.crphys.2023.100111.
18. Budatha M, Roshanravan S, Zheng Q, Weislander C, Chapman SL, Davis EC, Starcher B, Word RA, Yanagisawa H. Extracellular matrix proteases contribute to progression of pelvic organ prolapse in mice and humans. J Clin Invest. 2011;121:2048–59. https://doi.org/10.1172/JCI45636.
19. Carlson K, Nguyen H. Genitourinary syndrome of menopause. In: StatPearls. Treasure Island: StatPearls Publishing; 2025.
20. Casale J, Crane JS. Biochemistry, glycosaminoglycans. In: StatPearls. Treasure Island: StatPearls Publishing; 2025.
21. Cellai I, Filippi S, Comeglio P, Cipriani S, Maseroli E, Di Stasi V, Todisco T, Marchiani S, Tamburrino L, Villanelli F, Vezzani S, Corno C, Fambrini M, Guarnieri G, Sarchielli E, Morelli A, Rastrelli G, Maggi M, Vignozzi L. Testosterone positively regulates vagina NO-induced relaxation: an experimental study in rats. J Endocrinol Investig. 2022;45:1161–72. https://doi.org/10.1007/s40618-022-01743-4.
22. Chen B, Dave B. Challenges and future prospects for tissue engineering in female pelvic medicine and reconstructive surgery. Curr Urol Rep. 2014;15:425. https://doi.org/10.1007/s11934-014-0425-2.
23. Chen B, Wen Y, Polan ML. Elastolytic activity in women with stress urinary incontinence and pelvic organ prolapse. Neurourol Urodyn. 2004;23:119–26. https://doi.org/10.1002/nau.20012.
24. Chen J, Sun T, You Y, Wu B, Wang X, Wu J. Proteoglycans and Glycosaminoglycans in stem cell homeostasis and bone tissue regeneration. Front Cell Dev Biol. 2021;9:760532. https://doi.org/10.3389/fcell.2021.760532.
25. Cheng S-C, Chen K, Chiu C-Y, Lu K-Y, Lu H-Y, Chiang M-H, Tsai C-K, Lo C-J, Cheng M-L, Chang T-C, Lin G. Metabolomic biomarkers in cervicovaginal fluid for detecting endometrial cancer through nuclear magnetic resonance spectroscopy. Metabolomics. 2019;15:146. https://doi.org/10.1007/s11306-019-1609-z.
26. Chi N, Lozo S, Rathnayake RAC, Botros-Brey S, Ma Y, Damaser M, Wang RR. Distinctive structure, composition and biomechanics of collagen fibrils in vaginal wall connective tissues associated with pelvic organ prolapse. Acta Biomater. 2022;152:335–44. https://doi.org/10.1016/j.actbio.2022.08.059.
27. Chow L, Tsui BQ, Bahrami S, Masamed R, Memarzadeh S, Raman SS, Patel MK. Gynecologic tumor board: a radiologist's guide to vulvar and vaginal malignancies. Abdom Radiol (NY). 2021;46:5669–86. https://doi.org/10.1007/s00261-021-03209-2.

28. Clark GL, Pokutta-Paskaleva AP, Lawrence DJ, Lindsey SH, Desrosiers L, Knoepp LR, Bayer CL, Gleason RL, Miller KS. Smooth muscle regional contribution to vaginal wall function. Interface Focus. 2019;9:20190025. https://doi.org/10.1098/rsfs.2019.0025.
29. Clark-Patterson GL, Roy S, Desrosiers L, Knoepp LR, Sen A, Miller KS. Role of fibulin-5 insufficiency and prolapse progression on murine vaginal biomechanical function. Sci Rep. 2021;11:20956. https://doi.org/10.1038/s41598-021-00351-1.
30. Clark–Patterson G, Domingo M, Miller KS. Biomechanics of pregnancy and vaginal delivery. Curr Opin Biomed Eng. 2022;22:100386. https://doi.org/10.1016/j.cobme.2022.100386.
31. Colon-Caraballo M, Lee N, Nallasamy S, Myers K, Hudson D, Iozzo RV, Mahendroo M. Novel regulatory roles of small leucine-rich proteoglycans in remodeling of the uterine cervix in pregnancy. Matrix Biol. 2022;105:53–71. https://doi.org/10.1016/j.matbio.2021.11.004.
32. Crouch M-L, Alderete JF. Trichomonas vaginalis interactions with fibronectin and laminin. Microbiology. 1999;145:2835–43. https://doi.org/10.1099/00221287-145-10-2835.
33. Cunha GR, Robboy SJ, Kurita T, Isaacson D, Shen J, Cao M, Baskin LS. Development of the human female reproductive tract. Differentiation. 2018;103:46–65. https://doi.org/10.1016/j.diff.2018.09.001.
34. Dahal S, Kuang M, Rietsch A, Butler RS, Ramamurthi A, Damaser MS. Quantitative morphometry of elastic fibers in pelvic organ prolapse. Ann Biomed Eng. 2021;49:1909–22. https://doi.org/10.1007/s10439-021-02760-9.
35. Daucher JA, Clark KA, Stolz DB, Meyn LA, Moalli PA. Adaptations of the rat vagina in pregnancy to accommodate delivery. Obstet Gynecol. 2007;109:128–35. https://doi.org/10.1097/01.AOG.0000246798.78839.62.
36. De Landsheere L, Munaut C, Nusgens B, Maillard C, Rubod C, Nisolle M, Cosson M, Foidart J-M. Histology of the vaginal wall in women with pelvic organ prolapse: a literature review. Int Urogynecol J. 2013;24:2011–20. https://doi.org/10.1007/s00192-013-2111-1.
37. De Landsheere L, Brieu M, Blacher S, Munaut C, Nusgens B, Rubod C, Noel A, Foidart J-M, Nisolle M, Cosson M. Elastin density: link between histological and biomechanical properties of vaginal tissue in women with pelvic organ prolapse? Int Urogynecol J. 2016;27:629–35. https://doi.org/10.1007/s00192-015-2901-8.
38. DeLancey JOL. The anatomy of the pelvic floor. Current Opinion in Obstetrics and Gynecology 6 N2-The pelvic organs are suspended by the pelvic ligaments and supported by the levator ani muscles. Breaks in the connective tissue, and neuromuscular damage affecting the pelvic floor muscles cause pelvic organ prolapse. Magnetic resonance imaging and ultrasound have begun to define the dynamics of the pelvic floor and document the specific tissue lesions involved in this process. 1994. Copyright © 1994 YEAR Wolters Kluwer Health, Inc. All rights reserved.
39. Dicker KT, Gurski LA, Pradhan-Bhatt S, Witt RL, Farach-Carson MC, Jia X. Hyaluronan: a simple polysaccharide with diverse biological functions. Acta Biomater Biol Mater. 2014;10:1558–70. https://doi.org/10.1016/j.actbio.2013.12.019.
40. Downing KT, Billah M, Raparia E, Shah A, Silverstein MC, Ahmad A, Boutis GS. The role of mode of delivery on elastic fiber architecture and vaginal vault elasticity: a rodent model study. J Mech Behav Biomed Mater. 2014;29:190–8. https://doi.org/10.1016/j.jmbbm.2013.08.025.
41. Drewes PG, Marinis SI, Acevedo J, Keller P, Schaffer JI, Word RA. Paper 17: regulation of lysyl oxidase in the Vaginal Wall: role of estrogen, progesterone, and pregnancy. J Pelvic Med Surg. 2005;11:S8–9. https://doi.org/10.1097/01.spv.0000176091.92426.fa.
42. Drewes PG, Yanagisawa H, Starcher B, Hornstra I, Csiszar K, Marinis SI, Keller P, Word RA. Pelvic organ prolapse in Fibulin-5 knockout mice. Am J Pathol. 2007;170:578–89. https://doi.org/10.2353/ajpath.2007.060662.
43. Egorov V, van Raalte H, Shobeiri SA. Tactile and ultrasound image fusion for functional assessment of the female pelvic floor. Open J Obstet Gynecol. 2021;11:674–88. https://doi.org/10.4236/ojog.2021.116063.

44. Elenius K, Jalkanen M. Function of the syndecans – a family of cell surface proteoglycans. J Cell Sci. 1994;107:2975–82. https://doi.org/10.1242/jcs.107.11.2975.
45. Emmerson S, Young N, Rosamilia A, Parkinson L, Edwards SL, Vashi AV, Davies-Tuck M, White J, Elgass K, Lo C, Arkwright J, Werkmeister JA, Gargett CE. Ovine multiparity is associated with diminished vaginal muscularis, increased elastic fibres and vaginal wall weakness: implication for pelvic organ prolapse. Sci Rep. 2017;7:45709. https://doi.org/10.1038/srep45709.
46. Farage M, Maibach H. Lifetime changes in the vulva and vagina. Arch Gynecol Obstet. 2006;273:195–202. https://doi.org/10.1007/s00404-005-0079-x.
47. Feola A, Moalli P, Alperin M, Duerr R, Gandley RE, Abramowitch S. Impact of pregnancy and vaginal delivery on the passive and active mechanics of the rat vagina. Ann Biomed Eng. 2011;39:549–58. https://doi.org/10.1007/s10439-010-0153-9.
48. Ferruzzi J, Collins MJ, Yeh AT, Humphrey JD. Mechanical assessment of elastin integrity in fibrillin-1-deficient carotid arteries: implications for Marfan syndrome. Cardiovasc Res. 2011;92:287–95. https://doi.org/10.1093/cvr/cvr195.
49. Fitzgerald S, Akhtar J, Schartner E, Ebendorff-Heidepriem H, Mahadevan-Jansen A, Li J. Multimodal Raman spectroscopy and optical coherence tomography for biomedical analysis. J Biophotonics. 2023;16:e202200231. https://doi.org/10.1002/jbio.202200231.
50. Flores SA, Hall CA. Atrophic vaginitis. In: StatPearls. Treasure Island: StatPearls Publishing; 2025.
51. Gandhi NS, Mancera RL. The structure of glycosaminoglycans and their interactions with proteins. Chem Biol Drug Des. 2008;72:455–82. https://doi.org/10.1111/j.1747-0285.2008.00741.x.
52. Gelse K. Collagens—structure, function, and biosynthesis. Adv Drug Deliv Rev. 2003;55:1531–46. https://doi.org/10.1016/j.addr.2003.08.002.
53. Gimenez C, Alperin M, De Vita R. The effect of menopause on vaginal tissue mechanics: a brief review. J Biomech Eng. 2024;146:060903. https://doi.org/10.1115/1.4063101.
54. Goh JT. Biomechanical and biochemical assessments for pelvic organ prolapse. Curr Opin Obstet Gynecol. 2003;15:391–4. https://doi.org/10.1097/00001703-200310000-00007.
55. Gold EB. The timing of the age at which natural menopause occurs. Obstet Gynecol Clin N Am. 2011;38:425–40. https://doi.org/10.1016/j.ogc.2011.05.002.
56. Gospodarowicz D, Vlodavsky I, Greenburg G, Johnson L. Cellular shape is determined by the extracellular matrix and is responsible for the control of cellular growth and function. Hormones Cell Culture. 1979;6:561–92.
57. Guler Z, Roovers JP. Role of fibroblasts and myofibroblasts on the pathogenesis and treatment of pelvic organ prolapse. Biomolecules. 2022;12:94. https://doi.org/10.3390/biom12010094.
58. Gustilo-Ashby AM, Lee U, Vurbic D, Sypert D, Kuang M, Daneshgari F, Barber MD, Damaser MS. The impact of cesarean delivery on pelvic floor dysfunction in lysyl oxidase like-1 knockout mice. Female Pelvic Med Reconstr Surg. 2010;16:21–30. https://doi.org/10.1097/SPV.0b013e3181d00035.
59. Hadi THS, Hardianto G, Kurniawati EM, Parathon H, Yudaniayanti IS, Utomo B, Santoso BI. The effects of quercetin on the expression of collagen I, collagen III and elastin in vaginal: an experimental animal study. Clin Exp Obstet Gynecol. 2024;51:217. https://doi.org/10.31083/j.ceog5110217.
60. Hardingham TE, Fosang AJ. Proteoglycans: many forms and many functions. FASEB J. 1992;6:861–70.
61. Haukipuro K. Synthesis of collagen types I and III in reincised wounds in humans. J Br Surg. 1991;78:708–12. https://doi.org/10.1002/bjs.1800780624.
62. Haylen BT, Vu D, Wong A, Livingstone S. Surgical anatomy of the mid-vagina. Neurourol Urodyn. 2022;41:1293–304. https://doi.org/10.1002/nau.24994.
63. Henninger HB, Valdez WR, Scott SA, Weiss JA. Elastin governs the mechanical response of medial collateral ligament under shear and transverse tensile loading. Acta Biomater. 2015;25:304–12. https://doi.org/10.1016/j.actbio.2015.07.011.

64. Herschorn S. Female pelvic floor anatomy: the pelvic floor, supporting structures, and pelvic organs. Rev Urol. 2004;6(Suppl 5):S2–S10.
65. Hoffman KL, Rueda Morales RI, González-Mariscal G. Relevance of mating-associated stimuli, ovulation, and the progesterone receptor for the post-coital inhibition of estrous behavior in the female rabbit. Horm Behav. 2010;58:747–53. https://doi.org/10.1016/j.yhbeh.2010.07.007.
66. Hooper NM, editor. Zinc metalloproteases in health and disease. Boca Raton: CRC Press, Taylor & Francis Group; 1996.
67. Hu Y, Wu R, Li H, Gu Y, Wei W. Expression and significance of metalloproteinase and collagen in Vaginal Wall tissues of patients with pelvic organ prolapse. Ann Clin Lab Sci. 2017;47:698–705.
68. Huang AJ, Gregorich SE, Kuppermann M, Nakagawa S, Van Den Eeden SK, Brown JS, Richter HE, Walter LC, Thom D, Stewart AL. Day-to-day impact of vaginal aging questionnaire: a multidimensional measure of the impact of vaginal symptoms on functioning and Well-being in postmenopausal women. Menopause. 2015;22:144–54. https://doi.org/10.1097/GME.0000000000000281.
69. Huntington A, Donaldson K, De Vita R. Contractile properties of vaginal tissue. J Biomech Eng. 2020;142:080801. https://doi.org/10.1115/1.4046712.
70. Hympanova L, Rynkevic R, Urbankova I, Blacher S, de Landsheere L, Mackova K, Krofta L, Deprest J. Morphological and functional changes in the vagina following critical lifespan events in the ewe. Gynecol Obstet Investig. 2019;84:360–8. https://doi.org/10.1159/000495348.
71. Inki P. Expression of syndecan-1 in female reproductive tract tissues and cultured keratinocytes. Mol Hum Reprod. 1997;3:299–305. https://doi.org/10.1093/molehr/3.4.299.
72. Iozzo RV, Schaefer L. Proteoglycans in health and disease: novel regulatory signaling mechanisms evoked by the small leucine-rich proteoglycans. FEBS J. 2010;277:3864–75. https://doi.org/10.1111/j.1742-4658.2010.07797.x.
73. Jelovsek JE, Maher C, Barber MD. Pelvic organ prolapse. Lancet. 2007;369:1027–38. https://doi.org/10.1016/S0140-6736(07)60462-0.
74. Jiang Y, Zong W, Luan H, Liu J, Zhang A, Li X, Liu S, Zhang S, Gao J. Decreased expression of elastin and lysyl oxidase family genes in urogenital tissues of aging mice. J Obstet Gynaecol Res. 2014;40:1998–2004. https://doi.org/10.1111/jog.12425.
75. Kabakova I, Zhang J, Xiang Y, Caponi S, Bilenca A, Guck J, Scarcelli G. Brillouin microscopy. Nat Rev Methods Primers. 2024;4:8. https://doi.org/10.1038/s43586-023-00286-z.
76. Kalamajski S, Oldberg Å. The role of small leucine-rich proteoglycans in collagen fibrillogenesis. Matrix Biol. 2010;29:248–53. https://doi.org/10.1016/j.matbio.2010.01.001.
77. Karam JA, Vazquez DV, Lin VK, Zimmern PE. Elastin expression and elastic fibre width in the anterior vaginal wall of postmenopausal women with and without prolapse. BJU Int. 2007;100:346–50. https://doi.org/10.1111/j.1464-410X.2007.06998.x.
78. Kati LM, Feldner PC, De Castro RA, Kobayashi EY, Sartori MGF, Nader HB, Castello Girão MJB. Analysis of glycosaminoglycans in the parametrium and vaginal apex of women with and without uterine prolapse. J Women's Health. 2010;19:1341–4. https://doi.org/10.1089/jwh.2009.1567.
79. Kerkhof MH, Hendriks L, Brölmann HAM. Changes in connective tissue in patients with pelvic organ prolapse—a review of the current literature. Int Urogynecol J. 2009;20:461–74. https://doi.org/10.1007/s00192-008-0737-1.
80. Kerkhof MH, Ruiz-Zapata AM, Bril H, Bleeker MCG, Belien JAM, Stoop R, Helder MN. Changes in tissue composition of the vaginal wall of premenopausal women with prolapse. Am J Obstet Gynecol. 2014;210:168.e1–9. https://doi.org/10.1016/j.ajog.2013.10.881.
81. Kim NN, Min K, Pessina MA, Munarriz R, Goldstein I, Traish AM. Effects of ovariectomy and steroid hormones on vaginal smooth muscle contractility. Int J Impot Res. 2004;16:43–50. https://doi.org/10.1038/sj.ijir.3901138.

82. Kleinman HK, Weeks BS. Laminin: structure, functions and receptors. Curr Opin Cell Biol. 1989;1:964–7. https://doi.org/10.1016/0955-0674(89)90066-5.
83. Knuuti E, Kauppila S, Kotila V, Risteli J, Nissi R. Genitourinary prolapse and joint hypermobility are associated with altered type I and III collagen metabolism. Arch Gynecol Obstet. 2011;283:1081–5. https://doi.org/10.1007/s00404-010-1518-x.
84. Kow N, Ridgeway B, Kuang M, Butler RS, Damaser MS. Vaginal expression of LOXL1 in premenopausal and postmenopausal women with pelvic organ prolapse. Female Pelvic Med Reconstr Surg. 2016;22:229–35. https://doi.org/10.1097/spv.0000000000000251.
85. Krantz KE. The gross and microscopic anatomy of the human vagina. Ann N Y Acad Sci. 1959;83:89–104. https://doi.org/10.1111/j.1749-6632.1960.tb40886.x.
86. Krstić RV. Human microscopic anatomy: an atlas for students of medicine and biology. Berlin/New York: Springer-Verlag; 1991.
87. Krusius T, Ruoslahti E. Primary structure of an extracellular matrix proteoglycan core protein deduced from cloned cDNA. Proc Natl Acad Sci USA. 1986;83:7683–7. https://doi.org/10.1073/pnas.83.20.7683.
88. Li G, Yu P, Hu Y, Hu Z, Li J, Zhan X, Su Y, Yu C, Wen J, Liu H, He R. Establishment of rat model of female genital sexual arousal disorder. Sex Med. 2022;10:100530. https://doi.org/10.1016/j.esxm.2022.100530.
89. Lin S-Y, Tee Y-T, Ng S-C, Chang H, Lin P, Chen G-D. Changes in the extracellular matrix in the anterior vagina of women with or without prolapse. Int Urogynecol J. 2007;18:43–8. https://doi.org/10.1007/s00192-006-0090-1.
90. Lindau ST, Dude A, Gavrilova N, Hoffmann JN, Schumm LP, McClintock MK. Prevalence and correlates of vaginal estrogenization in postmenopausal women in the United States. Menopause. 2017;24:536–45. https://doi.org/10.1097/GME.0000000000000787.
91. Liu S-L, Bae YH, Yu C, Monslow J, Hawthorne EA, Castagnino P, Branchetti E, Ferrari G, Damrauer SM, Puré E, Assoian RK. Matrix metalloproteinase-12 is an essential mediator of acute and chronic arterial stiffening. Sci Rep. 2015;5:17189. https://doi.org/10.1038/srep17189.
92. Liu Z, Ai Y, Wang W, Zhou K, He L, Dong G, Fang J, Fu W, Su T, Wang J, Wang R, Yang J, Yue Z, Zang Z, Zhang W, Zhou Z, Xu H, Wang Y, Liu Y, Zhou J, Yang L, Yan S, Wu J, Liu J, Liu B. Acupuncture for symptoms in menopause transition: a randomized controlled trial. Am J Obstet Gynecol. 2018;219:373.e1–373.e10. https://doi.org/10.1016/j.ajog.2018.08.019.
93. Lowe JS, Anderson PG, Anderson SI. Female reproductive system. In: Stevens & Lowe's human histology. Philadelphia: Elsevier; 2024. p. 345–69.
94. Luczynska E, Zbigniew K. Diagnostic imaging in gynecology. Ginekol Pol. 2022;93:63–9. https://doi.org/10.5603/GP.a2021.0209.
95. Mac Bride MB, Rhodes DJ, Shuster LT. Vulvovaginal atrophy. Mayo Clin Proc. 2010;85:87–94. https://doi.org/10.4065/mcp.2009.0413.
96. Malavaki CJ, Theocharis AD, Lamari FN, Kanakis I, Tsegenidis T, Tzanakakis GN, Karamanos NK. Heparan sulfate: biological significance, tools for biochemical analysis and structural characterization. Biomed Chromatogr. 2011;25:11–20. https://doi.org/10.1002/bmc.1536.
97. Manabe Y, Yoshida Y. Collagenolysis in human vaginal tissue during pregnancy and delivery: a light and electron microscopic study. Am J Obstet Gynecol. 1986;155:1060–6. https://doi.org/10.1016/0002-9378(86)90350-9.
98. Mao M, Li Y, Zhang Y, Kang J, Zhu L. Tissue composition and biomechanical property changes in the Vaginal Wall of Ovariectomized Young rats. Biomed Res Int. 2019;2019:1–10. https://doi.org/10.1155/2019/8921284.
99. Masson LE, O'Brien CM, Gautam R, Thomas G, Slaughter JC, Goldberg M, Bennett K, Herington J, Reese J, Elsamadicy E, Newton JM, Mahadevan-Jansen A. In vivo Raman spectroscopy monitors cervical change during labor. Am J Obstet Gynecol. 2022;227:275.e1–275.e14. https://doi.org/10.1016/j.ajog.2022.02.019.

100. Mecham RP. Elastin in lung development and disease pathogenesis. Matrix Biol. 2018;73:6–20. https://doi.org/10.1016/j.matbio.2018.01.005.
101. Meester JAN, Vandeweyer G, Pintelon I, Lammens M, Van Hoorick L, De Belder S, Waitzman K, Young L, Markham LW, Vogt J, Richer J, Beauchesne LM, Unger S, Superti-Furga A, Prsa M, Dhillon R, Reyniers E, Dietz HC, Wuyts W, Mortier G, Verstraeten A, Van Laer L, Loeys BL. Loss-of-function mutations in the X-linked biglycan gene cause a severe syndromic form of thoracic aortic aneurysms and dissections. Genet Med. 2017;19:386–95. https://doi.org/10.1038/gim.2016.126.
102. Miao Y, Sudol NT, Li Y, Chen JJ, Arthur RA, Qiu S, Jiang Y, Tadir Y, Lane F, Chen Z. Optical coherence tomography evaluation of vaginal epithelial thickness during CO2 laser treatment: a pilot study. J Biophotonics. 2022;15:e202200052. https://doi.org/10.1002/jbio.202200052.
103. Mikami T, Kitagawa H. Biosynthesis and function of chondroitin sulfate. Biochim Biophys Acta Gen Subj. 2013;1830:4719–33. https://doi.org/10.1016/j.bbagen.2013.06.006.
104. Mitteroecker P, Fischer B. Evolution of the human birth canal. Am J Obstet Gynecol. 2024;230:S841–55. https://doi.org/10.1016/j.ajog.2022.09.010.
105. Mosier E, Lin VK, Zimmern P. Extracellular matrix expression of human prolapsed vaginal wall. Neurourol Urodyn. 2010;29:582–6. https://doi.org/10.1002/nau.20806.
106. Mouritsen L, Hulbæk M, Brostrøm S, Bogstad J. Vaginal pressure during daily activities before and after vaginal repair. Int Urogynecol J. 2007;18:943–8. https://doi.org/10.1007/s00192-006-0267-7.
107. Murphy G. Tissue inhibitors of metalloproteinases. Genome Biol. 2011;12:233. https://doi.org/10.1186/gb-2011-12-11-233.
108. Nappi RE, Martini E, Cucinella L, Martella S, Tiranini L, Inzoli A, Brambilla E, Bosoni D, Cassani C, Gardella B. Addressing vulvovaginal atrophy (VVA)/genitourinary syndrome of menopause (GSM) for healthy aging in women. Front Endocrinol. 2019;10:561. https://doi.org/10.3389/fendo.2019.00561.
109. Nguyen JD, Duong H. Anatomy, abdomen and pelvis: female external genitalia. In: StatPearls. Treasure Island: StatPearls Publishing; 2025.
110. O'Brien CM, Herington JL, Brown N, Pence IJ, Paria BC, Slaughter JC, Reese J, Mahadevan-Jansen A. In vivo Raman spectral analysis of impaired cervical remodeling in a mouse model of delayed parturition. Sci Rep. 2017;7:6835. https://doi.org/10.1038/s41598-017-07047-5.
111. O'Dell KK, Morse AN, Crawford SL, Howard A. Vaginal pressure during lifting, floor exercises, jogging, and use of hydraulic exercise machines. Int Urogynecol J. 2007;18:1481–9. https://doi.org/10.1007/s00192-007-0387-8.
112. Oliphant S, Canavan T, Palcsey S, Meyn L, Moalli P. Pregnancy and parturition negatively impact vaginal angle and alter expression of vaginal MMP-9. Am J Obstet Gynecol. 2018;218:242.e1–7. https://doi.org/10.1016/j.ajog.2017.11.572.
113. Ouni E, Bouzin C, Dolmans MM, Marbaix E, Pyr Dit Ruys S, Vertommen D, Amorim CA. Spatiotemporal changes in mechanical matrisome components of the human ovary from prepuberty to menopause. Hum Reprod. 2020;35:1391–410. https://doi.org/10.1093/humrep/deaa100.
114. Oyelowo T. Infections. In: Mosby's guide to women's health. Elsevier; 2007. p. 125–37. https://doi.org/10.1016/B978-032304601-5.50021-6.
115. Ozsvar J, Yang C, Cain SA, Baldock C, Tarakanova A, Weiss AS. Tropoelastin and elastin assembly. Front Bioeng Biotechnol. 2021;9:643110. https://doi.org/10.3389/fbioe.2021.643110.
116. Pendergrass PB, Belovicz MW, Reeves CA. Surface area of the human vagina as measured from vinyl polysiloxane casts. Gynecol Obstet Investig. 2003;55:110–3. https://doi.org/10.1159/000070184.
117. Puetzer JL, Ma T, Sallent I, Gelmi A, Stevens MM. Driving hierarchical collagen fiber formation for functional tendon, ligament, and meniscus replacement. Biomaterials. 2021;269:120527. https://doi.org/10.1016/j.biomaterials.2020.120527.

118. Rahaman A, Anantharaju A, Jeyachandran K, Manideep R, Pal UM. Optical imaging for early detection of cervical cancer: state of the art and perspectives. J Biomed Opt. 2023;28:080902. https://doi.org/10.1117/1.JBO.28.8.080902.
119. Ramachandran GN, Kartha G. Structure of collagen. Nature. 1955;176:593–5. https://doi.org/10.1038/176593a0.
120. Ricard-Blum S. The collagen family. Cold Spring Harb Perspect Biol. 2011;3:a004978. https://doi.org/10.1101/cshperspect.a004978.
121. Robbins JB, Broadwell C, Chow LC, Parry JP, Sadowski EA. Müllerian duct anomalies: embryological development, classification, and MRI assessment. Magn Reson Imaging. 2015;41:1–12. https://doi.org/10.1002/jmri.24771.
122. Ross R, Bornstein P. The elastic fiber. J Cell Biol. 1969;40:366–81. https://doi.org/10.1083/jcb.40.2.366.
123. Ruiz-Zapata AM, Kerkhof MH, Ghazanfari S, Zandieh-Doulabi B, Stoop R, Smit TH, Helder MN. Vaginal fibroblastic cells from women with pelvic organ prolapse produce matrices with increased stiffness and collagen content. Sci Rep. 2016;6:22971. https://doi.org/10.1038/srep22971.
124. Ruiz-Zapata AM, Heinz A, Kerkhof MH, Van De Westerlo-van Rijt C, Schmelzer CEH, Stoop R, Kluivers KB, Oosterwijk E. Extracellular matrix stiffness and composition regulate the myofibroblast differentiation of vaginal fibroblasts. IJMS. 2020;21:4762. https://doi.org/10.3390/ijms21134762.
125. Rynkevic R, Martins P, Hympanova L, Almeida H, Fernandes AA, Deprest J. Biomechanical and morphological properties of the multiparous ovine vagina and effect of subsequent pregnancy. J Biomech. 2017;57:94–102. https://doi.org/10.1016/j.jbiomech.2017.03.023.
126. Santoro N, Komi J. Prevalence and impact of vaginal symptoms among postmenopausal women. J Sex Med. 2009;6:2133–42. https://doi.org/10.1111/j.1743-6109.2009.01335.x.
127. Schönherr E, Hausser H, Beavan L, Kresse H. Decorin-type I collagen interaction: presence of separate core protein-binding domains. J Biol Chem. 1995;270:8877–83. https://doi.org/10.1074/jbc.270.15.8877.
128. Semmelink HJF, De Wilde PCM, Van Houwelingen JC, Vooijs GP. Histomorphometric study of the lower urogenital tract in pre- and post-menopausal women. Cytometry. 1990;11:700–7. https://doi.org/10.1002/cyto.990110607.
129. Shaikh R, Daniel A, Lyng FM. Raman spectroscopy for early detection of cervical cancer, a global women's health issue-a review. Molecules. 2023;28:2502. https://doi.org/10.3390/molecules28062502.
130. Sherman S. Defining the menopausal transition. Am J Med. 2005;118:3–7. https://doi.org/10.1016/j.amjmed.2005.11.002.
131. Shynlova O, Bortolini MAT, Alarab M. Genes responsible for vaginal extracellular matrix metabolism are modulated by women's reproductive cycle and menopause. Int Braz J Urol. 2013;39:257–67. https://doi.org/10.1590/S1677-5538.IBJU.2013.02.15.
132. Sicari BM, Londono R, Dziki JL, Badylak SF. Chapter 5 – Extracellular matrix as a bioscaffold for tissue engineering. In: De Boer J, Blitterswijk CAV, Uquillas JA, Malik N, editors. Tissue engineering. 3rd ed. Academic; 2023. p. 137–72. https://doi.org/10.1016/B978-0-12-824459-3.00005-6.
133. Siddique SA. Vaginal Anatomy and Physiology. J Pelvic Med Surg. 2003;9:263–72. https://doi.org/10.1097/01.spv.0000094481.95144.3d.
134. Slavkin HC. Extracellular matrix influences on gene expression. Oxford: Elsevier Science; 1975.
135. Snell RS. Clinical anatomy: an illustrated review with questions and explanations. 4th ed. Philadelphia: Lippincott Williams & Wilkins; 2004.
136. Soderberg MW, Bystrom B, Kalamajski S, Malmstrom A, Ekman-Ordeberg G. Gene expressions of small leucine-rich repeat proteoglycans and fibulin-5 are decreased in pelvic organ prolapse. Mol Hum Reprod. 2009;15:251–7. https://doi.org/10.1093/molehr/gap011.

137. Sridharan I, Ma Y, Kim T, Kobak W, Rotmensch J, Wang R. Structural and mechanical profiles of native collagen fibers in vaginal wall connective tissues. Biomaterials. 2012;33: 1520–7. https://doi.org/10.1016/j.biomaterials.2011.11.005.
138. Stinson MW, Liu S, Laurenson AJ, Rotty JD. Macrophage migration is differentially regulated by fibronectin and laminin through altered adhesion and myosin II localization. MBoC. 2024;35:ar22. https://doi.org/10.1091/mbc.e23-04-0137.
139. Suarez AC, Gimenez CJ, Russell SR, Wang M, Munson JM, Myers KM, Miller KS, Abramowitch SD, De Vita R. Pregnancy-induced remodeling of the murine reproductive tract: a longitudinal in vivo magnetic resonance imaging study. Sci Rep. 2024;14:586. https://doi.org/10.1038/s41598-023-50437-1.
140. Tavakoli J, Diwan AD, Tipper JL. The ultrastructural organization of elastic fibers at the interface of the nucleus and annulus of the intervertebral disk. Acta Biomater. 2020;114:323–32. https://doi.org/10.1016/j.actbio.2020.07.021.
141. Theocharis A, Gialeli C, Hascall V, Karamanos NK. 1.1 Extracellular matrix: a functional scaffold. In: Karamanos N, editor. Extracellular matrix: pathobiology and signaling. DE GRUYTER; 2012. p. 3–20. https://doi.org/10.1515/9783110258776.3.
142. Tian Z, Li Q, Wang X, Sun Z. The difference in extracellular matrix metabolism in women with and without pelvic organ prolapse: a systematic review and meta-analysis. BJOG. 2024;131:1029–41. https://doi.org/10.1111/1471-0528.17768.
143. Ulrich D, Edwards SL, Su K, White JF, Ramshaw JAM, Jenkin G, Deprest J, Rosamilia A, Werkmeister JA, Gargett CE. Influence of reproductive status on tissue composition and biomechanical properties of ovine vagina. PLoS One. 2014;9:e93172. https://doi.org/10.1371/journal.pone.0093172.
144. Valenta C. The use of mucoadhesive polymers in vaginal delivery. Adv Drug Deliv Rev. 2005;57:1692–712. https://doi.org/10.1016/j.addr.2005.07.004.
145. Vergeldt TFM, Weemhoff M, IntHout J, Kluivers KB. Risk factors for pelvic organ prolapse and its recurrence: a systematic review. Int Urogynecol J. 2015;26:1559–73. https://doi.org/10.1007/s00192-015-2695-8.
146. Vodegel EV, Guler Z, Ras L, Mackova K, Groeneveld ACHM, Bezuidenhout D, Deprest J, Jeffery ST, Roovers JWR. Vaginal changes after ovariectomy in ewes: a large animal model for genitourinary syndrome of menopause. Intl J Gynecol Obstet. 2023;162:1042–9. https://doi.org/10.1002/ijgo.14816.
147. Wagenseil JE, Mecham RP. New insights into elastic fiber assembly. Birth Defects Res Pt C. 2007;81:229–40. https://doi.org/10.1002/bdrc.20111.
148. Wang X, Liu J, Zou J, Luo C, Wei D. The study of vaginal wall thickness in adults based on histopathological measurements. Sci Rep. 2024;14:18644. https://doi.org/10.1038/s41598-024-69308-4.
149. Weber IT, Harrison RW, Iozzo RV. Model structure of decorin and implications for collagen Fibrillogenesis. J Biol Chem. 1996;271:31767–70. https://doi.org/10.1074/jbc.271.50.31767.
150. Wenger MPE, Bozec L, Horton MA, Mesquida P. Mechanical properties of collagen fibrils. Biophys J. 2007;93:1255–63. https://doi.org/10.1529/biophysj.106.103192.
151. White SE, Kiley JX, Visniauskas B, Lindsey SH, Miller KS. Biaxial murine vaginal remodeling with reproductive aging. J Biomech Eng. 2022;144:061010. https://doi.org/10.1115/1.4054362.
152. White SE, Karbasion N, Snider JC, Florian-Rodriguez M, Bersi MR, Miller KS. Remodeling of murine vaginal smooth muscle function with reproductive age and elastic fiber disruption. Acta Biomater. 2024;175:186–98. https://doi.org/10.1016/j.actbio.2023.12.035.
153. Wieslander CK, Marinis SI, Drewes PG, Keller PW, Acevedo JF, Word RA. Regulation of elastolytic proteases in the mouse vagina during pregnancy, parturition, and puerperium1. Biol Reprod. 2008;78:521–8. https://doi.org/10.1095/biolreprod.107.063024.
154. Wise SG, Yeo GC, Hiob MA, Rnjak-Kovacina J, Kaplan DL, Ng MKC, Weiss AS. Tropoelastin: a versatile, bioactive assembly module. Acta Biomater. 2014;10:1532–41. https://doi.org/10.1016/j.actbio.2013.08.003.

155. Woessner J. Catabolism of collagen and non-collagen protein in the rat uterus during post-partum involution. Biochem J. 1962;83:304–14. https://doi.org/10.1042/bj0830304.
156. Yamada KM. Fibronectin and other cell interactive glycoproteins. In: Hay ED, editor. Cell biology of extracellular matrix: Second Edition. Boston: Springer; 1991. p. 111–46. https://doi.org/10.1007/978-1-4615-3770-0_5.
157. Yanagisawa H, Davis EC, Starcher BC, Ouchi T, Yanagisawa M, Richardson JA, Olson EN. Fibulin-5 is an elastin-binding protein essential for elastic fibre development in vivo. Nature. 2002;415:168–71. https://doi.org/10.1038/415168a.
158. Yanagishita M. Function of proteoglycans in the extracellular matrix. Acta Pathol Jpn. 1993;43:283–93. https://doi.org/10.1111/j.1440-1827.1993.tb02569.x.
159. Yang D, Zhang M, Liu K. Tissue engineering to treat pelvic organ prolapse. J Biomater Sci Polym Ed. 2021;32:2118–43. https://doi.org/10.1080/09205063.2021.1958184.
160. Yoon H, Chung W, Park Y, Shim B, Han W, Kwon S. Effects of estrogen on nitric oxide synthase and histological composition in the rabbit clitoris and vagina. Int J Impot Res. 2001;13:205–11. https://doi.org/10.1038/sj.ijir.3900687.
161. Zhou L, Lee JH, Wen Y, Constantinou C, Yoshinobu M, Omata S, Chen B. Biomechanical properties and associated collagen composition in vaginal tissue of women with pelvic organ prolapse. J Urol. 2012;188:875–80. https://doi.org/10.1016/j.juro.2012.05.017.
162. Zulfiqar M, Shetty A, Yano M, McGettigan M, Itani M, Naeem M, Ratts VS, Siegel CL. Imaging of the vagina: spectrum of disease with emphasis on MRI appearance. Radiographics. 2021;41:1549–68. https://doi.org/10.1148/rg.2021210018.
163. Zvietcovich F, Larin KV. Wave-based optical coherence elastography: the 10-year perspective. Prog Biomed Eng (Bristol). 2022;4:012007. https://doi.org/10.1088/2516-1091/ac4512.

Vaginal Tissue Engineering: Biomaterial Strategies and Opportunities

Samantha G. Zambuto

Abstract Tissue engineering is an interdisciplinary field that combines techniques and principles from biology, engineering, and the life sciences to develop biological substitutes that can restore, maintain, or improve tissue function. In this chapter, we will discuss tissue engineering of the female reproductive system ("reproductive tissue engineering") in the context of vaginal tissue engineering. This chapter serves to outline what we currently know in the field of vaginal tissue engineering, to delineate key engineering design criteria for vaginal tissue engineering, and to highlight future opportunities for the field. In recent years, women's health research has seen explosive growth; however, many questions remain in this space that should receive attention, including how we can prevent and target gynecological injuries. Quality of life is negatively impacted by gynecologic conditions and obstetric injuries, including congenital malformations, childbirth injuries, bacterial vaginosis, vulvovaginal candidiasis, sexually transmitted infections, and the genito-urinary syndrome of menopause. The creation of tissue-engineered models of the female reproductive system allows generation of basic science data, which can then be used to inform the creation of neo-organs, specifically neovaginas, for eventual transplantation into patients.

Keywords Women's health · Vagina · Biomaterials · Tissue engineering · Regenerative medicine · Gynecology · In vitro · Three dimensional

1 Tissue Engineering and Regenerative Medicine

Largely attributed to Vacanti and Langer, tissue engineering is an interdisciplinary field that combines techniques and principles from biology, engineering, and the life sciences to develop biological substitutes that can restore, maintain, or improve tissue function [1]. Tissue engineering seeks to complement, and eventually replace,

S. G. Zambuto (✉)
Department of Mechanical and Aerospace Engineering, University of Kentucky, Lexington, KY, USA
e-mail: samantha.zambuto@uky.edu

S. G. Zambuto, M. L. Oyen (eds.), *Biomaterials for Women's Health Engineering*,
https://doi.org/10.1007/978-3-032-10745-9_3

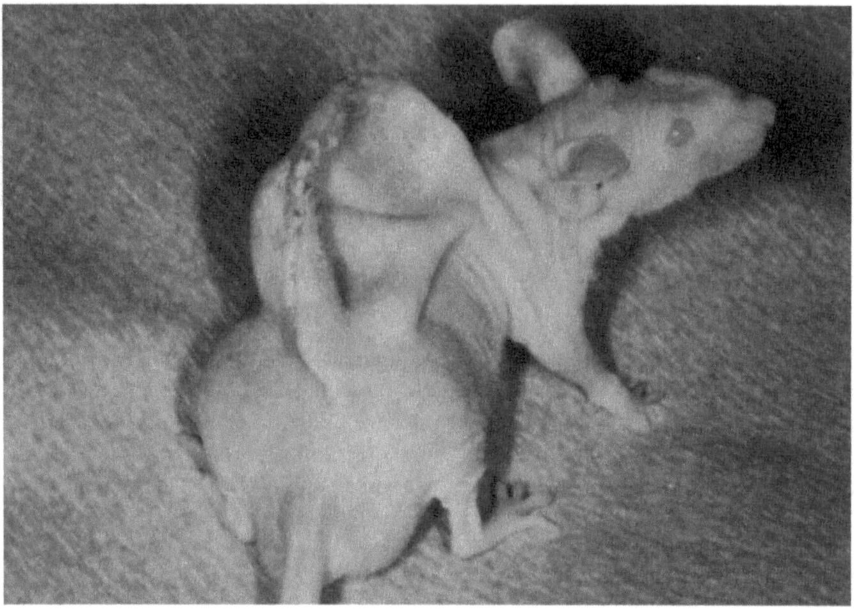

Fig. 1 The Vacanti Mouse or Auriculosaurus. (Image adapted from Cao et al. [3])

current gold standards of tissue replacement, including artificial medical devices (e.g., artificial hips), allografts (tissue from a living or deceased donor), or autografts (tissue from another site on the same patient). With tissue engineering, clinicians can regenerate, reconstruct, and replace tissue that is designed for the specific patient and specific application.

Tissue engineering came into being in the late 1980s and early 1990s [2]. The most infamous example of tissue engineering that comes to mind is the "auriculosaurus," or the mouse with the ear on its back, from Dr. Charles Vacanti's laboratory (Fig. 1). In this example, chondrocytes were seeded onto porous polymer fibers and then shaped into the shape of a 3-year-old child's auricle [3]. The year 1991 marked the first implantation of a tissue-engineered construct into a human patient: a human patient with Poland syndrome received a tissue-engineered implant consisting of a synthetic polymer implant seeded with autologous chondrocytes [3]. These examples highlight key principles of tissue engineering, notably how functional tissue could be regenerated using cells and a scaffold.

The core principles of tissue engineering can be distilled down to the tissue engineering triad of biomaterials/scaffolds, cells, and signals (Fig. 2). By combining these three constituents, a tissue engineer can begin to design and engineer a simplistic tissue. Through modular approaches, the complexity of the system can increase until eventually, a new or replacement organ is created ("regenerative medicine"). Regenerative medicine is a larger umbrella term that includes not only tissue engineering but also cell transplantation and stem cell biology [4]. As advances in science and technology continue to propel scientific discovery forward,

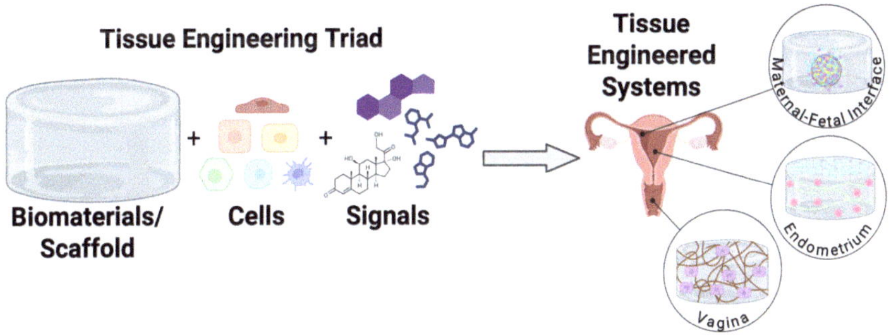

Fig. 2 Principles of reproductive tissue engineering

tissue engineering principles can also be combined with these other techniques. Ultimately, the goal of tissue engineering and regenerative medicine is to replace tissue.

Early pioneers in tissue engineering began by attempting to generate new connective tissue, including cartilage and skin [2]. Tissue engineering has resulted in excellent progress toward engineering more complex tissue and organ systems, including bladder, liver, and others. Although, as we will discuss in this chapter, tissue engineering of the female reproductive system ("reproductive tissue engineering") remains limited.

Because women have been previously understudied and excluded in basic and translational scientific research [5, 6], there is a dearth of sex- and gender-specific basic science information [7–10]. As such, the creation of neo-organs of the female reproductive system is aspirational. On one hand, the creation of tissue-engineered models of the female reproductive system allows generation of basic science data, which can then be used to inform the creation of neo-organs. On the other hand, regenerative medicine applications in female reproduction remain a distant dream. In this chapter, we explore principles of vaginal tissue engineering and propose future opportunities for the field to develop advanced tissue-engineered constructs for vaginal tissue engineering and regenerative medicine.

2 The Vagina

The vagina is a fibromuscular tube-shaped organ spanning from the hymenal ring to the cervix that plays critical roles in menstruation, pregnancy, and female sexual health [11, 12]. The vagina is approximately 6–10 cm in length, with wall length and diameter varying from posterior to anterior direction and cervix to introitus [11, 12].

Vaginal tissue is composed of four distinct layers (Fig. 3): epithelium, lamina propria, muscularis, and adventitia [13–15]. In women of reproductive age, the vaginal epithelium contains approximately 28 layers of non-keratinized stratified squamous epithelium that are entirely replaced every 96 h. The lamina propria is

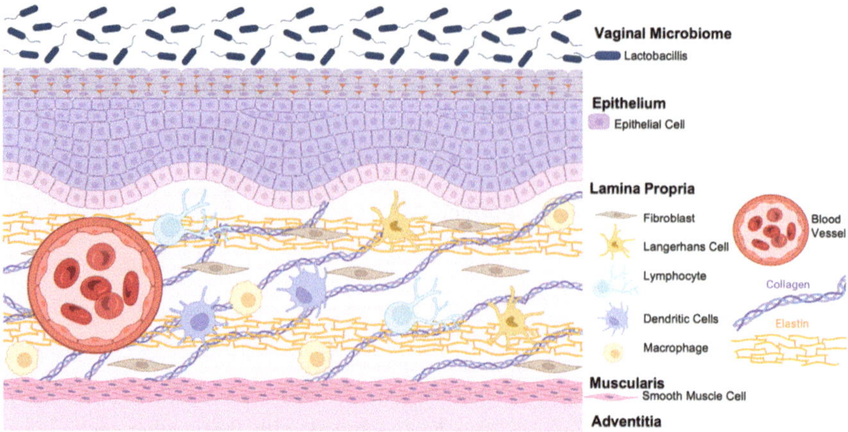

Fig. 3 The vaginal tissue microenvironment

vascularized and contains fibroblasts, immune cells (e.g., Langerhans cells, macrophages, dendritic cells, lymphocytes), and extracellular matrix (ECM) components—primarily collagen, which gives the vagina high tensile strength, and elastin, which enables the tissue to withstand deformation, especially in childbirth [13, 14]. The muscularis contains smooth muscle cells organized into bundles oriented in circular and longitudinal directions [16]. The adventitia connects the vaginal tissue to surrounding structures. Another important vaginal component is the vaginal microbiome. It is composed primarily of lactobacilli, which play an essential role in maintaining the low pH of the vaginal microenvironment and protecting the tissue against various infections, and reducing susceptibility to certain sexually transmitted diseases [17–20].

Of note, vaginal features are affected by menopausal status. Although beyond the scope of this chapter, the pre-versus postmenopausal features of the vagina are important to consider when designing tissue-engineered vaginal systems. We direct the reader to an excellent review on how vaginal features are affected by menopause [15].

3 Tissue Engineering of the Vagina

As mentioned, we are still far away from creating neovaginal constructs. In this chapter, however, we will focus on the application of basic tissue engineering principles to vaginal tissue engineering. The generation of basic science data pertaining to female gynecology has strong potential to fuel innovations in this space by providing crucial basic science information on gynecological anatomy and physiology. Additionally, in turn, this information can then be used to inform neovagina creation. Neovagina creation is relevant for a variety of conditions,

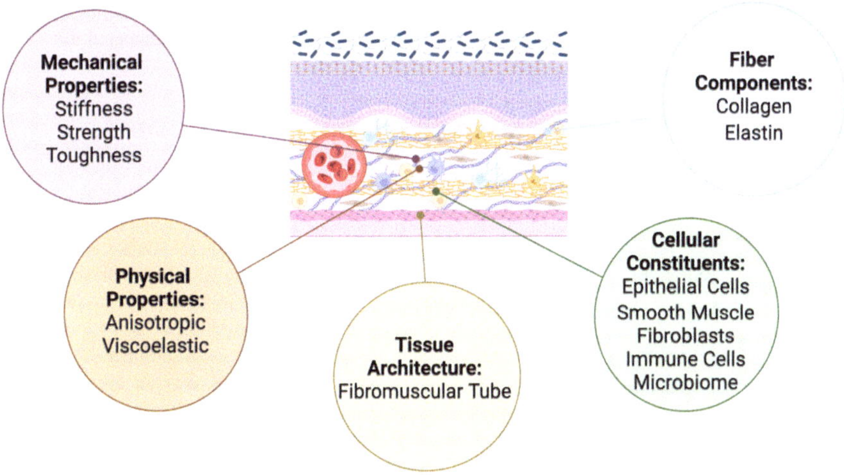

Fig. 4 Engineering criteria for the design of a tissue engineered vagina

including congenital malformations, Mayer-Rokitansky-Küster-Hauser syndrome, radiation damage from cancer treatments, and gender-affirming surgery. We hope this chapter will serve as a blueprint for researchers to use to begin the development of constructs for vaginal tissue engineering.

Design criteria for tissue engineering of the vagina should focus on the following major areas (Fig. 4): mechanical properties, physical properties, tissue architecture, cellular constituents, and fiber components. These core areas relate to the biomaterial/scaffold, cells, and signals of the tissue engineering triad. In Table 1, we provide a summary of these key features from the literature.

3.1 *Biomaterials and Scaffolds*

An optimal biomaterial for vaginal tissue engineering should recapitulate the mechanical properties, physical properties, and fiber components of the tissue. Vaginal features (e.g., tissue structure, cellular composition, extracellular matrix components) across all length scales (e.g., cm–nm) play critical roles in vaginal structure, function, and injury. The underlying microstructure of the vagina is essential in dictating the tissue's function. In particular, the cells and extracellular matrix fibers in the vagina contribute to the elastic performance and recovery of the tissue in childbirth. As such, an optimal biomaterial system will consider vaginal features across all length scales.

Mechanical properties are a necessary feature of tissue engineered vagina models. This relates to ensuring that mechanical properties of the biomaterial match that of the native tissue. The vagina exhibits both passive and active mechanical behavior, without or with smooth muscle activation, respectively [15]. Collagen and elastin

Table 1 Key engineering design criteria for tissue engineering of the vagina, including cited information from the literature and future opportunities for advancing tissue engineered models

Engineering design criteria	Feature	From the literature	Future opportunities
Mechanical properties	Stiffness	*Premenopausal*: 6.65 ± 1.48 MPa *Postmenopausal*: 10.26 ± 1.10 MPa	Hydrogel composites for enhanced mechanical properties Additional studies needed to quantify additional mechanical properties of the vagina (e.g., toughness)
	Strength	Conferred from elastin and collagen fibers	
Physical properties	Anisotropy	Fiber alignment	Advanced biomaterial techniques to create anisotropic structures (e.g., electrospinning) and to ensure viscoelasticity of biomaterials
	Viscoelasticity	Tissues, including the vagina, are viscoelastic	
Tissue architecture	Fibromuscular tube	The vagina is a fibromuscular tube-shaped organ	Advanced engineering to mimic shape and cellular distribution (e.g., bioprinting, patterning)
Cellular constituents	Various cell types	Multiple cell types exist in the vagina, including vaginal microbiome	Isolation and increased availability of additional vaginal cell types Co-cultures of vaginal cells and vaginal microbiome cells
Fiber components	Collagen and elastin fibers	The vagina contains predominantly collagen and elastin fibers that influence its mechanical abilities	Advanced biomaterials science and chemistry to ensure incorporation of nanoscale fibers Quantification of relative amounts of collagen and elastin in human vagina has not yet been performed

fibers ultimately determine passive mechanical properties of the tissue, including strength and distensibility [15]. Smooth muscle cells in the muscularis largely drive the active mechanical properties of the vagina, including contractility [15].

During childbirth, the vagina stretches significantly to almost five times its diameter to accommodate the delivery of the fetus [21]. A 9 cm fetal head experiences approximately 16 N of force at rest from the uterus, 54 N during a uterine contraction, and 120 N during a deliberate push, which in turn exposes vaginal tissue to these stresses required to deliver the fetus [12, 21]. Given the remarkable ability of the vagina to deform during childbirth and then return to its original structure, these biomechanical properties are critical tissue features that should be added to the tissue engineered construct.

In terms of stiffness, the ability to resist deformation from applied loads, the elastic modulus of premenopausal women is approximately 6.65 ± 1.48 MPa as determined from uniaxial tensile testing on vaginal tissue (Table 1) [15]. When considering what biomaterial scaffold to choose, a tissue engineer should preferentially select biomaterials with stiffness in the MPa regime. Hydrogels are usually the biomaterial system of interest for tissue engineering due to their excellent biocompatibility, ability to absorb high concentrations of water, and porosity, rendering them similar to native tissues. However, hydrogels are soft and compliant, which is not conducive to mimicking stiffer tissues like the vagina. Engineering strategies to improve the robustness of hydrogels, such as creating reinforced hydrogels with other materials and other chemistry techniques [22]. In terms of building hydrogel composites, combining hydrogels with nanometer-scale features (e.g., collagen and elastin fibers) will capture material properties across length scales. Other considerations for vaginal tissue engineering are the biomaterial strength, or the tissue's ability to withstand forces without experiencing failure, and toughness, the ability of a material to absorb energy when deforming prior to facture. Both collagen and elastin confer tissue strength. During menopause, production of collagen decreases and likely affects key mechanical properties of the vagina, including elastic modulus and ultimate stress and strain, as well as structural properties like stiffness, ultimate load, and ultimate elongation [15].

The vagina demonstrates some key physical properties such as anisotropy and viscoelasticity. Anisotropy, the property of being directionally dependent, applies to fibers and cells in the vagina. The muscularis layer contains smooth muscle cells organized into bundles oriented in circular and longitudinal directions. Advanced biomaterial strategies such as electrospinning or patterning can be used to create anisotropic biomaterials for vaginal tissue engineering. Vaginal tissue also has viscoelastic properties [15] and as such, viscoelastic biomaterials should be considered for vaginal tissue engineering. This includes a variety of hydrogels, including gelatin methacryloyl (GelMA) for which we have extensively characterized its viscoelastic properties using microindentation [23].

Finally, the vagina is a tube-shaped organ. As tissue-engineered constructs become larger and more complex, consideration should be taken to create tube-shaped structures to accurately mimic the native tissue architecture. This includes advanced engineering techniques such as 3D printing, the use of molds, electrospinning, and others.

3.2 Cells

Cell sources for tissue engineering include cell lines, primary cells, or stem cells. Cell lines have been immortalized using various techniques like human telomerase reverse transcriptase (hTERT) immortalization. Primary cells are derived directly from patients. Stem cells can be derived from a variety of sources although iPSCs (induced pluripotent stem cells) have become popular over the years. Although there are pros and cons to each cell source, here we will focus on primary vaginal cells. Primary vaginal cells offer an unaltered cell source unlike cell lines and because they are patient-derived, they allow for consideration of person-to-person heterogeneity in biological response. Compared to stem cell sources, these cells are cheaper and easier to culture.

Tissue-engineering models of the vagina should consider incorporating heterogeneous populations of vaginal cell types. However, a current limitation in the field is that only one primary vaginal cell type is commercially available: primary vaginal epithelial cells (LifeLine Cell Technology). Availability of commercially available vaginal cells or cells from collaborators would ensure that tissue engineered vaginal constructs can incorporate more than one cell type. For example, a key cellular feature of the vagina is smooth muscle cells. Unfortunately, these are not yet currently commercially available.

Other in vitro systems have also begun to incorporate bacterial cells from the vaginal microbiome [24]. Lactobacilli play an essential role in maintaining the low pH of the vaginal microenvironment. As tissue-engineered constructs of increased complexity are built, incorporation of the vaginal microbiome will be necessary not only to assess bacteria–cell interactions but also to ensure crucial immunity features conferred from the vaginal microbiome are not lost.

3.3 Signals

The final constituent of the tissue engineering triad is signals. Signals can range from bioactive molecules to hormones to drugs and more. The relevant signals that come to mind for vaginal tissue engineering are hormones and drugs.

The vagina is exposed to a variety of hormone states that affect the tissue, including pregnancy, menopause, and the use of vaginally applied contraceptives. However, much remains unknown regarding the effects of endogenous and exogenous hormones on vaginal tissue. Regardless, representation of the hormonal state of native tissue will be a key feature to incorporate in advanced tissue-engineered constructs.

Beyond contraceptives, other drugs are administered vaginally, including estrogen for treating lower urinary tract symptoms. Future studies may be interested in using these tissue-engineered constructs to investigate the potential of the vagina as a drug delivery site.

3.4 Existing Tissue-Engineered Systems of the Vagina

As mentioned earlier in this chapter, tissue-engineered systems of the vagina are limited. Although some in vitro models exist, they are lacking key tissue-engineered features such as use of a biomaterial scaffold or they utilize animal cells and not human cells.

Table 2 Summary of biomaterials implanted in patients (clinical) and tested with human vaginal cells (in vitro)

Biomaterial	Use
Decellularized porcine small intestinal submucosa	Clinical
Acellular human cadaver dermal matrix	Clinical
Collagen and collagen derivatives	Clinical
Alginate + chitosan	In vitro
Cellulose	Clinical
Poly-lactic acid (PLA)	Clinical
Decellularized porcine vagina	In vitro
Decellularized human vaginal ECM	None
Gelatin methacryloyl reinforced with electrospun fibers	In vitro

More information can be found in Ref. [25]

A 2022 systematic review by Francés-Herrero et al. [25] identified studies from 2000 to 2021 that used bioengineering strategies for studying the female reproductive system. In this review, 33 studies were identified that utilized bioengineering approaches to model the cervicovaginal region of the female reproductive system. The following biomaterials were identified to have been used in humans or with human vaginal cells (Table 2): decellularized porcine small intestinal submucosa, acellular human cadaver dermal matrix, collagen, alginate and chitosan, cellulose, poly-lactic acid (PLA), and decellularized porcine vagina [25]. Since this 2022 systematic review, there have been two additional studies that employ biomaterials for tissue engineered and regeneration of the human vagina [24, 26]. Sueters et al. utilized decellularized human vaginal ECM for vaginal reconstruction. This study did not test the biomaterials in cells; however, it was confirmed that structural features, minimal cellular residue, and biomechanics of the decellularized human vaginal ECM were maintained in these materials, so they show promise for further applications. Additionally, our group created fiber-reinforced hydrogel composites for vaginal tissue engineering. Nonetheless, additional studies since 2022 have used the following other types of biomaterials in animal models that may have potential to be used with human cells or in humans, but further studies are warranted: MatriStem™ (ECM scaffold derived from porcine urinary bladder) [27], silk fibroin [28, 29], and porcine vaginal ECM-gelatin methacrylate-silk fibroin composite bioink [30]. Although the following paper does not utilize biomaterials but instead utilizes emulate microfluidic chips to model the vaginal epithelium [24], organ-on-a-chip devices combined with biomaterials can result in sophisticated tissue engineering models of the vagina.

4 Perspectives and Future Outlook

In this chapter, we discussed tissue engineering of the female reproductive system ("reproductive tissue engineering") in the context of vaginal tissue engineering. We outlined what we currently know in the field of vaginal tissue engineering, delineated key engineering design criteria for vaginal tissue engineering, and highlighted future opportunities for the field.

The creation of a neovagina for individuals with congenital malformations, including Mayer–Rokitansky–Küster–Hauser syndrome, or individuals undergoing gender-affirming surgery is still limited, and the use of non-vaginal tissues for reconstruction is associated with complications such as graft rejection, lubrication issues, and excessive vaginal discharge [31]. Biomechanical problems associated with neovaginal tissue, including vaginal stenosis, dyspareunia, and vaginal prolapse, can negatively affect the performance of the tissue [31]. As researchers continue engineering efforts for creating a tissue-engineered vagina, we have the potential to target these issues and develop neovaginal constructs for vaginal reconstruction with enhanced features that reduce these complications and challenges. Through combined use of autologous cells and tissue, biomaterials can be used to support the mechanical loads of the neovaginal tissue and replicate the vaginal tissue architecture.

Acknowledgments Figures were created in BioRender. Zambuto, S. (2025) https://BioRender.com/14cimm5. The author thanks Dr. Marley Dewey for her thoughtful comments and review of this chapter. This publication was supported by the National Institutes of Health T32 Clinical Outcomes Research Training Program in Female Lower Urinary Tract Disorders [NIH T32DK120497] (SGZ) and the National Center for Research Resources and the National Center for Advancing Translational Sciences, National Institutes of Health, through Grant KL2TR001996. The content is solely the responsibility of the authors and does not necessarily represent the official views of the NIH.

References

1. Vacanti JP, Langer R. Tissue engineering: the design and fabrication of living replacement devices for surgical reconstruction and transplantation. Lancet. 1999;354:S32–4. https://doi.org/10.1016/s0140-6736(99)90247-7.
2. Vacanti CA. The history of tissue engineering. J Cell Mol Med. 2006;10:569–76. https://doi.org/10.1111/j.1582-4934.2006.tb00421.x.
3. Cao Y, Vacanti JP, Paige KT, Upton J, Vacanti CA. Transplantation of chondrocytes utilizing a polymer-cell construct to produce tissue-engineered cartilage in the shape of a human ear. Plast Reconstr Surg. 1997;100:297–302. https://doi.org/10.1097/00006534-199708000-00001.
4. Atala A. Regenerative medicine strategies. J Pediatr Surg. 2012;47:17–28. https://doi.org/10.1016/j.jpedsurg.2011.10.013.
5. Fisk N, Atun R. Systematic analysis of research underfunding in maternal and perinatal health. BJOG. 2009;116:347–56. https://doi.org/10.1111/j.1471-0528.2008.02027.x.
6. Mirin AA. Gender disparity in the funding of diseases by the U.S. National Institutes of Health. J Women's Health. 2021;30:956–63. https://doi.org/10.1089/jwh.2020.8682.

7. Schubert KG, Bird CE, Kozhimmanil K, Wood SF. To address women's health inequity, it must first be measured. Health Equity. 2022;6:881–6. https://doi.org/10.1089/heq.2022.0107.
8. Kalidasan D, Goshtasebi A, Chrisler J, Brown HL, Prior JC. Prospective analyses of sex/gender-related publication decisions in general medical journals: editorial rejection of population-based women's reproductive physiology. BMJ Open. 2022;12:e057854. https://doi.org/10.1136/bmjopen-2021-057854.
9. Hallam L, Vassallo A, Pinho-Gomes A-C, Carcel C, Woodward M. Does journal content in the field of women's health represent women's burden of disease? A review of publications in 2010 and 2020. J Women's Health. 2022;31:611–9. https://doi.org/10.1089/jwh.2021.0425.
10. White J, Clayton J. The gender health innovation gap: a perspective from the NIH Office of Research on Women's Health. Med. 2022;3:298–301. https://doi.org/10.1016/j.medj.2022.04.010.
11. Barnhart KT, et al. Baseline dimensions of the human vagina. Hum Reprod. 2006;21:1618–22. https://doi.org/10.1093/humrep/del022.
12. Ashton-Miller JA, Delancey JOL. On the biomechanics of vaginal birth and common sequelae. Annu Rev Biomed Eng. 2009;11:163–76. https://doi.org/10.1146/annurev-bioeng-061008-124823.
13. McCracken JM, et al. Animal models and alternatives in vaginal research: a comparative review. Reprod Sci. 2021;28:1759–73. https://doi.org/10.1007/s43032-021-00529-y.
14. Mazloomdoost D, et al. Histologic anatomy of the anterior vagina and urethra. Female Pelvic Med Reconstr Surg. 2017;23:329–35. https://doi.org/10.1097/SPV.0000000000000387.
15. Gimenez C, Alperin M, De Vita R. The effect of menopause on vaginal tissue mechanics: a brief review. J Biomech Eng. 2024;146:1–16. https://doi.org/10.1115/1.4063101.
16. Boreham MK, Wai CY, Miller RT, Schaffer JI, Word RA. Morphometric analysis of smooth muscle in the anterior vaginal wall of women with pelvic organ prolapse. Am J Obstet Gynecol. 2002;187:56–63. https://doi.org/10.1067/mob.2002.124843.
17. Amabebe E, Anumba DOC. The vaginal microenvironment: the physiologic role of lactobacilli. Front Med. 2018;5. https://doi.org/10.3389/fmed.2018.00181.
18. Ma B, Forney LJ, Ravel J. Vaginal microbiome: rethinking health and disease. Ann Rev Microbiol. 2012;66:371–89. https://doi.org/10.1146/annurev-micro-092611-150157.
19. Martin DH. The microbiota of the vagina and its influence on women's health and disease. Am J Med Sci. 2012;343:2–9. https://doi.org/10.1097/maj.0b013e31823ea228.
20. Hugon AM, Golos TG. Non-human primate models for understanding the impact of the microbiome on pregnancy and the female reproductive tractdagger. Biol Reprod. 2023;109:1–16. https://doi.org/10.1093/biolre/ioad042.
21. Clark–Patterson G, Domingo M, Miller KS. Biomechanics of pregnancy and vaginal delivery. Curr Opin Biomed Eng. 2022;22:100386. https://doi.org/10.1016/j.cobme.2022.100386.
22. Means AK, Grunlan MA. Modern strategies to achieve tissue-mimetic, mechanically robust hydrogels. ACS Macro Lett. 2019;8:705–13. https://doi.org/10.1021/acsmacrolett.9b00276.
23. Zambuto SG, et al. Evaluation of gelatin bloom strength on gelatin methacryloyl hydrogel properties. J Mech Behav Biomed Mater. 2024;154:106509. https://doi.org/10.1016/j.jmbbm.2024.106509.
24. Mahajan G, et al. Vaginal microbiome-host interactions modeled in a human vagina-on-a-chip. Microbiome. 2022;10:201. https://doi.org/10.1186/s40168-022-01400-1.
25. Francés-Herrero E, et al. Bioengineering trends in female reproduction: a systematic review. Hum Reprod Update. 2022;28:798–837. https://doi.org/10.1093/humupd/dmac025.
26. Zambuto SG, et al. Vaginal tissue engineering via gelatin-elastin fiber-reinforced hydrogels. Cold Spring Harbor Laboratory. 2024. https://doi.org/10.1101/2024.09.09.611932.
27. Liang R, et al. Towards rebuilding vaginal support utilizing an extracellular matrix bioscaffold. Acta Biomater. 2017;57:324–33. https://doi.org/10.1016/j.actbio.2017.05.015.
28. Chang Y, et al. Silk fibroin scaffold as a potential choice for female pelvic reconstruction: a study on the biocompatibility in abdominal wall, pelvic, and vagina. Microsc Res Tech. 2017;80:291–7. https://doi.org/10.1002/jemt.22653.

29. Nguyen T, Gundogdu G, Bottini C, Chaudhuri AK, Mauney JR. Evaluation of bi-layer silk fibroin grafts for inlay vaginoplasty in a rat model. Tissue Eng Regener Med. 2024;21:985–94. https://doi.org/10.1007/s13770-024-00653-1.
30. Zheng J, et al. Enhancing vaginal reconstruction through 3D bioprinted scaffolds using a novel vECM-GelMA-SF bioink. Biofabrication. 2025;17:015030. https://doi.org/10.1088/1758-5090/ad95bf.
31. Sueters J, et al. Tissue engineering neovagina for vaginoplasty in Mayer–Rokitansky–Küster–Hauser syndrome and gender dysphoria patients: a systematic review. Tissue Eng Part B Rev. 2023;29:28–46. https://doi.org/10.1089/ten.teb.2022.0067.

Biomaterials for Prolapse Repair

Sophya Breedlove, Amanda Artsen, and Katrina Knight

Abstract Biomaterials (both synthetic and biologically derived) are widely used in the repair of pelvic organ prolapse (prolapse), with roles in many nonsurgical and surgical solutions. This chapter will provide a comprehensive overview of both established and experimental biomaterials, beginning with those used in nonsurgical management such as pessaries, followed by those used in surgical interventions, for example, synthetic meshes and biologic grafts. Particular attention will be given to how specific properties of synthetic meshes, including textile properties, structural properties, and mechanical behavior, influence the host response, as well as how this response can be modulated using coatings and therapeutic agents. Additionally, we will discuss the challenges associated with absorbable synthetic meshes relative to traditional permanent synthetic meshes. We will provide insights into biologic grafts, a reemerging area in prolapse repairs, and discuss the strengths and limitations of various experimental, biologic materials. Finally, we will identify opportunities for innovation in future biomaterial development for prolapse repairs.

S. Breedlove
Department of Bioengineering, Swanson School of Engineering, University of Pittsburgh, Pittsburgh, PA, USA
e-mail: sob65@pitt.edu

A. Artsen
Department of Obstetrics, Gynecology, and Reproductive Sciences, University of Pittsburgh, Pittsburgh, PA, USA

Division of Urogynecology & Reconstructive Pelvic Surgery, University of Pittsburgh Medical Center Magee-Womens Hospital, Pittsburgh, PA, USA

Magee-Womens Research Institute, Pittsburgh, PA, USA
e-mail: artsenam@upmc.edu

K. Knight (✉)
Department of Bioengineering, Swanson School of Engineering, University of Pittsburgh, Pittsburgh, PA, USA

Magee-Womens Research Institute, Pittsburgh, PA, USA
e-mail: kmk144@pitt.edu

S. G. Zambuto, M. L. Oyen (eds.), *Biomaterials for Women's Health Engineering*,
https://doi.org/10.1007/978-3-032-10745-9_4

Keywords Synthetic mesh · Biologic grafts · Biomaterials · Host response · Pelvic floor disorders · Pelvic organ prolapse

1 Introduction

Pelvic organ prolapse (prolapse) is a common gynecologic condition characterized by the pathologic descent of the pelvic organs, including the bladder, rectum, or uterus, from their normal anatomic position into the vagina. The female pelvic floor is a complex structure composed of muscles, ligaments, and connective tissues that work in conjunction to support the pelvic organs. The levator ani muscles—the puborectalis, pubococcygeus, and illiococcygeus—play a crucial role in maintaining the structural positioning of the pelvic organs as they are essentially the shelf upon which the pelvic organs rest; they relax in order to open the bony pelvis for urination, defecation, and intercourse and keep the pelvis closed the remainder of the time. When the pelvic muscles and/or connective tissues become weakened or damaged, often due to childbirth, aging, or chronic strain, pelvic organ prolapse can occur, leading to the descent of one or more pelvic organs into the vaginal canal; in severe cases, this can result in the protrusion of the pelvic organs outside the body. Prolapse symptoms include, but are not limited to, the presence of a vaginal bulge, a sensation of vaginal pressure, urinary or fecal incontinence, and discomfort. An estimated one-third of women over the age of 20 have some degree of prolapse [1]. Risk factors for prolapse include obstetric factors such as parity and vaginal delivery [2–7], as well as age and BMI [2, 6–9].

Treatment of prolapse largely depends on the severity of prolapse and the patient's desire and health. Mild cases of prolapse can often be managed with conservative, nonsurgical treatments aimed at strengthening the pelvic floor, alleviating symptoms, and preventing the progression of prolapse. Pelvic floor muscle training, such as Kegel exercises, is often prescribed as a first-line treatment with the goal of strengthening the levator ani muscles, thus improving pelvic support and reducing symptoms. Vaginal pessaries, which are removable intravaginal medical devices designed to provide structural support for prolapsed pelvic organs, are also widely used in conservative treatments and can be considered one of the first biomaterials used in the repair of prolapse. By mechanically supporting the vaginal walls and adjacent pelvic structures, pessaries help to alleviate symptoms and contribute to improved quality of life for patients. They are particularly valuable for patients who are not surgical candidates, those who prefer to delay or avoid surgery, or as a temporary management tool during preoperative assessment. Pessaries come in a variety of shapes and sizes, are typically fit by a healthcare provider, and require regular cleaning and follow-up visits to prevent complications [10, 11].

For more severe cases of prolapse, surgical intervention may be necessary. Roughly 13% of women will undergo surgery to repair prolapse, and the cost of these surgeries exceeds \$1.5 billion annually [12–14]. Surgical repairs of prolapse can involve suturing the patient's own connective tissues to reinforce the vaginal walls or top of the vagina (referred to as a native tissue repair) or the implantation of biomaterials to restore pelvic support. Though advantageous in avoiding the foreign body response to a biomaterial, many native tissue repairs often fall short in providing durability and have a high risk of prolapse recurrence (40% risk of recurrence within 2 years and 70% risk within 5 years) [15, 16]. Although only about half of these patients will be symptomatic from this recurrence, these disappointing results have prompted the growing use of biomaterials such as synthetic meshes and biologic grafts in prolapse repairs.

The use of biomaterials in prolapse repairs aims to reinforce weakened tissues while simultaneously enhancing long-term support, thereby reducing the recurrence rate of prolapse. Thus, biomaterials play a crucial role in providing additional strength and durability beyond what the host tissues can provide. However, the unacceptable rates of mesh-related complications underscore the importance of advancing biomaterial design for prolapse treatment. Ultimately, this has led to a surge in research to understand the pathogenesis of mesh complications and to develop alternative devices, with the fundamental end goal of providing a device (s) that can be implanted using a minimally invasive approach and is well-tolerated. Thus, thoughtful material selection, device design, and thorough testing are essential for minimizing complications. This chapter will explore the role of biomaterials across both nonsurgical and surgical treatment modalities, beginning with an overview of pessaries and the biomaterials used in their design. We will then examine the various categories of surgical biomaterials, including synthetic meshes and biologic grafts, discussing their design, impact on the host response, and efforts to modulate the host response using innovative strategies. Finally, we will provide clinical perspectives and highlight potential future directions for innovation in the development of safer, more effective biomaterials for prolapse repair.

2 Biomaterials for Nonsurgical Treatment of Prolapse: Pessaries

2.1 *Overview and History of Pessaries*

Pessary-like solutions have been used for many years, predating the time of Hippocrates (400 BC). Similar nonsurgical treatments precede Hippocrates, with references to "remedies to allow the womb of a woman to slip into its place" in early Egyptian papyruses from around 1550 BC, in which honey and petroleum were used to push the uterus, and the uterine cavity was fumigated in an attempt to restore support [17]. At the time of Hippocrates, one treatment included succussion, in which the patient was hung upside down and shaken for 3–5 min so that gravity could restore the organ positioning [18]. Others believed that strong herbal odors and fumigation would cause the uterus to repel back into the cavity [19]. Eventually, early precursors to the modern pessary were developed, progressing from half a pomegranate soaked in lukewarm wine [20] to bronze cone-shaped pessaries secured with a band [21, 22]. By the Middle Ages, advancements included tampon-like pessaries made from cotton or wool [19, 23] and ball pessaries made of strips of linen, which were later followed by tightly bound sponges dipped in wax and oil or butter, oval-shaped pessaries made of hammered brass or waxed cork, and pear- and ring-shaped devices made of gold, silver, or brass [24]. In the 1600s, one of the first pessary complications was documented, in which a wax pessary obstructed a patient's lochia. Thus, a cork pessary was developed with a hole in the center to allow the passage of fluids and prevent similar complications [22]. To build upon this concept while also reducing the incidence of vaginal wall injuries that were common complications of pessaries at the time, a soft rubber pessary was developed in the 1700s with a perforated gold tip to allow for the passage of cervical secretions [24]. Eventually, prevalent materials such as sponge, cork, wood, and wax were discarded altogether and replaced by metals, glass, and porcelain. This was followed by hard rubbers, which were later replaced by polystyrene in the 1950s [25]. Today, pessaries are generally made from soft, sterilizable, relatively inert materials such as silicone, Lucite, rubber, and plastics [25, 26].

Throughout history, the development of pessary design has been driven by the need for effective support and guided toward reducing the complications associated with the pessary designs of the time. In 1860, a book titled *Diseases Peculiar to Women* postulated that pessary complications arise from three factors: the material, form (or shape), and size of the pessary [27]. Thus, the next section will explore these design considerations, addressing the biocompatibility, flexibility, and durability of the material; the range of pessary shapes; and how proper fit plays a crucial role in clinical outcomes.

2.2 Current Materials and Design Considerations for Pessary Manufacturing

Biocompatibility remains a fundamental requirement for any long-term vaginally inserted device; thus, materials used in the manufacture of pessaries are generally nontoxic, with material and surface properties that do not induce excessive inflammation, irritation, or infection. The structural strength and pliability of a pessary are also key material properties; pessaries generally need to be rigid enough to provide effective organ support and maintain their shape while also being flexible enough to allow for comfortable insertion and removal without causing discomfort, pressure necrosis, or ulceration. Finally, the mechanical integrity of pessaries should be maintained over extended periods without the pessary undergoing deformation or degradation in response to dynamic loading (i.e., changes in loading resulting from daily activities like walking, standing, or with coughing and sneezing) or during the cleaning process. As a result of these material requirements, modern pessaries tend to be made of medical-grade silicone, which offers excellent biocompatibility, flexibility, and durability. Silicone is inert, nonabsorbent, and can be sterilized, making it suitable for long-term intravaginal use. Other materials used to manufacture pessaries include latex, Lucite, and rubber, although latex pessaries are less common due to higher rates of allergic reactions and less-favorable mechanical properties [26].

From a design perspective, pessaries must accommodate a wide range of anatomical variations; so, they are manufactured in a variety of shapes, tailored to the degree and type of prolapse and to the patient's anatomy, with conventional shapes including ring, Gellhorn, donut, and cube pessaries [10, 26, 28] (Fig. 1). Most pessaries must be manually fit by a trained clinician. Although the initial size can be estimated from measurements made during a gynecologic exam, approximately 2–3 trials are often required before the optimal sizing is selected [29–32]. Due to anatomic variability, a range which widens considerably with prolapse, and limited sizes of pessaries for prolapse, challenges remain in achieving an ideal fit for all patients across the full range of pelvic anatomy. Factors associated with unsuccessful fittings include a short vaginal length, wide vaginal introitus [29], a history of pelvic surgery [31, 33], hysterectomy [32], stress urinary incontinence [30, 34], obesity [33], and younger age [35], while factors associated with satisfactory retention include hormone use [31], sexual activity [32], and a shorter perineal body at rest [30]. Poorly fitting pessaries have resulted in patients experiencing discomfort,

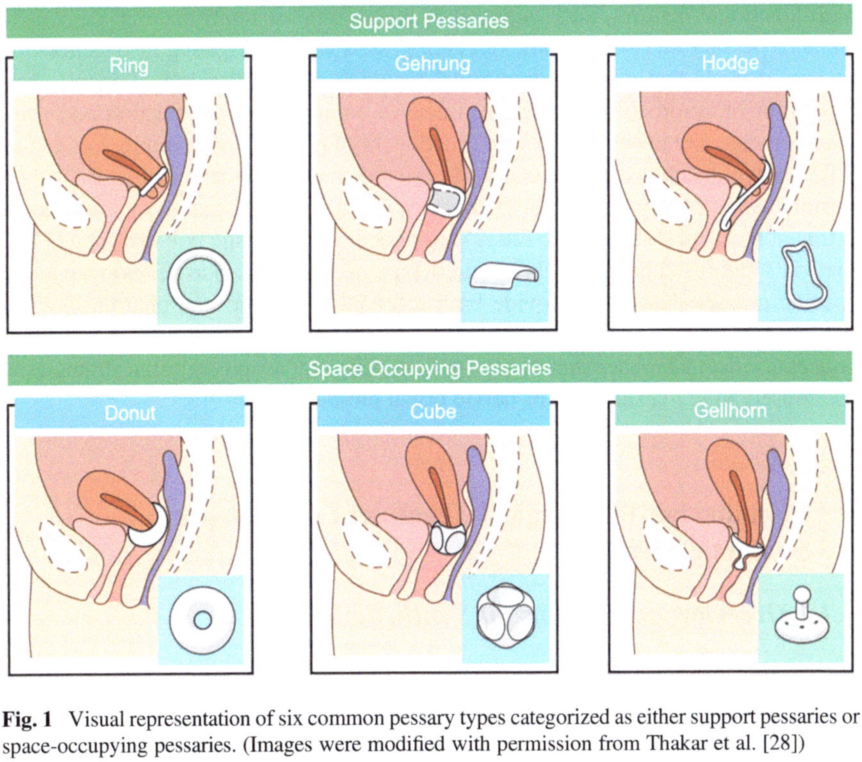

Fig. 1 Visual representation of six common pessary types categorized as either support pessaries or space-occupying pessaries. (Images were modified with permission from Thakar et al. [28])

difficulty with pessary retention, and increased risk of complications such as vaginal irritation, discharge, and odor. More severe, but less commonly reported, complications associated with pessary use include erosion, fistula, impaction, and fibrosis; therefore, it is important that pessaries be checked regularly [10, 11, 36–39]. As the limitations of current pessary shapes and materials become apparent, particularly in terms of patient-specific customization, research is turning toward the development of new materials and manufacturing methods aimed at enhancing pessary performance.

2.3 *Recent Advancements in Pessary Design*

In recent years, there has been a surge of innovation in the field of pessary design and material science. Emerging technologies such as 3D printing offer promising solutions to issues with fit and provide the opportunity for patient-specific customization. With the aid of imaging techniques like transvaginal ultrasound, it is feasible to generate custom pessaries that match a patient's unique vaginal topography, with potential for improving fit and retention, thus reducing the rate of complications associated with poor fit and enhancing overall patient satisfaction and clinical outcomes [40]. Additionally, additive manufacturing enables the integration of multifunctional features, such as creating more complex multi-material devices to enhance pessary outcomes. Some research groups are investigating next-generation pessary designs that combine traditional materials with antimicrobial agents, hormones, or bioresorbable polymers to improve comfort, reduce infection and complication risk, and to enhance device functionality [41, 42]. For example, Long et al. (2022) have developed a medicated 3D printed silicone pessary with slow-release estriol to simultaneously address the issue of vaginal atrophy caused by low vaginal estrogen levels [41]. Eder et al. (2022) have used thermoplastic polyurethane (TPU) materials and fused filament fabrication (a type of 3D printing) to develop a patient-specific pessary that could provide both mechanical support and pharmacological therapy via controlled drug release [42]. Although still in the early stages, such concepts reflect a broader shift toward patient-centered, adaptive design strategies in the conservative management of pelvic organ prolapse.

3 Biomaterials for Surgical Treatment of Prolapse: Synthetic Meshes

3.1 *Overview and History of Synthetic Meshes*

3.1.1 From Hernia Mesh to Prolapse Mesh

Synthetic plastics, which are made from man-made materials, are frequently used to manufacture synthetic meshes for prolapse repairs. Plastics are common for these

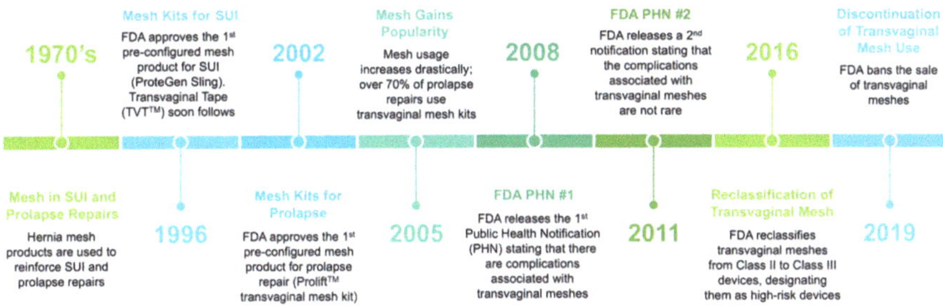

Fig. 2 Timeline of mesh product development and usage in the surgical repairs of pelvic organ prolapse

meshes due to their balance of strong mechanical properties sufficient to support a weakened pelvic floor, lightweight nature, and ability to be extruded into flexible filaments. The most common synthetic plastic used is polypropylene, a durable material with a high tensile strength, good handleability, biocompatibility, and heat and chemical resistance, and it can be extruded into a monofilament to be knit or woven into a strong, flexible mesh. Other synthetic materials that have been used for prolapse meshes include expanded polytetrafluorethylene (ePTFE) [43–45], polyethylene terephthalate (PET) [43], and polyvinylidene fluoride (PVDF) [46, 47].

The use of synthetic meshes for prolapse repairs dates to the 1970s (Fig. 2). At that time, there were no FDA-approved meshes for the surgical repair of prolapse. Thus, in the 1990s, to reinforce support to prolapsed pelvic organs beyond what native tissue could provide, surgeons began utilizing synthetic hernia meshes, which were effective at reinforcing weakened abdominal tissues. Given the high rates of prolapse recurrence following native tissue repair and the consequently high demand for a surgical mesh product for urogynecology applications, companies started remarketing their hernia products for prolapse applications. It is important to note that synthetic mesh is also used in the surgical treatment of stress urinary incontinence (SUI); however, this chapter will focus on synthetic mesh used in the context of prolapse. The interested reader should refer to Gomelsky et al. (2007) for an in-depth discussion regarding mesh and SUI [48].

To remarket hernia meshes for prolapse applications, manufacturers leveraged the 510(k) clearance pathway established by the U.S. Food and Drug Administration (FDA), which allows medical devices to enter the market without extensive clinical trials if they are deemed "substantially equivalent" to a previously approved device. Because the proposed prolapse meshes were essentially the same as hernia meshes and because hernia products were in existence before the 1976 Medical Device Amendments Act, companies were able to bypass the rigorous premarket approval (PMA) process. Thus, synthetic prolapse meshes entered the market without comprehensive clinical testing in the pelvic environment. Not surprisingly, synthetic mesh impacts vaginal tissue differently than abdominal tissue [49], and because these meshes were not designed for the unique anatomy and dynamic environment of the pelvic floor, the lack of testing ultimately contributed to clinical complications [50].

3.1.2 Synthetic Mesh Kits

To adapt the shape of mesh to the pelvic environment and improve the ease of surgical placement, mesh "kits" were developed for pelvic floor repair applications. In 1998, tension-free vaginal tape (TVT; Ethicon, Somerville, NJ, United States) was developed as one of the first commercially marketed mesh "kits" to treat SUI. The design of these kits improved the ease of surgical placement and meant that surgery could be performed under intravenous sedation rather than general anesthesia. It was an immediate success, and other manufacturers began producing their own versions of the design, resulting in an increasingly competitive environment for mesh kits.

Building upon a similar concept, transvaginal prolapse mesh kits were developed. Rather than requiring an abdominal incision for mesh implantation, transvaginal mesh could be implanted through a small incision in the vaginal tissue. This resulted in a procedure for prolapse repair that was less difficult, less invasive, and had a shorter operation time than the traditional transabdominal approaches. Thus, Prolift (Ethicon, Somerville, NJ, United States), a transvaginal mesh kit based on the commonly used transabdominal mesh, Gynemesh PS, became the first preconfigured mesh for prolapse repair. It was approved for use by the FDA in 2002, and other transvaginal mesh kit designs soon followed [50].

3.1.3 The Rise of Synthetic Mesh Usage and Complications

Although synthetic meshes had been used for decades in transabdominal repair, with the introduction of transvaginal mesh kits, the use of synthetic mesh in prolapse repair skyrocketed; by 2005, over 70% of mesh-augmented prolapse procedures used transvaginal mesh kits. The overall popularity of synthetic mesh for prolapse repair increased as well, leading to a massive surge in both transvaginal and transabdominal mesh use; by 2010, over one-third of the 300,000 prolapse surgeries performed annually used some form of synthetic mesh [51].

Unfortunately, this dramatic increase in mesh usage was accompanied by a subsequent increase in the number of mesh-related complications, with pain and mesh exposure through the vaginal epithelium being the most reported. Alarmed by the number of these complications, the FDA released a public health notification (PHN) in 2008 warning the public of complications associated with transvaginal meshes. In 2011, with reports of complications continuing to rise, the FDA issued a second notification stating that these complications are not rare, occurring in approximately 20% of cases [50].

3.1.4 The Discontinuation of Transvaginal Mesh

As a result of the PHNs, transvaginal mesh use declined dramatically, although there was no significant change in the use of synthetic mesh for transabdominal repairs of prolapse [52]. As complications with transvaginal mesh repairs continued to increase, the FDA reclassified transvaginal meshes from Class II to Class III devices in 2016, meaning that clinical trials were required before devices could be approved for use. In 2019, the FDA determined that the benefits of transvaginal mesh did not outweigh the risks of post-surgical complications, and they ordered the discontinuation of production, sales, and distribution of transvaginal mesh products. Similarly, countries such as the United Kingdom, Canada, Australia, New Zealand, and France also discontinued the use of transvaginal mesh products [50]. Despite the issues with transvaginal meshes, synthetic meshes continue to be used in transabdominal repairs of prolapse and are also associated with complications, albeit at a lower rate than those of transvaginal meshes. Complications associated with synthetic mesh used in transabdominal procedures are reported to occur at a rate of about 10.5% over 7 years, and this rate is expected to increase with time [53, 54].

3.2 *Design Considerations for Synthetic Meshes*

Ultimately, the discontinuation of transvaginal mesh and the revelation of the mesh-related complications associated with pelvic surgeries had a profound impact on the way prolapse mesh was viewed, calling into question the regulatory pathways and clinical testing requirements, or lack thereof, for approval of prolapse meshes. These events also altered the way the scientific community approached solutions for prolapse repair and shifted emphasis toward research-driven biomaterial selection and device design. In the past decade, there has been a dramatic increase in studies investigating the mechanisms of mesh complications, which has led to the identification of key factors contributing to mesh complications, as well as potential pathways toward more effective solutions. Thus, the etiology of mesh complications appears to be multifactorial, with research suggesting that host factors (e.g., smoking, diabetes, age, obesity) and mesh-specific factors such as the textile properties, structural properties, and mechanical behavior of the mesh contribute to the pathogenesis of mesh complications. In the next section, we will focus on the impact of the mesh-specific factors on the host response and discuss potential strategies for modulating the off-target effects of synthetic mesh.

3.2.1 Textile Properties and the Host Response

Synthetic meshes used in prolapse repairs are fundamentally textile materials and are composed of fibers, which themselves can be formed from either a single filament (monofilament) or multiple intertwined filaments (multifilament). These fibers are then typically knit or woven together, although newer techniques such as 3D printing are being explored. The spaces between the fibers, known as pores, vary in size and shape and are critical for biological integration and immune cell migration. Overall, the textile properties of prolapse mesh, including filament type, knit pattern, pore size and porosity, pore shape, and edge features, impact the structural properties of mesh and the host response, particularly in terms of tissue integration, infection risk, and compatibility with vaginal tissue. It is worth noting that these mesh characteristics, such as weight, pore size, and stiffness, are closely linked—modifying one will inevitably influence the others. As a result, isolating the biological response to a single property is challenging.

Filament Type and Surface Area

Synthetic mesh is generally constructed from fibers, which are made from filaments. As a result, meshes can either be monofilament (a single strand of material per mesh fiber) or multifilament (multiple braided or interwoven strands per mesh fiber). The structure of mesh fibers (monofilament versus multifilament) has significant clinical implications in prolapse repair, primarily affecting the risk of infection. Multifilament fibers are associated with a greater risk of infection. The presence of multiple filaments within a single fiber increases the total surface area of multifilament fibers by at least 1.57 times compared to monofilaments [55], providing ample surface for bacterial adhesion. Additionally, the interwoven structure likely creates small interstitial spaces (potentially $<10\ \mu m$) within multifilament fibers that would allow bacteria to enter but are too small for immune cells such as macrophages and neutrophils to access [56], thus creating reservoirs for bacterial proliferation [57]. Indeed, it has been shown that multifilament meshes are associated with higher bacterial colonization rates [58]. As a result, current prolapse meshes are predominantly manufactured using monofilament fibers, which offer reduced infection risk, better immune cell accessibility, and greater potential for tissue integration.

Similarly, the local surface area, a measure of the amount of material in contact with the surrounding tissue, is another key factor influencing the host response to mesh [59, 60]. Fibers with greater local surface area tend to invoke a more robust and active inflammatory response compared to those with smaller surface areas [61, 62]. Consequently, this issue is particularly pronounced for multifilament meshes, which have a surface area that is approximately 50% greater than monofilament meshes, offering a larger surface for bacterial adherence and proliferation [55]. It is important to note that this surface area refers to the local surface area of the mesh fibers rather than that of the entire mesh; for example, the issues caused by greater local surface area would not be mitigated by creating an overall narrower strip of mesh.

Knit Pattern

The knit pattern, or the way in which the mesh fibers are interconnected, plays a critical role in determining mechanical behavior, porosity, flexibility, and the biological response to mesh. Commercially available prolapse meshes are commonly fabricated by knitting or weaving. In knit meshes, a single fiber is continuously looped together, creating a flexible, extensible structure with relatively large pores and high porosity. This promotes better tissue integration, immune cell infiltration, and reduces infection risk [63–65]. Due to their flexibility, knitted meshes also conform to the dynamic movement of the underlying tissue, which reduces mechanical irritation. However, they generally have lower strength compared to woven meshes. Woven meshes involve two sets of fibers interlaced perpendicular to each other, forming a more rigid structure with higher strength but smaller pores and reduced porosity. Although mechanically robust with strong shape memory, woven meshes are less flexible, more prone to fraying when cut [62], and more prone to promoting encapsulation, poor tissue integration, and mechanical complications like wrinkling. Thus, woven meshes are not preferred for prolapse repair applications.

To overcome the limitations of knit or woven meshes, additive manufacturing (3D printing) is a promising solution. Specifically, additive manufacturing allows for precise control over pore size, shape, and distribution, enabling customizable designs that balance mechanical strength and flexibility while maintaining large, stable pores for tissue ingrowth. Irrespective of the manufacturing process, well-designed meshes that support tissue integration are key to improving the safety and efficacy of prolapse meshes.

Pore Size and Porosity

Pore size and porosity are critical parameters in mesh design for prolapse repair, as they directly influence tissue integration and the biological response to the implant. Pore size defines the dimensions of the individual void spaces within a mesh, while porosity refers to the proportion of the mesh structure composed of void spaces. These properties will vary depending on the specific mesh design (Table 1). Similar to multifilament meshes, pore sizes smaller than 10 μm can harbor unchecked bacterial proliferation [56], and small-pore, low-porosity meshes tend to be associated with increased inflammation, scarring, and adhesion risk [55, 60, 66–68]. Alternatively, meshes with larger pore sizes and greater porosity allow for better vascularization, better immune cell infiltration, and promote more effective tissue integration [69]. Pore size has also been shown to be inversely proportional to bridging fibrosis, a phenomenon in which scarring tissue forms that bridges across the pores of the mesh [70]. To prevent bridging fibrosis, the pore size for polypropylene meshes should be larger than 1 mm [55, 71]. Optimizing pore size and porosity remains a major goal in the development of meshes for pelvic organ prolapse repair.

Edge Features

The edge of synthetic meshes can have various features, including roughness (smooth or serrated) and tendency to fray, depending on the knit pattern, pore shape, number of filaments, and cutting methods. When knit or woven meshes are

Table 1 Properties of various synthetic prolapse meshes as reported by manufacturers

		Material	Manufacturer	Approved or introduced	Withdrawn	Weight (g/m^2)	Stiffness (N/mm)	Porosity (%)
Sacrocolpopexy mesh products	Gynecare Gynemesh PS	Polypropylene	Ethicon	01/08/2002		42	0.3–0.45	62%
	Restorelle	Polypropylene	Coloplast	08/04/2009		19	0.16–0.41	78%
	Upsylon	Polypropylene	Boston Scientific	12/18/2012		25	0.2	72%
	Artisyn	Poliglecaprone 25/Polypropylene	Ethicon	06/11/2012		28	0.08–0.49	68%
Transvaginal mesh products	Prolift	Polypropylene	Ethicon	03/01/2005	08/15/2012	42	0.29–1.37	62%
	Prolift+M	Poliglecaprone 25/Polypropylene	Ethicon	05/15/2008	08/15/2012	28	0.01–0.24	67%
	Uphold	Polypropylene	Boston Scientific	12/13/2012	04/16/2019	25	0.2	72%
	Avaulta Solo	Polypropylene	Bard Medical	03/12/2007	07/02/2012	18	0.16	75%
	Avaulta Plus/Biosynthetic	Type 1 polypropylene with acellular cross-linked collagen		03/12/2007	07/02/2012	100		
	Exair	Polypropylene	Coloplast	05/08/2009	01/07/2014	19	0.072	67%
	Ascend	Polypropylene	Caldera Medical	03/31/2009	10/15/2012	33	0.72–1.66	51%

Stiffness is given as a range from low stiffness to high stiffness when available mechanically cut to size during manufacturing or surgery, this can disrupt and loosen the mesh knots, creating frayed edges. To overcome this, mesh can be laser-cut or heat-sealed, which, in turn, can alter the mechanical properties. For example, in an ex vivo study that used an apparatus to generate erosion in porcine muscle, it was found that the meshes with laser-cut and heat-formed edges resulted in higher exposure rates through the tissue compared to those with mechanically cut edges [72]. It was also found that polypropylene sheets with serrated edges (mechanically cut serrations with depths of either 0.8 mm or 2.5 mm) yielded higher exposure rates than those with smooth edges [72]. These results suggest that the method used to cut and seal synthetic surgical mesh could potentially impact tissue damage, although the effects in vaginal tissue specifically have yet to be investigated. Thus, further research is necessary to better understand how mesh edge features impact in vivo outcomes in prolapse repair applications.

Mesh Weight

Mesh weight is defined by the specific gravity (g/m^2), also referred to as the relative density, and is generally categorized as ultralightweight (<20 g/m^2), lightweight (<45 g/m^2), or heavyweight (>45 g/m^2). Lightweight meshes tend to have larger pores and higher porosity than heavyweight meshes [69]. Subsequently, lightweight meshes typically translate to overall better biocompatibility, exhibiting less fibrosis, less inflammation, a higher affinity for tissue incorporation within the mesh pores, reduced potential for adhesion and pain, and a reduced number of mesh-related complications [60, 73–78]. On the other hand, heavyweight meshes are associated with an increase in the number of apoptotic cells surrounding the mesh fibers, a more pronounced and prolonged inflammatory response, and a higher turnover of the tissues surrounding the mesh fibers [75, 79–84]. Thus, heavyweight meshes are more prone to mesh complications and reinterventions for mesh-related complications compared to lightweight meshes [78].

Generally, lighter weight meshes perform better than heavyweight, but this is not always the case, and contrasting results have been observed. In a study comparing a heavyweight (large-pore, knitted) and lightweight (small-pore, woven) polypropylene mesh implanted in the abdomen of rats, the heavyweight mesh was associated with a reduced fibrotic reaction, improved tissue integration, and significantly fewer macrophages at the implant surface than the lightweight mesh [85], suggesting that pore size and knit pattern are more important than weight and can be tuned to offset the negative effects of mesh weight. Additionally, while lightweight mesh can reduce the rate of mesh complications, the mesh needs to be strong enough to support physiologic loads. Ultralightweight mesh can be associated with an earlier time to anterior vaginal recurrence, although there is no difference in the proportion of recurrences [86, 87]. Nevertheless, minimizing complications involves considerations of both mesh strength and weight.

3.2.2 Stiffness and the Host Response

The stiffness of mesh—both structural stiffness and material stiffness—is a key mechanical consideration in the design of prolapse meshes. Material stiffness refers to the property of the base material itself, independent of form, whereas structural stiffness accounts for the structural factors of the final device, including knit pattern, filament type, and porosity. Structurally, if an implant is significantly stiffer than the surrounding tissue, it can lead to a phenomenon known as stress shielding. Stress shielding occurs when an implant bears a disproportionate amount of mechanical load, reducing the normal physiological load experienced by the native biological tissue and because many tissues are designed to adapt to mechanical loads (Wolff's law), this can result in degeneration and atrophy of the adjacent tissue. Stress shielding is well documented in orthopedic applications, such as hip replacements. For example, if a metallic hip implant is much stiffer than the surrounding bone, it can shield the bone from normal mechanical stresses, resulting in bone resorption, atrophy, and implant loosening or failure [88]. The concept of stress shielding is equally relevant in the context of prolapse meshes.

Structural Stiffness and the Host Response

Studies implanting synthetic prolapse meshes onto the vagina of nonhuman primates (*Rhesus macaques*) with varying structural stiffnesses demonstrated that all mesh implantations negatively impacted the vaginal tissue; particularly, the mesh with the highest structural stiffness was associated with the greatest deterioration [82, 89–92]. Stress shielding was observed as thinning of the subepithelium and vaginal smooth muscle layers, decreased amounts of collagen and elastin, and increased apoptosis surrounding the mesh fibers [82]. An increase in active-matrix metalloproteinases (MMPs) MMP-1, MMP-8, and MMP-13, and increased total MMP-2 and MMP-9 were also observed, indicating that tissue degradation was active and ongoing [89]. In addition to impacting the structure of the tissue, the stiffest mesh detrimentally impaired vaginal contractile function [90–92]. Collectively, these results suggest that stress shielding induced by the implantation of stiff polypropylene mesh results in degeneration and atrophy, and that some of these adverse outcomes could potentially be mitigated by matching the mechanical properties of the mesh, particularly the material stiffness, to that of vaginal tissue [93].

Material Stiffness and the Host Response

The material stiffness of the mesh also appears to be an important factor in prolapse repair. Polypropylene is the most common material used to manufacture prolapse meshes due to its ease of manufacturing, biocompatibility, and durability in a biological environment. But relative to the stiffness of vaginal tissue ($\sim$6–34 MPa), polypropylene is significantly stiffer ($\sim$1–2 GPa), resulting in a

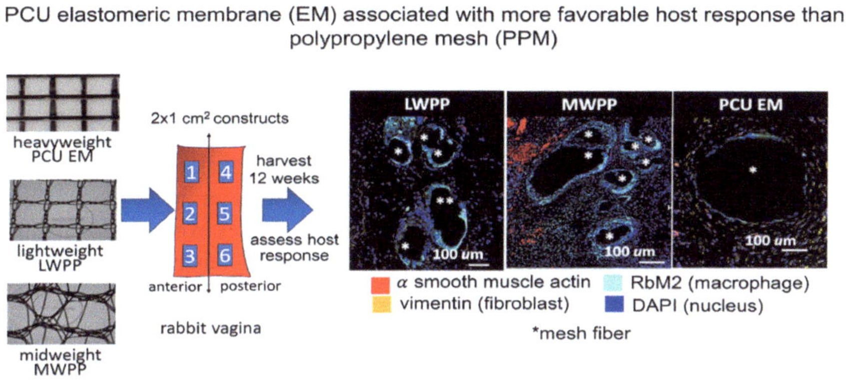

Fig. 3 Graphical abstract of Knight et al. [97]. A marked reduction in the macrophage response to the PCU EM was observed as compared to LWPP and MWPP meshes despite the increased weight of the PCU EM. (Figure was obtained with permission from Knight et al. [97])

mechanical mismatch [94–96]. Polycarbonate urethane (PCU) is an example of a soft elastomeric material that is being evaluated to address the mismatch in material stiffness between mesh material and vaginal tissue. Specifically, in an in vivo rabbit study, small constructs (2 cm × 1 cm) of high-stiffness polypropylene meshes (a lightweight mesh and a midweight mesh) and small constructs made from two different grades (i.e., stiffnesses) of polycarbonate urethane (stiffnesses of 8–65 MPa and 28–149 MPa) were implanted (in the absence of tension) onto the vagina of New Zealand White rabbits (Fig. 3) [97]. Results of this study showed that the low-stiffness PCU constructs had an overall superior host response compared to the high-stiffness polypropylene constructs. Overall, the PCU constructs had favorable preservation of vaginal smooth muscle morphology, a decreased cellular response to the construct fibers, and a reduced percentage of macrophages. However, all constructs had a detrimental impact on vaginal contractile function and glycosaminoglycan (GAG) content, regardless of material stiffness, but the PCU constructs had less of a negative impact on GAGs than the polypropylene constructs. These results suggest that devices with lower material stiffness have the potential to elicit a more favorable vaginal response compared to higher stiffness materials [97]. Future studies are needed to assess the host response to PCU membranes implanted on tension and at the dimensions that are comparable to human implantations.

3.2.3 Mechanics and the Host Response

Pore Shape and Planar Deformation

In vivo prolapse meshes are subjected to primarily uniaxial loads, and as a result, the pores of these meshes tend to collapse (i.e., pore size decreases). Previously, notable pore collapse and a significant loss of porosity were observed in the arms and central body (between the superior arms) of transvaginal meshes [98, 99] in response to relatively minimal tensile loads. Clinically, these areas have been associated with mesh complications, including mesh shrinkage, tenderness upon palpation of contracted mesh, pain, and dyspareunia [100]. Similarly, Barone et al. [101] observed a dramatic decline in pore size in response to uniaxial loading (up to 10 N) of commercially available meshes used in transabdominal repairs of prolapse. The shape of the mesh pores had a major influence on whether the pores remained open or collapsed. Overall, the mesh with square-shaped pores experienced minimal pore collapse, whereas the meshes with hexagon- and diamond-shaped pores experienced dramatic pore collapse and a significant reduction in porosity, reducing to nearly 0% (Fig. 4).

For polypropylene meshes, pore diameters that are or have collapsed to less than 1 mm can lead to poor tissue integration, bridging fibrosis, encapsulation, and pain. Thus, meshes with stable pore shapes (e.g., square-shaped pores) are preferred, as they allow for better tissue integration and ingrowth as compared to meshes with unstable pore shapes (e.g., hexagon and diamond). It is therefore essential that the architecture of the mesh pores is carefully considered for enhancing the long-term success of prolapse meshes. Knight et al. (2018) have explored auxetic designs, which are structures that expand in response to an applied force, for the pores of

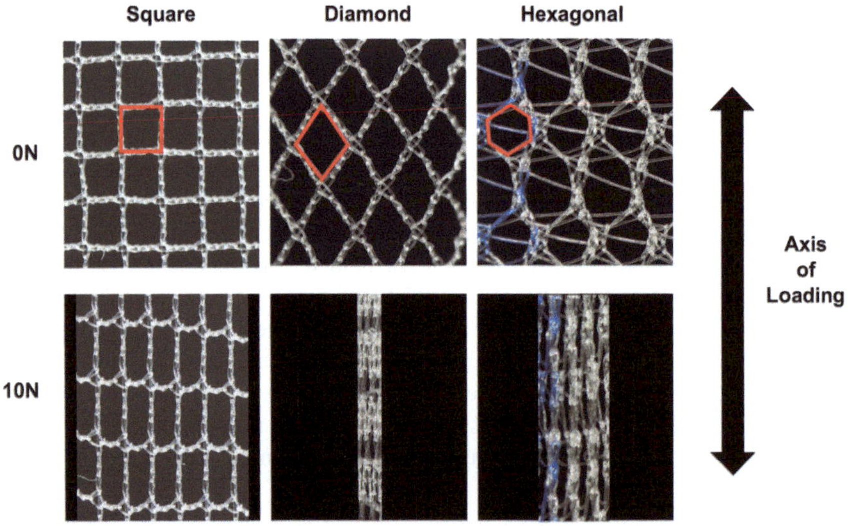

Fig. 4 Close-up images of meshes uniaxially loaded to 0N and 10N. Images include square pores (Restorelle, 0-degree offset), diamond pores (Restorelle, 45-degree offset), and hexagonal pores (Gynemesh) showing (1) that the 2D deformation (pore collapse) of mesh increases with increasing load, and (2) that the pore shape of a mesh affects its deformation behavior in response to tension. The square geometry is the most stable, deforming little with tension; however, when rotated by 45° to form a diamond shape, it becomes drastically less stable. All images are 10 mm × 10 mm. (Images were obtained with permission from Barone et al. [101])

prolapse meshes [102]. Auxetic pore shapes, mechanically, show promise for eliciting improved host responses due to the improved pore shape stability and sustained or increased porosity with loading of these structures. However, in vivo studies are needed to investigate the impact of auxetically designed prolapse meshes on the host response.

Boundary Conditions and Nonplanar Deformation

In addition to planar deformation (i.e., pore collapse), synthetic mesh can experience non-planar deformation, referred to as mesh wrinkling or bunching. When a mesh is loaded or deformed, the amount of wrinkling is influenced by the boundary conditions (i.e., how the mesh is physically constrained). In vivo boundary conditions are applied to synthetic meshes via sutures, in which sutures are used to attach the mesh to the vagina, sacrum, and/or the pelvic side wall. To simulate how these boundary conditions (i.e., sutures) influence mesh wrinkling, Barone et al. (2015) conducted a mechanical and computational evaluation of mesh curvature. Specifically, a low-stiffness and a high-stiffness mesh were subjected to three different boundary conditions: (1) clamped at opposing ends, (2) clamped at one end with two-point loads applied at the opposing end, and (3) two-point loads applied at opposing ends (Fig. 5).

The results of this study demonstrated that boundary conditions significantly influenced mesh surface curvature—that is, the amount of mesh wrinkling [103, 104]. Specifically, increasing the number of point loads (from 0 to 4) and the magnitude of the applied load led to increased mesh wrinkling. Additionally, these wrinkled regions contained a higher amount of mesh (i.e., a higher mesh burden), which is hypothesized to amplify the foreign body response [103, 104]. Indeed, mesh wrinkling is commonly observed in mesh explants removed from women with complications and following the implantation of mesh onto the vagina of New Zealand White rabbits (Fig. 6) [105, 106].

Mesh Deformation In Vivo

Hypotheses generated from ex vivo mechanical testing and computational modeling studies of mesh have led to in vivo studies to evaluate the association between mesh deformation and mesh complications. Knight et al. (2022) implanted lightweight polypropylene mesh in three predefined pore configurations onto the vagina of nonhuman primates via a sacrocolpopexy: stable (flat, square pore), unstable (flat, pores collapsed, diamond pore), and pre-deformed (pores intentionally collapsed and mesh wrinkled, diamond pore). The deformed configurations (pores collapsed with or without mesh wrinkling) had detrimental impacts on vaginal structure and function, resulting in clinical observations of mesh exposures and a complete loss of vaginal rugae as seen clinically (Fig. 7) [107].

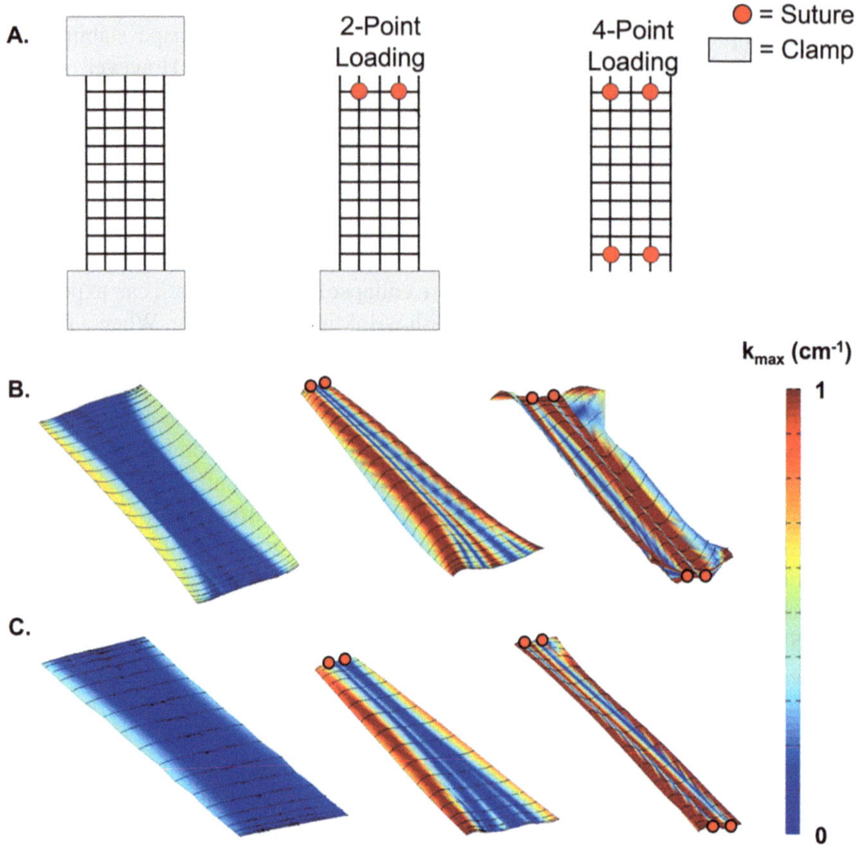

Fig. 5 Schematic representation of three boundary conditions applied to synthetic mesh: (1) clamped on opposing ends, (2) one end clamped and two sutures on the opposing end, and (3) two sutures on opposing ends (**a**). Contour maps of the maximum curvature (k_{max}) of Gynemesh loaded to 10 N with the three boundary conditions (**b**). Contour maps of the maximum curvature of Restorelle loaded to 10 N with the three boundary conditions (**c**). Red circles represent sutures, and solid black lines represent the direction of curvature. The location and type of attachments resulted in altered mesh wrinkling (k_{max}) for Gynemesh and Restorelle. (Images were obtained with permission from Barone et al. [104])

Conversely, when mesh was implanted flat with square pores and remained relatively flat throughout the duration of implantation, it did not lead to mesh complications. The structural and functional signs of degeneration observed for the deformed configurations included vaginal thinning, accelerated apoptosis, reduced collagen content, increased proteolysis, deterioration of mechanical integrity, and loss of vaginal contractile function. In addition, mesh deformation was associated with increased mesh burden (the number of mesh fibers per area), abnormal matrix deposition, and myofibroblast proliferation consistent with fibrosis, a likely mechanism of pain. Thus, mesh deformation appears to be associated with both mesh

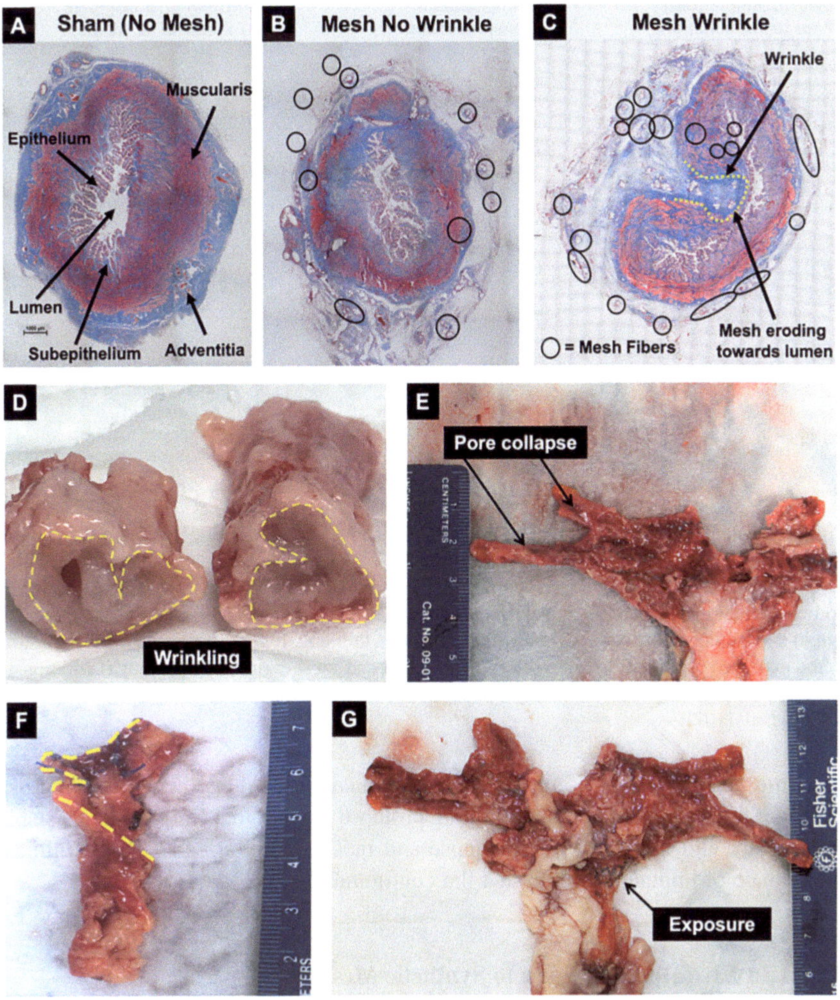

Fig. 6 Microgram of Sham vaginal tissue section from a rabbit stained with Masson's trichrome and depicting the layers of the vagina—the adventitia, muscularis (smooth muscle), subepithelium, epithelium, and the central lumen (**a**). Microgram of rabbit vaginal tissue with mesh implanted on the adventitia (no wrinkle). Black circles highlight the locations of mesh fibers; for aesthetic purposes, not all mesh fibers are circled (**b**). Microgram of rabbit vaginal tissue in which the mesh has wrinkled inward (dashed yellow line), and the underlying tissue has thinned (**c**). Cross-sectional view of a mesh-vagina complex removed from a rabbit demonstrating mesh wrinkling (dashed yellow line) (**d**). Image of a mesh explant removed from a patient with mesh exposure showing thin bands of mesh consistent with pore collapse (**e**). Image of a mesh explant removed from a patient for indications of pain (dashed yellow line depicts mesh wrinkling) (**f**). Image of a mesh explant removed from a patient with mesh exposures (**g**). (Images were modified with permission from Knight et al. [106])

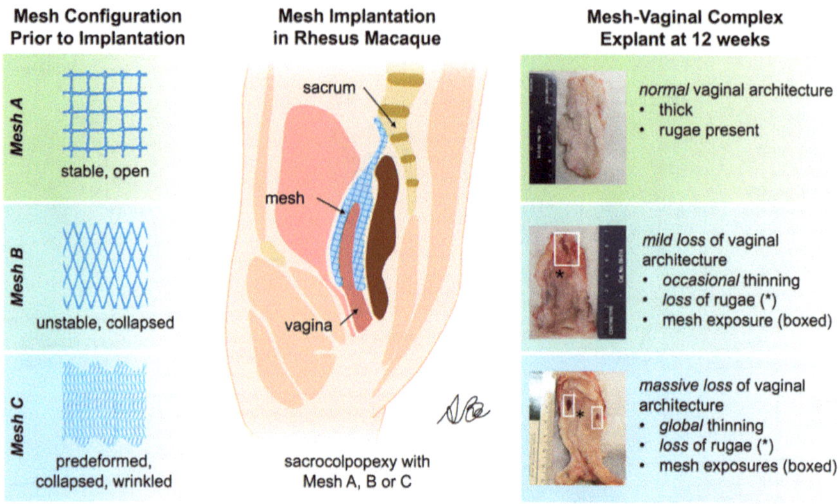

Fig. 7 Graphical abstract of Knight et al. [107], evaluating the impact of pore collapse and mesh wrinkling on vaginal tissue following 12 weeks of implantation in a nonhuman primate model (*Rhesus macaque*). Overall, the stable mesh (without pore collapse or mesh wrinkling) displayed normal vaginal architecture with thick tissue and rugae. When pore collapse was present, there was a mild loss of the vaginal architecture with some tissue thinning, loss of rugae, and mesh exposure. In the extreme case of deformed mesh (pore collapse and mesh wrinkling), there was widespread tissue thinning, loss of rugae, and mesh exposures. (This figure was obtained with permission from Knight et al. [107])

exposure and pain, two common mesh complications. Altogether, these findings highlight the importance of (1) designing prolapse meshes that can maintain a stable architecture and minimize pore collapse and mesh wrinkling, and (2) the clinical importance of implanting mesh in a flat configuration.

3.2.4 In Vivo Host Response to Synthetic Mesh

Our understanding of how the vagina responds to synthetic mesh has advanced significantly over the years due to a growing body of research using both animal models and human samples. These investigations have also provided valuable insight into the biological mechanisms that may underlie common mesh-related complications. The following sections will highlight key findings from these studies, with particular emphasis on basic science research that examines the host response to synthetic mesh implanted on the vagina.

Macrophages and the Immune Response to Synthetic Mesh

Once implanted, synthetic meshes are recognized by the body as foreign materials, triggering an innate immune response. Macrophages play a central role in shaping the long-term biological response to mesh implantation and can significantly influence clinical outcomes [108–111]. They can adopt a continuum of phenotypes in response to local microenvironmental cues, ranging from M1 to M2 phenotypes. M1 macrophages are considered part of a pro-inflammatory response; as such, they produce high levels of toxic reactive oxygen species, inducible nitric oxide synthase, and proinflammatory cytokines such as TNF-α, IL-1β, and IL-6. M2 macrophages, on the other hand, are part of a constructive remodeling phase; they release cytokines that facilitate tissue repair and remodeling, including high molecular weight IL-10, low molecular weight IL-12, IL-23, and other proremodeling mediators [112–116]. Both phenotypes are essential for a balanced immune response, but dysregulation of the M1 or M2 responses can be detrimental; excessive M1 activity can lead to chronic inflammation and tissue damage, while prolonged M2 dominance may result in excessive extracellular matrix deposition and drive fibrosis [117].

In a nonhuman primate (*Rhesus macaque*) study with polypropylene mesh implanted onto the vagina via sacrocolpopexy, M1 (CD86+) macrophages were the predominant phenotype at the mesh–tissue interface [83, 118]. Notably, lighter-weight, higher-porosity meshes were associated with an increased M2/M1 (CD206+/CD86+) ratio compared to heavier, lower-porosity meshes. Additionally, the percentage of both M1 (CD86+) and M2 (CD206+) macrophages was positively correlated with mesh perimeter, indicating that mesh burden—determined by pore size and fiber density—impacts the magnitude of the immune response [83]. Similarly, in human vaginal tissue removed for indications of pain or mesh exposure, macrophages were the predominant immune cells surrounding mesh fibers, reinforcing their pivotal role in the host response to mesh [84, 119].

Additionally, Therriault et al. (2025) investigated how mesh burden and pore collapse influence the macrophage response following the implantation of polypropylene mesh onto nonhuman primate vaginas with three predefined pore configurations as discussed previously (section "Mesh Deformation In Vivo"): stable (flat, square pore), unstable (flat, pores collapsed, diamond pore), and pre-deformed (pores intentionally collapsed and mesh wrinkled, diamond pore). This study found that greater mesh deformation was linked to a dominant M1 (CD86+) pro-inflammatory macrophage response and a disorganized cellular response. Notably, nearly half of the macrophages co-expressed M1 (CD86+) and M2 (CD206+) markers, indicating ongoing recruitment and polarization up to 12 weeks postimplantation, suggestive of unresolved inflammation or repeated microinjury [118]. In addition, increased mesh burden in this model, which increases with mesh deformation, was associated with an increased macrophage response, subepithelial apoptosis, and malondialdehyde, a marker of oxidative damage, indicating that reactive oxygen species produced by macrophages may be contributing to tissue damage and exposure [49].

As immune cells, macrophages interact with an assortment of other immune cells, such as T cells, as well as signaling molecules like cytokines and chemokines. In addition to the macrophages concentrated around mesh fibers, Tennyson et al. (2019) identified a distinct population of T cells positioned away from the mesh–

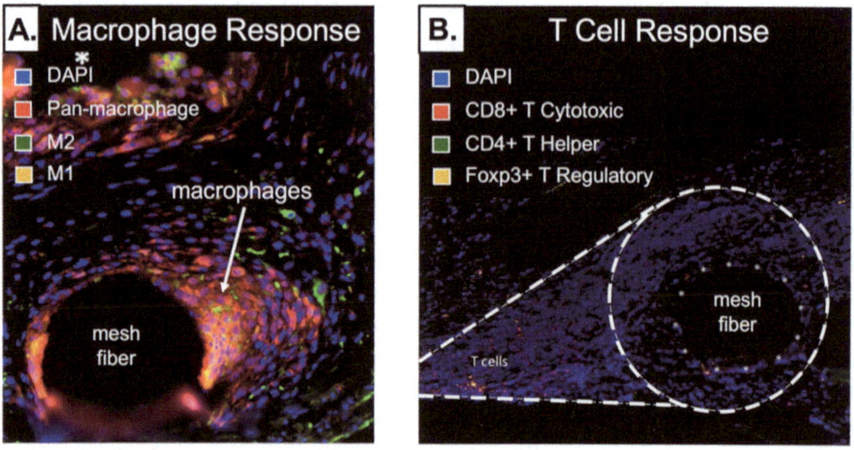

Fig. 8 Immunofluorescent micrographs of mesh explants removed from patients with complications, showing the typical (**a**) macrophage and (**b**) T cell responses. (**a**) Macrophages (predominately M1) closely surround mesh fibers, whereas (**b**) T cells localize away from mesh fibers. (**a**) Markers include 4′, 6-diamidino-2-phenylindole (DAPI, blue), pan-macrophage marker (red), M2 pro-remodeling macrophage marker CD206 (green), and M1 pro-inflammatory macrophage marker CD86 (yellow). (**b**) Markers include 4′, 6-diamidino-2-phenylindole (DAPI, blue), $CD8^+$ T cytotoxic (red), $CD4^+$ T helper (green), and Foxp3+ T regulatory (yellow). Original magnification, ×200. (Images were modified with permission from Nolfi et al. [84] and Tennyson et al. [119])

tissue interface, forming a characteristic teardrop shape in explants removed from patients (Fig. 8) [119]. Across all explants, regardless of the indication for removal, high levels of both pro-remodeling cytokines (IL-4, IL-10) and proinflammatory cytokines (TNF-α, IL-12p40p70, IL-12p70) were detected, along with chemokines such as the proinflammatory chemokine CXCL10 and the proremodeling chemokine CCL17 [84]. Importantly, the specific nature of the immune response differed based on the clinical indication for mesh removal. In exposure cases, elevated levels of pro–MMP-9 and increased numbers of CD8+ cytotoxic T cells were observed, consistent with enhanced tissue degradation, compared to meshes removed for pain [84, 119]. In contrast, explants removed due to pain showed a positive correlation between IL-10 and the proportion of M2 macrophages, as well as between TGF-β and collagen type I and III. These samples also exhibited thicker, more mature collagen fibers. Collectively, these findings highlight the complexity and context-dependence of the immune response to mesh implants.

The Protective Role of T Regulatory Cells

In recent years, the adaptive immune response has been increasingly shown to play an important role in the host response to biomaterials. Regulatory T (T_{reg}) cells, a subset of $CD4^+$ T cells within the adaptive immune system, are critical for modulating immune responses. They exert immunomodulatory effects by influencing macrophage differentiation, suppressing $CD8^+$ effector cell activity, and dampening chronic inflammation. In prolapse mesh explants removed from patients for pain or exposure, Artsen et al. (2019) observed a distinct spatial distribution of T cells, specifically $CD8^+$ cytotoxic T cells and T_{reg} cells, surrounding mesh fibers in a teardrop shape, mirroring earlier observations by Tennyson et al. (2019) [120]. Unlike macrophages, which were closely surrounding the mesh fibers, the T cells were in the "cap" of the teardrop (Fig. 8). Importantly, an inverse correlation was found between the concentration of T_{reg} cells and the amount of fibrosis, supporting a protective, antifibrotic role for T_{reg} cells. Additionally, the concentration of T_{reg} cells was inversely correlated with TGF-β1, implicating TGF-β1 in mesh-associated fibrosis [120]. Further highlighting the importance of T_{reg} cells, Artsen et al. (2020) found that women who experienced symptomatic improvement after mesh removal ("responders") had higher concentrations of T_{reg} cells in the mesh area as compared to "nonresponders," whose symptoms persisted [121]. Remarkably, the T_{reg} cell response was found to persist up to 12 years after mesh implantation, indicating a long-lasting adaptive immune response, underscoring the protective role that T_{reg} cells play in the long-term host response to synthetic mesh [120].

Dysregulated Wound Healing

Appropriate and tightly regulated inflammation is critical for wound healing but is only one component of tissue incorporation after mesh implantation. Following the implantation of synthetic mesh, proper wound healing is essential to ensure adequate tissue ingrowth and integration. Under physiological conditions, wound healing proceeds through a regulated sequence of phases. The initial inflammatory phase serves to seal the wound and protect against infection through the recruitment of immune cells and the initiation of pro-inflammatory signaling. This is followed by a proliferative phase, during which fibroblasts become activated and, under the influence of transforming growth factor-beta (TGF-β), differentiate into myofibroblasts. These cells are responsible for depositing a provisional extracellular matrix across the wound bed. The final phase of wound healing involves remodeling, during which inflammation resolves, myofibroblasts undergo apoptosis, and the deposited matrix is gradually replaced and organized, resulting in the maturation of collagen and restoration of tissue strength and structure. If the wound healing process is dysregulated, particularly if the tissue fails to transition into the remodeling phase, chronic inflammation, impaired matrix resolution, and excessive fibrosis can occur. Many features of mesh-related complications parallel those seen in dysregulated wound healing, prompting a growing body of research into the connections between these processes.

Artsen et al. (2023) investigated markers of inflammation, neuroinflammation, angiogenesis, and extracellular matrix remodeling in vaginal secretions from women with and without mesh complications. This study identified several biomarkers associated with mesh complications, demonstrating evidence of dysregulated wound healing. Elevated levels of basic fibroblast growth factor (bFGF), fibronectin, thrombospondin-2, tumor necrosis factor-beta (TNF-β), and vascular endothelial growth factor (VEGF) were strongly linked to the presence of complications. Specifically, individuals with high levels of any one of the identified markers had an odds ratio of 11.8 of being in the mesh-complication group. More strikingly, patients with elevated levels of at least three of the previously mentioned markers demonstrated an odds ratio of 237, despite controlling for confounding factors such as age, body mass index, and smoking status. The combination of high bFGF, thrombospondin-2, and fibronectin was perfectly predictive of mesh-related complications ($p < 0.0001$) [122]. While this study provides compelling evidence of an association between dysregulated wound healing and mesh complications, further research is necessary to determine whether these dysregulated pathways are causally involved and when in the healing process they become disrupted (i.e., a prospective study is warranted).

Angiogenesis, which is the formation of new blood vessels, also plays a pivotal role in the proliferative phase of wound healing by ensuring adequate oxygenation and nutrient delivery to regenerating tissues. Abnormalities in angiogenic signaling can contribute to chronic wound states. To evaluate the role of angiogenesis in synthetic mesh complications, Kowalski et al. (2020) examined both the expression of vascular endothelial growth factor A (VEGFA) and microvessel density in the vaginal tissue of patients who had undergone synthetic mesh implantation. VEGFA is a key mediator of angiogenesis, promoting the growth of preexisting blood vessels and the development of new vascular networks. The study found that VEGFA expression was decreased in patients with mesh compared to those without mesh, while microvessel density was increased in those with mesh-related complications compared to those without mesh [123]. These unusual findings in VEGFA expression and microvessel density indicate abnormal angiogenesis associated with synthetic mesh implantation, particularly in cases with mesh complications. Together, these data support the hypothesis that impaired or dysregulated wound healing, including abnormal angiogenesis, is associated with mesh-related complications.

3.3 *Strategies to Modulate the Host Response to Synthetic Mesh*

To modulate the host response to synthetic mesh, strategies such as coating meshes, utilizing composite materials, and functionalizing devices are being considered. Overall, these approaches aim to address critical impairments in traditional prolapse repair, including poor tissue healing, poor integration, and foreign body reactions, offering a more biologically supportive solution and enhancing the therapeutic potential of meshes beyond mechanical support. For example, surface modifications and coatings can either be used alone or as a means for drug release. Researchers have experimentally coated meshes with collagen or extracellular matrix [124–129], and grafts such as urinary bladder matrix have been investigated as barriers between synthetic mesh and the host tissue; these strategies will be discussed in greater detail in Sect. 5.

Investigators have tested coating meshes with anti-inflammatory, antimicrobial, and other drugs to promote mesh integration, to provide a more targeted treatment, and to improve the overall postsurgical response to mesh implantation. Prudente et al. (2017) investigated a polypropylene mesh coated with crosslinked poly(vinyl alcohol) (PVA) that was used as a method for releasing S-nitrosoglutathione (GSNO). This coated mesh resulted in an alteration of the wound healing response in a subcutaneous rat model by increasing angiogenesis, reducing the inflammatory response, and reducing apoptosis [130].

With the knowledge of the impact of synthetic mesh on the immune response, coatings that involve cytokine modulation offer another targeted approach for tuning the host response. Hachim et al. have investigated a mesh that can release IL-4, an M2 polarizing cytokine, at early stages of the host response. They found that the release time of IL-4 was dependent on the number of coatings, and that the release strategies could be tuned based on the expected host response [131]. Overall, the IL-4 eluting coating promoted M2 polarization in vitro, increased the M2/M1 ratio in a mouse model, diminished the fibrotic capsule response to polypropylene mesh, and resulted in improved tissue integration [132]. When looking specifically at the macrophage populations in mouse tissue in response to the IL-4 eluting mesh, Hachim et al. found that $F4/80^+$, $CD68^+$, and $CD11b^+$ macrophages were particularly susceptible to the M2 transition, that there was a significant reduction in $F4/80^+$ macrophages in coated samples, and that there was increased proteolytic activity and diminished matrix deposition, potentially explaining the decreased fibrotic response [133].

Growth factors play a major role in vaginal wound healing and have the potential to improve surgical outcomes via growth factor-supplemented therapies. Additionally, to further optimize the biological performance and therapeutic efficacy of prolapse meshes, some researchers are integrating cells, such as fibroblasts and stem cells [134], into the mesh to make it more functionally interactive with the host tissue. Basic fibroblast growth factor (bFGF) is an example of a growth factor that promotes proliferation, differentiation, and collagen types I and III production in vitro and has been shown to promote vaginal collagen production in vivo [135]. An experimental mesh has been investigated based on this concept, which incorporated three components: a silk fibroin (SF) knitted mesh (for mechanical support) coated with basic fibroblast growth factor (bFGF) (for its regenerative capabilities) and adipose-derived stem cells (ADSCs) (for the immune regulation and angiogenic capabilities). The mesh was able to achieve sustained release of bFGF, and promote cell proliferation and extracellular matrix synthesis. After 6 months of implantation in a rat abdominal model, the extracellular matrix reorganization, angiogenesis, immunomodulatory effects, and mechanical properties of the tissue were improved, suggesting this combination could prove beneficial

[136]. Similarly, connective tissue growth factor (CTGF) has been shown to be beneficial for improving the vaginal wound healing response [135]. An electrospun mesh made of polycaprolactone (PCL) coated with a combination of connective tissue growth factor (CTGF) and PEG-fibrinogen (PF) and seeded with rat mesenchymal stem cells was implanted in an abdominal rat model. After 53 weeks, it showed reduced collagen III, a diminished foreign body response, altered histological appearance, and comparable mechanical properties relative to a 24-week implantation, although future work is needed to compare these results to uncoated mesh [137]. Furthermore, it is important to note that the aforementioned studies evaluating meshes coated with bFGF and CTGF were completed in abdominal repair models in rats [136, 137]. Thus, studies are needed to evaluate the impact of these growth factor-loaded meshes on vaginal tissue in the context of prolapse repair.

Endometrial mesenchymal stem cells are another cell type being investigated for modulating the host response. In one study, an electrospun polycaprolactone (PCL) mesh loaded with endometrial mesenchymal stem cells (eMSCs) encapsulated in an aloe vera-sodium alginate (AV-ALG) hydrogel showed improved tissue integration, eMSC retention, and an anti-inflammatory M2 macrophage phenotype with F4/80$^+$CD206$^+$ colocalization [138]. This study highlights the potential for cell-seeded meshes to suppress the foreign body response and begin addressing the challenges associated with synthetic meshes in prolapse treatment.

Investigators have also considered the use of hormones, such as estrogen, to aid in wound repair and mesh integration. Estrogen is a sex hormone that plays a crucial role in the maintenance of the female reproductive system. During menopause, estrogen levels naturally decline, and one adverse outcome is decreased blood flow in vaginal tissue, which could slow wound healing and mesh integration. Estrogen replacement has been shown to improve vaginal blood flow in postmenopausal women, in addition to stimulating neo-collagen synthesis and inhibiting matrix metalloproteinases (MMPs) [139]. Thus, an estradiol-eluting mesh made by electrospinning PLA was developed by Mangır et al. in 2019 with the goal of promoting a well-vascularized wound site [140]. Preliminary results in an in vitro chick model showed that the estradiol-releasing mesh induced the formation of new blood vessels (angiogenesis) and increased the production of extracellular matrix in a human adipose-derived mesenchymal stem cell (ADMSC) model across 2 weeks. These results suggest that the use of estrogen in prolapse mesh could aid in the initial healing and integration phase following mesh implantation, although future studies in longer-term animal models are needed to support this work [140].

In conclusion, the approaches discussed in this section can begin to address longstanding challenges with the host response, including chronic inflammation, fibrosis, and dysregulated wound healing associated with conventional synthetic mesh. While many of these studies have demonstrated promising results in preclinical models, particularly in abdominal repair settings, further research is necessary, especially in in vivo vaginal models.

4 Biomaterials for Surgical Treatment of Prolapse: Absorbable Synthetic Meshes

4.1 Overview of Absorbable Synthetic Meshes

The synthetic meshes discussed in the previous section were non-absorbable permanent meshes with minimal to no degradation. However, synthetic meshes that degrade in the body have also been explored as an option for reducing the long-term response to a foreign implant. The degradation kinetics of an absorbable mesh, which refers to the rate at which the material breaks down and is absorbed by the body, can influence the extent of the foreign body response, the ability for tissue to integrate into the mesh, and the duration of support. A key challenge with absorbable meshes is the need to precisely balance the timing of mesh degradation with tissue integration and remodeling. Given that material breakdown impacts the mechanical integrity of the mesh, the degradation process directly influences the duration of mechanical support provided by the mesh. If the mesh degrades too quickly, the duration of structural support may be too short or remodeling of the tissue insufficient, likely increasing the risk of recurrent prolapse. Conversely, if degradation is too slow, it could increase rather than decrease the foreign body response. Thus, timing is a critical factor to consider in the design and manufacturing of an absorbable synthetic mesh.

4.2 Experimental Absorbable Synthetic Meshes

To date, few studies have begun investigating potential applications for absorbable materials in prolapse repair, either as the base material for mesh, a coating for a nonabsorbable mesh, or to create a partially absorbable composite mesh. Polylactic acid (PLA) and polyglycolic acid (PGA) are both absorbable polymers that have been used in hernia repair and have been used in some prolapse repair applications due to their biocompatible properties and degradation via hydrolysis and enzymatic activity [62, 140–142]. Compared to polypropylene (PP) mesh, a PLA mesh has shown favorable biocompatibility, with a milder inflammatory response, greater vascularization, more organized collagen deposition, and comparable strength and elongation when implanted for 90 days in a rat abdominal model [141]. In a longer-term subcutaneous rabbit model, a PLA mesh showed similar tissue integration, faster recovery, less inflammation, and greater tissue thickness relative to a PP mesh after 6 months of implantation [142]. Additionally, PLA has been used to develop drug-eluting meshes, which can aid prolapse repair by stimulating tissue integration and wound repair, for example [140]. Similarly, polyglycolic acid (PGA) mesh (marketed as Dexon) has been used in both hernia and prolapse repair [62], but tends to degrade more quickly and lose its mechanical properties faster than PLA.

Building on the individual properties of PLA and PGA, copolymers have been developed to optimize the material properties. For example, the mechanical and degradation properties of mesh can be tuned by combining PGA and PLA to create the copolymer poly(lactic-co-glycolic acid) (PLGA). Ethicon, a medical device company, produces an absorbable mesh made of PLGA (a specific copolymer of 90% PGA and 10% PLA and the same material as Vicryl sutures), which can be used for wound containment and temporary organ support [143]. Mesh made from these copolymers tends to degrade faster than either PGA or PLA alone. For example, while PGA mesh typically absorbs across 90 days, the absorption of Vicryl mesh starts after a few weeks, with nearly full absorption and no contribution to mechanical support after just 30 days [62].

Poly ε-caprolactone (PCL) is another absorbable material which has tunable mechanical properties and is compatible with modern fabrication techniques such as 3D printing [138, 144]. The properties of PCL can also be tuned by combining it with other polymers or biologic agents. For example, poly(l-lactide-co-ε-caprolactone) (PLCL) is a combination of PLA and PCL that is relatively biocompatible [145]. Additionally, studies have further combined PLCL with biologic materials to enhance mesh properties or for drug-release [146, 147]. For example, PLCL was combined with gelatin to enhance the material's biocompatibility properties and with silk fibroin to increase the mechanical performance for prolapse repair [146]. Additionally, an ascorbic acid-releasing PLCL mesh has been shown to enhance the cell proliferation and collagen production of human vaginal fibroblasts for prolapse repair applications [147]. These advancements demonstrate the versatility of PCL-based composites and their potential to be tailored for prolapse repair applications; however, more work is needed to evaluate this material via vaginal implantation.

4.3 Partially Absorbable Composite Synthetic Meshes

To offset the limitations of absorbable materials, while taking advantage of the benefits of both absorbable and non-absorbable materials, partially absorbable synthetic composite meshes have been investigated. Composites provide a path for prolapse meshes with both enhanced biocompatibility and long-term structural support. For example, composites of polypropylene (PP) and poliglecaprone (PG) have been used in both hernia and prolapse repair (marketed as VyPro and UltraPro for prolapse) [46, 143, 148]. Similarly, absorbable materials have been used as coatings or barriers for permanent meshes, taking advantage of the drug-releasing capabilities of absorbable materials, while maintaining the mechanical support provided by a permanent mesh, as previously described in Sect. 3.3 and later described in Sect. 5.3 [124–129, 134, 149]. This dual-material approach offers a potential compromise between long-term durability and compatibility with the host tissue.

5 Biomaterials for Surgical Treatment of Prolapse: Biologic Grafts

5.1 Overview of Biologic Grafts

With adverse events increasingly being reported from existing synthetic meshes, biologic materials are regaining popularity in the world of prolapse repair. Unlike synthetic materials, which are derived from man-made materials, biologic grafts are derived from natural materials (including human tissues, animal tissues, and plant-based materials) and are commonly processed to remove cells and antigens, leaving behind a scaffold material. This scaffold may be seeded with new cells or drugs, or it may be left bare to allow the patient's own cells to integrate and remodel the graft over time.

The main types of biologically derived grafts include (1) autologous grafts, which are typically harvested from rectus fascia or fascia lata and carry a low risk of foreign body reaction but are associated with longer operative time and donor site morbidity [150], (2) allografts, derived from cadaveric sources, and (3) xenografts, derived from animals, typically from bovine or porcine sources (Fig. 9). Both allografts and xenografts undergo extensive processing to reduce immunogenicity and have been used as uniform acellular scaffolds, cell-seeded composites, and grafts functionalized with growth factors or antibodies. These grafts are selected for their biocompatibility and potential to integrate with host tissue while minimizing foreign

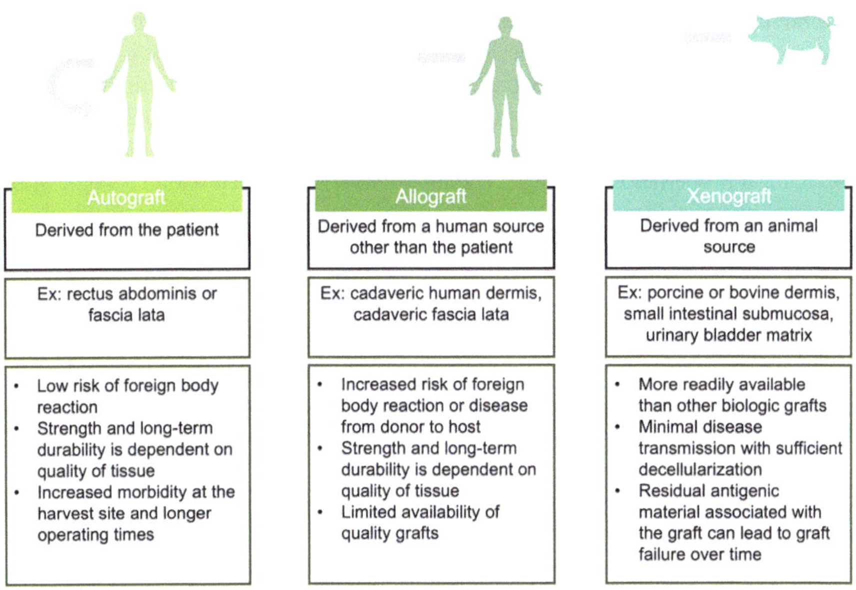

Fig. 9 Overview of the types of biologic grafts, including autograft, allograft, and xenograft. (Figure was created using BioRender.com)

body reactions. The host response to xenografts is primarily influenced by two factors: chemical cross-linking and porosity. Non-crosslinked xenografts serve as scaffolds that support cellular ingrowth and eventually degrade to be replaced by host connective tissue. However, a key concern with these resorbable materials is the potential loss of mechanical strength at the repair site during and following the remodeling process. Chemical cross-linking can be employed to improve durability by making the graft more resistant to degradation. Despite this benefit, the long-term behavior of cross-linked xenografts in vivo remains uncertain and could potentially be associated with adverse outcomes [151].

Biologic grafts offer many benefits over synthetic meshes. Although biologic grafts tend not to be as strong as their synthetic counterparts, their mechanical properties, such as stiffness and elasticity, tend to be much more compatible with vaginal tissue. Additionally, when properly decellularized, biologic grafts have a lower risk of evoking a harmful inflammatory response or long-term foreign body reactions than synthetic meshes. Biologic grafts can also be used as a natural coating or barrier to form a protective interface between a synthetic mesh and the host tissue. Moreover, biologic grafts can act as a natural scaffold for integration with the host cells and tissues, or they can act as a vehicle for the delivery of new cells and drugs.

5.2 *Limitations of Biologic Grafts*

While biologic grafts offer a natural alternative to synthetic mesh, they come with several limitations that can affect their reliability and effectiveness. Generally, biologic grafts degrade over time, and if their regenerative capacity is not enough to compensate for the loss of support, it can lead to inherent strength limitations and prolapse reoccurrence [152]. Another major concern is sample-to-sample variability; as biologic grafts are derived from human or animal tissues, their structural and mechanical properties can vary depending on the source. Even within a single graft, there can be variability in collagen content, fiber orientation, and porosity, which can lead to inconsistencies in mechanical strength and the degradation rate. Additionally, if the decellularization process—which removes cellular content to minimize immune rejection—is not thorough, the remaining biological material may trigger an inflammatory response, leading to fibrosis, graft degradation, or failure to properly integrate with native tissues. As is the case with many other medical devices, one challenge in biologic graft development is the uncertainty in translating results from animal studies to human use—a graft that performs well in preclinical animal models may provoke unexpected reactions in human patients, although animals with similar tissue properties to humans, such as nonhuman primates, can typically provide more assurance prior to clinical translation [153]. These factors make biologic grafts less predictable than synthetic alternatives, requiring careful selection and processing to ensure safety and effectiveness in prolapse repair. Investigators are working to develop solutions to overcome these limitations. For example, if the structure and bioactive factors in biologic grafts can encourage sufficient (mechanically and biologically) tissue growth, biologic grafts can begin to address concerns about the loss of support following degradation that are associated with many synthetic absorbable meshes. Building upon the growing interest in biologically derived alternatives, a wide array of biologic materials is being explored for use in prolapse repair, including materials derived from human and animal sources like collagen and other decellularized extracellular matrix (ECM) components, as well as materials derived from non-animal sources, such as cellulose, chitosan, and alginate.

5.3 *Experimental Biologic Grafts*

5.3.1 Cadaveric and Animal-Derived Biomaterials

Collagen, the most abundant protein in the human body and the main structural protein in the extracellular matrix (ECM), is at the forefront of biologic graft design. Collagen has been investigated as a coating for synthetic mesh, allowing the benefits of both synthetic materials and biologic materials to be leveraged. The combination of synthetic and biologic materials appears to be more effective than biologic or synthetic materials alone. For example, in a study by Tayrac et al. in 2007, collagen-coated polypropylene (PP) and non-coated PP meshes were compared in an ovine vaginal model [124]. Although not statistically significant ($p = 0.4$), vaginal erosions were observed at a lower rate in the coated PP group (16.7%, 3/18) compared to those with non-coated PP meshes (33.3%, 6/18). The lower erosion rate associated with the coated mesh may be explained by its reduced tendency to develop adhesions on the healing vaginal tissue during the early stages of recovery. Both mesh types, however, demonstrated comparable results in terms of mesh contraction, tissue integration, local inflammatory activity, and anatomical positioning within the vaginal wall [124]. In a rat abdominal model, polypropylene mesh coated with purified collagen gel resulted in increased tissue adherence, a milder inflammatory response, and enhanced structural organization and compaction of collagen fibers during the later stages of implantation compared to an uncoated polypropylene mesh [125]. These biological advantages appear to translate into measurable differences in the tissue response over time. The coated group also yielded a higher vessel density after 14 days and a decrease in the MMP-2 density after 21 and 90 days compared to the uncoated polypropylene group [126]. The polypropylene group had greater fluctuations in the behavior of MMP-3 across timepoints; the reactive area percentage of MMP-3 significantly decreased after 14 and 90 days, and the average density of MMP-3 significantly decreased after 21 days [126]. Together, these findings suggest that a highly purified collagen coating leads to alterations in the host response to synthetic mesh, and if such effects can be controlled in vaginal tissue, this strategy could offer a promising solution for enhancing mesh biocompatibility in prolapse repair.

In addition to collagen, the ECM contains other structural proteins (i.e., fibronectin, laminins, and elastin), ground substance components (i.e., proteoglycans and glycosaminoglycans), growth factors and other signaling molecules, and it has a distinct tissue-specific mechanical structure [154]. Tissue can be decellularized to leave behind the ECM structure without significant DNA content or other immunogenic cell components. This allows for implantation of a material with tissue-specific structure that won't elicit as severe of a host response. The intrinsic biochemical and mechanical cues of the ECM have the potential to aid in tissue regeneration, an important characteristic of absorbable meshes to ensure that support is maintained following the loss of mechanical contribution from the original graft material. The ECM can be converted into a hydrogel and used as a mesh coating for prolapse repair. Studies have shown that the chronic foreign body response and resultant fibrosis caused by synthetic PP mesh can be mitigated by an ECM coating [127]. For example, an ECM-coated polypropylene mesh showed a markedly reduced number of M1 macrophages (CD86+) immediately surrounding mesh fibers in a rat abdominal model after 14 days [127, 128], an increase in the ratio of M2/M1 macrophages (CD206+/CD86+ ratio), reduced number of foreign body giant cells at 14 and 35 days [127], and decreased density of collagen after 180 days compared to polypropylene mesh alone [128].

ECM grafts can also be derived from several tissue sources, including the small intestinal submucosa, pericardium, dermis, or urinary bladder (UBM). The small intestinal submucosa (SIS) in particular has shown promise for prolapse applications due to its biocompatibility and structural similarities to vaginal ECM, and it has FDA approval for soft tissue applications, such as the repair of hernias or body wall defects. SIS has also been extensively evaluated for other applications, including skin, abdominal wall, bladder, and tendon [155–159], bone regeneration, reproduction, valve replacement, tympanic membrane, meniscus, vocal cord, and trachea. Research is ongoing to optimize SIS products for prolapse repair, particularly with respect to decellularization protocols, crosslinking materials, and functionalization [160]. A study by Konstantinovic et al. in 2005, which evaluated a porcine-derived, non-crosslinked small intestinal submucosa (SIS) graft (Surgisis), found that the SIS graft resulted in overall less of an inflammatory response and differences in collagen deposition compared to polypropylene in a rat abdominal model. Initially, collagen formation had better organization and was more fibrous in the polypropylene groups, but by 90 days, the SIS group had more organized collagen formation. The tensile strength of the mesh-tissue explants followed a similar trend; after 30 days, the polypropylene group had a greater tensile strength than the SIS, but the tensile strength was comparable between groups after 90 days [161]. Despite the promise of SIS biocompatibility and mechanical properties shown in some testing of SIS, the clinical outcomes of a prolapse repair SIS graft, Surgisis, could be improved upon, and other biologic solutions continue to be investigated [162].

Crosslinking is one attempt at improving the mechanical properties of biologic grafts, and while it can prevent rapid degradation and improve the mechanical properties, it has also been associated with adverse effects. Cross-linked grafts derived from the pericardium and dermis have illustrated this effect. An acellular collagen matrix (ACM) derived from bovine pericardium and cross-linked with 0.05% of monomeric glutaraldehyde (GAD) was evaluated in a vaginal ovine model and compared to an uncoated-polypropylene mesh. After 180 days of implantation, the ACM samples were associated with several local adverse effects (most commonly palpable induration), comparable biomechanical properties to polypropylene mesh, and decreased vaginal contractility following partial degradation of the ACM [163]. Additionally, Pelvicol and PelviSoft, both cross-linked grafts derived from porcine dermis, have illustrated some of the effects of cross-linking and the variability of biologic grafts. In one study, PelviSoft Acellular Collagen BioMesh, (C.R. Bard Inc., Covington, GA), was evaluated in both the abdomen and vagina in a rabbit model. The porcine dermis elicited a stronger and more variable response than the polypropylene mesh, and it was degraded after 9 months of implantation. The degradation of PelviSoft was associated with decreased stiffness and ultimate tensile strength. Although crosslinked grafts are considered more permanent, this study illustrates how cross-linked materials can also lose strength and degrade over time during graft remodeling and because of the foreign body response [151]. Claerhout et al. (2008) compared polypropylene, SIS, and porcine dermis (Pelvicol) using a rabbit abdominal wall repair model. While polypropylene integrated quickly and SIS remodeled into native tissue within 2 months, Pelvicol, contrastingly, remained unchanged for 6 months, eventually degrading but remaining stiff even after 720 days. Histology revealed persistent chronic inflammation with Pelvicol, unlike the transient response seen with SIS [164]. These differences align with prior evidence that crosslinked biologics provoke prolonged foreign body reactions, whereas non-crosslinked materials support constructive remodeling [165].

Urinary bladder matrix (UBM) is a well-characterized candidate graft material for prolapse repair applications. It has been evaluated for tissue engineering applications for the urethra, larynx, esophagus, and heart, and has also been formed into hydrogels for applications in abdominal wall repair and neural research [166–171]. A UBM-derived device, MatriStem, is commercially available for wound management applications. Investigations of non-crosslinked UBM/SIS composite meshes compared to a SIS-alone mesh have elucidated the added benefits of a UBM/SIS composite for prolapse repair. In a rabbit vaginal defect model spanning 180 days, the UBM/SIS mesh elicited a milder inflammatory response, earlier cell infiltration, angiogenesis, collagen production, more orderly collagen, greater tensile strength, and greater elongation at break compared to the SIS mesh [172]. Crosslinking has been utilized in experimental UBM grafts to optimize mechanical properties; a 12-week study of cross-linked UBM showed favorable biocompatibility, good tissue integration, and maintenance of mechanical properties in rabbit vaginal and abdominal implants compared to synthetic PP mesh [173]. Additionally, using a nonhuman primate model, it was shown that a UBM matrix has favorable compatibility with vaginal tissue across 12 weeks, exhibiting comparable functional, morphological, and biochemical properties relative to a no-graft control in a vaginal model [149]. In addition to using UBM matrix alone, a UBM matrix that acts as a barrier between synthetic PP mesh and vaginal tissue has shown an ability to attenuate the degenerative effects of synthetic mesh in a nonhuman primate vaginal model, particularly with respect to the smooth muscle layer of vaginal tissue [149].

To achieve even greater tissue-specificity, ECM scaffolds can be derived from vaginal tissue. Sueters et al. [129] have shown the ability to recapitulate the vaginal tissue architecture and matrix composition via decellularization of human vaginal tissue, overall preserving the structural proteins with only moderate alterations to biomechanical properties [129].

5.3.2 Plant- and Bacterial-Derived Biomaterials

In addition to materials derived from animal and human tissues, products from other natural sources such as plants and bacteria are being investigated. Cellulose, which is a major fibrous component of plant cell walls, can also be produced by certain bacteria, and has been synthesized as a prosthetic mesh for prolapse repair. Upon benchtop mechanical evaluation, bacterial cellulose meshes were found to have much greater rigidity than polypropylene mesh, but they had sufficient softness to prevent mesh deformation while allowing for smooth conformability [174]. In a study comparing bacterial cellulose mesh with collagen-coated bacterial cellulose mesh, investigators found favorable biocompatibility and only minimal inflammation for bacterial cellulose meshes in a subcutaneous rabbit model after 1 week [174]. Following a 90-day implantation on the posterior vagina of a ewe model, bacterial cellulose meshes showed promising tissue integration without infection, exposure, or contracture, indicating their potential as a candidate for new prolapse repair devices. In vivo comparisons of bacterial cellulose meshes to currently available synthetic meshes (i.e., polypropylene mesh) would be beneficial [174].

Chitosan is another natural material that has been shown to be beneficial in a broad range of applications due to its biological properties, including nontoxicity, affinity for protein adsorption, antibacterial, hemostatic, fungistatic, and antitumoral properties [175]. A study using an abdominal rat model showed that the chitosan coating on a polypropylene mesh yielded the restoration of functional muscle, histomorphologic characteristics resembling native muscle, and an early macrophage phenotypic response that has been associated with more functional outcomes. The results of this study demonstrate the potential of chitosan coating for prolapse repair meshes, although more studies are needed in a vaginal model to support these findings [176].

Poly-4-hydroxybutyrate (P4HB) is a biodegradable material produced by bacterial fermentation that has been introduced for clinical use in ventral hernia repairs, tendon and ligament repair, and plastic and reconstructive surgery [177–179], and it is a promising biomaterial for prolapse repair [180–182]. P4HB forms exceptionally strong fibers that resorb in 12–18 months and are replaced by collagen, and unlike other biologic meshes, the degradation kinetics are not influenced by factors such as pH, making P4HB a more predictable method of support than other biologic meshes [183, 184]. In prolapse applications, P4HB has shown a favorable cellular response compared to polypropylene mesh, with greater attachment, proliferation, and collagen deposition from vaginal fibroblasts isolated from patients with prolapse in an in vitro model [185]. In a ewe vaginal model with 60- and 180-day implantations, a P4HB scaffold exhibited excellent tissue integration, favorable biomechanical properties, a moderate host response, and tissue remodeling compared to polypropylene mesh [180]. The P4HB scaffold exhibited a gradual degradation profile and load transfer to vaginal tissue, but longer timepoints are necessary to evaluate the long-term efficacy following complete scaffold degradation [180]. Additionally, P4HB can be functionalized; for example, one study found improved outcomes when incorporating estradiol into an electrospun P4HB mesh [181]. Overall, this biologically derived mesh material shows potential for use in prolapse repair.

In addition to single-source biologic scaffolds, multiple biologics can be combined to form biologic composites. For example, aloe vera is a biomaterial with antimicrobial and antioxidant properties. It has been shown to regulate the immune response and has been used in topical creams for vaginal applications [186–188], but has not been extensively used in tissue engineering applications. Alginate, on the other hand, has been used extensively as a bioink or hydrogel in tissue engineering applications [189]. An aloe vera-sodium alginate (AV-ALG) composite-based hydrogel coating has been used to encapsulate stem cells and to attach them to a synthetic mesh, showing promise for enhanced tissue integration and reduced inflammation in a mouse abdominal model [190].

5.3.3 Biologic Strategies for Mesh Fixation

In addition to their use in prolapse mesh and as mesh coatings, biologic materials are also being investigated as alternatives to traditional suture materials used in prolapse mesh repair. Gelatin methacrylol (GelMA) hydrogel, a gelatin-based material that has been chemically modified with methacrylic anhydride, has been evaluated in the vaginal wall of a guinea pig model [191]. This study compared mesh fixation using traditional polyglactin 910 suture to mesh fixation with the gelatin methacrylol hydrogel. The study found that fixation with the GelMA hydrogel resulted in less inflammation, lower vessel density, and a greater abundance of thick collagen fibers throughout the implanted mesh after 4 weeks compared to traditional suture fixation, as well as minimal profibrotic encapsulation of the mesh fibers relative to traditional suture after 3 months [191].

Overall, biologically derived materials represent a rapidly evolving area in prolapse repair research, spanning a diverse range of sources to achieve unique properties, and offering potential alternatives to traditional synthetic materials. As the field advances, these biologic materials could provide more tailored solutions to match the needs and properties of the pelvic environment, with the potential to improve long-term patient outcomes and minimize post-surgical complications. Continued research and clinical validation will be key to translating promising experimental findings into widely adopted clinical practices.

6 Outlook and Opportunities for Innovation

Overall, prolapse repair solutions have sought to better accommodate anatomical complexities and surgical needs through research-driven approaches, with biomaterials that help reinforce the vaginal walls, reduce tension on host tissues, minimize symptoms, and improve patient quality of life. Fundamentally, prolapse repair devices should (1) provide mechanical support to prolapsed organs and weakened connective tissues and muscles, (2) ensure secure and long-term support (usually via tissue integration or new tissue growth), and (3) have the capacity to remain compatible within the body without adverse reactions. Within these criteria, there is room for innovation to continue advancing the field of prolapse treatment.

Despite decades of clinical use, the development of safe and effective biomaterials for prolapse repair remains a significant challenge. When selecting an appropriate mesh, multiple design and performance factors must be carefully weighed and thoroughly tested before clinical implementation. The first step in addressing this challenge is to gain a clear understanding of the mechanisms behind mesh complications. Research using computational models and simulations, in vitro models, and in vivo models, as well as human samples and clinical trials, is essential for improving our understanding of mesh complications. Despite enhanced knowledge regarding the etiology of mesh complications, logistical challenges remain in biomaterial development. For example, one of the biggest challenges currently is finding a balance between the mechanical strength of the mesh and mechanical compatibility with the vagina—that is, an ideal mesh needs to be strong enough to support prolapsed organs and sufficiently soft and elastic to conform to the tissue and minimize degeneration caused by stress shielding.

In terms of manufacturing advancements, nonwoven methods such as electrospinning, 3D printing, and meltwriting techniques could provide cost-effective options for producing mesh-like constructs [97], allowing for fine control over fiber size and pore geometry, customization of device shape, and the possibility of gradient patterns or multi-material structures. Additionally, creating prolapse repair solutions that incorporate multiple materials or variance in structure could help to optimize the tissue response. In most prolapse meshes, material properties are designed to be homogeneous across the entire device, and the mesh is typically fabricated from a single material with consistent fiber diameters, pore sizes, knit patterns, and material properties throughout. This uniformity simplifies manufacturing and provides predictable mechanical behavior, ensuring consistency across all regions. However, meshes designed with heterogeneous properties could have the potential to better match the diverse mechanical and biological demands of different anatomical pelvic regions. A gradient structure, for example, could feature gradual variations in pore size, pore shape, fiber thickness, or material density across the mesh to account for varying requirements for tissue integration, flexibility, and load-bearing capabilities. Similarly, multi-material mesh designs, where different regions of the mesh incorporate distinct materials, such as coatings or blends of multiple materials in different ratios, could allow the device to combine the advantageous properties of multiple materials.

Similarly, there is an opportunity for increasing mesh customization based on an individual patient's anatomy. Anatomical variation across patients, such as location and size of pelvic organs, type and severity of prolapse, and overall pelvic morphology, can influence surgical outcomes. A device with improved customizability of size, shape, material properties, and fixation options would allow surgeons to better tailor prolapse repair to individual patient needs. Similarly, variations in vaginal tissue robustness (influenced by factors such as age or hormonal status) may warrant different material or textile properties to minimize trauma. Customizable mesh devices that consider these factors could offer more precise, patient-specific solutions, reducing complications associated with poorly sized implants.

An often overlooked yet critical aspect of prolapse repair is the method of fixation to the tissue. The location and type of mesh fixation can influence the amount of localized tissue trauma, the degree of mesh deformation, and the overall distribution of stress. Experimental fixation strategies, such as alternative suture materials or surgical adhesives, have the potential to simplify surgical procedures and decrease the risk of suture-related effects. However, research is needed to ensure sufficient mechanical support, biocompatibility, and adequate integration with vaginal tissue and mesh materials.

Because of the biocompatibility issues experienced with current synthetic meshes, emerging trends in prolapse mesh design are moving toward more biologically attuned approaches. Biologically derived materials, such as collagen-based materials and decellularized extracellular matrix, offer potential for enhancing biocompatibility, tissue integration, and reducing foreign body responses. In parallel, there is growing interest in functionalized meshes capable of delivering cells, drugs, or other therapeutic agents to promote healing, reduce inflammation and the foreign body response, and prevent infection. Drug-eluting prolapse meshes have the potential to advance pelvic organ prolapse repair by combining structural support with targeted therapeutic delivery. Their ability to provide localized, sustained treatment could minimize systemic side effects while addressing key challenges associated with traditional mesh implants. However, further research is needed to evaluate specific therapeutic agents, refine drug-loading techniques and release mechanisms, tailor release profiles, and ensure long-term safety and efficacy. As innovation in biomaterials and drug delivery continues to evolve, drug-eluting meshes have the potential to offer more personalized and effective solutions for improved patient outcomes. Collectively, these strategies represent a shift from purely structural implants to multifunctional biomaterials that experience bidirectional interactions with the biological environment.

Expanding upon mesh functionalization, the delivery of therapeutic agents introduces the opportunity for devices with regenerative capabilities, shifting mesh design away from permanent structural implants and toward bioactive, degradable scaffolds that restore native tissue integrity and function. Emerging biomaterials hold promise for these regenerative applications, especially when combined with therapeutic agents or cell-based therapies that could enhance tissue remodeling and healing by guiding host cell infiltration, stimulating extracellular matrix production, restoring tissue structure, and strengthening muscle function. This would allow implants to be absorbed over time, leaving behind strengthened native tissue capable of maintaining pelvic support without the risk of prolapse recurrence, and it could mitigate complications associated with permanent implants and a persistent foreign body response, such as mesh exposure and fibrosis.

Finally, future advancements in biomaterials for prolapse repair should keep regulatory requirements in mind. Bridging the gap between innovation and regulation requires not only rigorous testing but also interdisciplinary collaboration among material scientists, engineers, clinicians, and regulatory personnel. As we move toward the next generation of prolapse repair materials, integrating translational research with a comprehensive regulatory strategy will be essential to advance the field of prolapse repair.

In conclusion, the field of biomaterials for prolapse repair is rapidly advancing. Continued interdisciplinary collaboration between clinicians, materials scientists, and biomedical engineers is essential to drive innovation and improve patient outcomes. By designing meshes that balance mechanical demands with biological compatibility, and by harnessing new materials and technologies, the next generation of prolapse repair strategies has the potential to minimize the risk of post-surgical complications and improve the quality of life of patients. As part of the broader theme of this book—exploring the role of biomaterials in women's health—this chapter underscores the vital role that thoughtful, research-driven, patient-focused biomaterial design can play in addressing complex conditions like pelvic organ prolapse.

References

1. Samuelsson EC, Victor FT, Tibblin G, Svärdsudd KF. Signs of genital prolapse in a Swedish population of women 20 to 59 years of age and possible related factors. Am J Obstet Gynecol. 1999;180(2 Pt 1):299–305. https://doi.org/10.1016/s0002-9378(99)70203-6.
2. Whitcomb EL, Rortveit G, Brown JS, et al. Racial differences in pelvic organ prolapse. Obstet Gynecol. 2009;114(6):1271–7. https://doi.org/10.1097/AOG.0b013e3181bf9cc8.
3. Nygaard I, Bradley C, Brandt D. Pelvic organ prolapse in older women: prevalence and risk factors. Obstet Gynecol. 2004;104(3):489–97. https://doi.org/10.1097/01.AOG.0000136100.10818.d8.
4. Glazener C, Elders A, MacArthur C, et al. Childbirth and prolapse: long-term associations with the symptoms and objective measurement of pelvic organ prolapse. BJOG. 2013;120(2):161–8. https://doi.org/10.1111/1471-0528.12075.
5. Yeniel A, Ergenoglu AM, Askar N, Itil IM, Meseri R. How do delivery mode and parity affect pelvic organ prolapse? Acta Obstet Gynecol Scand. 2013;92(7):847–51. https://doi.org/10.1111/aogs.12129.
6. Risk factors for genital prolapse in non-hysterectomized women around menopause. Results from a large cross-sectional study in menopausal clinics in Italy. Progetto Menopausa Italia Study Group. Eur J Obstet Gynecol Reprod Biol. 2000;93(2):135–40.
7. Kudish BI, Iglesia CB, Gutman RE, et al. Risk factors for prolapse development in white, black, and Hispanic women. Female Pelvic Med Reconstr Surg. 2011;17(2):80–90. https://doi.org/10.1097/SPV.0b013e31820e5d06.

8. Swift S, Woodman P, O'Boyle A, et al. Pelvic Organ Support Study (POSST): the distribution, clinical definition, and epidemiologic condition of pelvic organ support defects. Am J Obstet Gynecol. 2005;192(3):795–806. https://doi.org/10.1016/j.ajog.2004.10.602.
9. Vergeldt TFM, Weemhoff M, IntHout J, Kluivers KB. Risk factors for pelvic organ prolapse and its recurrence: a systematic review. Int Urogynecol J. 2015;26(11):1559–73. https://doi.org/10.1007/s00192-015-2695-8.
10. Jones KA, Harmanli O. Pessary use in pelvic organ prolapse and urinary incontinence. Rev Obstet Gynecol. 2010;3(1):3–9.
11. Bash KL. Review of vaginal pessaries. Obstet Gynecol Surv. 2000;55(7):455–60.
12. Wu JM, Matthews CA, Conover MM, Pate V, Jonsson FM. Lifetime risk of stress urinary incontinence or pelvic organ prolapse surgery. Obstet Gynecol. 2014;123(6):1201–6.
13. Wu JM, Vaughan CP, Goode PS, et al. Prevalence and trends of symptomatic pelvic floor disorders in U.S. women. Obstet Gynecol. 2014;123(1):141–8.
14. St Martin B, Markowitz MA, Myers ER, Lundsberg LS, Ringel N. Estimated national cost of pelvic organ prolapse surgery in the United States. Obstet Gynecol. 2024;143(3):419–27. https://doi.org/10.1097/aog.0000000000005485.
15. Barber MD, Brubaker L, Burgio KL, et al. Comparison of 2 transvaginal surgical approaches and perioperative behavioral therapy for apical vaginal prolapse: the OPTIMAL randomized trial. JAMA. 2014;311(10):1023–34.
16. Jelovsek JE, Barber MD, Brubaker L, et al. Effect of uterosacral ligament suspension vs sacrospinous ligament fixation with or without perioperative behavioral therapy for pelvic organ vaginal prolapse on surgical outcomes and prolapse symptoms at 5 years in the OPTIMAL randomized clinical trial. JAMA. 2018;319(15):1554–65. https://doi.org/10.1001/jama.2018.2827.
17. Bryan C. The Ebers Papyrus. London: Geoffrey Bles; 1930.
18. de Citium A. Apollonius von Kitium Illustrierter Kommentar zu der Hippokrateischen Schrift "Peri arthrōn": mit 31 Tafeln in Lichtdruck. Teubner; 1896.
19. Emge LA, Durfee R. Pelvic organ prolapse: four thousand years of treatment. Clin Obstet Gynecol. 1966;9(4):997–1032.
20. McKay WJS. The history of ancient gynaecology. London: Baillière, Tindall and Cox; 1901.
21. Novak E. Genealogy of gynaecology. Obstet Gynecol Surv. 1950;5(5):775.
22. Clanerani T. A short history of obstetrics and gynecology. Springfield: Charles C Thomas; 1960.
23. Leonardo RA. History of gynecology. New York: Froben Press; 1944.
24. Miller S. Contemporary use of the pessary. Gynecol Obstet. 1991;39:1–12.
25. Deger R, Menzin A, Mikuta J. The vaginal pessary: past and present. Postgrad Obstet Gynecol. 1993;13(18):1–8.
26. Shah SM, Sultan AH, Thakar R. The history and evolution of pessaries for pelvic organ prolapse. Int Urogynecol J Pelvic Floor Dysfunct. 2006;17(2):170–5. https://doi.org/10.1007/s00192-005-1313-6.
27. Hodge HL. On diseases peculiar to women: including displacements of the uterus. Philadelphia: Blanchard and Lea; 1860.
28. Thakar R, Stanton S. Management of genital prolapse. BMJ. 2002;324(7348):1258–62.
29. Clemons JL, Aguilar VC, Tillinghast TA, Jackson ND, Myers DL. Patient satisfaction and changes in prolapse and urinary symptoms in women who were fitted successfully with a pessary for pelvic organ prolapse. Am J Obstet Gynecol. 2004;190(4):1025–9.
30. Jones K, Yang L, Lowder JL, et al. Effect of pessary use on genital hiatus measurements in women with pelvic organ prolapse. Obstet Gynecol. 2008;112(3):630–6.
31. Donnelly MJ, Powell-Morgan S, Olsen AL, Nygaard IE. Vaginal pessaries for the management of stress and mixed urinary incontinence. Int Urogynecol J. 2004;15:302–7.
32. Hanson L-AM, Schulz JA, Flood CG, Cooley B, Tam F. Vaginal pessaries in managing women with pelvic organ prolapse and urinary incontinence: patient characteristics and factors contributing to success. Int Urogynecol J. 2006;17:155–9.

33. Mutone MF, Terry C, Hale DS, Benson JT. Factors which influence the short-term success of pessary management of pelvic organ prolapse. Am J Obstet Gynecol. 2005;193(1):89–94.
34. Brincat C, Kenton K, Fitzgerald MP, Brubaker L. Sexual activity predicts continued pessary use. Am J Obstet Gynecol. 2004;191(1):198–200.
35. Wu V, Farrell SA, Baskett TF, Flowerdew G. A simplified protocol for pessary management. Obstet Gynecol. 1997;90(6):990–4.
36. Fernando RJ, Sultan AH, Thakar R, Jeyanthan K. Management of the neglected vaginal ring pessary. Int Urogynecol J. 2007;18:117–9.
37. Russell JK. The dangerous vaginal pessary. Br Med J. 1961;2(5267):1595.
38. Esin S, Harmanli O. Large vesicovaginal fistula in women with pelvic organ prolapse: the role of colpocleisis revisited. Int Urogynecol J. 2008;19:1711–3.
39. Grody M, Nyirjesy P, Chatwani A. Intravesical foreign body and vesicovaginal fistula: a rare complication of a neglected pessary. Int Urogynecol J. 1999;10:407–8.
40. Lin YH, Lim CK, Chang SD, Chiang CC, Huang CH, Tseng LH. Tailor-made three-dimensional printing vaginal pessary to treat pelvic organ prolapse: a pilot study. Menopause. 2023;30(9):947–53. https://doi.org/10.1097/gme.0000000000002223.
41. Long J, Zidan G, Seyfoddin A, Tong S, Brownfoot FC, Chowdary P. An estriol-eluting pessary to treat pelvic organ prolapse. Sci Rep. 2022;12(1):20021. https://doi.org/10.1038/s41598-022-23791-9.
42. Eder S, Wiltschko L, Koutsamanis I, et al. Toward a new generation of vaginal pessaries via 3D-printing: concomitant mechanical support and drug delivery. Eur J Pharm Biopharm. 2022;174:77–89. https://doi.org/10.1016/j.ejpb.2022.04.001.
43. Kanagarajah P, Ayyathurai R, Gomez C. Evaluation of current synthetic mesh materials in pelvic organ prolapse repair. Curr Urol Rep. 2012;13(3):240–6. https://doi.org/10.1007/s11934-012-0247-z.
44. Clavero PA, Guerrero JA, Salamanca A. Gore-Tex mesh pelvic occlusion and secondary colpopexy: a new surgical technique for posthysterectomy vaginal vault prolapse. Eur J Obstet Gynecol Reprod Biol. 2006;126(1):113–5. https://doi.org/10.1016/j.ejogrb.2005.07.032.
45. Takeyama M, Kuwata T, Kashihara H, Kato C, Watanabe M. Is transvaginal mesh surgery with polytetrafluoroethylene mesh ORIHIME(®) feasible for anterior pelvic organ prolapse?-Randomized comparative study between ORIHIME(®) and Polyform™. Int J Urol. 2024;31(9):1017–21. https://doi.org/10.1111/iju.15506.
46. Callewaert G, Housmans S, Cattani L, et al. Medium-term outcome of laparoscopic sacrocolpopexy using polivinylidene fluoride as compared to a hybrid polyglecaprone and polypropylene mesh: a matched control study. Neurourol Urodyn. 2019;38(7):1874–82. https://doi.org/10.1002/nau.24083.
47. Klinge U, Klosterhalfen B, Öttinger AP, Junge K, Schumpelick V. PVDF as a new polymer for the construction of surgical meshes. Biomaterials. 2002;23(16):3487–93.
48. Gomelsky A, Dmochowski RR. Biocompatibility assessment of synthetic sling materials for female stress urinary incontinence. J Urol. 2007;178(4):1171–81. https://doi.org/10.1016/j.juro.2007.05.123.
49. Artsen AM, Mayr CA, Weber K, Rytel K, Moalli PA. Polypropylene surgical mesh induces lipid oxidation in a nonhuman primate model. Acta Biomater. 2025;198:207–18. https://doi.org/10.1016/j.actbio.2025.04.003.
50. Food, Administration D. Urogynecologic surgical mesh. update on the safety and effectiveness of transvaginal placement for pelvic organ prolapse. 2011. http://www.fda.gov/downloads/MedicalDevices/Safety/AlettsandNotices/UCM262760.pdf.
51. Shah AD, Kohli N, Rajan SS, Hoyte L. The age distribution, rates, and types of surgery for pelvic organ prolapse in the USA. Int Urogynecol J. 2008;19:421–8.
52. Clemons JL, Weinstein M, Guess MK, et al. Impact of the 2011 FDA transvaginal mesh safety update on AUGS members' use of synthetic mesh and biologic grafts in pelvic reconstructive surgery. Urogynecology. 2013;94(4):191–8.

53. Nygaard I, Brubaker L, Zyczynski HM, et al. Long-term outcomes following abdominal sacrocolpopexy for pelvic organ prolapse. JAMA. 2013;309(19):2016–24. https://doi.org/10.1001/jama.2013.4919.
54. Bretschneider CE, Myers ER, Geller EJ, Kenton KS, Henley BR, Matthews CA. Long-term mesh exposure 5 years following minimally invasive total hysterectomy and sacrocolpopexy. Int Urogynecol J. 2024;35(4):901–7.
55. Klinge U, Junge K, Spellerberg B, Piroth C, Klosterhalfen B, Schumpelick V. Do multifilament alloplastic meshes increase the infection rate? Analysis of the polymeric surface, the bacteria adherence, and the in vivo consequences in a rat model. J Biomed Mater Res. 2002;63(6):765–71. https://doi.org/10.1002/jbm.10449.
56. Amid P. Classification of biomaterials and their related complications in abdominal wall hernia surgery. Hernia. 1997;1(1):15–21.
57. Iglesia CB, Fenner DE, Brubaker L. The use of mesh in gynecologic surgery. Int Urogynecol J Pelvic Floor Dysfunct. 1997;8(2):105–15.
58. Engelsman AF, van Dam GM, van der Mei HC, Busscher HJ, Ploeg RJ. In vivo evaluation of bacterial infection involving morphologically different surgical meshes. Ann Surg. 2010;251(1):133–7. https://doi.org/10.1097/SLA.0b013e3181b61d9a.
59. Leveen HH, Barberio JR. Tissue reaction to plastics used in surgery with special reference to teflon. Ann Surg. 1949;129(1):74–84. https://doi.org/10.1097/00000658-194901000-00008.
60. Conze J, Rosch R, Klinge U, et al. Polypropylene in the intra-abdominal position: influence of pore size and surface area. Hernia. 2004;8(4):365–72.
61. Klosterhalfen B, Klinge U, Schumpelick V. Functional and morphological evaluation of different polypropylene-mesh modifications for abdominal wall repair. Biomaterials. 1998;19(24):2235–46. https://doi.org/10.1016/s0142-9612(98)00115-x.
62. Cosson M, Debodinance P, Boukerrou M, et al. Mechanical properties of synthetic implants used in the repair of prolapse and urinary incontinence in women: which is the ideal material? Int Urogynecol J. 2003;14:169–78.
63. Chen CC, Ridgeway B, Paraiso MF. Biologic grafts and synthetic meshes in pelvic reconstructive surgery. Clin Obstet Gynecol. 2007;50(2):383–411. https://doi.org/10.1097/GRF.0b013e31804b184c.
64. Cobb W, Peindl R, Zerey M, Carbonell A, Heniford B. Mesh terminology 101. Hernia. 2009;13:1–6.
65. Wohlrab KJ, Erekson EA, Myers DL. Postoperative erosions of the Mersilene suburethral sling mesh for antiincontinence surgery. Int Urogynecol J Pelvic Floor Dysfunct. 2009;20(4):417–20. https://doi.org/10.1007/s00192-008-0787-4.
66. Greca FH, de Paula JB, Biondo-Simões ML, et al. The influence of differing pore sizes on the biocompatibility of two polypropylene meshes in the repair of abdominal defects. Experimental study in dogs. Hernia. 2001;5(2):59–64. https://doi.org/10.1007/s100290100001.
67. Greca FH, Souza-Filho ZA, Giovanini A, et al. The influence of porosity on the integration histology of two polypropylene meshes for the treatment of abdominal wall defects in dogs. Hernia. 2008;12(1):45–9. https://doi.org/10.1007/s10029-007-0276-6.
68. Orenstein SB, Saberski ER, Kreutzer DL, Novitsky YW. Comparative analysis of histopathologic effects of synthetic meshes based on material, weight, and pore size in mice. J Surg Res. 2012;176(2):423–9.
69. Patel H, Ostergard DR, Sternschuss G. Polypropylene mesh and the host response. Int Urogynecol J. 2012;23(6):669–79. https://doi.org/10.1007/s00192-012-1718-y.
70. Orenstein SB, Saberski ER, Kreutzer DL, Novitsky YW. Comparative analysis of histopathologic effects of synthetic meshes based on material, weight, and pore size in mice. J Surg Res. 2012;176(2):423–9. https://doi.org/10.1016/j.jss.2011.09.031.
71. Klinge U, Klosterhalfen B. Modified classification of surgical meshes for hernia repair based on the analyses of 1,000 explanted meshes. Hernia. 2012;16(3):251–8. https://doi.org/10.1007/s10029-012-0913-6.

72. Schmidt A, Taylor D. Erosion of soft tissue by polypropylene mesh products. J Mech Behav Biomed Mater. 2021;115:104281. https://doi.org/10.1016/j.jmbbm.2020.104281.
73. Klinge U, Klosterhalfen B, Conze J, et al. Modified mesh for hernia repair that is adapted to the physiology of the abdominal wall. Eur J Surg. 1998;164(12):951–60. https://doi.org/10.1080/110241598750005138.
74. Klinge U, Klosterhalfen B, Müller M, Ottinger AP, Schumpelick V. Shrinking of polypropylene mesh in vivo: an experimental study in dogs. Eur J Surg. 1998;164(12):965–9. https://doi.org/10.1080/110241598750005156.
75. Klinge U, Junge K, Stumpf M, Ap AP, Klosterhalfen B. Functional and morphological evaluation of a low-weight, monofilament polypropylene mesh for hernia repair. J Biomed Mater Res. 2002;63(2):129–36. https://doi.org/10.1002/jbm.10119.
76. Klinge U, Klosterhalfen B, Birkenhauer V, Junge K, Conze J, Schumpelick V. Impact of polymer pore size on the interface scar formation in a rat model. J Surg Res. 2002;103(2):208–14. https://doi.org/10.1006/jsre.2002.6358.
77. O'Dwyer PJ, Kingsnorth AN, Molloy RG, Small PK, Lammers B, Horeyseck G. Randomized clinical trial assessing impact of a lightweight or heavyweight mesh on chronic pain after inguinal hernia repair. Br J Surg. 2005;92(2):166–70. https://doi.org/10.1002/bjs.4833.
78. Page AS, Cattani L, Pacquée S, et al. Long-term data on graft-related complications after sacrocolpopexy with lightweight compared with heavier-weight mesh. Obstet Gynecol. 2023;141(1):189–98. https://doi.org/10.1097/aog.0000000000005021.
79. Rosch R, Junge K, Schachtrupp A, Klinge U, Klosterhalfen B, Schumpelick V. Mesh implants in hernia repair. Inflammatory cell response in a rat model. Eur Surg Res. 2003;35(3):161–6. https://doi.org/10.1159/000070045.
80. Costello C, Bachman S, Grant S, Cleveland D, Loy T, Ramshaw B. Characterization of heavyweight and lightweight polypropylene prosthetic mesh explants from a single patient. Surg Innov. 2007;14(3):168–76.
81. Novitsky YW, Cristiano JA, Harrell AG, et al. Immunohistochemical analysis of host reaction to heavyweight-, reduced-weight-, and expanded polytetrafluoroethylene (ePTFE)-based meshes after short- and long-term intraabdominal implantations. Surg Endosc. 2008;22(4):1070–6. https://doi.org/10.1007/s00464-007-9737-3.
82. Liang R, Abramowitch S, Knight K, et al. Vaginal degeneration following implantation of synthetic mesh with increased stiffness. BJOG. 2013;120(2):233–43.
83. Brown BN, Mani D, Nolfi AL, Liang R, Abramowitch SD, Moalli PA. Characterization of the host inflammatory response following implantation of prolapse mesh in rhesus macaque. Conference Paper. Am J Obstet Gynecol. 2015;213(5):668e1–668e10. https://doi.org/10.1016/j.ajog.2015.08.002.
84. Nolfi AL, Brown BN, Liang R, et al. Host response to synthetic mesh in women with mesh complications. Am J Obstet Gynecol. 2016;215(2):206.e1–8. https://doi.org/10.1016/j.ajog.2016.04.008.
85. Weyhe D, Schmitz I, Belyaev O, et al. Experimental comparison of monofile light and heavy polypropylene meshes: less weight does not mean less biological response. World J Surg. 2006;30(8):1586–91. https://doi.org/10.1007/s00268-005-0601-0.
86. Askew AL, Visco AG, Weidner AC, Truong T, Siddiqui NY, Bradley MS. Does mesh weight affect time to failure after robotic-assisted laparoscopic sacrocolpopexy? Female Pelvic Med Reconstr Surg. 2020;26(9):536–40. https://doi.org/10.1097/spv.0000000000000632.
87. Giugale LE, Hansbarger MM, Askew AL, Visco AG, Shepherd JP, Bradley MS. Assessing pelvic organ prolapse recurrence after minimally invasive sacrocolpopexy: does mesh weight matter? Int Urogynecol J. 2021;32(8):2195–201. https://doi.org/10.1007/s00192-021-04681-6.
88. Goel VK, Lim TH, Gwon J, et al. Effects of rigidity of an internal fixation device. A comprehensive biomechanical investigation. Spine. 1991;16(3 Suppl):S155–61.

89. Liang R, Zong W, Palcsey S, Abramowitch S, Moalli PA. Impact of prolapse meshes on the metabolism of vaginal extracellular matrix in rhesus macaque. Am J Obstet Gynecol. 2015;212(2):174.e1–7. https://doi.org/10.1016/j.ajog.2014.08.008.
90. Feola A, Abramowitch S, Jallah Z, et al. Deterioration in biomechanical properties of the vagina following implantation of a high-stiffness prolapse mesh. BJOG. 2013;120(2):224–32.
91. Jallah Z, Liang R, Feola A, et al. The impact of prolapse mesh on vaginal smooth muscle structure and function. BJOG. 2016;123(7):1076–85. https://doi.org/10.1111/1471-0528.13514.
92. Shaffer RM, Liang R, Knight K, Carter-Brooks CM, Abramowitch S, Moalli PA. Impact of polypropylene prolapse mesh on vaginal smooth muscle in rhesus macaque. Am J Obstet Gynecol. 2019;221(4):330.e1–9. https://doi.org/10.1016/j.ajog.2019.05.008.
93. Maurer MM, Röhrnbauer B, Feola A, Deprest J, Mazza E. Mechanical biocompatibility of prosthetic meshes: a comprehensive protocol for mechanical characterization. J Mech Behav Biomed Mater. 2014;40:42–58. https://doi.org/10.1016/j.jmbbm.2014.08.005.
94. Lei L, Song Y, Chen R. Biomechanical properties of prolapsed vaginal tissue in pre-and postmenopausal women. Int Urogynecol J. 2007;18:603–7.
95. Knight KM, Moalli PA, Nolfi A, Palcsey S, Barone WR, Abramowitch SD. Impact of parity on ewe vaginal mechanical properties relative to the nonhuman primate and rodent. Int Urogynecol J. 2016;27:1255–63.
96. Goh J. Biomechanical properties of prolapsed vaginal tissue in pre-and postmenopausal women. Int Urogynecol J. 2002;13:76–9.
97. Knight K, Breedlove S, Obisesan T, et al. Vaginal host response to polycarbonate urethane, an alternative material for the repair of pelvic organ prolapse. Acta Biomater. 2024;189:298–310. https://doi.org/10.1016/j.actbio.2024.09.040.
98. Otto J, Kaldenhoff E, Kirschner-Hermanns R, Mühl T, Klinge U. Elongation of textile pelvic floor implants under load is related to complete loss of effective porosity, thereby favoring incorporation in scar plates. J Biomed Mater Res A. 2014;102(4):1079–84.
99. Barone WR, Knight KM, Moalli PA, Abramowitch SD. Deformation of transvaginal mesh in response to multiaxial loading. J Biomech Eng. 2019;141(2):021001.
100. Feiner B, Maher C. Vaginal mesh contraction: definition, clinical presentation, and management. Obstet Gynecol. 2010;115(2 Pt 1):325–30. https://doi.org/10.1097/AOG.0b013e3181cbca4d.
101. Barone WR, Moalli PA, Abramowitch SD. Textile properties of synthetic prolapse mesh in response to uniaxial loading. Am J Obstet Gynecol. 2016;215:326.e1–9.
102. Knight KM, Moalli PA, Abramowitch SD. Preventing mesh pore collapse by designing mesh pores with auxetic geometries: a comprehensive evaluation via computational modeling. J Biomech Eng. 2018;140(5):0510051–8. https://doi.org/10.1115/1.4039058.
103. Barone WR. Mechanical characterization of synthetic mesh for pelvic organ prolapse repair. Doctoral Dissertation, University of Pittsburgh. 2015.
104. Barone WR, Amini R, Maiti S, Moalli PA, Abramowitch SD. The impact of boundary conditions on surface curvature of polypropylene mesh in response to uniaxial loading. J Biomech. 2015;48(9):1566–74.
105. Svabík K, Martan A, Masata J, El-Haddad R, Hubka P, Pavlikova M. Ultrasound appearances after mesh implantation—evidence of mesh contraction or folding? Int Urogynecol J. 2011;22(5):529–33. https://doi.org/10.1007/s00192-010-1308-9.
106. Knight KM, Artsen AM, Routzong MR, King GE, Abramowitch SD, Moalli PA. New Zealand white rabbit: a novel model for prolapse mesh implantation via a lumbar colpopexy. Int Urogynecol J. 2020;31(1):91–9. https://doi.org/10.1007/s00192-019-04071-z.
107. Knight KM, King GE, Palcsey SL, Suda A, Liang R, Moalli PA. Mesh deformation: a mechanism underlying polypropylene prolapse mesh complications in vivo. Acta Biomater. 2022;148:323–35. https://doi.org/10.1016/j.actbio.2022.05.051.
108. Anderson JM. Biological responses to materials. Annu Rev Mater Res. 2001;31(1):81–110.

109. Anderson JM, Rodriguez A, Chang DT. Foreign body reaction to biomaterials. Semin Immunol. Elsevier. 2008;20:86–100.
110. Brown BN, Londono R, Tottey S, et al. Macrophage phenotype as a predictor of constructive remodeling following the implantation of biologically derived surgical mesh materials. Acta Biomater. 2012;8(3):978–87.
111. Brown BN, Ratner BD, Goodman SB, Amar S, Badylak SF. Macrophage polarization: an opportunity for improved outcomes in biomaterials and regenerative medicine. Biomaterials. 2012;33(15):3792–802.
112. Mills CD, Kincaid K, Alt JM, Heilman MJ, Hill AM. M-1/M-2 macrophages and the Th1/Th2 paradigm. J Immunol. 2000;164(12):6166–73. https://doi.org/10.4049/jimmunol.164.12.6166.
113. Mantovani A, Sica A, Sozzani S, Allavena P, Vecchi A, Locati M. The chemokine system in diverse forms of macrophage activation and polarization. Trends Immunol. 2004;25(12):677–86. https://doi.org/10.1016/j.it.2004.09.015.
114. Mosser DM, Edwards JP. Exploring the full spectrum of macrophage activation. Nat Rev Immunol. 2008;8(12):958–69. https://doi.org/10.1038/nri2448.
115. Brown BN, Badylak SF. Expanded applications, shifting paradigms and an improved understanding of host–biomaterial interactions. Acta Biomater. 2013;9(2):4948–55.
116. Gundra UM, Girgis NM, Ruckerl D, et al. Alternatively activated macrophages derived from monocytes and tissue macrophages are phenotypically and functionally distinct. Blood. 2014;123(20):e110–22. https://doi.org/10.1182/blood-2013-08-520619.
117. Murray PJ, Wynn TA. Protective and pathogenic functions of macrophage subsets. Nat Rev Immunol. 2011;11(11):723–37. https://doi.org/10.1038/nri3073.
118. Therriault MA, Kottapalli S, Artsen A, et al. Profiling of the macrophage response to polypropylene mesh burden in vivo. Biomaterials. 2025;318:123177. https://doi.org/10.1016/j.biomaterials.2025.123177.
119. Tennyson L, Rytel M, Palcsey S, Meyn L, Liang R, Moalli P. Characterization of the T-cell response to polypropylene mesh in women with complications. Am J Obstet Gynecol. 2019;220(2):187.e1–8. https://doi.org/10.1016/j.ajog.2018.11.121.
120. Artsen AM, Rytel M, Liang R, et al. Mesh induced fibrosis: the protective role of T regulatory cells. Acta Biomater. 2019;96:203–10.
121. Artsen AM, Liang R, Meyn L, et al. T regulatory cells and TGF-β1: predictors of the host response in mesh complications. Acta Biomater. 2020;115:127–35.
122. Artsen AM, Liang R, Meyn L, Bradley MS, Moalli PA. Dysregulated wound healing in the pathogenesis of urogynecologic mesh complications. Sci Rep. 2023;13(1):21437.
123. Kowalski JT, Goodheart MJ, Genadry R, Bhattarai A, Bradley CS. Alterations of vascular endothelial growth factor a expression and microvessel density associated with polypropylene vaginal mesh. Female Pelvic Med Reconstr Surg. 2020;26(1):73–9. https://doi.org/10.1097/spv.0000000000000593.
124. Tayrac R, Alves A, Thérin M. Collagen-coated vs noncoated low-weight polypropylene meshes in a sheep model for vaginal surgery. A pilot study. Int Urogynecol J. 2007;18(5):513–20. https://doi.org/10.1007/s00192-006-0176-9.
125. Siniscalchi RT, Melo M, Palma PCR, Fabbro IMD, De Campos Vidal B, Riccetto CLZ. Highly purified collagen coating enhances tissue adherence and integration properties of monofilament polypropylene meshes. Int Urogynecol J. 2013;24(10):1747–54. https://doi.org/10.1007/s00192-013-2109-8.
126. Dias FGF, Prudente A, Siniscalchi RT, de Vidal BC, Riccetto CLZ. Can highly purified collagen coating modulate polypropylene mesh immune-inflammatory and fibroblastic reactions? Immunohistochemical analysis in a rat model. Int Urogynecol J Pelvic Floor Dysfunct. 2015;26(4):569–76. https://doi.org/10.1007/s00192-014-2529-0.
127. Wolf MT, Dearth CL, Ranallo CA, et al. Macrophage polarization in response to ECM coated polypropylene mesh. Biomaterials. 2014;35(25):6838–49. https://doi.org/10.1016/j.biomaterials.2014.04.115.

128. Faulk DM, Londono R, Wolf MT, et al. ECM hydrogel coating mitigates the chronic inflammatory response to polypropylene mesh. Biomaterials. 2014;35(30):8585–95. https://doi.org/10.1016/j.biomaterials.2014.06.057.
129. Sueters J, Xiao F, Roovers J-P, et al. Creation of a decellularized vaginal matrix from healthy human vaginal tissue for potential vagina reconstruction: experimental studies. Int J Surg. 2023;109(12):3905–18.
130. Prudente A, Favaro WJ, Reis LO, Riccetto CL. Nitric oxide coating polypropylene mesh increases angiogenesis and reduces inflammatory response and apoptosis. Int Urol Nephrol. 2017;49(4):597–605. https://doi.org/10.1007/s11255-017-1520-3.
131. Hachim D, Iftikhar A, LoPresti ST, et al. Distinct release strategies are required to modulate macrophage phenotype in young versus aged animals. J Control Release. 2019;305:65–74. https://doi.org/10.1016/j.jconrel.2019.05.020.
132. Hachim D, LoPresti ST, Yates CC, Brown BN. Shifts in macrophage phenotype at the biomaterial interface via IL-4 eluting coatings are associated with improved implant integration. Biomaterials. 2017;112:95–107. https://doi.org/10.1016/j.biomaterials.2016.10.019.
133. Hachim D, LoPresti ST, Rege RD, et al. Distinct macrophage populations and phenotypes associated with IL-4 mediated immunomodulation at the host implant interface. Biomater Sci. 2020;8(20):5751–62. https://doi.org/10.1039/d0bm00568a.
134. Gao Y, Liu LJ, Blatnik JA, et al. Methodology of fibroblast and mesenchymal stem cell coating of surgical meshes: a pilot analysis. J Biomed Mater Res B Appl Biomater. 2014;102 (4):797–805. https://doi.org/10.1002/jbm.b.33061.
135. van Velthoven MJJ, Gudde AN, Struijs F, et al. The effect of growth factors on vaginal wound healing: a systematic review and meta-analysis. Tissue Eng Part B Rev. 2023;29(4):429–40. https://doi.org/10.1089/ten.TEB.2022.0225.
136. Wu X, Guo H, Jia Y, et al. Adipose mesenchymal stem cell-based tissue engineering mesh with sustained bFGF release to enhance tissue repair. Biomater Sci. 2022;10(12):3110–21. https://doi.org/10.1039/d1bm01893k.
137. Laursen SH, Hansen SG, Taskin MB, et al. Electrospun nanofiber mesh with connective tissue growth factor and mesenchymal stem cells for pelvic floor repair: Long-term study. J Biomed Mater Res B Appl Biomater. 2023;111(2):392–401. https://doi.org/10.1002/jbm.b.35158.
138. Paul K, Darzi S, McPhee G, et al. 3D bioprinted endometrial stem cells on melt electrospun poly ε-caprolactone mesh for pelvic floor application promote anti-inflammatory responses in mice. Acta Biomater. 2019;97:162–76. https://doi.org/10.1016/j.actbio.2019.08.003.
139. Moalli PA, Klingensmith WL, Meyn LA, Zyczynski HM. Regulation of matrix metalloproteinase expression by estrogen in fibroblasts that are derived from the pelvic floor. Am J Obstet Gynecol. 2002;187(1):72–9. https://doi.org/10.1067/mob.2002.124845.
140. Mangır N, Hillary CJ, Chapple CR, MacNeil S. Oestradiol-releasing biodegradable mesh stimulates collagen production and angiogenesis: an approach to improving biomaterial integration in pelvic floor repair. Eur Urol Focus. 2019;5(2):280–9. https://doi.org/10.1016/j.euf.2017.05.004.
141. de Tayrac R, Oliva-Lauraire MC, Guiraud I, Henry L, Vert M, Mares P. Long-lasting bioresorbable poly(lactic acid) (PLA94) mesh: a new approach for soft tissue reinforcement based on an experimental pilot study. Int Urogynecol J Pelvic Floor Dysfunct. 2007;18(9): 1007–14. https://doi.org/10.1007/s00192-006-0270-z.
142. Lu Y, Dong S, Zhang P, Liu X, Wang X. Preparation of a polylactic acid knitting mesh for pelvic floor repair and in vivo evaluation. J Mech Behav Biomed Mater. 2017;74:204–13. https://doi.org/10.1016/j.jmbbm.2017.05.034.
143. Gigliobianco G, Regueros SR, Osman NI, et al. Biomaterials for pelvic floor reconstructive surgery: how can we do better? Biomed Res Int. 2015;2015:968087. https://doi.org/10.1155/2015/968087.
144. Vaz MFR, Martins JAP, Pinheiro F, et al. Medical- and non-medical-grade polycaprolactone mesh printing for prolapse repair: establishment of melt electrowriting prototype parameters. Appl Sci. 2024;14(21):9670.

145. Jeong SI, Kim SH, Kim YH, et al. Manufacture of elastic biodegradable PLCL scaffolds for mechano-active vascular tissue engineering. J Biomater Sci Polym Ed. 2004;15(5):645–60. https://doi.org/10.1163/156856204323046906.
146. Wu J, Yao H, Yu L, et al. A novel 3D printed type II silk fibroin/polycaprolactone mesh for the treatment of pelvic organ prolapse. Biomater Sci. 2023;11(21):7203–15. https://doi.org/10.1039/d3bm01158e.
147. Kurki A, Paakinaho K, Hannula M, et al. Promoting cell proliferation and collagen production with ascorbic acid 2-phosphate-releasing poly(l-lactide-co-ε-caprolactone) membranes for treating pelvic organ prolapse. Regen Biomater. 2024;11:rbae060. https://doi.org/10.1093/rb/rbae060.
148. Lim YN, Muller R, Corstiaans A, Hitchins S, Barry C, Rane A. A long-term review of posterior colporrhaphy with Vypro 2 mesh. Int Urogynecol J Pelvic Floor Dysfunct. 2007;18(9):1053–7. https://doi.org/10.1007/s00192-006-0290-8.
149. Liang R, Knight K, Barone W, et al. Extracellular matrix regenerative graft attenuates the negative impact of polypropylene prolapse mesh on vagina in rhesus macaque. Am J Obstet Gynecol. 2017;216(2):153.e1–9. https://doi.org/10.1016/j.ajog.2016.09.073.
150. Bang S-L, Belal M. Autologous pubovaginal slings: back to the future or a lost art? Res Rep Urol. 2016;8:11–20.
151. Pierce LM, Grunlan MA, Hou Y, Baumann SS, Kuehl TJ, Muir TW. Biomechanical properties of synthetic and biologic graft materials following long-term implantation in the rabbit abdomen and vagina. Am J Obstet Gynecol. 2009;200(5):549.e1–8. https://doi.org/10.1016/j.ajog.2008.12.041.
152. Dora CD, Dimarco DS, Zobitz ME, Elliott DS. Time dependent variations in biomechanical properties of cadaveric fascia, porcine dermis, porcine small intestine submucosa, polypropylene mesh and autologous fascia in the rabbit model: implications for sling surgery. J Urol. 2004;171(5):1970–3. https://doi.org/10.1097/01.ju.0000121377.61788.ad.
153. Abramowitch SD, Feola A, Jallah Z, Moalli PA. Tissue mechanics, animal models, and pelvic organ prolapse: a review. Eur J Obstet Gynecol Reprod Biol. 2009;144(Suppl 1):S146–58. https://doi.org/10.1016/j.ejogrb.2009.02.022.
154. Liu C, Pei M, Li Q, Zhang Y. Decellularized extracellular matrix mediates tissue construction and regeneration. Front Med. 2022;16(1):56–82. https://doi.org/10.1007/s11684-021-0900-3.
155. Prevel CD, Eppley BL, McCarty M, et al. Experimental evaluation of small intestinal submucosa as a microvascular graft material. Microsurgery. 1994;15(8):586–91; discussion 592–3. https://doi.org/10.1002/micr.1920150812.
156. Prevel CD, Eppley BL, Summerlin DJ, Jackson JR, McCarty M, Badylak SF. Small intestinal submucosa: utilization for repair of rodent abdominal wall defects. Ann Plast Surg. 1995;35(4):374–80.
157. Badylak SF, Tullius R, Kokini K, et al. The use of xenogeneic small intestinal submucosa as a biomaterial for Achilles tendon repair in a dog model. J Biomed Mater Res. 1995;29(8):977–85. https://doi.org/10.1002/jbm.820290809.
158. Jelodari S, Sadroddiny E. Decellularization of small intestinal submucosa. Adv Exp Med Biol. 2021;1345:71–84. https://doi.org/10.1007/978-3-030-82735-9_7.
159. Kropp BP, Eppley BL, Prevel CD, et al. Experimental assessment of small intestinal submucosa as a bladder wall substitute. Urology. 1995;46(3):396–400. https://doi.org/10.1016/s0090-4295(99)80227-1.
160. Zhao J, Chao T, Zhou M, et al. Decellularization techniques pave the way for tissue engineering and regenerative medicine: a narrative review. Regen Med Rep. 2024;1(2):117–30. https://doi.org/10.4103/regenmed.Regenmed-d-24-00016.
161. Konstantinovic ML, Lagae P, Zheng F, Verbeken EK, De Ridder D, Deprest JA. Comparison of host response to polypropylene and non-cross-linked porcine small intestine serosal-derived collagen implants in a rat model. BJOG. 2005;112(11):1554–60. https://doi.org/10.1111/j.1471-0528.2005.00688.x.

162. Alexandridis V, Teleman P, Rudnicki M. Efficacy and safety of pelvic organ prolapse surgery with porcine small intestinal submucosa graft implantation. Eur J Obstet Gynecol Reprod Biol. 2021;267:18–22.
163. Endo M, Urbankova I, Vlacil J, et al. Cross-linked xenogenic collagen implantation in the sheep model for vaginal surgery. Gynecol Surg. 2015;12(2):113–22. https://doi.org/10.1007/s10397-015-0883-7.
164. Claerhout F, Verbist G, Verbeken E, Konstantinovic M, De Ridder D, Deprest J. Fate of collagen-based implants used in pelvic floor surgery: a 2-year follow-up study in a rabbit model. Am J Obstet Gynecol. 2008;198(1):94.e1–6.
165. Brown BN, Badylak SF. Extracellular matrix as an inductive scaffold for functional tissue reconstruction. Transl Res. 2014;163(4):268–85.
166. Medberry CJ, Crapo PM, Siu BF, et al. Hydrogels derived from central nervous system extracellular matrix. Biomaterials. 2013;34(4):1033–40.
167. Zhang L, Zhang F, Weng Z, et al. Effect of an inductive hydrogel composed of urinary bladder matrix upon functional recovery following traumatic brain injury. Tissue Eng Part A. 2013;19(17–18):1909–18.
168. Ghuman H. Intracerebral implantation of ECM hydrogel for the treatment of stroke. Doctoral Dissertation: University of Pittsburgh; 2019.
169. Crapo PM, Tottey S, Slivka PF, Badylak SF. Effects of biologic scaffolds on human stem cells and implications for CNS tissue engineering. Tissue Eng Part A. 2014;20(1–2):313–23. https://doi.org/10.1089/ten.TEA.2013.0186.
170. Faust A, Kandakatla A, van der Merwe Y, et al. Urinary bladder extracellular matrix hydrogels and matrix-bound vesicles differentially regulate central nervous system neuron viability and axon growth and branching. J Biomater Appl. 2017;31(9):1277–95. https://doi.org/10.1177/0885328217698062.
171. Kao CY, Nguyen HQ, Weng YC. Characterization of porcine urinary bladder matrix hydrogels from sodium dodecyl sulfate decellularization method. Polymers (Basel). 2020;12(12). https://doi.org/10.3390/polym12123007.
172. Wang Y, Zhang K, Yang J, et al. Outcome of a novel porcine-derived UBM/SIS composite biological mesh in a rabbit vaginal defect model. Int Urogynecol J. 2023;34(7):1501–11.
173. Fan X, Wang Y, Wang Y, Xu H. Comparison of polypropylene mesh and porcine-derived, cross-linked urinary bladder matrix materials implanted in the rabbit vagina and abdomen. Int Urogynecol J. 2014;25(5):683–9. https://doi.org/10.1007/s00192-013-2283-8.
174. Lai C, Zhang SJ, Chen XC, Sheng LY, Qi TW, Yan LP. Development of a cellulose-based prosthetic mesh for pelvic organ prolapse treatment: in vivo long-term evaluation in an ewe vagina model. Mater Today Bio. 2021;12:100172. https://doi.org/10.1016/j.mtbio.2021.100172.
175. Kim I-Y, Seo S-J, Moon H-S, et al. Chitosan and its derivatives for tissue engineering applications. Biotechnol Adv. 2008;26(1):1–21.
176. Udpa N, Iyer SR, Rajoria R, et al. Effects of chitosan coatings on polypropylene mesh for implantation in a rat abdominal wall model. Tissue Eng Part A. 2013;19(23–24):2713–23. https://doi.org/10.1089/ten.tea.2012.0739.
177. Tran DH, Rubarth C, Leeds SG, et al. The use of poly-4-hydroxybutyrate (P4HB, Phasix™) mesh in ventral hernia repair: a systematic review and meta-analysis. Hernia. 2024;28(4):989–1004.
178. Mellia JA, Othman S, Naga HI, et al. Outcomes of poly-4-hydroxybutyrate mesh in ventral hernia repair: a systematic review and pooled analysis. Plast Reconstr Surg Glob Open. 2020;8(12):e3158.
179. Williams SF, Rizk S, Martin DP. Poly-4-hydroxybutyrate (P4HB): a new generation of resorbable medical devices for tissue repair and regeneration. Biomed Tech/Biomed Eng. 2013;58(5):439–52.

180. Diedrich CM, Guler Z, Hympanova L, et al. Evaluation of the short-term host response and biomechanics of an absorbable poly-4-hydroxybutyrate scaffold in a sheep model following vaginal implantation. BJOG. 2022;129(7):1039–49. https://doi.org/10.1111/1471-0528.17040.
181. Verhorstert K, Gudde A, Weitsz C, Bezuidenhout D, Roovers JP, Guler Z. Absorbable electrospun poly-4-hydroxybutyrate scaffolds as a potential solution for pelvic organ prolapse surgery. ACS Appl Bio Mater. 2022;5(11):5270–80. https://doi.org/10.1021/acsabm.2c00691.
182. Deeken CR, Chen DC, Lopez-Cano M, Martin DP, Badhwar A. Fully resorbable poly-4-hydroxybutyrate (P4HB) mesh for soft tissue repair and reconstruction: a scoping review. Systematic review. Front Surg. 2023;10. https://doi.org/10.3389/fsurg.2023.1157661.
183. Fowler CC, Klifto KM, Wietlisbach LE, et al. Poly-4-hydroxybutyrate mesh for ventral hernia repairs: a single-surgeon experience. Eplasty. 2023;23:e48.
184. Martin DP, Williams SF. Medical applications of poly-4-hydroxybutyrate: a strong flexible absorbable biomaterial. Biochem Eng J. 2003;16(2):97–105.
185. Diedrich CM, Roovers JP, Smit TH, Guler Z. Fully absorbable poly-4-hydroxybutyrate implants exhibit more favorable cell-matrix interactions than polypropylene. Mater Sci Eng C Mater Biol Appl. 2021;120:111702. https://doi.org/10.1016/j.msec.2020.111702.
186. Hayat M, Kumar T, Ahmad N, Jan S, Sajjad W, Faisal S, Gao, B-X, Khan K, Rahman Z, Abbasi B. In vitro antimicrobial activity of Aloe vera L. extracts against pathogenic bacteria and fungi. Mycopath. 2016;14(1):21–27.
187. Sahu PK, Giri DD, Singh R, et al. Therapeutic and medicinal uses of Aloe vera: a review. Pharmacol Pharm. 2013;4(08):599.
188. Rajeswari R, Umadevi M, Rahale CS, et al. Aloe vera: the miracle plant its medicinal and traditional uses in India. J Pharmacogn Phytochem. 2012;1(4):118–24.
189. Mei Y. Alginate hydrogel for 3D bioprinting. Microsc Microanal. 2016;22(S3):1764–5.
190. Paul K, Darzi S, Del Borgo MP, et al. Vaginal delivery of tissue engineered endometrial mesenchymal stem/stromal cells in an aloe vera-alginate hydrogel alleviates maternal simulated birth injury. Appl Mater Today. 2021;22:100890.
191. Jackson LA, Shi H, Acevedo J, et al. Effect of gelatin methacryloyl hydrogel on healing of the guinea pig vaginal wall with or without mesh augmentation. Int Urogynecol J. 2022;33(8):2223–32. https://doi.org/10.1007/s00192-021-05031-2.

Uterus and Cervix

The Structure and Function of the Uterus and Cervix Across the Reproductive Lifespan: Considerations for Biomaterial Design

Daniella M. Fodera and Erin M. Louwagie

Abstract The uterus and cervix are dynamic, multilayered organs within the female reproductive tract that undergo remarkable structural, compositional, and functional transformations throughout a woman's lifespan. This chapter provides a comprehensive overview of the structural and compositional features of the human uterus and cervix across cell, tissue, and organ length scales at different stages of the reproductive lifespan, including reproductive age, pregnancy, postpartum, and menopause. The isthmus, the transition region between the uterus and cervix, is also discussed. Finally, this chapter concludes by highlighting the importance of multiscale structure–function relationships of the uterus and cervix in the design of biomaterials that replicate physiologic conditions.

Keywords Uterus · Cervix · Isthmus · Growth and remodeling · Pregnancy · Postpartum · Aging · Women's health · Obstetrics · Gynecology

1 Introduction

The uterus and cervix are central organs of the female reproductive tract, each fulfilling fundamental roles in gynecologic and obstetric health. The uterus, situated between the urinary bladder and rectum, is a thick-walled organ with a single fluid-filled cavity (Fig. 1) [1]. The cervix, Latin for "neck," is located at the base of the uterus and is roughly cylindrical in shape [1]. The cervix acts as a pathway and barrier between the vaginal canal and intrauterine cavity [1]. Connecting the uterus and cervix is a transition region known as the isthmus [1].

D. M. Fodera (✉)
Department of Biomedical Engineering, Columbia University, New York, NY, USA
e-mail: dmf2194@columbia.edu

E. M. Louwagie
Department of Mechanical Engineering, Columbia University, New York, NY, USA
e-mail: eml2218@columbia.edu

S. G. Zambuto, M. L. Oyen (eds.), *Biomaterials for Women's Health Engineering*,
https://doi.org/10.1007/978-3-032-10745-9_5

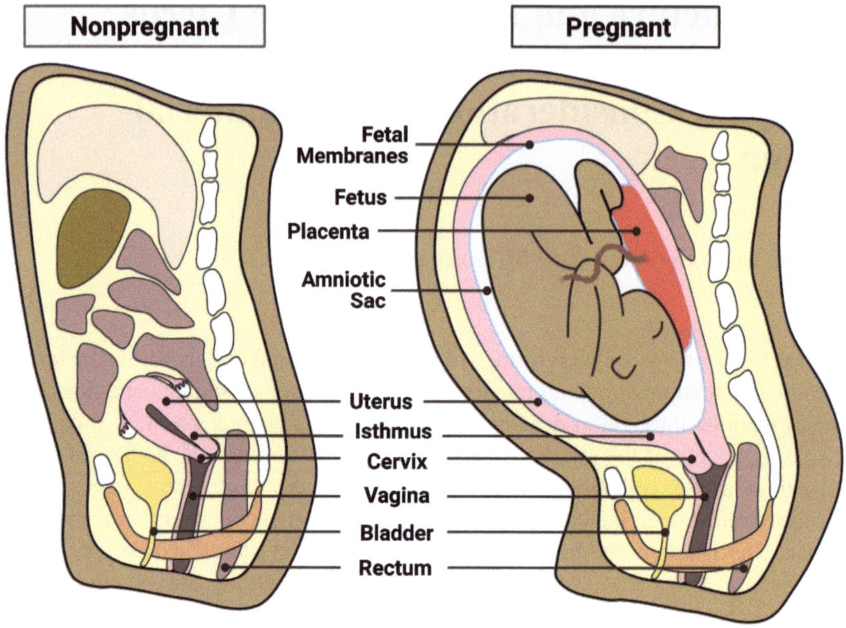

Fig. 1 Schematic of the female reproductive anatomy in nonpregnant and third-trimester pregnant states. The illustration highlights major reproductive and pelvic structures, including the uterus, cervix, isthmus, and surrounding organs (Adapted from Clark-Patterson et al. [7]. Created with https://Biorender.com)

The uterus and cervix undergo dramatic structural and compositional changes in pregnancy (Fig. 1). Over the course of gestation, the human uterus expands dramatically to accommodate the size of the growing fetus, exhibiting a 14-fold increase in wet weight (70 g to 1000 g) and 500-fold increase in intrauterine volume (10 mL to 5 L) from nonpregnancy to term [1–3]. In contrast, the cervix softens and shortens throughout gestation, finally dilating to 10 cm to allow for vaginal birth [1, 4–6]. In this chapter, we will discuss the constituents, structure, and function of the *human* uterus and cervix in nonpregnancy, pregnancy, postpartum, and aging.

2 Uterus

2.1 Nonpregnancy

2.1.1 Shape and Size

In nonpregnancy, the uterus is pyriform in shape, decreasing in width toward the utero-cervical junction (Figs. 1 and 2) [1, 8]. Total uterine volume ranges from

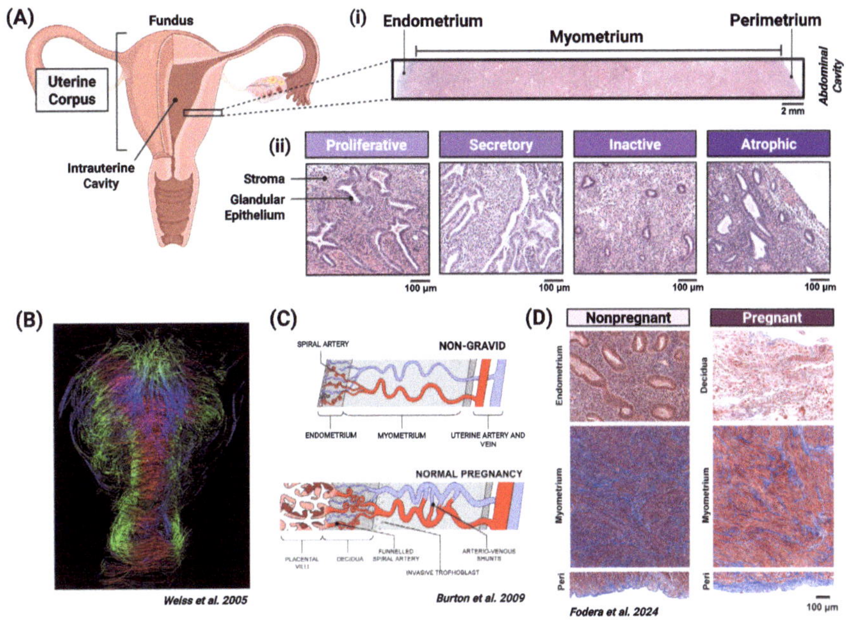

Fig. 2 Constituents and architecture of the human uterus. **(a)** Diagram of the human uterus. **(i)** Cross-section of the uterine wall containing endometrium, myometrium, and perimetrium layers visualized with a hematoxylin & eosin (H&E) stain (blue/purple = nuclei; pink = extracellular matrix and cytoplasm). **(ii)** Histology of endometrium depicting proliferative, secretory, inactive, and atrophic states. The stroma and glandular epithelium are marked. Images courtesy of the Myers Lab (Columbia University). **(b)** Fiber architecture of the nonpregnant uterus with directionality of individual fiber components indicated by distinct colors (red = left to right; green = through-plane; blue = top-down direction). Scale not provided by source (Reprinted from Weiss et al. [19] with permission [19]). **(c)** Diagram of vascular remodeling of the uterus in pregnancy (red = arterial; blue = venous). Adapted from [20]. Image licensed under CC-BY 4.0. **(d)** Histology of nonpregnant and third-trimester pregnant uterine tissue layers stained with Masson's Trichrome (blue = collagen; red = muscle fibers, cytoplasm; black = nuclei). Third-trimester decidua vera tissue is shown. Adapted from Fodera et al. [21] with permission from Elsevier [21]. (Created with https://Biorender.com)

15 to 56 cm^3 on average [9]. The average dimensions of the reproductive-aged uterus are 8 cm in length (superior–inferior plane) and 5 cm in width (anterior–posterior plane), with a mean length-to-width ratio of 1.6 [8, 10, 11]. The uterine body to cervix ratio is 2:1 [8]. The uterine wall thickness ranges from 3 to 40 mm, with a median value of 12 mm, and exhibits slight regional variations [8, 12–14].

Within the pelvic cavity, the orientation of the uterus relative to the bladder and rectum can be variable, thereby changing the angle of attachment between the uterus and cervix [15, 16]. Most commonly, the uterus is anteverted (tilted forward toward the bladder), yet, in 15% of the population, it is retroverted (tilted back toward the rectum) [16–18].

Notably, Müllerian duct anomalies occurring during fetal development can give rise to a spectrum of uterine and cervical malformations, affecting an estimated 5% of the general population [22]. In such cases, the following developmental anomalies may arise: (i) the incomplete formation of one or both Müllerian ducts can lead to agenesis or a unicornuate uterus, (ii) failure of ductal fusion may result in a bicornuate uterus (characterized by two uterine cavities and/or cervical canals) or uterine didelphys (two fully formed uteri and cervices), and (iii) incomplete resorption of the tissue between the fused ducts can lead to a septate or arcuate uterus [22–24].

2.1.2 Constituents and Architecture

The nonpregnant uterine wall is composed of three structurally and functionally distinct tissue layers: (i) endometrium, (ii) myometrium, and (iii) perimetrium (i.e., serosa) [1, 8, 25]. The nonpregnant endometrium is the innermost uterine layer consisting of epithelial, stromal, and vascular endothelial cells embedded in a collagen-dense extracellular matrix (ECM) (Fig. 2a) [1, 26]. On its surface, the endometrium is lined with a single layer of ciliated luminal epithelial cells that adopt a columnar shape (Fig. 2a) [27, 28]. Glandular epithelial cells extend from the luminal surface through the full thickness of the endometrium, creating tubular structures with both winding and branching morphologies (Fig. 2a) [1, 11, 29]. Residing at the base of these epithelial glands are stem cells that enable tissue regeneration [27, 30]. Within the endometrium, its vasculature, termed spiral arteries, consists of terminal branches of larger uterine arteries and exhibits a distinct coiled morphology, extending radially across the endometrium (Fig. 2c) [1, 20, 31]. Immune cells, including natural killer cells, macrophages, neutrophils, and dendritic cells, are also present in the endometrium but to a lesser degree [1, 28, 32]. Within the endometrium, there are two histologically distinct regions: (i) the stratum basalis and (ii) the stratum functionalis [1, 11, 33]. The stratum functionalis occupies the upper two thirds of the endometrium adjacent to the intrauterine cavity, while the deeper stratum basalis layer lies adjacent to the myometrium at the uterine junctional zone (Fig. 2a) [1, 11, 33, 34].

In nonpregnancy, the endometrium undergoes cyclic cellular and molecular changes throughout the menstrual cycle in response to hormonal fluctuations (Fig. 2a) [11, 26, 35]. These changes are largely isolated to the stratum functionalis layer [1, 11]. The menstrual cycle, dictated by fluctuations in the release of ovarian hormones, is approximately 28 days long and consists roughly of three phases: (i) the proliferative phase, (ii) the secretory phase, and (iii) menstruation (i.e., menses) [1, 11, 35]. In the early proliferative phase, the glandular epithelium forms narrow, straight tubular structures, accompanied by elongation of the spiral arteries and proliferation of stromal cells (Fig. 2a,ii) [1]. By the late proliferative phase, the endometrium thickens through glandular hyperplasia and further stromal proliferation (Fig. 2a,ii) [1]. The stroma appears loosely packed, the glands become longer and pseudostratified, and the luminal epithelium acquires microvilli and cilia (Fig. 2a,ii) [1, 11]. The secretory phase is marked by extensive coiling of the glandular epithelium, secretions by the luminal epithelium, mitosis and edema of the stroma, and elongation and coiling of the spiral arteries (Fig. 2a,ii) [1]. Uterine gland secretions, rich in growth factors, cytokines, and mucins, play a key role in promoting stromal decidualization and mediating uterine receptivity in preparation for pregnancy [36, 37]. At this stage, the stromal cells surrounding spiral arteries acquire a more conspicuous eosinophilic cytoplasm and are often referred to as predecidual cells [11]. In the immediate days preceding menstruation, the breakdown of endometrial tissue is facilitated by neutrophil infiltration and the subsequent release of matrix metalloproteases (MMPs) [1]. At the same time, vasoconstriction of the spiral arteries occurs in preparation for menstruation to limit subsequent menstrual bleeding [1]. At the point of menstruation, the functionalis layer is completely shed over the course of several days [1]. Menstrual efflux is comprised of blood, endometrial cells, vaginal secretions, and a host of biochemical molecules, including proteolytic enzymes and cytokines [38]. Endometrial cell autophagy and apoptosis are two mechanisms by which tissue degradation of the human endometrium is facilitated during menstruation [39]. These structural and cellular changes are accompanied by marked fluctuations in endometrial thickness across the menstrual cycle, increasing from 5–11 mm during the proliferative phase to 7–16 mm in the secretory phase, before declining to 2–4 mm during menstruation [11, 40]. It is important to note that the administration of exogenous hormones can notably alter the histomorphology of the endometrium [11, 41]. Often, the endometrium appears inactive or atrophic and the stroma exhibits a pseudo-decidual response (Fig. 2a) [11, 41].

The myometrium is the middle layer of the uterus and is primarily composed of smooth muscle fascicles interwoven with collagen and elastin fibers [1]. Vasculature extends radially along the width of the uterine wall (Fig. 2a, d) [1, 20]. To a lesser degree, immune cells, fibroblasts, and nerve fibers are also present in the myometrium [42–44]. The myometrium is the thickest uterine layer, with an average thickness of 1–2 cm (Fig. 2a) [45]. While some studies have reported cyclical changes in myometrial thickness that parallel those of the endometrium, other data suggest that myometrial thickness remains relatively constant throughout the menstrual cycle [46, 47]. Fiber directionality has been shown to vary across the myometrium; the inner and outer regions of the myometrium exhibit longitudinal fibers, running parallel to the uterus's long axis, while the middle region has circularly oriented fibers (Fig. 2c) [19, 48]. Additionally, three-dimensional fiber mapping of myometrial tissue has shown significant local fiber dispersion [49, 50]. Uterine vasculature exhibits both circumferential and radial branching with a decreasing gradient of vascular smooth muscle content from the outer to inner myometrium [51].

Lastly, the perimetrium (i.e., serosa) is a thin, collagen-dense connective tissue layer that envelops the uterine corpus and acts as a smooth, lubricated surface between the uterus and surrounding abdominal organs (Fig. 2a, d) [8]. The thickness of the perimetrium is reported to be on the order of 100 μm (Fig. 2a, d) [21]. Comparatively, not much is known about the function of the perimetrium in the literature.

2.1.3 Functional Aspects in Nonpregnancy

In addition to its passive mechanical functions, the myometrium exhibits active mechanical behavior, termed uterine peristalsis, which produces rhythmic, 'wave-like' contractions [52]. The direction and amplitude of these contractions change throughout the menstrual cycle to aid with sperm motility during ovulation and menstrual blood egress during menstruation [52, 53].

2.2 Changes During Pregnancy

Pregnancy is initiated following the successful implantation of a blastocyst into the decidualized endometrial layer during the ovulatory window [1]. In humans, pregnancy is customarily divided into three trimesters: 1st (0–14 weeks), 2nd (15–28 weeks), and 3rd (29–42 weeks) [1].

2.2.1 Size and Shape

The overall volume of the uterine body dramatically increases during pregnancy, but individual dimensions change in a nonuniform manner [1, 3, 54]. In pregnancy, the intrauterine volume reaches up to 5 L by the late third trimester due to the presence of amniotic fluid, a placenta, and a growing fetus [1–3, 54, 55]. In extreme cases, such as multiple pregnancies or pregnancies complicated by polyhydramnios (excess amniotic fluid), the volume may be more than fourfold normal quantities [55]. During the first few weeks of pregnancy, changes in uterine size occur predominantly in the anterior–posterior direction, until the uterus assumes a globular shape, approximately 8 cm in diameter, by 12 weeks of gestation [1]. Beyond the first trimester, the expansion of the uterus mimics that of an expanding balloon; there is a greater increase in intrauterine diameter in the inferior–superior plane compared to the anterior–posterior plane [3]. Further, the inferior region of the uterus (proximal to the cervix) expands to a lesser degree than the superior region (uterine fundus) [54]. Interestingly, a retroverted orientation of the uterus has been linked with decreased fertility rates, but does not appear to impact pregnancy progression once implantation has successfully occurred [56]. In most cases, retroversion of the uterus resolves itself by the second trimester [57].

Differential changes in uterine wall thickness are also observed by tissue layer in pregnancy. In the first trimester, the thickness of the decidua basalis increases to approximately 13–25 mm and is greater than that of the decidua parietalis, which remains rather unchanged in terms of thickness [1, 58, 59]. Beyond the first trimester, no studies to date have directly measured the thickness of the decidua. For the myometrium tissue layer, there appears to be a decrease in myometrial thickness from the first to second trimesters *in vivo* [60]. Beyond the second trimester, the thickness of the myometrium remains rather unchanged across gestation [54, 60, 61]. One notable exception is the lower uterine segment (i.e., isthmus), which normally thins over the course of pregnancy from the second to third trimesters; excessive thinning in this region has been linked to adverse obstetric outcomes, including preterm birth and uterine rupture [3, 54, 61–63]. At the time of labor, the myometrium is notably thinner than pre-labor measurements [64]. No changes in the thickness of the perimetrium have been shown to occur in pregnancy [21].

2.2.2 Constituents and Architecture

At the point of implantation, the endometrium transforms into what is known as the decidua under the influence of estrogen and progesterone secreted by the blastocyst [1]. The composition and structure of the decidua depend on its location relative to the placenta and fetus, as well as its corresponding gestational age [1]. At the site of implantation and subsequent placental formation lies the decidua basalis [1]. The decidua capsularis overlies the enlarging blastocyst and is opposite the placenta [1]. The decidua parietalis represents all other decidua tissue away from the site of implantation [1]. Beyond 14 weeks of gestation, the intrauterine cavity is obliterated, and the decidua capsularis and decidua parietalis merge to form the decidua vera [1]. The decidua parietalis, basalis, and vera tissues are each composed of three layers: (i) zona compacta, (ii) zona spongiosa, and (iii) zona basalis [1]. In early pregnancy, the zona spongiosa is characterized by distended glands and a sparse stromal matrix [1]. Within the decidua basalis, there is a notable influx of immune cells aiding in trophoblast invasion and angiogenesis [1, 65]. In addition, collagen deposition is elevated in the decidua basalis relative to the decidua parietalis in the first trimester, exhibiting increased collagen fibril diameter [66]. As gestation advances, the glandular epithelium gradually regresses and becomes less prominent (Fig. 2) [1]. The decidua basalis facilitates the formation of the placenta's basal plate and, as such, undergoes the greatest degree of spiral artery remodeling, exhibiting a five-to-tenfold increase in terminal luminal diameter, loss of elastic lamina, and deposition of a fibrinoid matrix (Fig. 2) [1, 67, 68]. Deeper spiral artery remodeling of the myometrium layer begins at around 12 weeks of gestation, coinciding with placental maturation (Fig. 2) [20, 69, 70].

Throughout pregnancy, the myometrium must undergo passive growth and stretch to accommodate the growing size of the fetus. This is achieved through two processes: (*i*) hyperplasia, an increase in cell number, and (*ii*) hypertrophy, an increase in cell size (Fig. 2) [1, 71, 72]. Accordingly, there is a relative increase in the ratio of smooth muscle to collagen content within the uterus by the third trimester of pregnancy (Fig. 2) [21]. Throughout gestation, myometrial cells remain largely quiescent, exhibiting minimal electrical activity [73]. At the time of labor, SMCs are responsible for producing and propagating active uterine contractions via bioelectrical impulses [53, 74].

Collectively, the total collagen content of the uterus increases by approximately seven to eightfold at term relative to nonpregnancy, with about 97% present in an insoluble form [2, 75]. Hydration of the uterus remains rather constant across gestation, ranging between 70 and 85% on an individual tissue layer basis [75, 76].

2.3 Changes During Postpartum

Postpartum, also known as puerperium, is the period of time between placental delivery and the return of the uterus toward its prepregnancy size, undergoing a process known as involution [1]. Immediately following delivery, the uterus rapidly contracts to minimize blood loss [1, 77]. Uterine size then continues to rapidly decrease in the first two weeks, returning close to its prepregnancy baseline within eight weeks of delivery [75, 78–81]. However, this regression is not strictly a return to the nulliparous state as the primiparous uterus remains measurably larger than that of a nulliparous uterus [82]. Additionally, the pace of uterine involution is influenced by the mode of delivery (i.e., vaginal or cesarean section) and breastfeeding status [78].

Accompanying gross changes in uterine size are structural and compositional changes to the ECM and cellular components of the uterus. During delivery, the decidua's zona compacta and spongiosa layers are shed; the zona basalis layer is retained, giving rise to a new endometrium layer [1]. Still, the shedding is not uniform, and this layer exhibits a jagged appearance histomorphologically [1]. Subsequent regeneration of the nonpregnant endometrium is rapid, except at the placental site, and occurs within 16 days postpartum [1, 83]. Within the myometrium, there is a decrease in the size of individual myocytes, but it is unclear whether the total number decreases from term [1, 84]. Of the studies demonstrating decreases in myocyte count, myocyte apoptosis and autophagy have been suggested as two mechanisms of uterine involution in the postpartum period [71, 84].

In addition to cellular changes, there is a rapid resorption of collagen; by day 8 of the postpartum period, there is a 72% decrease in total collagen relative to term [2, 75]. Similar trends have been shown for elastin content [2]. There is also evidence of interstitial edema within the myometrium, which is accompanied by increases in tissue hydration during this period [75].

2.4 *Effects of Aging*

2.4.1 Reproductive Age

During the reproductive period, uterine size does not vary as a direct result of age, but rather as a product of parity and the presence of certain gynecologic disorders (i.e., uterine fibroids and adenomyosis) [82, 85, 86]. The baseline size of the nonpregnant uterus increases with parity, with notable differences found across individuals that are nulliparous (zero prior pregnancies), primiparous (one prior pregnancy), and multiparous (two or more prior pregnancies) [82].

There is mixed data on the effect of age on uterine activity during a person's reproductive years. Experimentally, *ex vivo* uterine contractility appears to decrease with increasing patient age, but only to a significant extent in the nonpregnant state [87, 88]. Third-trimester pregnant uterine tissue exhibits no change in contractility as a function of age [87, 88]. Clinically, there is conflicting observational evidence on key indicators of myometrial function (i.e., duration of first stage of labor, duration of second stage of labor, and need for oxytocin augmentation) as a function of age [89, 90]. Globally, rates of cesarean section appear to increase with increasing maternal age for both nulliparous and multiparous women; however, it is presently unknown whether this trend reflects underlying biological mechanisms or social factors [91–94].

2.4.2 Perimenopause

Perimenopause is a time of great transition in the homeostasis of the female reproductive system [95]. Ovarian function diminishes, which induces functional, morphological, and cellular changes to the uterus [96–98]. The length, time of onset, and associated symptomology of perimenopause can vary drastically on an individual basis, and as such, the changes undergone by the uterus can be just as variable [95]. Irregularities in menstrual timing and flow are common phenomena in perimenopause, reflecting underlying functional changes within the uterus [95, 97]. Often, the endometrium is described as inactive—devoid of morphologic features indicative of active proliferation or secretion—and its thickness is on par with the early to mid-proliferative phase [41]. In individuals with abnormal uterine bleeding, the endometrium may exhibit normal secretory or proliferative patterns, benign pathologic states such as hyperplasia or atrophy, or malignancies in the form of carcinoma [99–101].

Overall, uterine volume has been shown to decrease slowly in perimenopause in the years prior to an individual's final menstrual period [102]. This is accompanied by age-related cellular changes in the myometrium, as evidenced by impaired cell–cell communication and gene expression of endothelial, smooth muscle, fibroblast, perivascular, and immune cells [42].

Interestingly, the symptoms of certain gynecologic conditions, such as uterine fibroids and adenomyosis, peak in the perimenopause years and decrease following the onset of menopause [103, 104].

2.4.3 Menopause

Menopause is a permanent state of menstrual cycle cessation, which occurs after the loss of ovarian activity [95]. Menopause is a condition that can only be diagnosed retrospectively, one year following an individual's last menstrual cycle [95]. Structurally, the size and shape of the uterus appear to rapidly change in the immediate years following an individual's final menstrual period, plateauing in the years thereafter [82, 102]. The uterine body to cervix ratio shifts to 1:2 in menopause, similar in size to the prepubertal uterus [8, 10]. During this time, uterine volume (cm^3) decreases by seven to eightfold on average [102]. Among the uterine layers, the myometrium exhibits the most pronounced shrinkage, which is accompanied by a decrease in endometrial thickness to approximately 5 mm or less [40, 82].

Cellular and compositional changes to the uterus accompany gross changes to uterine size [33]. By and large, the activity of the uterus wanes and becomes rather quiescent [33]. Cyclical changes to the endometrium no longer occur once menstruation has halted [33, 105]. The endometrium appears thin and atrophic, undergoing gradual degeneration (Fig. 2a,ii) [11, 105]. Often, the postmenopausal endometrium consists solely of the stratum basalis layer [11]. Within the endometrium, glandular epithelium is still present but varies morphologically from small, widely spaced atrophic tubules to cystically dilated glands (Fig. 2a,ii) [11, 33]. The endometrial stroma can appear as densely cellular or fibrous, depending on the individual (Fig. 2a,ii) [11, 33, 105]. Within the myometrium layer, aging has been shown to impair gene expression of endothelial, smooth muscle, fibroblast, perivascular, and immune cells and induce alterations to cell signaling pathways involving cell-to-cell communication pathways, endothelial function, and angiogenesis (i.e., de novo blood vessel formation) [42]. Calcification, the accumulation of calcium salts in biological tissues [106], has also been demonstrated to occur in myometrial blood vessels as well as the endometrium in postmenopausal women [107, 108].

3 Isthmus

The isthmus is the transition region where the uterus narrows into the cervix (Fig. 1) [109–111]. In nonpregnancy, the median thickness of the anterior isthmus has been found to be 13.45 mm (IQR: 11.03, 16.90) [112]. Its location is approximated at the lowest level of insertion of the uterine arteries, which are often used to demarcate the proximal end of the cervix [109–111]. The isthmus is also thought of as the region between the anatomical internal os and histological internal os [1, 109]. The histological internal os marks the region where endocervical epithelium changes to isthmic epithelium, or where the cervical mucosa ends [109, 113, 114]. The anatomical internal os is typically defined at the point where the base of the uterus narrows, approximately 6–10 mm above the histological internal os [109, 113]. Compared to the uterus and cervix, far less is known about the isthmus structure, function, and changes with aging.

3.1 Constituents and Architecture

Histomorphologically, the surface layer of the isthmus adjacent to the intrauterine cavity contains epithelial and stromal cells [11]. The glands appear small and ciliated with irregular distributions, while the stroma appears quite fibrous [11, 115]. Thick-walled vessels can also be found within the stroma [112]. The epithelium of the isthmus has been likened to that of the endometrial basalis using both standard histology stains and transmission electron microscopy [115, 116]. Further, Sorvari and Laakso [117] found that the mucin production of the isthmus was more analogous to that found in the endometrium compared to the cervical mucosa [117]. Despite these distinctions, the precise definitions of these regions remain debated and appear to vary on an individual patient basis [109, 114–116]. Hoogduin et al. [118] used morphometry and immunohistochemistry techniques to better define the isthmus and found the transition from endocervical epithelium to isthmus epithelium to be characterized by intense keratin 5, BCL2, and Ki-67 expression [118]. The transition zone of the isthmus has also been marked by differential changes in CD10 expression, a marker of endometrial stromal cells [118, 119]. At the transition from the isthmus to the uterus, the underlying stroma expresses CD10 across its full thickness [118]. However, the stroma in the isthmus itself exhibits increased CD10 expression [118]. The level of smooth muscle cell content in the isthmus has been investigated by Schwalm and Dubrausky [120], finding a near-linear increase across the isthmus from the cervix to the uterus [120]. The amount of collagen in the isthmus also lies between the levels observed in the uterus and cervix, as found by Petersen et al. [121] through hydroxyproline assays [121]. Danforth [109] described this transition from the fibrous cervix to muscular uterus as the fibromuscular junction, which in some cases was abrupt and in others was gradual over a distance of 5–10 mm [109].

The isthmus has been reported to be hormonally responsive, exhibiting morphological and biochemical changes throughout the menstrual cycle [115]. Still, such hormone-induced changes are lessened for the isthmus relative to endometrium tissue sourced from the fundus [115].

3.2 Functional Aspects in Nonpregnancy

Similar to the uterus, the isthmus experiences peristaltic contractions in nonpregnancy [122]. Youssef [122] found contractions at the level of the isthmus to be variable depending on the menstrual cycle phase, with the internal os appearing longer and tightly closed during the luteal phase and relaxed (shorter and wider) in the days preceding [122]. This is reflected in measurements of internal os diameter, which was found to be the largest in the first days of menstruation (days 1–3) and the smallest during the luteal phase (days 22–28) [123].

3.3 Changes During Pregnancy

In early pregnancy, the isthmus elongates, thickens, and softens [1, 109]. The elongation of the isthmus is proportional to the thickening of the muscular uterine tissue during the first trimester [109]. The softening of the isthmus has historically been a sign of early pregnancy, known as "Hegar's sign" [1, 124]. By the end of the first trimester (10–13 weeks of gestation), the median length of the isthmus was found to be 13.8 mm (range: 0–49.4) [125]. As pregnancy progresses, the isthmus opens and shortens and is hereafter referred to as the lower uterine segment [54, 109]. By 20–24 weeks of gestation, the length of the isthmus was found to be 7.8 mm (range: 0–51.0) [125]. In a subset of pregnancies (15–25%), the early opening of the uterine isthmus can occur, but this event does not appear to adversely affect placental development or perinatal outcomes [126].

During pregnancy, the isthmus retains its ability to contract [127]. Isthmic contractions are common after bladder voiding, occurring in 43% of pregnant individuals [127]. During labor, the lower uterine segment is mostly passive, where it dilates, distends, and thins due to contractions from the upper uterine segment [1].

3.4 Effects of Aging

There are few studies reporting the effects of aging on the uterine isthmus. Youssef [122] found the isthmus of postmenopausal individuals to be wider and more relaxed when compared to individuals of childbearing age and attributed this change to the musculature atrophy and decreased ovarian function [122]. Schweppe and Wynn [115] investigated the mucosa of the isthmus in postmenopausal uterine specimens and found that it migrates toward the uterine corpus, extending above the level of the anatomical internal os [115]. Changes to the isthmus stroma with age remain unknown.

4 Cervix

In humans, the cervix is roughly cylindrical in shape, containing a single, straight endocervical canal, which provides a pathway and barrier between the vaginal canal and intrauterine cavity [1]. In nonpregnancy, the cervix is approximately 3 cm in length and 3 cm in diameter, though the size of the cervix is both age and parity dependent [128]. The cervical openings at the uterine cavity and vaginal junctions are identified as the internal os (IO) and external os (EO), respectively [1]. In nulliparous individuals, the external os appears as a circular pinhole, and in parous individuals, it has a slit-like appearance [1, 129].

4.1 Constituents and Architecture

Like the uterus, the cervix is a heterogeneous structure composed of multiple distinct tissue layers (Fig. 3a). The endocervical canal is lined by a layer of epithelial cells, which fold and create crypt-like structures along its length [129, 130]. The endocervical epithelium is also known as the cervical mucosa, as these cells secrete mucus [129, 130]. These cells are columnar and contain a finely granular cytoplasm with droplets of mucous (Fig. 3b,i) [129]. The distal end of the cervix which protrudes into the vaginal canal is known as the ectocervix or exocervix [129]. The ectocervix is covered by a layer of squamous epithelium that appears as flat, sheet-like cells (Fig. 3b,iii) [129]. The shapes of these cells vary from the basal layer to the surface of the ectocervix: basal cells are the smallest, containing minimal cytoplasm and relatively large nuclei, whereas the superficial flattened cells have abundant cytoplasm and smaller nuclei [129]. Between the endocervical and ectocervical epithelium lies the epithelial transformation zone, also known as the squamocolumnar junction (Fig. 3b,ii) [129]. Squamous metaplasia occurs within this transformation zone, where the columnar cells of the endocervical canal are replaced by layered squamous epithelium [129]. The ECM components of the cervical epithelium include a basement membrane of type IV collagen, proteoglycans, and glycoproteins, among other components [131–133].

Beneath the epithelial surface of the cervix lies a thick, stromal layer (Fig. 3a). The ECM of the stroma is composed mainly of collagen (predominantly type I and type III), accounting for 70% of the tissue's dry weight [4, 141–143]. The structure of the collagen within the ECM is distinct across three zones: (1) the innermost zone, where the collagen fibers run parallel to the cervical canal, (2) the mid-stroma, in which collagen is circumferentially oriented, and (3) the outermost zone, with fibers again parallel to the cervical canal (Fig. 3b,vi) [138, 143, 144]. Still, there is a considerable amount of dispersion of fiber directionality about the primary directions [139, 145]. The level of collagen fiber dispersion is location dependent, with more dispersion found near the IO compared to the EO [145]. The ECM also contains a substantial amount of elastin fibers (0.9–2.4%), which is hypothesized to give the

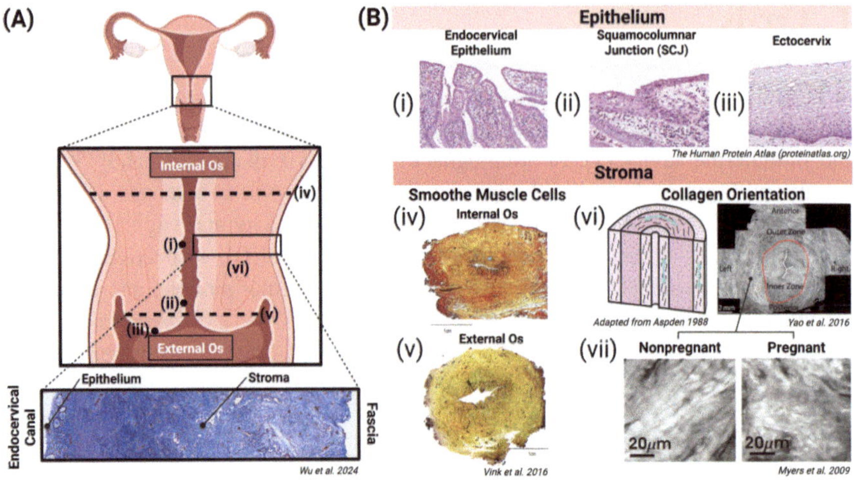

Fig. 3 Anatomy of the human cervix. **(a)** The cervix is located at the base of the uterus, with the internal os and the external os marking its ends. The main layers of the cervix are the epithelium and stroma. A radial cross section of the mid-cervix stained with Masson's Trichrome (blue = collagen; red = muscle fibers, cytoplasm; black = nuclei) is shown [134]. Image licensed under CC-BY 4.0. **(b)** Structure of the epithelium and stroma, visualized with a hematoxylin & eosin (H&E) stain, showing distinct components: (i) endocervical epithelium, (ii) squamocolumnar junction, and (iii) ectocervix (blue/purple = nuclei; pink = extracellular matrix and cytoplasm). Images courtesy of The Human Protein Atlas via a CC BY-SA 4.0 license; scales not provided by source [135–137]. In the stroma, the concentration of smooth muscle cells is location dependent, with a higher concentration at the (iv) internal os than the (v) external os, as shown by Vink et al. [110] using Movat pentachrome staining (red = smooth muscle; yellow = collagen) [110] (Reprinted from Vink et al. [110] with permission from Elsevier [110]). (vi) Collagen within the cervical stroma is organized into three zones, where the inner and outer zones have longitudinal collagen fibers and the middle zone has circumferential collagen fibers [138]. Reprinted from Aspden [138] with permission from Elsevier [138]. Optical coherence tomography of cervical slices demonstrates the structure of the collagen fibers in the mid stroma [139]. Image reprinted from Yao et al. [139] under the CC-BY 4.0 license [139]. (vii) The collagen fibers are wavier and more disorganized in the pregnant state compared to the nonpregnant state, as captured via second harmonic generation imaging [140]. (Reprinted from Myers et al. [140] with permission from Elsevier. Created with https://BioRender.com)

cervix the ability to recoil quickly after being fully effaced and stretched during birth [146]. Glycosaminoglycans (GAGs), proteoglycans, and matricellular proteins are also present in the ECM [5]. In its nonpregnant state, the cervix exhibits a high degree of hydration, with water content typically between 75% and 80% [140]. Together, these ECM components play an important role in modulating tissue mechanical properties. For a detailed review of these components and their functions, refer to [5].

The stromal cell population of the cervix includes smooth muscle cells, fibroblasts, immune cells, vascular endothelial cells, and neurons [143, 147]. The density and architecture of these cells vary along the length of the cervix. For instance, smooth muscle content increases proximally along the cervix, from about 10% at the external os to 50–60% at the internal os (Fig. 3b,iv–v) [110, 120]. Vasculature within the cervix is also variable by location, demonstrating four zones of vessel organization [148]. From the outer cervix to the inner endocervical canal, the outermost zone contains large blood vessels, which feed into the middle zone of arterioles and venules [148]. Near the endocervical canal, there is a network of capillaries which are disorganized near the internal os, but run parallel to the endocervical canal closer to the external os [148]. Lining the endocervical canal are small subepithelial blood vessels [148]. Additionally, in comparison to the uterus, the cervix is highly innervated, with nerve fibers found throughout the stroma [147].

4.2 Functional Changes Across the Menstrual Cycle

In nonpregnancy, the cervix has a dual role of acting as both a barrier and passageway between the vaginal canal and intrauterine cavity [1]. The epithelial layer of the cervix secretes mucus, which aids in preventing ascending infection into the sterile, anaerobic intrauterine microenvironment [1, 149]. The composition, consistency, and amount of mucus secreted by the endothelial mucosa change during the menstrual cycle, exhibiting lower viscosity during ovulation, allowing for easier passage of sperm [150, 151]. These observed differences in cervical mucus can be attributed to variations in mucus composition and concentration during the menstrual cycle [150, 152].

Beyond the epithelium, the underlying cervical stroma also undergoes cyclical remodeling. In the late secretory phase, Bradburn and Webb [153] first reported pronounced stromal edema [153]. However, subsequent studies have yielded conflicting reports regarding the hormonal responsiveness of cervical tissue constituents [153–155].

4.3 Changes During Pregnancy and Postpartum

Throughout the course of gestation, the cervix must act as both a physical and immunological barrier to retain the fetus *in utero* and prevent the migration of infectious pathogens [1, 5, 156]. In support of this function, a thick, viscous mucus plug forms within the endocervical canal during early gestation and remains in place until the onset of labor [1, 5, 157, 158]. The mucosa lining the cervical canal also increases during pregnancy, so much so that it makes up about half of the total mass of the cervix at term [1]. At the time of labor, the cervix must then transform into a compliant structure, undergoing extensive dilation and effacement, to permit fetal delivery [1, 5, 156].

Unlike the uterus, the cervix does not grow dramatically during pregnancy [3, 54, 140]. Rather, its dimensions, namely length, decrease in pregnancy once the third trimester has been reached [3, 54, 140]. The cervical stroma undergoes dramatic remodeling throughout gestation, accompanied by an increase in hydration at term by approximately 5% [140]. Increased vascularity in the pregnant cervix compared to nonpregnancy is also evidenced [1]. In the first and early second trimesters, the cervix dramatically softens [3, 159]. However, the length of the cervix does not begin to significantly decrease until the beginning of the third trimester [3, 159]. Cervical remodeling has been studied extensively in rodents, where cervical softening has been attributed to changes in intermolecular cross-links between collagen molecules [160]. These cross-links form and organize the collagen molecules into fibrils, being constantly synthesized, assembled, and degraded during pregnancy [160]. The dispersion of collagen also changes across gestation, becoming more dispersed about the original principal direction in term cervices compared to nonpregnant ones (Fig. 3b,vi) [139, 161]. At the time of labor, the cervix undergoes ripening, where it rapidly becomes more compliant to allow for vaginal delivery [5]. The authors recommend the review paper by Timmons et al. [5] for a detailed account of the role of different cervical components in this process [5]. In combination with this material softening, the cervix is thought to dilate by radial tension placed on the cervix by uterine contractions [162]. The dilation of the compliant cervix is a critical step in the labor process [1]. During parturition, the cervix must dilate to a diameter of 10 cm to allow for vaginal birth [1]. Cervical dilation is accompanied by cervical effacement, where the cervix thins and the IO is taken up into the lower uterine segment [1].

In the postpartum period, the cervix undergoes repair to recover from the large deformation imposed during parturition and return to its nonpregnant state [5]. To facilitate this repair, inflammatory cells, such as neutrophils and macrophages, play an important role in ECM degradation [5]. Using sonographic and aspiration-based methods, stiffness measurements of the *in vivo* postpartum cervix indicate that it remains measurably softer than the nonpregnant cervix during the first 6–16 weeks postpartum [159, 163, 164]. Concurrently, the concentration of collagen (as a percentage of tissue dry weight) has been shown to increase in the months following birth, from 50% at 3 months to 65% at 9 months postpartum, with no statistically significant changes observed after 9 months [165].

4.4 Effects of Aging

Few studies have explored the effects of aging on cervical constituents, architecture, and function. It has been shown that the cervical diameter is significantly decreased in individuals over 55 years of age when compared to those younger than 55 (2.6 cm vs 3.5 cm, respectively) [128]. Parity also influences cervical diameter, with a larger cervical diameter found in parous (3.4 cm) versus nulliparous (3.0 cm) individuals [128].

Histomorphologically, the glandular epithelium has been described as sparse and simple in postmenopausal individuals by Bradburn and Webb [153]. Further,

Najmabadi et al. [166] evaluated the effect of age and parity on cervical mucous quantity and quality [166]. Parous individuals were found to have more days of "fertility-favorable" cervical mucus compared to nulliparous individuals [166]. Among nulliparous individuals, those under 30 years of age exhibited more "fertile" mucus days than their older counterparts [166]. Roberts et al. [167] investigated differences in collagen and water content in biopsies collected at the squamocolumnar junction from pre- and postmenopausal individuals [167]. While the premenopausal samples contained more water and collagen than the postmenopausal biopsies, samples from deeper in the stroma did not exhibit these differences [167]. Similarly, Oxlund et al. [168] found that collagen concentration increased with age, but decreased with parity for cervical biopsy specimens [168].

5 Relevance for Biomaterial Design

A thorough understanding of the constituents, structure, and function of uterine and cervical tissues is fundamental to advancing biomaterial design for reproductive applications. The uterus and cervix are heterogeneous, multilayered organs that continuously remodel throughout a woman's reproductive lifespan in response to hormonal, cellular, and physiological cues. The dynamic, multiscale remodeling of these organs encompasses molecular, cellular, and tissue-level transformations, providing valuable biological templates for designing materials that can support, repair, replicate, or augment the physiologic functions of the human uterus and cervix.

Biomimetic materials that emulate the microenvironments of the uterus and cervix are essential for capturing their inherent structural and functional complexity. Incorporating region-specific patterns of extracellular matrix proteins, distinct cell types, and vascular networks may better recapitulate physiological function. Applications of these biomaterials extend across the entire translational science spectrum. For example, tissue-engineered scaffolds may facilitate reconstruction of the uterus or cervix to treat congenital anomalies or full/partial hysterectomies. Bioengineered matrices can also support endogenous repair and remodeling processes following surgical manipulation (e.g., myomectomy, dilation and curettage (D&C), or endometriosis excision) or during the postpartum period.

Ultimately, the multiscale organization and dynamic nature of the uterus and cervix provide powerful design principles for creating biomaterials that are biologically informed, hormonally responsive, and capable of replicating innate tissue function across the reproductive lifespan.

For further reading on efforts in tissue engineering for the uterus and cervix, we recommend the respective chapters by Campo et al. [169] and Koullali and House [170] in *Handbook of Tissue Engineering Scaffolds: Volume Two.*

Conflicts of Interest
The authors declare no conflicts of interest.

Author Contributions
E.L. and D.F. contributed equally to the conception, literature review, writing, and visualization of this work. D.F. was responsible for all content related to the uterus; E.L. was responsible for all content related to the cervix and isthmus. Both authors reviewed, edited, and approved the final version.

Acknowledgements The authors gratefully acknowledge the library services of Columbia University and Wayne State University for their assistance in accessing source literature. This work was supported by the Eunice Kennedy Shriver National Institute of Child Health & Human Development of the National Institutes of Health (NIH) under award number 1F31HD114449-01 (DMF). The content is solely the responsibility of the authors and does not necessarily represent the official views of the NIH.

References

1. Cunningham F, et al. Williams Obstetrics 26e. Columbus: McGraw Hill LLC; 2022. ISBN: 978-1-260-46274-6. https://books.google.com/books?id=2HVKEAAAQBAJ.
2. Woessner JF, Brewer TH. Formation and breakdown of collagen and elastin in the human uterus during pregnancy and post-partum involution. Biochem J. 1963;89:75–82. ISSN: 0264-6021. https://www.ncbi.nlm.nih.gov/pmc/articles/PMC1202274/ (2023).
3. Louwagie EM, et al. The biomechanical evolution of the uterus and cervix and fetal growth in human pregnancy. npj Women's Health. 2024;2:1–9. ISSN: 2948-1716. https://www.nature.com/articles/s44294-024-00038-8 (2025).
4. Leppert PC. Anatomy and physiology of cervical ripening. Clin Obstet Gynecol. 1995;38: 267–79. ISSN: 0009-9201.
5. Timmons B, Akins M, Mahendroo M. Cervical remodeling during pregnancy and parturition. Trends Endocrinol Metabol TEM. 2010;21:353–61. ISSN: 1043-2760. https://www.ncbi.nlm.nih.gov/pmc/articles/PMC2880223/ (2025).
6. First and Second Stage Labor Management: ACOG Clinical Practice Guideline No. 8. Obstet Gynecol. 2024;143:144–62. ISSN: 1873-233X.
7. Clark–Patterson G, Domingo M, Miller KS. Biomechanics of pregnancy and vaginal delivery. Curr Opin Biomed Eng. 2022;22:100386. ISSN: 24684511. https://linkinghub.elsevier.com/retrieve/pii/S2468451122000198 (2025).
8. Ameer MA, Fagan SE, Sosa-Stanley JN, Peterson DC. StatPearls. Treasure Island: StatPearls Publishing; 2023. http://www.ncbi.nlm.nih.gov/books/NBK470297/ (2023).
9. Sheth SS, Hajari AR, Lulla CP, Kshirsagar D. Sonographic evaluation of uterine volume and its clinical importance. J Obstet Gynaecol Res. 2017;43:185–9. ISSN: 1447-0756. https://onlinelibrary.wiley.com/doi/abs/10.1111/jog.13189 (2025).
10. Verguts J, Ameye L, Bourne T, Timmerman D. Normative data for uterine size according to age and gravidity and possible role of the classical golden ratio. Ultrasound Obstet Gynecol. 2013;42:713–7. ISSN: 1469-0705. https://onlinelibrary.wiley.com/doi/abs/10.1002/uog.12538 (2025).
11. Lastra RR, McCluggage WG, Hedrick Ellenson L. In: Kurman RJ, Hedrick Ellenson L, Ronnett BM, editors. Blaustein's pathology of the female genital tract. Cham: Springer International Publishing; 2019, p. 375–437. ISBN: 978-3-319-46334-6. https://doi.org/10.1007/978-3-319-46334-6_7 (2025).
12. Chen F, et al. Assessment of key parameters of normal uterus in women of reproductive age. Scientific Rep. 2023;13:17794. ISSN: 2045-2322. https://www.nature.com/articles/s41598-023-44489-6 (2025).

13. Madani T, et al. Association between myometrial thickness and assisted reproductive technologies outcomes: a prospective cohort study. Int J Fert Steril. 2024;18:123–7. ISSN: 2008-076X. https://pmc.ncbi.nlm.nih.gov/articles/PMC10875306/ (2025).
14. Gergolet M, et al. Defining the "normal uterus" by ultrasound measurement of uterine lengths, thicknesses, and angles in a population of nulliparous women: the Normal UteRus asSEssment study. Fertil Steril. 2025;125:127–36. ISSN: 00150282. https://linkinghub.elsevier.com/retrieve/pii/S0015028225017972 (2026).
15. Appelbaum AH, Tirandaz M, Ricci G, Levi D'Ancona R. Alignment of the cervix with the vagina in uterine retroversion: a possible risk factor in uterine prolapse. Diagnostics. 2022;12: 1428. ISSN: 2075-4418. https://www.ncbi.nlm.nih.gov/pmc/articles/PMC9222133/ (2025).
16. Stewart WW. Ante and Retro-positions of the uterus—their pathology, symtomatology and treatment. South Med Rec. 1893;13.
17. Fidan U, Keskin U, Ulubay M, Öztürk M, Bodur S. Value of vaginal cervical position in estimating uterine anatomy. Clin Anat. 2017;30:404–408. ISSN: 1098-2353. https://onlinelibrary.wiley.com/doi/abs/10.1002/ca.22854 (2025).
18. Refaey M, Sicaja M, Kearns C. In: Radiopaedia.org (Radiopaedia.org) 2008. https://radiopaedia.org/articles/4570 (2025).
19. Weiss S, et al. Three-dimensional fiber architecture of the nonpregnant human uterus determined ex vivo using magnetic resonance diffusion tensor imaging. Anatom Rec Part A: Discov Mol Cell Evolut Biol. 2005;288A:84–90. ISSN: 1552-4892. https://onlinelibrary.wiley.com/doi/abs/10.1002/ar.a.20274 (2025).
20. Burton GJ, Woods AW, Jauniaux E, Kingdom JCP. Rheological and physiological consequences of conversion of the maternal spiral arteries for utero-placental blood flow during human pregnancy. Placenta 2009;30:473–82. ISSN: 1532-3102.
21. Fodera DM, et al. Material properties of nonpregnant and pregnant human uterine layers. J Mech Behav Biomed Mater. 2024;151:106348. ISSN: 1751-6161. https://www.sciencedirect.com/science/article/pii/S1751616123007026 (2025).
22. Bortoletto P, Romanski PA, Pfeifer SM. Müllerian anomalies: presentation, diagnosis, and counseling. Obstetr Gynecol. 2024;143:369. ISSN: 0029-7844. https://journals.lww.com/greenjournal/fulltext/2024/03000/m_llerian_anomalies__presentation,_diagnosis,_and.8.aspx (2025).
23. Chandler TM, Machan LS, Cooperberg PL, Harris AC, Chang SD. Müllerian duct anomalies: from diagnosis to intervention. Br J Radiol. 2009;82:1034–42. ISSN: 0007-1285. https://www.ncbi.nlm.nih.gov/pmc/articles/PMC3473390/ (2025).
24. Pfeifer S, et al. Uterine septum: a guideline. Fert Steril. 2016;106:530–540. ISSN: 0015-0282. https://www.sciencedirect.com/science/article/pii/S0015028216612815 (2025).
25. Myers KM, Elad D. Biomechanics of the human uterus. Wiley Interdiscip Rev Syst Biol Med. 2017;9. ISSN: 1939-005X.
26. Critchley HOD, Maybin JA, Armstrong GM, Williams ARW. Physiology of the endometrium and regulation of menstruation. Physiol Rev. 2020;100:1149–79. ISSN: 1522-1210.
27. Marečková M, et al. An integrated single-cell reference atlas of the human endometrium. Nat Genet. 2024;56:1925–37. ISSN: 1546-1718. https://www.nature.com/articles/s41588-024-01873-w (2025).
28. Garcia-Alonso L, et al. Mapping the temporal and spatial dynamics of the human endometrium in vivo and in vitro. Nat Genet. 2021;53:1698–711. ISSN: 1546-1718. https://www.nature.com/articles/s41588-021-00972-2 (2025).
29. Yamaguchi M, et al. Three-dimensional understanding of the morphological complexity of the human uterine endometrium. iScience. 2021;24:102258. ISSN: 2589-0042. https://www.sciencedirect.com/science/article/pii/S2589004221002261 (2025).
30. Gargett CE, Chan RWS, Schwab KE. Endometrial stem cells. Curr Opin Obstet Gynecol. 2007;19:377–83. ISSN: 1040-872X.

31. Espinoza J, et al. Normal and abnormal transformation of the spiral arteries during pregnancy. J Perinat Med. 2006;34:447–58. ISSN: 0300-5577. https://www.ncbi.nlm.nih.gov/pmc/articles/PMC7062302/ (2025).
32. Robertson SA, Moldenhauer LM, Green ES, Care AS, Hull ML. Immune determinants of endometrial receptivity: a biological perspective. Fertil Steril. 2022;117:1107–20. ISSN: 0015-0282. https://www.sciencedirect.com/science/article/pii/S0015028222002679 (2025).
33. Swain M, Kulkarni AD. Endometrium at menopause: the Pathologist's view. J Mid-Life Health. 2021;12:310–5. ISSN: 0976-7800. https://www.ncbi.nlm.nih.gov/pmc/articles/PMC8849152/ (2025).
34. Fusi L, Cloke B, Brosens JJ. The uterine junctional zone. Best Pract Res Clin Obstet Gynaecol Adenomyosis. 2006;20:479–91. ISSN: 1521-6934. https://www.sciencedirect.com/science/article/pii/S1521693406000356 (2025).
35. Noyes RW, Hertig AT, Rock J. Dating the endometrial biopsy. Am J Obstet Gynecol. Trans Forty-second Ann Meet Centr Assoc Obstetr Gynecol. 1950;122:262–3. ISSN: 0002-9378. https://www.sciencedirect.com/science/article/pii/S0002937816335001 (2025).
36. Zhou M, Tian T, Wu C. Mechanism underlying the regulation of mucin secretion in the uterus during pregnancy. Int J Molecul Sci. 2023;24:15896. ISSN: 1422-0067. https://www.ncbi.nlm.nih.gov/pmc/articles/PMC10647571/ (2025).
37. Filant J, Spencer TE. Uterine glands: biological roles in conceptus implantation, uterine receptivity, and decidualization. Int J Develop Biol. 2014;58:107–16. ISSN: 0214-6282. https://www.ncbi.nlm.nih.gov/pmc/articles/PMC4199233/ (2025).
38. Yang H, Zhou B, Prinz M, Siegel D. Proteomic analysis of menstrual blood. Molecul Cell Proteomics: MCP. 2012;11:1024–35. ISSN: 1535-9484.
39. Choi J, Jo M, Lee E, Oh YK, Choi D. The role of autophagy in human endometrium. Biol Reproduct. 2012;86:70. ISSN: 1529-7268.
40. Weerakkody Y, Knipe H, Fahrenhorst-Jones T. In: Radiopaedia.org (Radiopaedia.org) 2010. https://radiopaedia.org/articles/8106 (2025).
41. Ferenczy A. en. In: Kurman RJ, editor. Blaustein's pathology of the female genital tract. New York: Springer; 1987, p. 257–291. ISBN: 978-1-4757-1942-0. https://doi.org/10.1007/978-1-4757-1942-0_9 (2025).
42. Punzon-Jimenez P, et al. Effect of aging on the human myometrium at single-cell resolution. Nat Commun. 2024;15:945. ISSN: 2041-1723. https://www.ncbi.nlm.nih.gov/pmc/articles/PMC10830479/ (2025).
43. Ji K, et al. Exploring myometrial microenvironment changes at the single-cell level from nonpregnant to term pregnant states. Physiol Genom. 2024;56:32–47. ISSN: 1094-8341. https://www.ncbi.nlm.nih.gov/pmc/articles/PMC11281821/ (2025).
44. Brauer MM. Cellular and molecular mechanisms underlying plasticity in uterine sympathetic nerves. Auton Neurosci. 2008;140:1–16. ISSN: 1566-0702. https://www.sciencedirect.com/science/article/pii/S1566070208000301 (2025).
45. Garcia D, et al. Myometrial wall thickness ratio-A nomogram reference for diagnosing myometrial wall asymmetry. J Clin Ultrasound: JCU. 2022;50:655–9. ISSN: 1097-0096.
46. Haynor DR, et al. Changing appearance of the normal uterus during the menstrual cycle: MR studies. Radiology. 1986;161:459–62. ISSN: 0033-8419.
47. McCarthy S, Tauber C, Gore J. Female pelvic anatomy: MR assessment of variations during the menstrual cycle and with use of oral contraceptives. Radiology. 1986;160:119–23. ISSN: 0033-8419.
48. Escalante N, Henriquez Pino J. Arrangement of muscle fibers in the myometrium of the human uterus: a mesoscopic study. MOJ Anatom Physiol. 2017;4. ISSN: 2471-139X. https://medcraveonline.com/MOJAP/MOJAP-04-00131.pdf (2025).
49. McLean JP, Fang S, Gallos G, Myers KM, Hendon CP. Three-dimensional collagen fiber mapping and tractography of human uterine tissue using OCT. Biomed Opt Exp. 2020;11:5518–41. ISSN: 2156-7085. https://opg.optica.org/boe/abstract.cfm?uri=boe-11-10-5518 (2023).

50. Fang S, et al. Anisotropic mechanical properties of the human uterus measured by spherical indentation. Ann Biomed Eng. 2021;49:1923–42. ISSN: 0090-6964. https://www.ncbi.nlm.nih.gov/pmc/articles/PMC8376808/ (2025).
51. Aitken E, Khaund A, Hamid SA, Millan D, Campbell S. The normal human myometrium has a vascular spatial gradient absent in small fibroids. Hum Reprod (Oxford, England). 2006;21:2669–78. ISSN: 0268-1161.
52. Kunz G, Leyendecker G. Uterine peristaltic activity during the menstrual cycle: characterization, regulation, function and dysfunction. Reproduct BioMed Online. 2002;4:5–9. ISSN: 1472-6483. https://www.sciencedirect.com/science/article/pii/S1472648312601084 (2025).
53. Wang S, et al. Noninvasive electrophysiological imaging identifies 4D uterine peristalsis patterns in subjects with normal menstrual cycles and patients with endometriosis. Res Square. 2023;rs.3.rs–2432192. ISSN: 2693-5015. https://www.ncbi.nlm.nih.gov/pmc/articles/PMC10029120/ (2025).
54. Louwagie EM, et al. Longitudinal ultrasonic dimensions and parametric solid models of the gravid uterus and cervix. PLOS ONE. 2021;16:e0242118. ISSN: 1932-6203. https://journals.plos.org/plosone/article?id=10.1371/journal.pone.0242118 (2023).
55. Moore TR. Clinical assessment of amniotic fluid. Clin Obstetr Gynecol. 1997;40:303. ISSN: 0009-9201. https://journals.lww.com/clinicalobgyn/fulltext/1997/06000/clinical_assessment_of_amniotic__fluid.7.aspx (2025).
56. Bachar G, et al. The impact of uterine position on conception modes and perinatal outcomes in nulliparous patients. Euro J Obstetr Gynecol Reproduct Biol. 2025;305:324–8. ISSN: 0301-2115. https://www.sciencedirect.com/science/article/pii/S0301211524007176 (2025).
57. Schneider ER, et al. Retroverted uterus in the first trimester and associated pregnancy outcomes. Am J Perinatol. 2024. ISSN: 1098-8785.
58. Moschos E, Twickler DM. Endometrial thickness predicts intrauterine pregnancy in patients with pregnancy of unknown location. Ultrasound Obstetr Gynecol. 2008;32:929–34. ISSN: 1469-0705. https://onlinelibrary.wiley.com/doi/abs/10.1002/uog.6248 (2025).
59. Wong HS, Cheung YK, Tait J. Sonographic study of the decidua basalis in the first trimester of pregnancy. Ultrasound Obstetr Gynecol. 2009;33:634–7. ISSN: 1469-0705. https://onlinelibrary.wiley.com/doi/abs/10.1002/uog.6311 (2025).
60. Durnwald CP, Mercer BM. Myometrial thickness according to uterine site, gestational age and prior cesarean delivery. J Mater-Fetal Neonat Med. 2008;21:247–50. ISSN: 1476-7058. https://doi.org/10.1080/14767050801926709 (2025).
61. Degani S, Leibovitz Z, Shapiro I, Gonen R, Ohel G. Myometrial thickness in pregnancy: longitudinal sonographic study. J Ultrasound Med Off J Am Instit Ultrasound Med. 1998;17:661–5. ISSN: 0278-4297.
62. Sokolowski P, et al. Human uterine wall tension trajectories and the onset of parturition. PLoS ONE. 2010;5:e11037. ISSN: 1932-6203. https://www.ncbi.nlm.nih.gov/pmc/articles/PMC2890413/ (2025).
63. Gotoh H, et al. Predicting incomplete uterine rupture with vaginal sonography during the late second trimester in women with prior cesarean. Obstetr Gynecol. 2000;95:596–600. ISSN: 0029-7844. https://www.sciencedirect.com/science/article/pii/S0029784499006201 (2023).
64. Buhimschi CS, Buhimschi IA, Malinow AM, Weiner CP. Myometrial thickness during human labor and immediately post partum. Am J Obstetr Gynecol. 2003;188:553–9. ISSN: 0002-9378.
65. Yang F, Zheng Q, Jin L. Dynamic function and composition changes of immune cells during normal and pathological pregnancy at the maternal-fetal interface. Front Immunol. 2019;10:2317. ISSN: 1664-3224. https://www.ncbi.nlm.nih.gov/pmc/articles/PMC6813251/ (2025).
66. Sinai Talaulikar V, Kronenberger K, Bax BE, Moss R, Manyonda I. Differences in collagen ultrastructure of human first trimester decidua basalis and parietalis: implications for trophoblastic invasion of the placental bed. J Obstetr Gynaecol Res. 2014;40:80–8. ISSN: 1447-0756. https://onlinelibrary.wiley.com/doi/abs/10.1111/jog.12127 (2025).

67. Roberts JM. Pathophysiology of ischemic placental disease. Semin Perinatol. 2014;38:139–145. ISSN: 01460005. https://linkinghub.elsevier.com/retrieve/pii/S0146000514000159 (2025).
68. Whitley GSJ, Cartwright JE. Cellular and molecular regulation of spiral artery remodelling: lessons from the cardiovascular field. Placenta. 2010;31:465–474. ISSN: 0143-4004. https://www.sciencedirect.com/science/article/pii/S0143400410001013 (2025).
69. Pijnenborg R, Vercruysse L, Hanssens M. The uterine spiral arteries in human pregnancy: facts and controversies. Placenta. 2006;27:939–58. ISSN: 0143-4004. https://www.sciencedirect.com/science/article/pii/S0143400405003206 (2025).
70. Burton GJ, Jauniaux E. The human placenta: new perspectives on its formation and function during early pregnancy. Proc R Soc B: Biol Sci. 2023;290:20230191. https://royalsocietypublishing.org/doi/full/10.1098/rspb.2023.0191 (2025).
71. Shynlova O, Tsui P, Jaffer S, Lye SJ. Integration of endocrine and mechanical signals in the regulation of myometrial functions during pregnancy and labour. Euro J Obstetr Gynecol Reproduct Biol. 2009;144:S2–10. ISSN: 0301-2115, 1872-7654. https://www.ejog.org/article/S0301-2115(09)00134-1/abstract (2026).
72. Jashnani K, Palve M. Uterine myometrial preischemia: yet another physiological change of pregnancy! J Laborat Phys. 2021;14:157–63. ISSN: 0974-2727. https://www.ncbi.nlm.nih.gov/pmc/articles/PMC9381321/ (2025).
73. Rabotti C, Mischi M. Propagation of electrical activity in uterine muscle during pregnancy: a review. Acta Physiol. 2015;213:406–16. ISSN: 1748-1716. https://onlinelibrary.wiley.com/doi/abs/10.1111/apha.12424 (2025).
74. Garfield RE, Maner WL. Physiology and electrical activity of uterine contractions. Semin Cell Develop Biol. 2007;18:289–95. ISSN: 1084-9521. https://www.ncbi.nlm.nih.gov/pmc/articles/PMC2048588/ (2023).
75. Morrione TG, Seifter S. Alteration in the collagen content of the human uterus during pregnancy and postpartum involution. J Exp Med. 1962;115:357–65. ISSN: 0022-1007.
76. Fodera DM, et al. Time-dependent material properties and composition of the nonhuman primate uterine layers through gestation. Scient Rep. 2025;15:23194. ISSN: 2045-2322. https://www.nature.com/articles/s41598-025-02986-w (2025).
77. Masuzawa Y, Yaeko, K. Uterine activity during the two hours after placental delivery among low-risk pregnancies: an observational study. eng. J Mater-Fetal Neonat Med Off J Euro Assoc Perinat Med Federat Asia Oceania Perinat Society Int Society Perinat Obstetr. 2017;30:2446–51. ISSN: 1476-4954.
78. Negishi H, et al. Changes in uterine size after vaginal delivery and cesarean section determined by vaginal sonography in the puerperium. Arch Gynecol Obstetr. 1999;263:13–6. ISSN: 1432-0711. https://doi.org/10.1007/s004040050253 (2025).
79. Lavery JP, Shaw LA. Sonography of the puerperal uterus. J Ultrasound Med Off J Am Instit Ultrasound Med. 1989;8:481–6. ISSN: 0278-4297.
80. Wachsberg RH, Kurtz AB, Levine CD, Solomon P, Wapner RJ. Real-time ultrasonographic analysis of the normal postpartum uterus: technique, variability, and measurements. J Ultrasound Med Off J Am Instit Ultrasound Med. 1994;13:215–21. ISSN: 0278-4297.
81. Belachew J, Axelsson O, Mulic-Lutvica A, Eurenius K. Longitudinal study of the uterine body and cavity with three-dimensional ultrasonography in the puerperium. Acta Obstetr Gynecol Scandinavica. 2012;91:1184–90. ISSN: 1600-0412. https://onlinelibrary.wiley.com/doi/abs/10.1111/j.1600-0412.2012.01418.x (2025).
82. Merz E, Miric-Tesanic D, Bahlmann F, Weber G, Wellek S. Sonographic size of uterus and ovaries in pre- and postmenopausal women. Ultrasound Obstetr Gynecol. 1996;7:38–42. ISSN: 1469-0705. https://onlinelibrary.wiley.com/doi/abs/10.1046/j.1469-0705.1996.07010038.x (2025).
83. Sharman A. Post-partum regeneration of the human endometrium. J Anatomy. 1953;87:1–10.4. ISSN: 0021-8782. https://www.ncbi.nlm.nih.gov/pmc/articles/PMC1244561/ (2025).

84. Hsu K-F, et al. Enhanced myometrial autophagy in postpartum uterine involution. Taiwan J Obstetr Gynecol. 2014;53:293–302. ISSN: 1028-4559. https://www.sciencedirect.com/science/article/pii/S102845591400120X (2025).
85. Antero MF, Ayhan A, Segars J, Shih I-M. Pathology and pathogenesis of adenomyosis. Semin Reproduct Med. 2020;38:108–18. ISSN: 1526-8004. https://www.ncbi.nlm.nih.gov/pmc/articles/PMC7987203/ (2025).
86. Stoelinga B, et al. The estimated volume of the fibroid uterus: a comparison of ultrasound and bimanual examination versus volume at MRI or hysterectomy. Euro J Obstetr Gynecol Reproduct Biol. 2015;184:89–96. ISSN: 0301-2115. https://www.sciencedirect.com/science/article/pii/S0301211514005946 (2025).
87. Arrowsmith S, Robinson H, Noble K, Wray S. What do we know about what happens to myometrial function as women age? J Muscle Res Cell Motil. 2012;33:209–17. ISSN: 0142-4319. https://www.ncbi.nlm.nih.gov/pmc/articles/PMC3413813/ (2025).
88. Crankshaw DJ, O'Brien YM, Crosby DA, Morrison JJ. Maternal age and contractility of human myometrium in pregnancy. Reproduct Sci. 2015;22:1229–35. ISSN: 1933-7191. https://doi.org/10.1177/1933719115572483 (2025).
89. Zaki MN, Hibbard JU, Kominiarek MA. Contemporary labor patterns and maternal age. Obstetr Gynecol. 2013;122:1018–24. ISSN: 1873-233X.
90. Main DM, Main EK, Moore DH. The relationship between maternal age and uterine dysfunction: a continuous effect throughout reproductive life. Am J Obstetr Gynecol. 2000;182:1312–20. ISSN: 0002-9378.
91. Martel M, Wacholder S, Lippman A, Brohan J, Hamilton E. Maternal age and primary cesarean section rates: a multivariate analysis. Am J Obstetr Gynecol. 1987;156:305–8. ISSN: 0002-9378. https://www.sciencedirect.com/science/article/pii/0002937887902730 (2025).
92. Šťastná A, Fait T, Kocourková J, Waldaufová E. Does advanced maternal age comprise an independent risk factor for caesarean section? A population-wide study. Int J Environ Res Pub Health. 2022;20:668. ISSN: 1660-4601.
93. Ganeriwal SA, Ryan GA, Geary M, Purandare NC. Caesarean section rates in primigravid women categorised by age and BMI. J Obstetr Gynaecol J Inst Obstetr Gynaecol. 2022;42: 941–5. ISSN: 1364-6893.
94. Bergholt T, et al. Maternal age and risk of cesarean section in women with induced labor at term-A Nordic register-based study. Acta Obstetr Gynecol Scand. 2020;99:283–9. ISSN: 1600-0412.
95. Practice Bulletin No. 141: Management of Menopausal Symptoms. Obstetr Gynecol. 2014;123:202. ISSN: 0029-7844. https://journals.lww.com/greenjournal/fulltext/2014/01000/practice_bulletin_no141management_of.37.aspx (2025).
96. Boon J, van de Putte SCJ, Scholten PC, Heintz APM. Histological patterns in endometrial samples from perimenopausal women. Maturitas. 1999;32:155–9. ISSN: 0378-5122. https://www.sciencedirect.com/science/article/pii/S0378512299000286 (2025).
97. Wang L, Wei W, Cai M. A review of the risk factors associated with endometrial hyperplasia during perimenopause. Int J Women's Health. 2024;16:1475–82. https://www.dovepress.com/a-review-of-the-risk-factors-associated-with-endometrial-hyperplasia-d-peer-reviewed-fulltext-article-IJWH (2025).
98. Selvam V, Lakshminarayanan P. A comprehensive approach: correlating ultrasound imaging with endometrial histopathological analysis in perimenopausal women with heavy menstrual bleeding. Cureus. 2024;16:e57201. ISSN: 2168-8184.
99. Mishra J, Nigam N, Rathod I. Study of histopathology of endometrium in perimenopausal women with abnormal uterine bleeding. Int J Reprod Contracept Obstetr Gynecol. 2023;12: 2750–5. ISSN: 2320-1789, 2320-1770. https://www.ijrcog.org/index.php/ijrcog/article/view/13365 (2025).
100. Dhakhwa R, Bhattarai R, Shah J, Shakya A, Pradhan S. Benign histopathologic findings of endometrium among perimenopausal women presenting with abnormal uterine bleeding: a

descriptive cross-sectional study. J Nepal Med Assoc. 2021;59:1141–5. ISSN: 1815-672X, 0028-2715. https://www.jnma.com.np/jnma/index.php/jnma/article/view/7146 (2025).
101. Hedrick Ellenson L, Ronnett BM, Kurman RJ. en. In: Kurman RJ, Hedrick Ellenson L, Ronnett BM. editors. Blaustein's pathology of the female genital tract. Cham: Springer International Publishing; 2019, p. 439–472. ISBN: 978-3-319-46334-6. https://doi.org/10.1007/978-3-319-46334-6_8 (2025).
102. Li J, et al. Changes in ultrasound uterine morphology and endometrial thickness during ovarian aging and possible associated factors: findings from a prospective study. Menopause. 2020;27:794. https://journals.lww.com/menopausejournal/fulltext/2020/07000/changes_in_ultrasound_uterine_morphology_and.12.aspx (2025).
103. Ulin M, Ali M, Chaudhry ZT, Al-Hendy A, Yang Q. Uterine fibroids in menopause and perimenopause. Menopause. 2020;27:238. https://journals.lww.com/menopausejournal/fulltext/2020/02000/uterine_fibroids_in_menopause_and_perimenopause.17.aspx (2025).
104. Naftalin J, et al. How common is adenomyosis? A prospective study of prevalence using transvaginal ultrasound in a gynaecology clinic. Hum Reprod. 2012;27:3432–9. ISSN: 0268-1161. https://doi.org/10.1093/humrep/des332 (2025).
105. Deligdisch L. Hormonal pathology of the endometrium. Mod Pathol. 2000;13:285–94. ISSN: 0893-3952. https://www.sciencedirect.com/science/article/pii/S0893395222040728 (2025).
106. Wen J, et al. Calcification: a disregarded or ignored issue in the gynecologic tumor microenvironments. Int J Gynecol Cancer. 2018;28:486–92. ISSN: 1048-891X. https://www.sciencedirect.com/science/article/pii/S1048891X24074991 (2025).
107. Hessler SC, et al. Myometrial artery calcifications and aging. Menopause (New York, NY). 2015;22:1285–88. ISSN: 1530-0374.
108. Truskinovsky AM, Gerscovich EO, Duffield CR, Vogt PJ. Endometrial microcalcifications detected by ultrasonography: clinical associations, histopathology, and potential etiology. Int J Gynecol Pathol Off J Int Soc Gynecol Pathol. 2008;27:61–7. ISSN: 0277-1691.
109. Danforth, D. The fibrous nature of the human cervix, and its relation to the isthmic segment in gravid and nongravid uteri. Am J Obstetr Gynecol. 1947;53:541–60. ISSN: 00029378. https://linkinghub.elsevier.com/retrieve/pii/0002937847902731 (2023).
110. Vink JY, et al. A new paradigm for the role of smooth muscle cells in the human cervix. eng. Am J Obstetr Gynecol. 2016;215:478.e1–11. ISSN: 1097-6868.
111. Banerjee A, et al. Reproducibility of assessment of full-dilatation Cesarean section scar in women undergoing second-trimester screening for preterm birth. Ultrasound Obstetr Gynecol. 2022;60:396–403. ISSN: 0960-7692, 1469-0705. https://obgyn.onlinelibrary.wiley.com/doi/10.1002/uog.26027 (2025).
112. Maudot C, et al. Caesarean section scar: histological analysis on hysterectomy specimen. A pilot study. Euro J Obstetr Gynecol Reprod Biol. 2024;303:236–43. ISSN: 03012115. https://linkinghub.elsevier.com/retrieve/pii/S0301211524005955 (2026).
113. Kagan KO, Sonek J. How to measure cervical length. Ultrasound Obstetr Gynecol. 2015;45:358–62. ISSN: 0960-7692, 1469-0705. https://obgyn.onlinelibrary.wiley.com/doi/10.1002/uog.14742 (2025).
114. Ober KG, Schneppenheim P, Hamperl H, Kaufmann C. Die Epithelgrenzen im Bereiche des Isthmus uteri. Archiv fur Gynakologie. 1958;190:346–83. ISSN: 0003-9128, 1432-0711. http://link.springer.com/10.1007/BF00672657 (2022).
115. Schweppe KW, Wynn RM. Ultrastructural studies of the mucosa of the human uterine isthmus. Gynecol Obstetr Investigat. 1981;12:225–44. ISSN: 0378-7346.
116. Danforth DN, Chapman JCF. The incorporation of the Isth-Mus uteri. Am J Obstetr Gynecol. 1950;59:979–88. ISSN: 0002-9378.
117. Sorvari TE, Laakso L. Histochemical investigation of epithelial mucosubstances in the uterine isthmus. Obstetr Gynecol. 1970;36:76–81. ISSN: 0029-7844.
118. Hoogduin KJ, Hopman ANH, Ramaekers FC, McCluggage WG, Smedts F. BCL2 and Keratin 5 define the Uterine-Cervix-Isthmus junction, a transition between endocervical and tubal-like

epithelium: Int J Gynecol Pathol. 2013;32:122–30. ISSN: 0277-1691. http://journals.lww.com/00004347-201301000-00014 (2022).
119. Toki T, Shimizu M, Takagi Y, Ashida T, Konishi I. CD10 is a marker for normal and neoplastic endometrial stromal cells. Int J Gynecol Pathol. 2002;21:41. ISSN: 0277-1691. https://journals.lww.com/intjgynpathology/fulltext/2002/01000/cd10_is_a_marker_for_normal_and_neoplastic.8.aspx (2025).
120. Schwalm H, Dubrauszky V. The structure of the musculature of the human uterus—muscles and connective tissue. Am J Obstetr Gynecol. 1966;94:391–404. ISSN: 00029378. https://linkinghub.elsevier.com/retrieve/pii/0002937866906612 (2023).
121. Petersen LK, Oxlund H, Uldbjerg N, Forman A. In vitro analysis of muscular contractile ability and passive biomechanical properties of uterine cervical samples from nonpregnant women. Obstetr Gynecol. 1991;77:772–6. ISSN: 0029-7844.
122. Youssef AF. The uterine isthmus and its sphincter mechanism, a radiographic study. I. The uterine isthmus under normal conditions. Am J Obstetr Gynecol. 1958;75:1305–19. ISSN: 0002-9378.
123. Johnstone FD, Boyd IE, McArthy TG, McClure Browne JC. The diameter of the uterine isthmus during the menstrual cycle, pregnancy and the puerperium. BJOG: Int J Obstetr Gynaecol. 1974;81:558–62. https://onlinelibrary.wiley.com/doi/pdf/10.1111/j.1471-0528.1974.tb00516.x. ISSN: 1471-0528. https://onlinelibrary.wiley.com/doi/abs/10.1111/j.1471-0528.1974.tb00516.x (2025).
124. Shampo MA. Tests, signs, and indications of pregnancy. J Pelvic Surgery. 2001;7:133–5.
125. Greco E, Lange A, Ushakov F, Calvo JR, Nicolaides KH. Prediction of spontaneous preterm delivery from endocervical length at 11 to 13 weeks. Prenat Diagnos. 2011;31:84–9. ISSN: 1097-0223. https://onlinelibrary.wiley.com/doi/abs/10.1002/pd.2640 (2023).
126. Hasegawa J, et al. Opening of the uterine isthmus at 11–13 weeks' gestation is not related to developmental abnormalities of the placenta. Early Hum Develop. 2013;89:973–6. ISSN: 03783782. https://linkinghub.elsevier.com/retrieve/pii/S0378378213002284 (2026).
127. Farràs A, et al. Real-time ultrasound demonstration of uterine isthmus contractions during pregnancy. Am J Obstetr Gynecol. 2024;230:89.e1–12. ISSN: 00029378. https://linkinghub.elsevier.com/retrieve/pii/S0002937823004763 (2025).
128. Harvey M-A. The size of the cervix and its relationship with age and parity. Urogynaecol Int J. 2016;29. ISSN: 1121-3086, 2038-8314. http://www.urogynaecologia.org/index.php/uij/article/view/171 (2025).
129. Ferenczy A, Wright TC. In: Kurman RJ, editor. Blaustein's pathology of the female genital tract. New York: Springer; 1994, p. 185–201. ISBN: 978-1-4757-3889-6. https://doi.org/10.1007/978-1-4757-3889-6_5 (2022).
130. Yoshida K. Bioengineering and the cervix: the past, current, and future for addressing preterm birth. Curr Res Physiol. 2023;6:100107. ISSN: 2665-9441. https://www.sciencedirect.com/science/article/pii/S266594412300010X (2025).
131. Bremer GL, Tiebosch ATMG, van der Putten HWHM, de Haan J, Arends JW. Basement membranes in cervical cancer: relationship to pelvic lymph node metastasis and prognosis. Gynecol Oncol. 1995;57:351–5. ISSN: 0090-8258. https://www.sciencedirect.com/science/article/pii/S0090825885711547 (2025).
132. Herbster S, Paladino A, de Freitas S, Boccardo E. Alterations in the expression and activity of extracellular matrix components in HPV-associated infections and diseases. Clinics. 2018;73:e551s. ISSN: 1807-5932. https://www.sciencedirect.com/science/article/pii/S1807593222011437 (2025).
133. Padežnik T, Oleksy A, Cokan A, Takač I, Sobočan M. Changes in the extracellular matrix in endometrial and cervical cancer: a systematic review. Int J Mol Sci. 2023;24:5463. ISSN: 1422-0067. https://www.mdpi.com/1422-0067/24/6/5463 (2025).
134. Wu W, et al. Whole cervix imaging of collagen, muscle, and cellularity in term and preterm pregnancy. Nat Commun. 2024;15:5942. ISSN: 2041-1723. https://www.nature.com/articles/s41467-024-48680-9 (2025).

135. Uhlén M, et al. Tissue-based map of the human proteome. Science. 2015;347:1260419. https://www.science.org/doi/10.1126/science.1260419 (2025).
136. The Human Protein Atlas. 2025. https://www.proteinatlas.org/ (2025).
137. Dictionary - Normal: Cervix - The Human Protein Atlas. 2025. https://www.proteinatlas.org/learn/dictionary/normal/cervix (2025).
138. Aspden RM. Collagen organisation in the cervix and its relation to mechanical function. Collagen Related Res. 1988;8:103–12. ISSN: 0174-173X. https://www.sciencedirect.com/science/article/pii/S0174173X88800220 (2025).
139. Yao W, et al. Collagen fiber orientation and dispersion in the upper cervix of non-pregnant and pregnant women. PloS One. 2016;11:e0166709. ISSN: 1932-6203.
140. Myers K, Socrate S, Tzeranis D, House M. Changes in the biochemical constituents and morphologic appearance of the human cervical stroma during pregnancy. Euro J Obstetr Gynecol Reproduct Biol. 2009;144:S82–9. ISSN: 03012115. https://linkinghub.elsevier.com/retrieve/pii/S0301211509001456 (2025).
141. Maillot KV, Zimmermann BK. The solubility of collagen of the uterine cervix during pregnancy and labour. Archiv Fur Gynakologie. 1976;220:275–80. ISSN: 0003-9128.
142. Myers KM, Paskaleva AP, House M, Socrate S. Mechanical and biochemical properties of human cervical tissue. Acta Biomater. 2008;4:104–16. ISSN: 1742-7061. https://www.sciencedirect.com/science/article/pii/S1742706107000682 (2025).
143. Vink J, Mourad M. The pathophysiology of human premature cervical remodeling resulting in spontaneous preterm birth: where are we now? Semin Perinatol Curr Preterm Birth Prevent Strateg. 2017;41:427–37. ISSN: 0146-0005. https://www.sciencedirect.com/science/article/pii/S0146000517300861 (2023).
144. Nott J, et al. Diffusion tensor imaging determines three-dimensional architecture of human cervix: a cross-sectional study. BJOG: Int J Obstetr Gynaecol. 2018;125:812–8. ISSN: 1471-0528. https://onlinelibrary.wiley.com/doi/abs/10.1111/1471-0528.15002 (2023).
145. Shi L, Hu L, Lee N, Fang S, Myers K. Three-dimensional anisotropic hyperelastic constitutive model describing the mechanical response of human and mouse cervix. Acta Biomater. 2022;150:277–94. ISSN: 1742-7061. https://www.sciencedirect.com/science/article/pii/S1742706122004640 (2022).
146. Leppert PC, Keller S, Cerreta J, Hosannah Y, Mandl I. The content of elastin in the uterine cervix. Arch Biochem Biophys. 1983;222:53–8. ISSN: 0003-9861. https://www.sciencedirect.com/science/article/pii/0003986183905015 (2025).
147. Bryman I, Norström A, Dahlström A, Lindblom B. Immunohistochemical evidence for preserved innervation of the human cervix during pregnancy. Gynecol Obstetr Invest. 1987;24:73–9. ISSN: 1423-002X, 0378-7346. https://karger.com/GOI/article/doi/10.1159/000298782 (2025).
148. Walocha JA, Litwin JA, Bereza T, Klimek-Piotrowska W, Miodonski AJ. Vascular architecture of human uterine cervix visualized by corrosion casting and scanning electron microscopy. Hum Reprod. 2012;27:727–32. ISSN: 0268-1161, 1460-2350. https://academic.oup.com/humrep/article-lookup/doi/10.1093/humrep/der458 (2025).
149. Nallasamy S, Mahendroo M. Distinct roles of Cervical Epithelia and stroma in pregnancy and parturition. Semin Reprod Med. 2017;35:190–200. ISSN: 1526-4564.
150. Wolf DP, Blasco L, Khan MA, Litt M. Human cervical mucus. II. Changes in viscoelasticity during the ovulatory menstrual cycle*. Fertil Steril. 1977;28:47–52. ISSN: 0015-0282. https://www.sciencedirect.com/science/article/pii/S0015028216423162 (2025).
151. Berek & Novaks Gynecology. Berek JS, editor. ISBN: 978-1-4963-8035-7. Philadelphia: Lippincott, Williams & Wilkins; 2020.
152. Van Kooij RJ, Roelofs HJM, Kathmann GAM, Kramer MF. Human cervical mucus and its mucous glycoprotein during the menstrual cycle*. Fertil Steril. 1980;34:226–33. ISSN: 0015-0282. https://www.sciencedirect.com/science/article/pii/S0015028216449526 (2025).

153. Bradburn GB, Webb CF. Cyclic variations in the endocervix. Am J Obstetr Gynecol. 1951;62: 997–1008. ISSN: 00029378. https://linkinghub.elsevier.com/retrieve/pii/0002937851910198 (2026).
154. Wollner A. The menstrual cycle in the human cervical mucosa and its clinical significance. Am J Surgery. 1942;57:331–5. ISSN: 0002-9610. https://www.sciencedirect.com/science/article/pii/S0002961042909917 (2026).
155. Topkins P. The histologic appearance of the endocervix during the menstrual cycle. Am J Obstetr Gynecol. 1949;58:654–63. ISSN: 0002-9378.
156. Myers KM, et al. The mechanical role of the cervix in pregnancy. J Biomech. 2015;48:1511–23. ISSN: 1873-2380.
157. Becher N, Waldorf KA, Hein M, Uldbjerg N. The cervical mucus plug: structured review of the literature. Acta Obstetr Gynecol Scandinavica. 2009;88:502–13. ISSN: 1600-0412. https://onlinelibrary.wiley.com/doi/abs/10.1080/00016340902852898 (2024).
158. Becher N, Hein M, Danielsen CC, Uldbjerg N. Matrix metalloproteinases in the cervical mucus plug in relation to gestational age, plug compartment, and preterm labor. Reprod Biol Endocrinol RB&E. 2010;8:113. ISSN: 1477-7827. https://www.ncbi.nlm.nih.gov/pmc/articles/PMC2954884/ (2024).
159. Badir S, Mazza E, Zimmermann R, Bajka M. Cervical softening occurs early in pregnancy: characterization of cervical stiffness in 100 healthy women using the aspiration technique. Prenatal Diagnos. 2013;33:737–41. ISSN: 1097-0223. https://onlinelibrary.wiley.com/doi/abs/10.1002/pd.4116 (2025).
160. Yoshida K, Jayyosi C, Lee N, Mahendroo M, Myers KM. Mechanics of cervical remodelling: insights from rodent models of pregnancy. Interf Focus. 2019;9:20190026. ISSN: 2042-8898, 2042-8901. https://royalsocietypublishing.org/doi/10.1098/rsfs.2019.0026 (2025).
161. Danforth D, Buckingham J, Roddick J. Connective tissue changes incident to cervical effacement. Am J Obstetr Gynecol. 1960;80:939–45. ISSN: 00029378. https://linkinghub.elsevier.com/retrieve/pii/0002937860904725 (2025).
162. Young RC. Myocytes, myometrium, and uterine contractions. Ann New York Acad Sci. 2007;1101:72–84. ISSN: 1749-6632. https://onlinelibrary.wiley.com/doi/abs/10.1196/annals.1389.038 (2025).
163. Villegas-Downs M, et al. Trajectory of postpartum cervical remodeling in women delivering full-term and spontaneous preterm: sensitivity to quantitative ultrasound biomarkers. Ultrasound Med Biol. 2024;50:1777–84. ISSN: 03015629. https://linkinghub.elsevier.com/retrieve/pii/S0301562924002618 (2025).
164. Badir S, et al. Aspiration technique-based device is more reliable in cervical stiffness assessment than digital palpation. BMC Pregnancy Childbirth. 2020;20:391. ISSN: 1471-2393.
165. Sundtoft I, Sommer S, Uldbjerg N. Cervical collagen concentration within 15 months after delivery. Am J Obstetr Gynecol. 2011;205:59.e1–3. ISSN: 0002-9378. https://www.sciencedirect.com/science/article/pii/S0002937811003747.
166. Najmabadi S, et al. Cervical mucus patterns and the fertile window in women without known subfertility: a pooled analysis of three cohorts. Hum Reprod. 2021;36:1784–95. ISSN: 0268-1161, 1460-2350. https://academic.oup.com/humrep/article/36/7/1784/6276047 (2025).
167. Roberts ADG, et al. The variation in cervical hydroxyproline and cervical water with age. BJOG: Int J Obstetr Gynaecol. 1988;95:1159–64. ISSN: 1470-0328, 1471-0528. https://obgyn.onlinelibrary.wiley.com/doi/10.1111/j.1471-0528.1988.tb06794.x (2025).
168. Oxlund BS, et al. Collagen concentration and biomechanical properties of samples from the lower uterine cervix in relation to age and parity in non-pregnant women. Reprod Biol Endocrinol. 2010;8:82. ISSN: 1477-7827. https://rbej.biomedcentral.com/articles/10.1186/1477-7827-8-82 (2025).

169. Campo H, Santamaria X, Cervelló I, Simón C. In: Handbook of tissue engineering scaffolds: volume two. Amsterdam: Elsevier; 2019, p. 283–316. ISBN: 978-0-08-102561-1. https://linkinghub.elsevier.com/retrieve/pii/B9780081025611000117 (2025).
170. Koullali B, House MD. Handbook of tissue engineering scaffolds: volume two. Amsterdam: Elsevier; 2019, p. 333–43. ISBN: 978-0-08-102561-1. https://linkinghub.elsevier.com/retrieve/pii/B9780081025611000130 (2025).

Biomechanics of the Uterus and Cervix Across Pregnancy and Disease: Considerations for Biomaterial Design

Erin M. Louwagie and Daniella M. Fodera

Abstract The uterus and cervix are dynamic, mechanically active organs that play central roles in reproductive function and disease. This chapter provides a comprehensive overview of the fundamental biomechanical principles and experimental methodologies used to characterize their material behavior across length scales, including compression, tension, indentation, and shear. A detailed synthesis of *ex vivo* mechanical properties measured for the human uterus and cervix in nonpregnant and pregnant states is presented, describing parameters of stiffness, strength, extensibility, and time dependence. This chapter further highlights notable obstetric and gynecologic disorders affecting the uterus and/or cervix in which mechanical factors are either characteristic features of the disease or implicated in its pathogenesis. This chapter concludes by outlining future research directions and underscoring the importance of biomechanical insights in guiding the design of biomaterials for therapeutic and investigative applications applied to reproductive health.

Keywords Uterus · Cervix · Biomechanics · Stiffness · Strength · Extensibility · Time dependence · Pregnancy · Gynecology · Obstetrics

1 Introduction

The uterus and cervix are dynamic, mechanically active organs that undergo profound structural and functional transformations across the reproductive lifespan. Their capacity to grow, stretch, remodel, and contract enables essential reproductive processes including menstruation, implantation, gestation, parturition, and postpartum involution. These mechanical functions are tightly regulated by their underlying

E. M. Louwagie (✉)
Department of Mechanical Engineering, Columbia University, New York, NY, USA
e-mail: eml2218@columbia.edu

D. M. Fodera
Department of Biomedical Engineering, Columbia University, New York, NY, USA
e-mail: dmf2194@columbia.edu

S. G. Zambuto, M. L. Oyen (eds.), *Biomaterials for Women's Health Engineering*,
https://doi.org/10.1007/978-3-032-10745-9_6

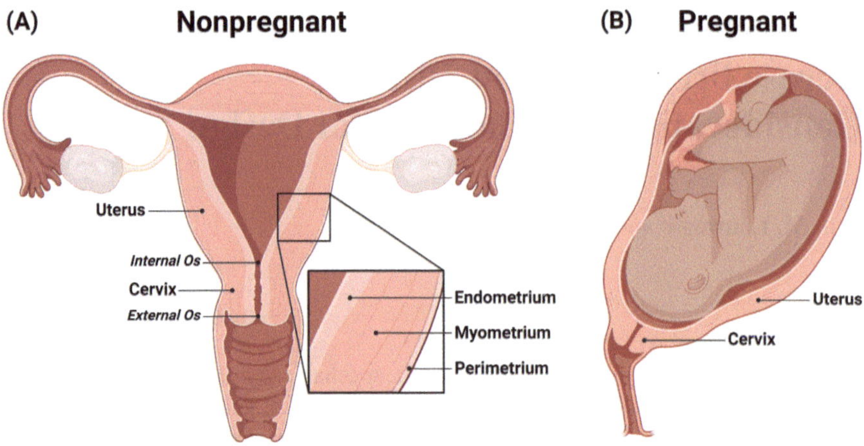

Fig. 1 Representative diagrams of the uterus and cervix under nonpregnant and pregnant conditions. (**a**) Uterus and cervix in nonpregnancy, highlighting the distinct uterine layers (endometrium, myometrium, and perimetrium). The internal os and external os of the cervix are marked. (**b**) Uterus and cervix in late pregnancy. Note that schematic representations of reproductive anatomy and are not drawn to scale relative to one another. (Created with https://Biorender.com)

tissue architectures, which together govern how these organs generate, transmit, and respond to internal and external loads. Understanding the biomechanical behavior of the uterus and cervix is therefore critical not only for elucidating the physiology of pregnancy but also for uncovering the mechanical basis of gynecologic and obstetric disorders.

Anatomically, the human uterus is an inverted, pear-shaped organ with a single uterine cavity [1–3]. The cervix is situated at the base of the uterus, extending into the vaginal canal, and is roughly cylindrical in shape, containing a single, straight endocervical canal [1]. The uterus and cervix are each composed of distinct tissue layers that function in concert to support normal homeostasis [1].

The uterine wall is composed of three structurally and functionally distinct tissue layers: (i) the nonpregnant endometrium and pregnant decidua, (ii) the myometrium, and (iii) the perimetrium (i.e., serosa) (Fig. 1) [1–3]. The nonpregnant endometrium and pregnant decidua together represent the innermost uterine layer consisting of luminal and glandular epithelial cells, stromal cells, and spiral arteries embedded in a collagen-dense extracellular matrix (ECM) [1, 4]. In nonpregnancy, the endometrium undergoes cyclic cellular and molecular changes throughout the menstrual cycle in response to hormonal fluctuations [4]. The decidua, the pregnant counterpart of the endometrium, forms the basis of the maternal-fetal interface, providing critical nutritional support and immunological protection for the developing fetus [1]. The myometrium, the middle and thickest layer of the uterus, is primarily composed of smooth muscle fascicles interwoven with collagen and elastin fibers and pocketed with blood vessels [1]. Throughout pregnancy, the myometrium undergoes active remodeling through smooth muscle cell hyperplasia and hypertrophy [1]. Exterior to the myometrium and adjacent to the abdominal cavity is the perimetrium, a thin collagen-dense tissue layer that acts as a smooth, lubricated barrier for the uterus [1, 2]. Beyond its ECM and cellular constituents, the uterus as a whole is a largely hydrated tissue (70–85% water content), with notable differences observed across the distinct tissue layers [5, 6]. Hydration of the uterus remains rather constant across gestation [6].

The main body of the cervix is known as the stroma and is comprised of dense connective tissue and smooth muscle cells arranged longitudinally and circumferentially around the endocervical canal (Fig. 1) [1, 7]. Along the length of the cervix, there exists a gradient in compositional features, with the internal os exhibiting a greater ratio of smooth muscle to collagen content compared to the external os [1, 7]. The cervix is a hydrated tissue, with water content ranging between 75% and 80% in nonpregnancy and increasing by another 5% during pregnancy [8]. The endocervical canal is lined on its surface with a layer of mucus-secreting columnar epithelium and functions primarily as an immunological barrier [1, 9, 10]. The portion of the cervix that extends into the vaginal canal is lined by a layer of stratified squamous epithelium known as the ectocervix [1].

Together, the uterus and cervix must accommodate large and rapidly changing mechanical loads to meet the physiologic demands of menstruation, pregnancy, parturition, and involution. The organization and composition of each tissue layer determine how forces are transmitted and dissipated across the uterus and cervix. In this chapter, we review fundamental biomechanical principles, summarize reported *ex vivo* mechanical properties of the human uterus and cervix, and discuss how these findings inform our understanding of reproductive health, disease, and biomaterial design.

2 Biomechanical Characterization of the Uterus and Cervix

At a fundamental level, the mechanical properties of biological tissues are governed by their underlying structure and composition, which in turn, influence cell behavior through mechanotransduction [11–14]. Alterations to these features can be a byproduct of normal physiologic processes, such as pregnancy and aging, or a contributor to disease pathogenesis and progression [11, 12]. The uterus and cervix must withstand a broad range of mechanical loads and experience complex loading profiles that evolve across pregnancy, postpartum, and age [3]. Understanding how these tissues respond to such forces requires careful characterization of their mechanical behavior. This section first outlines established *ex vivo* mechanical testing approaches and key mechanical parameters that can be extracted from such analyses, concluding with a detailed description of the mechanical properties of the uterus and cervix.

2.1 Mechanical Testing Methods

Mechanical tests quantify the relationship between a force or load applied to a material of known geometry and the level to which it deforms, enabling the characterization of a material's intrinsic mechanical properties (Fig. 2a)

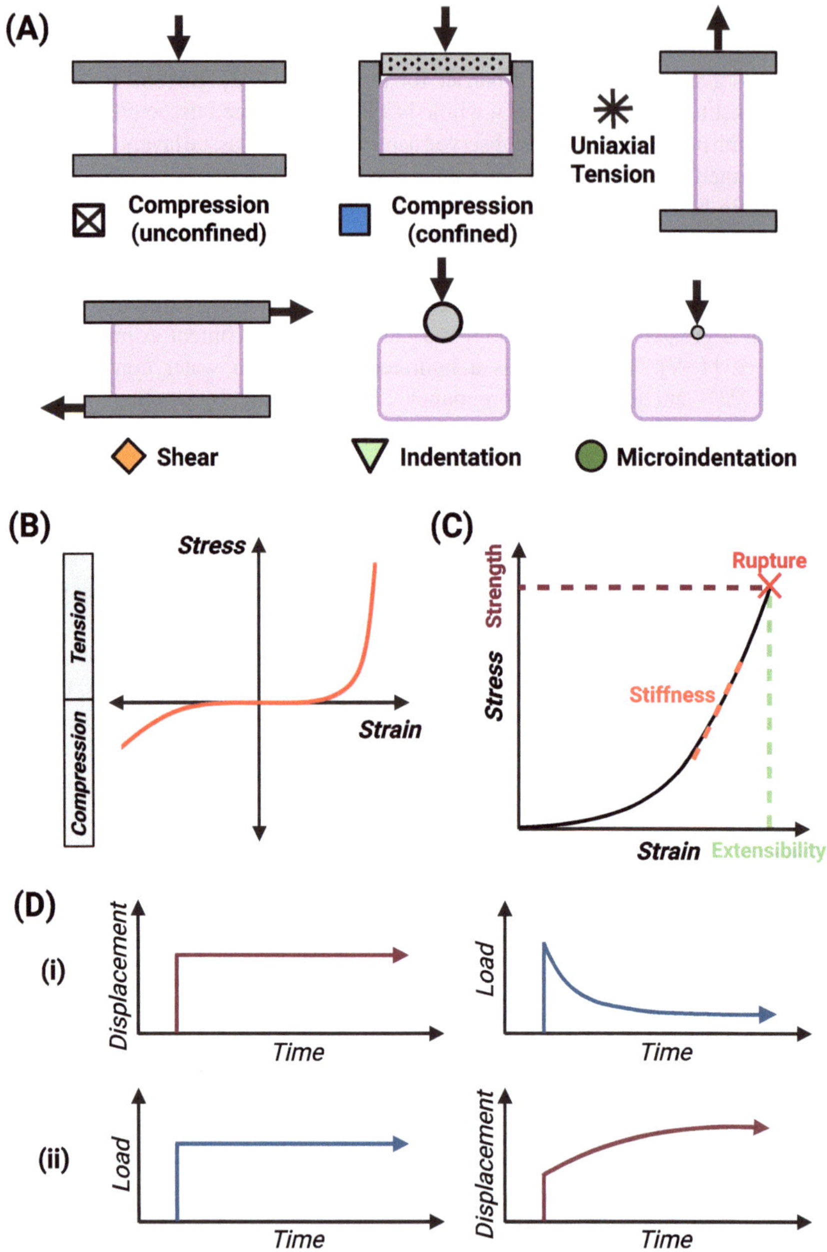

Fig. 2 **(a)** *Ex vivo* mechanical testing approaches used to evaluate the human uterus and cervix. Arrows indicate the direction of the applied load. Symbols correspond to those shown in Figs. 3 and 4. **(b)** Representative stress-strain response of a biological tissue demonstrating tension-compression asymmetry. **(c)** Example of resulting stress-strain "J" curve from a uniaxial tension test on biological tissue. Dashed lines indicate material parameters during loading (i.e., stiffness) and rupture (i.e., extensibility and strength) derived from this data. **(D)** Example of data generated from a (i) displacement-controlled mechanical test to evaluate stress relaxation, where the strain is held constant and the measured stress varies with time, and a (ii) load-controlled mechanical test to evaluate creep, where the load is held constant and displacement varies with time. (Created with https://Biorender.com)

[15]. These mechanical tests can be either load-controlled, in which a prescribed force is applied and the resulting deformation is measured, or displacement-controlled, in which a prescribed deformation is applied and the resulting force is measured (Fig. 2c) [16]. Additionally, the load or displacement can be applied perpendicular (normal) or parallel (shear) to the material face (Fig. 2a) [15]. The direction of the normal load or displacement can also be applied to elongate (i.e., tension) or compress (i.e., compression) the material in the direction of the applied force (Fig. 2a) [15]. Knowing the material's geometry, the stress (force acting over an area) and strain (relative deformation) can be calculated [15]. An important distinction is made between the true/Cauchy stress (force acting over deformed area) and the engineering stress (force acting over original area), which can greatly influence the reported stress [15]. Because most biological tissues are anisotropic, in that they exhibit direction-dependent properties due to structural variations, multiple mechanical testing approaches are required to fully characterize their behavior [15]. Here, we outline established *ex vivo* mechanical testing approaches that have been used to characterize the *passive* mechanical properties of the human uterus and cervix. Notably, no studies to date have directly measured the mechanical properties of the isthmus—the transition region between the uterus and cervix. In vivo mechanical tests, such as shear wave elastography and tissue aspiration, have not been included in the scope of this analysis.

2.1.1 Compression (Unconfined)

An unconfined compression test measures the mechanical response of a tissue as it is compressed between two opposing, rigid, non-permeable plates (i.e., platens) (Fig. 2a) [17, 18]. Unlike confined compression tests, unconfined compression does not constrain the tissue's lateral faces, and fluid is allowed to readily flow from the lateral tissue walls [17, 19]. The mechanical response of biological tissues under this loading modality is largely dictated by the properties of their nonfibrillar ground substance, which is provided, in large part, by glycosaminoglycans (GAGs) and proteoglycans [19, 20]. The fiber network constrains the lateral expansion of the ground matrix, but contributes little to the mechanical response under this mode of deformation [19].

2.1.2 Compression (Confined)

Confined compression mechanical tests assess a tissue's response to compressive loading under conditions that restrict lateral deformation (Fig. 2a) [17]. In confined compression tests, the tissue is cut to the exact dimensions of the testing chamber in which it is placed, with the top compressing platen, bottom platen, and/or lateral walls allowing for the flow of fluid out of the tissue [17]. Confined compression induces significant interstitial fluid pressurization, and the measured mechanical response can be influenced by the pore size of the platens [21, 22]. Confined compression is considered to be a more complex loading configuration, both in experimental setup and in subsequent time-dependent analysis, than unconfined compression [17].

2.1.3 Uniaxial Tension

Uniaxial tension tests measure the mechanical response of the tissue under a tensile load by extending the tissue in a single direction perpendicular to the tissue's face (Fig. 2a) [17, 19]. The tissue is attached to the mechanical testing machine at opposite ends and then extended to prescribed loads or deformations in one direction [23, 24]. In contrast to compression, the results from tensile mechanical tests are largely dictated by a material's fiber network, which primarily occurs through fiber uncrimping, alignment, and sliding [19, 20, 25].

2.1.4 Shear

Shear testing investigates the ability of tissues to resist forces applied parallel to the tissue face, distorting the internal angles of the tissue (Fig. 2) [15]. One approach to shear mechanical testing involves affixing the tissue to opposing platens, with prescribed loads or deformations applied parallel to the affixed face [26, 27]. There are several resulting elastic modulus (stiffness) parameters that can be reported [28]. The simple shear modulus can be found as the slope of the resulting stress vs. shear strain curve [28]. The complex shear modulus is the ratio of the maximum applied stress (or strain) to the measured strain (or stress) [28]. Additionally, rheological methods of measuring shear, or those that quantify the flow and deformation of materials, have been frequently used to characterize the viscoelastic behavior of biological tissues [29].

2.1.5 Indentation

Indentation is a mechanical characterization method in which a probe (indenter) is pressed into a material to measure its resistance to deformation (Fig. 2) [30]. Indenter shapes can vary widely and include spherical, conical, pyramidal, Berkovich, Knoop, and cube-corner geometries [31, 32]. The choice of probe geometry depends on both the material being tested and the mechanical parameters of interest [31]. For soft materials, spherical indenters are most commonly used [31]. An important exception is for hardness testing, in which pointed geometries, such as conical, pyramidal, Berkovich, Knoop, or cube-corner tips, are more appropriate [30–32].

Indentation induces a complex loading profile of compression, radial tension, and shear and can be used to determine the elastic, plastic, viscous, and fracture mechanical properties of a material [31]. Engagement of a material's macro-structure is achieved under this length scale [30–32]. Importantly, the measured mechanical properties are sensitive to certain testing parameters such as indentation depth, probe radius, and prescribed ramp time [31, 33–35].

2.1.6 Microindentation

Micro- and nanoindentation are variants of indentation and exert similar loading profiles to that of indentation, but at smaller length scales (Fig. 2a) [31]. Notably, atomic force microscopy (AFM) is a common type of microindentation/ nanoindentation technique that is often coupled with an imaging component [36]. Probes can be pyramidal, spherical, or colloidal in shape and range in size from a few nanometers to several hundred micrometers [31, 36]. Often, these probes are attached at the end of a cantilever; bending of the cantilever is then converted into force outputs [37]. Indentations can be performed on single molecules, single cells, or a collection of cells and ECM components [31, 37, 38]. The relative engagement of ECM and cellular components will vary depending on the probe size used [39, 40].

2.2 *Mechanical Properties*

The mechanical properties of materials are found based on the resulting stress vs. strain (or force vs. displacement) data from mechanical tests (Fig. 2b, c). Often, biological tissues exhibit a mechanical force response that varies in a nonlinear manner with strain, generating a canonical J-shaped curve (Fig. 2b, c) [11]. For the purposes of this review, we will consider the mechanical properties of the uterus and cervix in four broad categories of mechanical features: (i) stiffness, (ii) strength, (iii) extensibility, and (iv) time dependence. The stiffness of a material refers to its ability to resist deformation under an applied force [11]. Stiffness is often described by the elastic (Young's) modulus, which can be calculated from the slope of the linear portion of the stress vs. strain curve (Fig. 2c) [11, 41]. A material's strength refers to the amount of stress that can be applied before it is permanently damaged (Fig. 2c) [41]. Measures of strength include yield stress (stress at which a material is permanently deformed) and the ultimate tensile stress (tensile stress at which a material breaks) [41]. Similar to strength, extensibility refers to the amount of deformation (strain or stretch) a material can undergo without permanently deforming (Fig. 2c) [41, 42]. A material's extensibility is typically measured in tension and is the maximum strain or stretch at which the material fails (Fig. 2c) [42]. Time-dependent material features are those that consider how the mechanical response can change with sustained load or displacement over time (Fig. 2d) [11, 19, 43]. Time dependency consists of two distinct yet overlapping mechanisms: (i) viscoelasticity, the rearrangement of the solid matrix, and (ii) poroelasticity, fluid pressurization and subsequent migration through a porous matrix [44–46]. Under compression, time-dependent behavior is primarily governed by poroelasticity, while viscoelastity dominates the tensile response [19, 20, 25, 47]. There are numerous time-dependent features that measure the mechanical response of a material over a period of time. Creep (increase in strain under constant load), stress relaxation (decrease in load under constant displacement), and hysteresis (nonoverlapping loading and unloading stress-strain curves) are three types of time-dependent mechanical phenomena exhibited by soft biological tissues (Fig. 2d) [11, 19, 43].

2.3 Uterus

The stiffness and time dependence of the uterus have been characterized across its distinct tissue layers with compression (confined and unconfined), uniaxial tension, indentation, microindentation, and shear testing modalities [24, 26, 48–61]. Strength and extensibility measures exclusively represent the myometrium layer, as determined with confined compression and uniaxial tension testing [24, 52, 57, 58, 60, 62].

2.3.1 Stiffness

Notable changes have been demonstrated across distinct tissue layers [48] and as a product of pregnancy [48, 49, 49, 63] (Fig. 3a).

The stiffness of the nonpregnant endometrium in the secretory phase was first quantified by Abbas et al. [49], who, along with Fodera et al. [48], reported values in the range of 100–300 Pa (Fig. 3a) [48, 49]. In contrast, Wang et al. [61] measured the stiffness of the secretory-phase endometrium to be 4.726 ± 0.385 kPa with AFM, an order of magnitude greater than previous reports (Fig. 3a) [61]. Such discrepancies could have arisen from differences in sample preparation employed by Wang et al. [61], including the use of excessively thin samples, testing prior to achieving swelling equilibrium, and the unknown degree of sample hydration during measurement [61]. Further, Wang et al. [61] reported positive α-SMA staining in tissue labeled as normal endometrium, which raises questions regarding the identity and cellular purity of the tested "endometrium" samples [61].

The stiffness of the nonpregnant myometrium has been shown to span multiple orders of magnitude (10^2–10^8 Pa), with notable differences evidenced across mechanical deformation modes, demonstrating tension-compression asymmetry (Fig. 3a, Table 1) [24, 26, 48, 50–57, 59]. The largest values of myometrial stiffness were measured under confined compression and uniaxial tension (Fig. 3a) [52, 57, 59]. Stiffness measurements under confined compression were three orders of magnitude greater than those measured under unconfined compression (Fig. 3a) [51–53, 55]. This marked difference likely reflects the contribution of interstitial fluid pressurization and the effective incompressibility of the tissue under confined conditions, which can lead to elevated stiffness values [73]. The stiffness of the

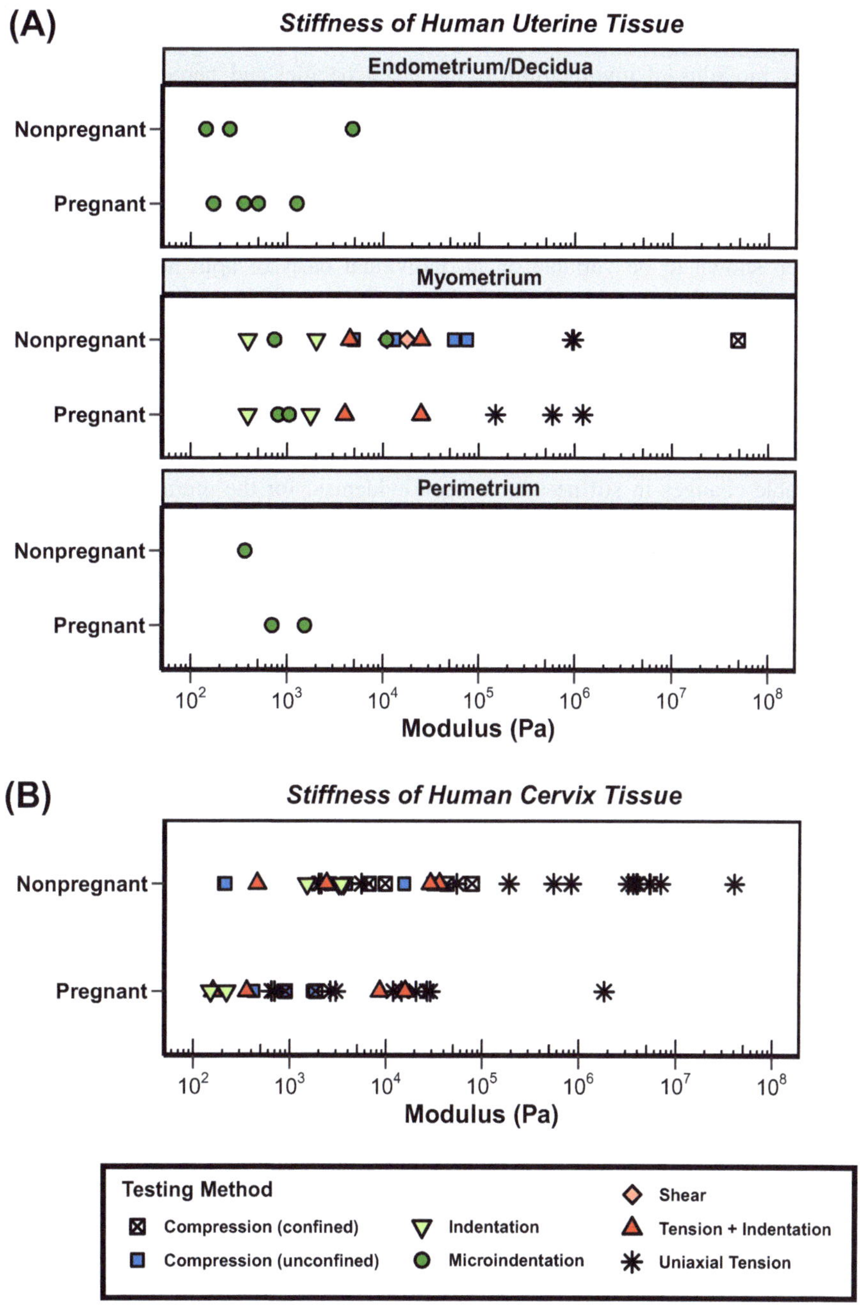

Fig. 3 Stiffness of the human **(a)** uterus [24, 26, 48–61] and **(b)** cervix stroma [20, 23, 53, 64–72] measured *ex vivo*. Uterine tissue is separated by tissue layers: nonpregnant endometrium/pregnant decidua, myometrium, and perimetrium. The shape of each symbol marks the mechanical testing method utilized, as shown in Fig. 2

myometrium has also been shown to be anisotropic, indicating preferential fiber directionality [24, 50, 53]. Kiss et al. [53] evaluated the frequency-dependent complex modulus of myometrium tissue taken parallel and perpendicular to the intrauterine cavity with unconfined compression; parallel-cut myometrium samples exhibited a greater complex modulus compared to perpendicular-cut samples [53]. Kiss et al. [53] also demonstrated that the stiffness of the myometrium varied with frequency and strain amplitude nonlinearly, akin to a power-law relationship [53]. The stiffness of different anatomic regions (i.e., anterior, posterior, and fundus) has been shown to be variable on an individual basis in both nonpregnant and pregnant states, but no systemic trends have been identified to date [48, 50, 74].

Comparisons across distinct tissue layers were conducted by Fodera et al. [48]. The myometrium was found to be significantly stiffer than the nonpregnant endometrium, thereby suggesting a gradient in material properties between the endometrium and myometrium layers [48]. The stiffness of the perimetrium did not markedly differ from that of the myometrium (Fig. 3a) [48].

Notable changes in stiffness have been evidenced for the uterus as a result of pregnancy. In the first trimester, the decidua basalis (at the site of implantation) was found to stiffen relative to the nonpregnant endometrium (1250 vs. 250 Pa) [49]. The decidua basalis was also significantly stiffer than the decidua parietalis (away from the implantation site) by an order of magnitude (171 Pa) [49]. No differences in stiffness between the nonpregnant endometrium and first-trimester decidua parietalis were found [49]. In the third trimester, Fodera et al. [48] found that the decidua parietalis, taken from two patient populations, stiffened (0.35–0.5 kPa) relative to the nonpregnant endometrium (0.143 ± 0.04 kPa) [48]. Taken together, the stiffness of the decidua parietalis/vera increases rather linearly across gestation [5]. No data currently exist on the mechanical properties of these tissues for mid-gestational time points in humans, but have been reported for nonhuman primates [5]. Mechanical testing of the human myometrium has revealed that pregnancy-associated softening is highly dependent on the mode and magnitude of applied strain [24]. A clear reduction in stiffness was observed in late pregnancy for strains exceeding 30%; however, at lower tensile strains and under indentation testing, no such differences were found between nonpregnant and pregnant tissues [24, 48, 50]. These modality-specific findings point to distinct roles of tissue components; the collagen fiber network is thought to primarily govern the tensile response, whereas indentation appears more sensitive to the properties of the ground substance (e.g., water, glycosaminoglycans, proteoglycans) [20, 24]. The requirement of high tensile strain to observe tissue softening suggests that collagen fiber engagement is a critical factor in detecting pregnancy-induced mechanical adaptations of the uterine myometrium.

2.3.2 Strength and Extensibility

Under uniaxial tensile loading, the maximum value of true strain (i.e., extensibility) was determined to be in the range of 30–55% and 30–95% for nonpregnant and pregnant myometrium tissues, respectively (Fig. 4b,i) [57, 58, 60, 62]. The strength

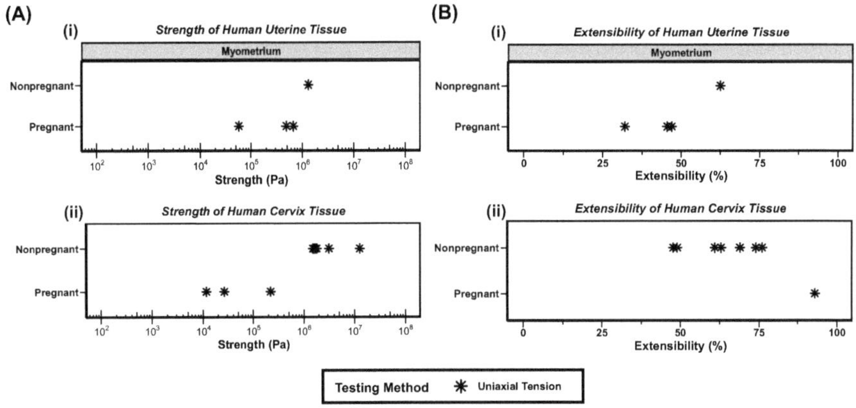

Fig. 4 **(a)** Strength and **(b)** extensibility of human (i) uterine myometrium [24, 57, 58, 60, 62] and (ii) cervix stroma tissue [23, 64–67, 75] measured *ex vivo*. The shape of each symbol marks the mechanical testing method utilized, as shown in Fig. 2

of nonpregnant myometrium tissue under uniaxial tension ranges from 9 kPa to 2 MPa (Fig. 4a,i) [57, 58, 60, 62]. When comparing values across studies, the pregnant myometrium appears to be slightly more extensible than nonpregnant tissue, with no corresponding differences in strength; however, no individual study to date has directly compared failure mechanics across pregnancy states [57, 58, 60, 62].

Locking stretch is another parameter that describes a material's extensibility, but specifically that of the non-Gaussian chain fiber network [24]. This parameter can also be described as the corresponding stretch/strain at the transition point along the "J" curve [76]. Fang et al. [24] evaluated the locking stretch of nonpregnant and third-trimester pregnant myometrial tissue and found this parameter to range from 2 to 3 on average; locking stretch was found to be greater for pregnant uterine tissue compared to nonpregnant samples [24].

2.3.3 Time Dependence

Collectively, uterine tissue exhibits time dependency, as evidenced by stress relaxation, hysteresis, and creep behaviors [24, 48, 50, 53, 55, 74, 77].

On an individual tissue layer basis, notable changes in the viscoelastic ratio were reported by Fodera et al. [48]. Viscoelastic ratio, defined as the ratio between equilibrium (E_∞) and instantaneous (E_0) elastic moduli, provides a measure of a material's viscoelastic behavior, ranging from purely elastic ($E_\infty/E_0 = 1$) to purely viscous ($E_\infty/E_0 = 0$) [48, 78]. On average, the human uterus exhibits a viscoelastic ratio of 0.5, indicating that this tissue behaves as both a viscous liquid and an elastic solid at the microscale [48]. Across tissue layers, the nonpregnant endometrium and pregnant decidua were found to be more viscous than the myometrium and perimetrium layers; no differences were found between the myometrium and perimetrium [48]. In pregnancy, the viscoelastic ratio of pregnant decidua parietalis tissue was found to be increased relative to the nonpregnant endometrium, suggesting that the decidua becomes less viscous in pregnancy [48].

Tan δ, also known as the loss factor, is a viscoelastic parameter that describes the relative energy dissipation or damping of a material and is a ratio of the storage to loss moduli [79]. Tan δ ranges from zero for an ideal elastic solid to infinity for an ideal liquid; the greater the value of tan δ, the greater the damping capacity of a material [79]. Both Kiss et al. [53] and Omari et al. [55] found the value of tan δ to be in the range of 0.3–0.45 for myometrium tissue [53, 55].

Lastly, a mathematical model describing the time-dependent creep behavior of the myometrium has been developed in Jelen et al. [77], reporting functions of tissue stiffness and viscosity as a function of load [77].

2.3.4 Other

Intrinsic permeability and diffusivity are two material properties that describe the flow of fluid through a porous medium with units of m^2 and m^2/s, respectively [48, 78, 80]. Fodera et al. [48] evaluated these parameters across distinct nonpregnant and third-trimester pregnant uterine tissue layers and found median intrinsic permeability and diffusivity to be in the range of 10^{-17}–10^{-15} m^2 and 10^{-12} –10^{-8} m^2/s, respectively [48]. The nonpregnant endometrium exhibited decreased permeability and diffusivity relative to the nonpregnant myometrium and perimetrium layers [48]. In late pregnancy, changes in permeability and diffusivity across tissue layers were patient-dependent and not consistent between the two patient cohorts, differing by surgical indication (i.e., placenta accreta or routine C-section) and gestational age (i.e., early and late third trimester) [48]. Permeability changes as a result of pregnancy were not statistically significant for all three uterine layers [48]. The pregnant decidua parietalis tissue exhibited increased diffusivity relative to the nonpregnant endometrium; pregnancy induced no changes to the diffusivity of the myometrium or perimetrium [48].

2.4 Cervix

The mechanical response of human cervical stroma tissue has been reported at various anatomical locations (internal os and external os) under a myriad of loading configurations, including compression (confined and unconfined), uniaxial tension, and indentation [20, 23, 53, 64–66, 68–72, 81–84]. Cervical tissue samples were collected both during nonpregnancy and pregnancy in the third trimester. The mechanical properties of the cervical epithelium have not been reported to date.

Table 1 Median stiffness (i.e., elastic modulus) values under uniaxial tension and compression/indentation mechanical tests for nonpregnant and pregnant uterine myometrium [24, 48, 50–53, 55–57, 59, 60] and cervical stroma [20, 23, 64–67, 69–72] tissue measured via *ex vivo* mechanical tests

Tissue type	Testing method	Nonpregnant (Pa)	Pregnant (Pa)
Uterine myometrium	Uniaxial tension	9.4×10^5	3.7×10^5
	Compression/indentation	7.9×10^3	1.0×10^3
Cervical stroma	Uniaxial tension	2.0×10^6	1.3×10^4
	Compression/indentation	3.4×10^3	5.4×10^2

2.4.1 Stiffness

The mechanical response of the human cervix is different under tensile and compressive loads, exhibiting tension-compression asymmetry (Fig. 3b, Table 1) [23, 70]. Under compression and indentation testing, the cervix has an apparent elastic modulus of $1.5 \times 10^2 - 3.9 \times 10^4$ Pa [20, 70–72]. Pregnant cervical samples have been found, on average, to be less stiff ($1.5 \times 10^2 - 1.7 \times 10^3$ Pa) than nonpregnant ($2.1 \times 10^2 - 3.9 \times 10^4$ Pa) under compression and indentation [20, 70–72]. A much larger range in cervical tissue stiffness has been documented under uniaxial tension, with reported elastic moduli between $2.1 \times 10^3 - 4.0 \times 10^7$ Pa (Fig. 3b, Table 1) [64–66, 69, 70, 81]. As with compression, larger stiffness values under tensile loads were found for nonpregnant ($2.1 \times 10^3 - 4.0 \times 10^7$ Pa) cervical tissue when compared to pregnant ($2.7 \times 10^3 - 1.8 \times 10^6$ Pa) counterparts [64–66, 69, 70, 81]. It is important to note that the cervix exhibits a nonlinear mechanical response, whereby the measured elastic modulus varies as a function of applied strain [23, 70]. This phenomenon is particularly apparent in tension, with reduced stiffness at low strains and increased stiffness at higher strains [23, 70]. The wide range of reported stiffness values across studies can be attributed to several factors. Methodological inconsistencies across studies, including sample geometries and rate of tissue deformation, can lead to greater degrees of variation in the reported stiffness values [85]. While mechanical tests often apply a deformation or load at a constant rate, the rates often differ between studies. This is a particularly important consideration as the mechanical properties of the cervix have been shown to be strain-dependent [53, 64, 65, 75, 81]. Additionally, the point at which stiffness is calculated (e.g., toe region, linear region, at equilibrium) can lead to variation across studies due to the time-dependent and nonlinear mechanical response exhibited by the cervix [23, 86]. At low levels of strain, the collagen fibers within the tissue are not fully engaged, resulting in smaller stiffness values [87]. At higher levels of strain, the collagen network is engaged, resulting in larger stiffness values [87]. These differences may also arise due to the time-dependent behavior of cervical tissue, particularly when comparing the instantaneous elastic modulus (stress measured immediately after deformation is held constant) and the elastic modulus at equilibrium (after energy is allowed to dissipate) [70]. These effects were quantified by Myers et al. [69], with an average instantaneous elastic modulus of 8.37×10^5 Pa and equilibrium elastic modulus of 5.54×10^5 Pa for the nonpregnant cervix

[69, 70]. In addition, differences in the calculation of stress can also act as a confounding factor, with some studies reporting the true stress [64–66, 81] and others reporting the engineering stress [70].

In order to capture the full nonlinearity of cervical tissue across tension and compression, a more sophisticated approach to understanding stiffness has been employed in several studies, which consider the tissue as a composite material, with a compliant ground substance and embedded fiber network [23, 71, 84]. For example, Myers et al. [69] found the stiffness of the ground substance in pregnant and nonpregnant cervical tissue to be of similar magnitude (6.5×10^2 Pa vs. 2.0×10^3 Pa, respectively) [84]. However, fiber stiffness was found to be much smaller in the pregnant cervix when compared to the nonpregnant state (7.0×10^2 Pa vs. 1.9×10^5 Pa) [84]. These trends are consistent with other work that considers the cervix as a composite material [23]. Finally, variations in reported cervical stiffness may also be affected by the variation within and between individual cervices [72, 88, 89].

2.4.2 Strength and Extensibility

Differences in strength values have been measured between nonpregnant and pregnant cervical tissue (Fig. 4). Strength values for nonpregnant cervical tissues have been measured in the range of $1.5 \times 10^6 - 1.3 \times 10^7$ Pa, whereas pregnant cervical tissues are in the range of $1.1 \times 10^4 - 2.2 \times 10^5$ Pa [64–67, 75]. Therefore, higher stresses are required to permanently damage nonpregnant cervical tissue compared to pregnant cervical tissue. The associated extensibility follows a reverse pattern, with the pregnant cervix being more extensible than the nonpregnant cervix (0.93 vs. 0.48–0.76, respectively) [65–67, 75]. Outside of the strain at rupture, another measure of extensibility is the locking stretch, which is specifically related to the maximum extensibility of a fibrous material [23]. Shi et al. [23] also found the pregnant cervix to be more extensible than the nonpregnant cervix, with respective locking stretch values of 2.4 and 1.3 [23].

2.4.3 Time Dependence

The biomechanical response of the cervix is highly time-dependent, which has been shown in experiments quantifying creep, hysteresis, and stress relaxation [66, 70]. Several studies have used various mathematical models to describe the time-dependent behavior of cervical tissue, including a 1D rheological model [70], a two-time constant Prony series [83], a poro-viscoelastic model [20], and a hyper-viscoelastic model [90]. In comparisons between pregnant and nonpregnant cervical tissue, no statistically significant changes in viscoelastic ratio were found [20]. The loss factor, tan δ, of cervical tissue was measured by Kiss et al. [53] and Dewall et al. [68], with both reporting average values between 0.3 and 0.5 [53, 68].

2.4.4 Other

While the ECM is thought to dominate the tensile mechanical response of cervical tissue, the tissue's time-dependent mechanical behavior, particularly under compressive loads, is also influenced by fluid dynamics [20]. Direct measurements of permeability have found the pregnant cervix to be more permeable than nonpregnant tissue, with average hydraulic permeability values of 3.2×10^{-13} $m^4/N{\cdot}s$ and 2.1×10^{-14} $m^4/N{\cdot}s$, respectively [82]. The same trend was found by Shi and Myers [20], though reported values were an order of magnitude larger and were obtained via indentation mechanical tests [20]. The permeability of ectocervical tissue was specifically measured by Sassi et al. [91], with fresh cervical tissue having an average apparent permeability coefficient of 8×10^{-5} cm/s [91].

3 Biomechanical Relevancy of Gynecologic and Obstetric Disorders

The following section highlights select obstetric and gynecologic disorders affecting the uterus and/or cervix in which mechanical factors are either characteristic features of the disease or implicated in its pathogenesis. Often, these conditions can be concomitant on an individual basis.

3.1 Gynecologic Disorders

3.1.1 Endometrial Polyps

Endometrial polyps are overgrowths of endometrial glands and stromal cells that protrude into the intrauterine cavity [92]. The overall prevalence of this condition is approximately 8%, a rate which increases with nulliparity, obesity, and menopause [93, 94]. Abnormal uterine bleeding is the most common symptom of endometrial polyps [92]. Endometrial polyps can vary in size from a few millimeters to several centimeters in diameter and can be pedunculated (hanging from a thin stalk) or sessile (flat, dome-shaped) [92]. Polyps are typically noncancerous; however, the risk of malignant transformation increases with age [92, 95]. Using *in vivo* shear wave elastography techniques, endometrial polyps have been mechanically characterized as soft tissue structures that are notably less stiff than patient-matched myometrium tissue [96, 97].

3.1.2 Endometriosis

Endometriosis is a chronic gynecological disorder, affecting approximately 10% of reproductive-aged women, and can cause severe pelvic pain, menorrhagia (heavy or prolonged menstrual bleeding), and infertility [98, 99]. This disease is characterized by the ectopic presence of endometrial-like tissue [99, 100]. Ectopic endometriosis lesions are most commonly attached to the pelvic peritoneum, but can also be found on the ovaries, rectum, bladder, and, more rarely, the heart, lungs, and brain [99–101]. Ectopic endometriosis lesions largely resemble the cellular components of eutopic endometrium tissue (glandular epithelial cells surrounded by stromal cells), but notable differences exist [102, 103]. Compared to patient-matched eutopic endometrial tissues, endometriosis lesions are more enriched in perivascular, endothelial, and immune cells and exhibit dysregulation of pro-inflammatory and angiogenesis pathways [102, 104]. The prevailing hypothesis for the etiology of endometriosis is retrograde menstruation: the reverse flow of menstrual blood through the fallopian tubes and into the pelvic cavity [99, 100, 105]. The occurrence of retrograde menstruation has been visualized laparoscopically [106] and via transvaginal ultrasound [107] in endometriosis patients at a rate ninefold greater than healthy controls [108]. Still, retrograde menstruation can occur regularly in healthy women and is not an exclusive biomarker of endometriosis [106, 108, 109]. A second theory has been proposed describing the atypical differentiation of cells from the Müllerian duct, a developmental precursor of the female reproductive system, to account for endometriosis diagnoses in men and hysterectomized women [110].

The passive mechanical characterization of endometriosis lesions is not well established. One study conducted by Batur et al. [111] demonstrated increased stiffness for endometriomas (i.e., endometriosis-derived ovarian cysts) compared to the hemorrhagic ovarian cysts, but how this compares to normal uterine and ovarian tissue is not presently known [110, 111]. From an active biomechanics standpoint, the pattern and amplitude of peristaltic contractions within the uterus appear to be altered for women diagnosed with endometriosis [112–114].

3.1.3 Uterine Fibroids

Uterine fibroids, also known as leiomyomas, are noncancerous tumors that form within the uterus and are present in up to 70–80% of women by age 50 [115–118]. Among those affected, 10–50% will experience clinically significant symptoms in their reproductive years [119–121]. Uterine fibroids can cause prolonged heavy menstrual bleeding, chronic pelvic pain, anemia, and infertility in nonpregnancy and increase the risk of pregnancy complications in the form of miscarriage, severe acute pelvic pain, preterm birth, and placental abnormalities [118, 120, 122, 123].

Uterine fibroids are known to exhibit an immense amount of heterogeneity, varying widely in size, location, and gross architecture within and across different patients. While all fibroids originate as "seedling" structures on the millimeter scale [120, 124], they can regularly grow beyond 5 cm in diameter [125, 126], occasionally reaching 50 cm [127–129]. Uterine fibroids are thought to be clonally derived, arising from a single cell mutation [118, 120, 130] and can be found in all three uterine layers as submucosal (endometrium), intramural (myometrium), and subserosal (perimetrium) tumors [120, 124, 131, 132]. In addition to smooth muscle cells, fibroblasts, leukocytes, macrophages, and endothelial cells can also be found within fibroid tissues [133–136].

Increased biomechanical stiffness and dense ECM structure are distinguishing hallmarks of this disease [26, 51–53, 56, 124]. Mechanically, uterine fibroids have been found to be consistently 1.5–5-fold stiffer than patient-matched myometrium tissue [26, 51–56, 124]. Both uterine fibroid and myometrium tissues have been shown to exhibit time-dependent material behavior [48, 50, 53, 55, 63, 137]. On the basis of structure and composition, abundant collagen deposition comprises a large degree of the ECM components in fibroid tissues [51, 52, 124, 138]. The exact ECM components that differ between fibroid and myometrium tissues, such as collagen subtypes, glycosaminoglycans, and proteoglycans, vary widely in the literature [51, 52, 124, 138–140]. Altered organization of fibrous ECM components is another key feature of fibroids. Uterine fibroid architecture has been classically described as whorled, but additional structural subtypes, including nodular, trabecular, and mixed, have been identified [124].

3.1.4 Adenomyosis

Adenomyosis is marked by the presence of ectopic endometrial basalis tissue, containing both glandular and stromal cells, beyond the junctional zone and within the myometrium tissue layer of the uterus [141–143]. The true incidence of adenomyosis is unknown due to fundamental diagnostic challenges, with reports varying widely from 8.8% to 61.5% in individuals undergoing total hysterectomy procedures [144]. Symptoms of adenomyosis include abnormal uterine bleeding, pelvic pain, and infertility, though approximately one third of individuals remain asymptomatic [141, 145].

Adenomyosis tissue most often represents endometrial tissue in the proliferative stage, but can exhibit morphological changes akin to the secretory and menstrual phases [142, 143]. The boundaries of adenomyosis tissue within the myometrium are poorly defined, as observed in both visual and ultrasonic assessments [143, 146]. The presence of adenomyosis is often accompanied by pathologic changes to myometrial tissue, as evidenced by smooth muscle cell hypertrophy (i.e., increase in cell size) and hyperplasia (i.e., increase in cell number), which contribute to alterations in fiber alignment [141, 143, 147]. Thickening of the junctional zone has also been reported [143, 148]. As such, uterine volume is often globally enlarged in cases of adenomyosis [143, 146, 149]. The exact pathogenesis of adenomyosis remains unknown; however, several competing theories have been proposed: (i) invagination of the endometrial basalis into the myometrium, (ii) metaplasia of displaced embryonic pluripotent Müllerian remnants, (iii) differentiation of adult endometrial progenitor cells, (iv) displacement of endometrial cells into the myometrium from eutopic endometriosis lesions, and (v) altered lymphatic drainage pathways [141–143].

The passive mechanical properties of adenomyosis tissue have been exclusively investigated with *in vivo* elastography techniques to date. However, tissue stiffness data are mixed, with some studies reporting a relative increase in stiffness [146, 149–151], others noting a decrease [152, 153], and some finding no significant change [154] when compared to normal myometrial tissue. There is some evidence to suggest that the pattern and amplitude of active peristaltic contractions within the uterus also appear to be altered for women diagnosed with adenomyosis [155, 156].

3.2 *Obstetric Disorders*

Biomechanical functions of the uterus and cervix are critical to ensuring a healthy pregnancy from conception to birth. The ability of the uterus and cervix to accommodate the physical demands of a growing fetus underscores the mechanical roles of these tissues. Mechanical, structural, and biochemical aberrations to these tissues are thought to lead to a host of obstetric disorders. Still, our understanding of the mechanical properties of the uterus and cervix in both normal homeostasis and disease pathophysiology is rather limited.

3.2.1 Preterm Birth

Globally, preterm birth (PTB), defined as birth before 37 weeks of gestation, affects approximately 10% of births [157]. PTB is the leading cause of death for newborns, and babies that do survive are at increased risk of lifelong morbidities [157]. The mechanical integrity of reproductive tissues is essential to a healthy pregnancy [158]. Clinically, many causes cited for preterm birth are mechanical in nature, including the preterm premature rupture of membranes (PPROM), uterine overdistention, and cervical insufficiency [159, 160]. PPROM is the rupture of fetal membranes before 37 weeks of gestation and is the cause of 40% of all spontaneous preterm births [161]. Uterine overdistention, as seen in multiple gestations (e.g., twins or triplets) and polyhydramnios (excess amniotic fluid), is thought to contribute to preterm labor (PTL) by increasing mechanical stress within the uterine wall [162]. Cervical insufficiency is defined as the inability of the cervix to retain the fetus due to a functional or structural defect in the absence of uterine contractions [163]. Due to a lack of objective findings and clear diagnostic criteria, diagnosing cervical insufficiency is difficult [164]. It is believed that the premature remodeling of cervical tissue is a key contributor of cervical insufficiency, and *in vivo* aspiration measurements of the cervix have shown the cervix to be less stiff in pregnancies at high-risk for PTB [165]. The pathophysiology and interplay of these conditions remains unknown, and 70–80% of PTB is spontaneous and unexplained [158, 166].

3.2.2 Post-term Birth

Post-term birth is defined as a pregnancy that extends beyond 42 weeks of gestation [167, 168]. This condition affects 7% of pregnancies and is associated with higher rates of cesarean deliveries and perinatal morbidity and mortality [167–169]. Delayed or inadequate cervical remodeling is thought to be the primary mechanism preventing normal timing for dilation of the cervix [167, 168]. The inability to initiate proper uterine contractions is another purported cause of post-term birth [7]. Many of the clinical methods to initiate labor involve mechanical intervention, such as membrane sweeps, Foley balloon catheters, and synthetic osmotic cervical dilators (e.g., Dilapan-S) [1, 167, 170]. Pharmacological methods can also be used to induce labor and stimulate uterine contractions, such as oxytocin and prostaglandins, which may also be used with mechanical labor induction methods [1, 167].

3.2.3 Placenta Accreta Spectrum Disorder

Placenta accreta spectrum (PAS) disorder, occurring in 0.3% of pregnancies, is defined by abnormal placental adherence or invasion of the placenta beyond the decidua into the myometrium (accreta and increta), and, in severe cases, through the perimetrium (percreta) [1, 171–173]. During labor, PAS placentas fail to appropriately detach from the uterine wall, which can lead to severe maternal hemorrhaging, permanent loss of fertility, and mortality for both mother and fetus [171–175]. Prior uterine surgeries, including cesarean sections, myomectomies, endometrial ablations, and dilation and curettage (D&C) procedures, are major risk factors for PAS in humans [1, 174, 176]. In fact, globally increasing rates of cesarean sections [177, 178] have largely contributed to the substantial rise in PAS incidence in modern years [1, 176, 179]. Consequently, uterine scar tissue is considered a key contributor to PAS pathogenesis [174, 176].

Uterine scar tissue is a biophysical modification to the uterus exhibiting increased collagen deposition and disrupted fiber architecture [180]. There is some evidence to suggest that uterine scar tissue exhibits increased stiffness compared to unaltered myometrium tissue via strain elastography imaging [181].

3.2.4 Uterine Rupture

Uterine rupture is defined as a disruption or tear in the uterine myometrium, often including the perimetrium [182–185]. This condition occurs in approximately 0.05–0.8% of all pregnancies, a rate that depends on an individual's obstetric history

[182–185]. Nearly all cases of uterine rupture occur in the third trimester, usually following a trial of labor after a previous cesarean section [182, 186]. Risk factors include (i) gross structural abnormalities (e.g., congenital Müllerian anomalies and distortion of uterine anatomy due to fibroids or adhesions), (ii) uterine surgeries that produce scar tissue (e.g., cesarean sections, myomectomies, endometrial ablations, etc.), (iii) connective tissue disorders (e.g., Ehlers-Danlos syndrome), and (iv) a prior ectopic pregnancy [187]. Together, these conditions reflect compromised structural integrity of the uterus, increasing the risk of mechanical failure under the substantial loads imposed by gestation and labor.

4 Conclusions

4.1 Future Research Avenues

Despite decades of research, major gaps remain in our understanding of uterine and cervical mechanics and how these properties contribute to distinct structure-function relationships. Many gynecologic and obstetric pathologies lack clearly defined etiologies, which hinders the development of effective prevention and treatment strategies. In many cases, the biomechanical underpinnings of such diseases have yet to be deeply explored. Future progress will require interdisciplinary collaboration, robust longitudinal study designs, and the development of high-fidelity *in vitro* and *in vivo* models that accurately recapitulate the dynamic mechanical environments of these tissues. While this chapter has focused on the baseline biomechanical properties of the uterus and cervix, it is important to recognize that current definitions of "normal" are often based on limited, nonrepresentative populations. Future research must prioritize inclusivity across age, race, ethnicity, geography, and parity to more fully capture the spectrum of physiologic variation.

4.2 Biomechanical Relevance for Biomaterial Design

The design of biomaterials for gynecologic and obstetric applications must be grounded in a rigorous understanding of the biomechanical properties of the uterus and cervix. Biomaterials can serve diverse roles across the translational science spectrum, from basic science tools to probe the pathophysiological mechanisms of normal and diseased tissue states to engineered implants intended to augment or treat structural or functional defects. In both contexts, the success of a biomaterial depends critically on its ability to replicate the native organ's ultrastructure and mechanical properties. The uterus and cervix are highly dynamic, viscoelastic tissues that undergo profound biomechanical and structural changes during menstruation, pregnancy, parturition, postpartum, and age. Biomaterials that fail to match a tissue's mechanical behavior risk functional failure of the biomaterial or injury to the organ itself.

For further reading on efforts to tissue engineer the uterus and cervix for basic science and translational applications, we recommend the respective chapters by Campo et al. [188] and Koullali and House [189] in *Handbook of Tissue Engineering Scaffolds: Volume Two.*

4.3 Concluding Remarks

The uterus and cervix are dynamic, mechanically active organs whose structure and function are tightly linked to reproductive health and disease. As outlined in this chapter, biomechanical characterization across multiple length scales has begun to reveal how the mechanical properties of the uterus and cervix evolve across pregnancy and in pathologic contexts. Still, despite these important contributions, fundamental gaps remain in our understanding of how uterine and cervical biomechanics change across the lifespan and under normal physiological conditions such as menstruation, pregnancy, and aging. Moreover, how mechanical forces integrate with molecular and cellular signaling to guide tissue remodeling, growth, and repair in the uterus and cervix remains largely understudied. Ultimately, a deeper understanding of uterine and cervical biomechanics holds the potential to transform therapeutic strategies, inform biomaterial design, and advance personalized approaches in gynecologic and obstetric care.

Conflicts of Interest The authors declare no conflicts of interest.

Author Contributions E.L. and D.F. contributed equally to the conception, literature review, writing, and visualization of this work. D.F. analyzed the literature review data and generated the matching visualization. D.F. was responsible for all content related to the uterus; E.L. was responsible for all content related to the cervix. Both authors reviewed, edited, and approved the final version.

Acknowledgements The authors gratefully acknowledge the library services of Columbia University and Wayne State University for their assistance in accessing source literature. This work was supported by the Eunice Kennedy Shriver National Institute of Child Health & Human Development of the National Institutes of Health (NIH) under award number 1F31HD114449-01A1 (DMF). The content is solely the responsibility of the authors and does not necessarily represent the official views of the NIH.

Data Availability The compiled dataset from the literature review has been made available on Columbia University's Academic Commons (https://doi.org/10.7916/5s1b-cs21). The code used for data analysis is available upon request to the corresponding author (EML).

References

1. Cunningham F. et al. Williams Obstetrics 26e. Columbus: McGraw Hill LLC; 2022. ISBN: 978-1-260-46274-6. https://books.google.com/books?id=2HVKEAAAQBAJ.
2. Ameer MA, Fagan SE, Sosa-Stanley JN, Peterson DC. StatPearls. Treasure Island: StatPearls Publishing; 2023. http://www.ncbi.nlm.nih.gov/books/NBK470297/ (2023).
3. Myers KM, Elad D. Biomechanics of the human uterus. Wiley Interdiscip Rev Syst Biol Med. 2017;9. ISSN: 1939-005X.
4. Critchley HOD, Maybin JA, Armstrong GM, Williams ARW. Physiology of the endometrium and regulation of menstruation. Physiol Rev. 2020;100:1149–79. ISSN: 1522–1210.
5. Fodera DM, et al. Time-dependent material properties and composition of the nonhuman primate uterine layers through gestation. Scient Rep. 2025;15:23194. ISSN: 2045-2322. https://www.nature.com/articles/s41598-025-02986-w (2025).
6. Morrione TG, Seifter S. Alteration in the collagen content of the human uterus during pregnancy and postpartum involution. J Exp Med. 1962;115:357–65. ISSN: 0022–1007.
7. Vink JY, et al. A new paradigm for the role of smooth muscle cells in the human cervix. eng. Am J Obstetr Gynecol. 2016;215:478.e1–11. ISSN: 1097-6868.
8. Myers K, Socrate S, Tzeranis D, House M. Changes in the biochemical constituents and morphologic appearance of the human cervical stroma during pregnancy. Euro J Obstetr Gynecol Reproduct Biol. 2009;144:S82–9. ISSN: 03012115. https://linkinghub.elsevier.com/retrieve/pii/S0301211509001456 (2025).
9. Nallasamy S, Mahendroo M. Distinct roles of Cervical Epithelia and stroma in pregnancy and parturition. Semin Reprod Med. 2017;35:190–200. ISSN: 1526–4564.
10. Wira CR, Grant-Tschudy KS, Crane-Godreau MA. Epithelial cells in the female reproductive tract: a central role as sentinels of immune protection. Am J Reprod Immunol (New York, N. Y.: 1989). 2005;53:65–76. ISSN: 1046-7408.
11. Fung YC. Biomechanics: mechanical properties of living tissues. Berlin: Springer Science & Business Media; 1981. ISBN: 978-1-4757-2257-4.
12. Ayad NME, Kaushik S, Weaver VM. Tissue mechanics, an important regulator of development and disease. Philos Trans R Soc B: Biol Sci. 2019;374:20180215. https://royalsocietypublishing.org/doi/10.1098/rstb.2018.0215 (2024).
13. Müller C, Müller A, Pompe T. Dissipative interactions in cell–matrix ad-hesion. Soft Matt. 2013;9:6207–6216. https://pubs.rsc.org/en/content/articlelanding/2013/sm/c3sm50803j (2024).
14. Cantini M, Donnelly H, Dalby MJ, Salmeron-Sanchez M. The plot thickens: the emerging role of matrix viscosity in cell mechanotransduction. Adv Healthc Mater 2020;9:1901259. ISSN: 2192–2659. https://onlinelibrary.wiley.com/doi/abs/10.1002/adhm.201901259 (2025).
15. Humphrey JD, O'Rourke SL. An introduction to biomechanics: solids and fluids, analysis and design. 2nd ed. New York: Springer; 2015. ISBN: 978-1-4939-2622-0.
16. Goel VK, Wilder DG, Pope MH, Edwards WT. Biomechanical testing of the spine: load-controlled versus displacement-controlled analysis. Spine. 1995;20:2354–7. ISSN: 0362-2436. http://journals.lww.com/00007632-199511000-00017 (2025).
17. Patel JM, Wise BC, Bonnevie ED, Mauck RL. A systematic review and guide to mechanical testing for articular cartilage tissue engineering. Tissue Eng Part C Methods. 2019;25:593–608. ISSN: 1937-3384. https://www.ncbi.nlm.nih.gov/pmc/articles/PMC6791482/ (2025).
18. Navindaran K, Kang JS, Moon K. Techniques for characterizing mechanical properties of soft tissues. J Mech Behav Biomed Mater. 2023;138:105575. ISSN: 17516161. https://linkinghub.elsevier.com/retrieve/pii/S1751616122004805 (2025).
19. Mow VC, Holmes MH, Lai WM. Fluid transport and mechanical properties of articular cartilage: a review. J Biomech 1984;17:377–94. ISSN:0021–9290.

20. Shi L, Myers K. A finite porous-viscoelastic model capturing mechanical behavior of human cervix under multi-step spherical indentation. J Mech Behav Biomed Mater. 2023;143: 105875. ISSN: 1751–6161. https://www.sciencedirect.com/science/article/pii/S175161612300228X (2023).
21. Soltz MA, Ateshian GA. Experimental verification and theoretical prediction of cartilage interstitial fluid pressurization at an impermeable contact interface in confined compression. J Biomech. 1998;31:927–34. ISSN: 0021–9290. https://www.sciencedirect.com/science/article/pii/S0021929098001055 (2025).
22. Gor GY, et al. Relation between pore size and the compressibility of a confined fluid. J Chem Phys. 2015;143:194506. ISSN: 0021–9606. https://www.ncbi.nlm.nih.gov/pmc/articles/PMC4697274/ (2025).
23. Shi L, Hu L, Lee N, Fang S, Myers K. Three-dimensional anisotropic hyperelastic constitutive model describing the mechanical response of human and mouse cervix. Acta Biomater. 2022;150:277–94. ISSN: 1742–7061. https://www.sciencedirect.com/science/article/pii/S1742706122004640 (2022).
24. Fang S, et al. Equilibrium mechanical properties of the human uterus in tension and compression. Acta Biomater. 2025. ISSN: 1742–7061. https://www.sciencedirect.com/science/article/pii/S1742706125000431 (2025).
25. Screen HRC, Lee DA, Bader DL, Shelton JC. An investigation into the effects of the hierarchical structure of tendon fascicles on micromechanical properties. Proc Inst Mech Eng Part H: J Eng Med. 2004;218:109–19. ISSN: 0954–4119. https://doi.org/10.1243/095441104322984004 (2024).
26. Jayes FL, et al. Loss of stiffness in collagen-rich uterine fibroids after digestion with purified collagenase Clostridium histolyticum. Am J Obstetr Gynecol. 2016;215:596.e1–8. ISSN: 1097–6868.
27. Budday S, et al. Mechanical characterization of human brain tissue. Acta Biomater. 2017;48: 319–40. ISSN: 1742–7061. https://www.sciencedirect.com/science/article/pii/S1742706116305633 (2025).
28. A Basic Introduction to Rheology White Paper. Worchestershire: Malvern Instruments; 2016, p. 1–20. https://cdn.technologynetworks.com/tn/resources/pdf/wp160620basicintrorheology.pdf (2025).
29. Barnes HA. A handbook of elementary rheology. Aberystwyth: University of Wales Institute of Non-Newtonian Fluid Mechanics; 2000. ISBN: 978-0-9538032-0-0.
30. VanLandingham M. Review of instrumented indentation. J Res Natl Inst Stand Technol. 2003;108:249. ISSN: 1044677X. https://nvlpubs.nist.gov/nistpubs/jres/108/4/j84vanl.pdf (2025).
31. Oyen ML, Cook RF. A practical guide for analysis of nanoindentation data. J Mech Behav Biomed Mater. Nanoindent Biol Mater. 2009;2:396–407. ISSN: 1751-6161. https://www.sciencedirect.com/science/article/pii/S1751616108000805 (2024).
32. Liu M, et al. Progress in indentation study of materials via both experimental and numerical methods. Crystals. 2017;7:258. ISSN: 2073-4352. https://www.mdpi.com/2073-4352/7/10/258 (2025).
33. Hu Y, Zhao X, Vlassak JJ, Suo Z. Using indentation to characterize the poroelasticity of gels. Appl Phys Lett. 2010;96:121904. ISSN: 0003-6951, 1077–3118. http://aip.scitation.org/doi/10.1063/1.3370354 (2023).
34. Islam MR, Oyen ML. Load-relaxation characteristics of chemical and physical hydrogels as soft tissue mimics. Experiment Mech. 2021;61:939–49. ISSN: 1741–2765. https://doi.org/10.1007/s11340-021-00712-x (2024).
35. Wang Q-M, Mohan AC, Oyen ML, Zhao X-H. Separating viscoelasticity and poroelasticity of gels with different length and time scales. Acta Mech Sin. 2014;30:20–7. ISSN: 0567–7718, 1614–3116. http://link.springer.com/10.1007/s10409-014-0015-z (2022).

36. Trache A, Meininger GA. Atomic Force Microscopy (AFM). Curr Protocols Microbiol. 2008;8:2C.2.1–17. ISSN: 1934–8533. https://onlinelibrary.wiley.com/doi/abs/10.1002/9780471729259.mc02c02s8 (2025).
37. Lekka M, Pabijan J. In: Santos NC, Carvalho FA. editors. Atomic force microscopy: methods and protocols. New York: Springer; 2019, p. 315–324. ISBN: 978-1-4939-8894-5. https://doi.org/10.1007/978-1-4939-8894-5_18 (2025).
38. Sumbul F, Rico F. In: Santos NC, Carvalho FA. editros. Atomic force microscopy: methods and protocols. New York: Springer; 2019. p. 163–189. ISBN: 978-1-4939-8894-5. https://doi.org/10.1007/978-1-4939-8894-5_9 (2025).
39. Arnold KM, Sicard D, Tschumperlin DJ, Westendorf JJ. Atomic force microscopy micro-indentation methods for determining the elastic modulus of murine articular cartilage. Sensors. 2023;23:1835. ISSN: 1424–8220. https://www.mdpi.com/1424-8220/23/4/1835 (2025).
40. Viji Babu PK, Rianna C, Mirastschijski U, Radmacher M. Nano-mechanical mapping of interdependent cell and ECM mechanics by AFM force spectroscopy. Scient Rep. 2019;9:12317. ISSN: 2045–2322. https://www.ncbi.nlm.nih.gov/pmc/articles/PMC6707266/ (2025).
41. Gdoutos E, Konsta-Gdoutos M. Mechanical testing of materials. Cham: Springer Nature Switzerland; 2024. ISBN: 978-3-031-45992-4. https://link.springer.com/10.1007/978-3-031-45990-0 (2025).
42. Rubinstein M, Colby RH. Polymer physics. Oxford: Oxford University Press; 2014. ISBN: 978-0-19-852059-7.
43. Knauss WG, Emri I, Lu H. In: Sharpe WN. editor. Springer handbook of experimental solid mechanics. Boston: Springer US; 2008. p. 49–96. ISBN: 978-0-387-30877-7. https://doi.org/10.1007/978-0-387-30877-7_3 (2025).
44. Mak AF. The apparent viscoelastic behavior of articular cartilage—the contributions from the intrinsic matrix viscoelasticity and interstitial fluid flows. J Biomech Eng. 1986;108:123–30. ISSN: 0148–0731. https://doi.org/10.1115/1.3138591 (2023).
45. Oftadeh R, Connizzo BK, Nia HT, Ortiz C, Grodzinsky AJ. Biological connective tissues exhibit viscoelastic and poroelastic behavior at different frequency regimes: application to tendon and skin biophysics. Acta Biomater. 2018;70:249–59. ISSN: 1742–7061. https://www.sciencedirect.com/science/article/pii/S1742706118300527 (2023).
46. Suh J-K, DiSilvestro MR. Biphasic poroviscoelastic behavior of hydrated biological soft tissue. J Appl Mech. 1999;66:528–35. ISSN: 0021–8936. https://doi.org/10.1115/1.2791079 (2023).
47. Li LP, Herzog W, Korhonen RK, Jurvelin JS. The role of viscoelasticity of collagen fibers in articular cartilage: axial tension versus compression. Med Eng Phys. 2005;27:51–7. ISSN: 1350–4533. https://www.sciencedirect.com/science/article/pii/S135045330400147X (2025).
48. Fodera DM, et al. Material properties of nonpregnant and pregnant human uterine layers. J Mech Behav Biomed Mater. 2024;151:106348. ISSN: 1751–6161. https://www.sciencedirect.com/science/article/pii/S1751616123007026 (2025).
49. Abbas Y, et al. Tissue stiffness at the human maternal–fetal interface. Hum Reprod (Oxford, England). 2019;34:1999–2008. ISSN: 0268–1161. https://www.ncbi.nlm.nih.gov/pmc/articles/PMC6809602/ (2025).
50. Fang S, et al. Anisotropic mechanical properties of the human uterus measured by spherical indentation. Ann Biomed Eng. 2021;49:1923–42. ISSN: 0090–6964. https://www.ncbi.nlm.nih.gov/pmc/articles/PMC8376808/ (2025).
51. Rogers R, et al. Mechanical homeostasis is altered in uterine leiomyoma. Am J Obstetr Gynecol. 2008;198:474.e1–11. ISSN: 1097–6868.
52. Norian JM, et al. Characterization of tissue biomechanics and mechanical signaling in uterine leiomyoma. Matrix Biol J Int Soc Matrix Biol. 2012;31:57–65. ISSN: 0945–053X. https://www.ncbi.nlm.nih.gov/pmc/articles/PMC3576015/ (2025).
53. Kiss MZ, et al. Frequency-dependent complex modulus of the uterus: preliminary results. Phys Med Biol. 2006;51:3683–95. ISSN: 0031-9155, 1361–6560. https://iopscience.iop.org/article/10.1088/0031-9155/51/15/006 (2025).

54. Brunengraber LN, Jayes FL, Leppert PC. Injectable clostridium histolyticum collagenase as a potential treatment for uterine fibroids. Reprod Sci. 2014;21:1452–9. ISSN: 1933–7191. https://www.ncbi.nlm.nih.gov/pmc/articles/PMC4231132/ (2024).
55. Omari EA, Varghese T, Kliewer MA, Harter J, Hartenbach EM. Dynamic and Quasi-Static mechanical testing for characterization of the viscoelastic properties of human uterine tissue. J Biomech. 2015;48:1730–6. ISSN: 0021–9290. https://www.ncbi.nlm.nih.gov/pmc/articles/PMC4582656/ (2025).
56. Purdy MP, et al. YAP/TAZ are activated by mechanical and hormonal stimuli in myometrium and exhibit increased baseline activation in uterine fibroids. Reprod Sci. 2020;27:1074–85. ISSN: 1933–7205. https://doi.org/10.1007/s43032-019-00106-4 (2024).
57. Pearsall GW, Roberts VL. Passive mechanical properties of uterine muscle (myometrium) tested *in vitro*. J Biomech. 1978;11:167–76. ISSN: 0021-9290. https://www.sciencedirect.com/science/article/pii/002192907890009X (2025).
58. Rupp JD, et al. Development and testing of a prototype pregnant abdomen for the small-female hybrid III ATD. Stapp Car Crash J. 2001;45:61–78. ISSN: 1532–8546.
59. Conrad JT, Johnson WL, Kuhn WK, Hunter CA. Passive stretch relationships in human uterine muscle. Am J Obstetr Gynecol. 1966;96:1055–9. ISSN: 00029378. https://linkinghub.elsevier.com/retrieve/pii/0002937866905138 (2025).
60. Wood C. Physiology of uterine contractions. J Obstetr Gynaecol Brit Commonw. 1964;71: 360–73. ISSN: 0022–3204.
61. Wang X. et al. The matrix stiffness is increased in the eutopic endometrium of adenomyosis patients: a study based on atomic force microscopy and histochemistry. Euro J Histochem: EJH 2024;68:4131. ISSN: 1121-760X. https://www.ncbi.nlm.nih.gov/pmc/articles/PMC11694501/ (2025).
62. Manoogian SJ, Bisplinghoff JA, Kemper AR, Duma SM. Dynamic material properties of the pregnant human uterus. J Biomech. 2012;45:1724–7. ISSN: 0021-9290. https://www.sciencedirect.com/science/article/pii/S0021929012002199 (2025).
63. Fang S. et al. Equilibrium mechanical properties of the nonhuman primate cervix. J Biomech Eng. 2024;146:081001. ISSN: 1528–8951.
64. Conrad JT, Ueland K. Reduction of the stretch modulus of human cervical tissue by prostaglandin E2. Am J Obstetr Gynecol. 1976;126:218–23. ISSN: 0002-9378, 1097-6868. https://www.ajog.org/article/0002-9378(76)90278-7/abstract (2025).
65. Rechberger T, Uldbjerg N, Oxlund H. Connective tissue changes in the cervix during normal pregnancy and pregnancy complicated by cervical incompetence. Obstetr Gynecol. 1988;71: 563–7. ISSN: 0029–7844.
66. Petersen LK, Oxlund H, Uldbjerg N, Forman A. In vitro analysis of muscular contractile ability and passive biomechanical properties of uterine cervical samples from nonpregnant women. Obstetr Gynecol. 1991;77:772–6. ISSN: 0029–7844.
67. Petersen LK, Vogel I, Oxlund H, Forman A, Uldbjerg N. No effects of human relaxin on the active and passive biomechanical properties of isolated cervical specimens from nonpregnant women. Euro J Obstetr Gynecol Reprod Biol. 1997;73:183–7. ISSN: 03012115. https://linkinghub.elsevier.com/retrieve/pii/S0301211597027322 (2025).
68. Dewall RJ, Varghese T, Kliewer MA, Harter JM, Hartenbach EM. Compression-dependent viscoelastic behavior of human cervix tissue. Ultrason Imaging. 2010;32:214–28. ISSN: 0161–7346. https://www.ncbi.nlm.nih.gov/pmc/articles/PMC3074596/ (2025).
69. Myers KM, et al. The mechanical role of the cervix in pregnancy. J Biomech. 2015;48:1511–23. ISSN: 1873–2380.
70. Myers KM, Socrate S, Paskaleva A, House M. A study of the anisotropy and tension/compression behavior of human cervical tissue. J Biomech Eng. 2010;132. ISSN: 0148–0731. https://doi.org/10.1115/1.3197847 (2025).
71. Shi L, et al. Anisotropic material characterization of human cervix tissue based on indentation and inverse finite element analysis. J Biomech Eng. 2019;141:0910171–3. ISSN: 1528–8951.

72. Myers KM, Paskaleva AP, House M, Socrate S. Mechanical and biochemical properties of human cervical tissue. Acta Biomater. 2008;4:104–16. ISSN: 1742-7061. https://www.sciencedirect.com/science/article/pii/S1742706107000682 (2025).
73. Bursać PM, Obitz TW, Eisenberg SR, Stamenović D. Confined and unconfined stress relaxation of cartilage: appropriateness of a transversely isotropic analysis. J Biomech. 1999;32: 1125–30. ISSN: 0021-9290. https://www.sciencedirect.com/science/article/pii/S0021929099001050 (2025).
74. Kauer M, Vuskovic V, Dual J, Szekely G, Bajka M. Inverse finite element characterization of soft tissues. Med Image Anal. Special Issue Med Image Comput Comput-Assist Intervent - MICCAI 2001 2002;6:275–87. ISSN: 1361-8415. https://www.sciencedirect.com/science/article/pii/S1361841502000853 (2025).
75. Oxlund BS, et al. Collagen concentration and biomechanical properties of samples from the lower uterine cervix in relation to age and parity in non-pregnant women. Reprod Biol Endocrinol 2010;8:82. ISSN: 1477-7827. https://rbej.biomedcentral.com/articles/10.1186/1477-7827-8-82 (2025).
76. Smith M. ABAQUS/standard user's manual, version 6.9. Johnston: Dassault Systèmes Simulia Corp, 2009. https://research.manchester.ac.uk/en/publications/abaqusstandard-users-manual-version-69 (2025).
77. Jelen K, Lopot F, Budka S, Novácek V, Sedlácek R. Rheological properties of myometrium: experimental quantification and mathematical modeling. Neuro Endocrinol Lett. 2008;29: 454–60. ISSN: 0172-780X.
78. Islam MR, Virag J, Oyen ML. Micromechanical poroelastic and viscoelastic properties of ex-vivo soft tissues. J Biomech 2020;113:110090. ISSN: 1873–2380.
79. Menczel JD, Prime RB. Thermal analysis of polymers: fundamentals and applications. Hoboken: John Wiley; 2009. ISBN: 978-0-471-76917-0.
80. Cummins BM, Chinthapatla R, Ligler FS, Walker GM. Time-dependent model for fluid flow in porous materials with multiple pore sizes. Anal Chem. 2017;89:4377–81. ISSN: 0003-2700. https://doi.org/10.1021/acs.analchem.6b04717 (2025).
81. Conrad JT, Ueland K. The stretch modulus of human cervical tissue in spontaneous, oxytocin-induced, and prostaglandin E2-induced labor. Am J Obstetr Gynecol. 1979;133:11–4. ISSN: 00029378. https://linkinghub.elsevier.com/retrieve/pii/0002937879904034 (2025).
82. Fernandez M, Vink J, Yoshida K, Wapner R, Myers KM. Direct measurement of the permeability of human cervical tissue. J Biomech Eng. 2013;135:021024. ISSN: 1528–8951.
83. Yao W, et al. Measuring the compressive viscoelastic mechanical properties of human cervical tissue using indentation. J Mech Behav Biomed Mater. 2014;34:18–26. ISSN: 1751-6161. https://www.sciencedirect.com/science/article/pii/S1751616114000174 (2025).
84. Myers KM, et al. A continuous fiber distribution material model for human cervical tissue. J Biomech. 2015;48:1533–40. ISSN: 1873–2380.
85. Lin AC, et al. Shape or size matters? Towards standard reporting of tensile testing parameters for human soft tissues: systematic review and finite element analysis. Front Bioeng Biotechnol. 2024;12. ISSN: 2296-4185. https://www.frontiersin.org/journals/bioengineering-and-biotechnology/articles/10.3389/fbioe.2024.1368383/full (2026).
86. Ma Y, Feng X, Rogers JA, Huang Y, Zhang Y. Design and application of 'J-shaped' stress-strain behavior in stretchable electronics: a review. Lab Chip. 2017;17:1689–1704. ISSN: 1473-0197. https://www.ncbi.nlm.nih.gov/pmc/articles/PMC5505255/ (2025).
87. Yoshida K, Jayyosi C, Lee N, Mahendroo M, Myers KM. Mechanics of cervical remodelling: insights from rodent models of pregnancy. Interf Focus. 2019;9:20190026. ISSN: 2042-8898, 2042-8901. https://royalsocietypublishing.org/doi/10.1098/rsfs.2019.0026 (2025).
88. Conrad JT, Tokarz RD, Williford JF. In: Dilatation of the uterine cervix: connective tissue biology and clinical management. New York: Raven Press Press; 1980. p. 255–264. ISBN: 978-0-89-004300-4.

89. Louwagie EM, et al. The biomechanical evolution of the uterus and cervix and fetal growth in human pregnancy. npj Women's Health. 2024;2:1–9. ISSN: 2948-1716. https://www.nature.com/articles/s44294-024-00038-8 (2025).
90. Shi L, Myers KM. Microstructure-informed hyper-viscoelastic model capturing soft tissue tensile behavior across large deformations. J Mech Phys Solids. 2026;206:106348. ISSN: 0022-5096. https://www.sciencedirect.com/science/article/pii/S0022509625003229 (2025).
91. Sassi AB, McCullough KD, Cost MR, Hillier SL, Rohan LC. Permeability of tritiated water through human cervical and vaginal tissue. J Pharmaceut Sci. 2004;93:2009–16. ISSN: 1520-6017. https://onlinelibrary.wiley.com/doi/abs/10.1002/jps.20107 (2025).
92. Nijkang NP, Anderson L, Markham R, Manconi F. Endometrial polyps: pathogenesis, sequelae and treatment. SAGE Open Med. 2019;7:2050312119848247. ISSN: 2050–3121.
93. Jang S, Hwang SO. The risk factors for premalignant and malignant endometrial polyps in premenopausal and postmenopausal women and trends over the past decade: a retrospective study in a single center, South Korea. Euro J Obstetr Gynecol Reprod Biol. 2024;295:118–23. ISSN: 03012115. https://linkinghub.elsevier.com/retrieve/pii/S0301211524000411 (2025).
94. Dreisler E, Stampe Sorensen S, Ibsen PH, Lose G. Prevalence of endometrial polyps and abnormal uterine bleeding in a Danish population aged 20–74 years. Ultrasound Obstetr Gynecol. 2009;33:102–8. ISSN: 0960-7692, 1469-0705. https://obgyn.onlinelibrary.wiley.com/doi/10.1002/uog.6259 (2025).
95. Hileeto D, Fadare O, Martel M, Zheng W. Age dependent association of endometrial polyps with increased risk of cancer involvement. World J Surg Oncol. 2005;3:8. ISSN: 1477–7819.
96. Vora Z, et al. Transvaginal shear wave elastography for assessment of endometrial and subendometrial pathologies: a prospective pilot study. J Ultrasound Med. 2022;41:61–70. ISSN: 0278-4297, 1550-9613. https://onlinelibrary.wiley.com/doi/10.1002/jum.15679 (2025).
97. Gultekin I, et al. Elastosonographic evaluation of patients with a sonographic finding of thickened endometrium. Euro J Obstetr Gynecol Reprod Biol. 2016;198:105–9. ISSN: 03012115. https://linkinghub.elsevier.com/retrieve/pii/S0301211516000191 (2025).
98. Buck Louis GM, et al. Incidence of endometriosis by study population and diagnostic method: the ENDO study. Fertil Steril. 2011;96:360–5. ISSN: 00150282. https://linkinghub.elsevier.com/retrieve/pii/S0015028211008739 (2025).
99. Giudice LC, Kao LC. Endometriosis. Lancet. 2004;364:1789–99. ISSN: 01406736. https://linkinghub.elsevier.com/retrieve/pii/S0140673604174035 (2025).
100. Bulun SE, et al. Endometriosis. Endocrine Rev. 2019;40:1048–79. ISSN: 0163-769X, 1945-7189. https://academic.oup.com/edrv/article/40/4/1048/5469279 (2025).
101. Brookmeyer C, Fishman EK, Sheth S. Emergent and unusual presentations of endometriosis: pearls and pitfalls. Emerg Radiol. 2023;30:377–85. ISSN: 1438-1435. https://link.springer.com/10.1007/s10140-023-02128-7 (2025).
102. Sarsenova M, et al. Endometriotic lesions exhibit distinct metabolic signature compared to paired eutopic endometrium at the single-cell level. Commun Biol. 2024;7:1026. ISSN: 2399-3642. https://www.nature.com/articles/s42003-024-06713-5 (2025).
103. Fonseca MAS, et al. Single-cell transcriptomic analysis of endometriosis. Nat Genet. 2023;55:255–67. ISSN: 1061-4036, 1546-1718. https://www.nature.com/articles/s41588-022-01254-1 (2025).
104. Zou G, et al. Cell subtypes and immune dysfunction in peritoneal fluid of endometriosis revealed by single-cell RNA-sequencing. Cell Biosci. 2021;11:98. ISSN: 2045-3701. https://cellandbioscience.biomedcentral.com/articles/10.1186/s13578-021-00613-5 (2025).
105. Sampson JA. Peritoneal endometriosis due to the menstrual dissemination of endometrial tissue into the peritoneal cavity. Am J Obstetr Gynecol. 1927;14:422–469. ISSN: 0002-9378. https://linkinghub.elsevier.com/retrieve/pii/S000293781530003X (2025).

106. Bulletti C, et al. Characteristics of uterine contractility during menses in women with mild to moderate endometriosis. Fertil Steril. 2002;77:1156–61. ISSN: 0015-0282. https://www.sciencedirect.com/science/article/pii/S001502820203087X (2025).
107. Salamanca A, Beltrán E. Subendometrial contractility in menstrual phase visualized by transvaginal sonography in patients with endometriosis. Fertil Steril. 1995;64:193–5. ISSN: 0015-0282. https://www.sciencedirect.com/science/article/pii/S0015028216576808 (2025).
108. Salmeri N, et al. Functional determinants of uterine contractility in endometriosis and adenomyosis: a systematic review and meta-analysis. Fertil Steril. 2024;122:1063–78. ISSN: 0015-0282. https://www.sciencedirect.com/science/article/pii/S0015028224006228 (2025).
109. Halme J, Hammond MG, Hulka JF, Raj SG, Talbert LM. Retrograde menstruation in healthy women and in patients with endometriosis. Obstetr Gynecol. 1984;64:151–4. ISSN: 0029-7844.
110. Vercellini P, Viganò P, Somigliana E, Fedele L. Endometriosis: pathogenesis and treatment. Nat Rev Endocrinol. 2014;10:261–75. ISSN: 1759-5029, 1759-5037. https://www.nature.com/articles/nrendo.2013.255 (2025).
111. Batur A, et al. The utility of ultrasound elastography in differentiation of endometriomas and hemorrhagic ovarian cysts. J Med Ultrason. 2016;43:395–400. ISSN: 1346-4523, 1613-2254. http://link.springer.com/10.1007/s10396-016-0701-5 (2025).
112. Kido A, et al. Cine MR imaging of uterine peristalsis in patients with endometriosis. Euro Radiol. 2007;17:1813–9. ISSN: 0938-7994.
113. Wang S, et al. Noninvasive electrophysiological imaging identifies 4D uterine peristalsis patterns in subjects with normal menstrual cycles and patients with endometriosis. Res Square. 2023;rs.3.rs–2432192. ISSN: 2693-5015. https://www.ncbi.nlm.nih.gov/pmc/articles/PMC10029120/ (2025).
114. Leyendecker G, Kunz G, Wildt L, Beil D, Deininger H. Uterine hyperperistalsis and dysperistalsis as dysfunctions of the mechanism of rapid sperm transport in patients with endometriosis and infertility. Hum Reprod. 1996;11:1542–51. ISSN: 0268-1161. https://doi.org/10.1093/oxfordjournals.humrep.a019435 (2025).
115. Cramer SF, Patel A. The frequency of uterine leiomyomas. Am J Clin Pathol. 1990;94:435–8. ISSN: 0002-9173.
116. Baird DD, Dunson DB, Hill MC, Cousins D, Schectman JM. High cumulative incidence of uterine leiomyoma in black and white women: ultrasound evidence. Am J Obstetr Gynecol. 2003;188:100–7. ISSN: 0002-9378. https://www.sciencedirect.com/science/article/pii/S0002937802714294 (2024).
117. Hartmann KE, et al. Management of uterine fibroids. Rockville: Agency for Healthcare Research and Quality (US); 2017. http://www.ncbi.nlm.nih.gov/books/NBK537742/ (2024).
118. Bulun SE. Uterine fibroids. New Engl J Med. 2013;369:1344–55. ISSN: 0028-4793 (2024).
119. Downes E, et al. The burden of uterine fibroids in five European countries. Euro J Obstetr Gynecol Reprod Biol. 2010;152:96–102. ISSN: 0301-2115. https://www.sciencedirect.com/science/article/pii/S0301211510002563 (2024).
120. Stewart EA, et al. Uterine fibroids. Nat Rev Dis Primers. 2016;2:16043. ISSN: 2056-676X. https://www.nature.com/articles/nrdp201643 (2024).
121. Marshall LM, et al. Variation in the incidence of uterine leiomyoma among premenopausal women by age and race. Obstetr Gynecol. 1997;90:967–73. ISSN: 0029-7844. https://www.sciencedirect.com/science/article/pii/S0029784497005346 (2024).
122. Guo XC, Segars JH. The impact and management of fibroids for fertility: an evidence-based approach. Obstetr Gynecol Clin North America. 2012;39:521–33. ISSN: 0889-8545. https://www.ncbi.nlm.nih.gov/pmc/articles/PMC3608270/ (2024).
123. Li H, Hu Z, Fan Y, Hao Y. The influence of uterine fibroids on adverse outcomes in pregnant women: a meta-analysis. BMC Pregnancy Childbirth. 2024;24:345. ISSN: 1471-2393. https://doi.org/10.1186/s12884-024-06545-5 (2024).
124. Jayes FL, et al. Evidence of biomechanical and collagen heterogeneity in uterine fibroids. PloS One. 2019;14:e0215646. ISSN: 1932-6203.

125. Moshesh M, Peddada SD, Cooper T, Baird D. Intra-observer variation in fibroid size measurements: estimated effects on assessing fibroid growth. J Ultrasound Med Off J Am Inst Ultrasound Med 2014;33:1217–24. ISSN: 0278-4297. https://www.ncbi.nlm.nih.gov/pmc/articles/PMC5452979/ (2025).
126. Bray MJ, Torstenson ES, Jones SH, Edwards TL, Velez Edwards DR. Evaluating risk factors for differences in fibroid size and number using a large electronic health record population. Maturitas. 2018;114:9–13. ISSN: 0378-5122. https://www.ncbi.nlm.nih.gov/pmc/articles/PMC6022822/ (2025).
127. Lim PT, Tan CH, Chia HL, Phoon J. Management of a giant uterine leiomyoma. BMJ Case Rep. 2018;2018:bcr2017224052. ISSN: 1757-790X. https://www.ncbi.nlm.nih.gov/pmc/articles/PMC6129052/ (2025).
128. Amber I, Kennedy G, Martinez H, Pearson JM, Jimenez E. A leiomyoma in a cachectic woman presenting as a giant abdominal mass. J Radiol Case Rep. 2009;3:23–9. ISSN: 1943-0922. https://www.ncbi.nlm.nih.gov/pmc/articles/PMC3303273/ (2025).
129. Viva W, et al. Massive uterine fibroid: a diagnostic dilemma: a case report and review of the literature. J Med Case Rep. 2021;15:344. ISSN: 1752–1947. https://doi.org/10.1186/s13256-021-02959-3 (2025).
130. Holdsworth-Carson SJ, Zaitseva M, Vollenhoven BJ, Rogers PA. Clonality of smooth muscle and fibroblast cell populations isolated from human fibroid and myometrial tissues. Molecul Hum Reprod. 2014;20:250–9. ISSN: 1360–9947. https://doi.org/10.1093/molehr/gat083 (2025).
131. Gomez E, Nguyen M-LT, Fursevich D, Macura K, Gupta A. MRI-based pictorial review of the FIGO classification system for uterine fibroids. Abdom Radiol. 2021;46:2146–55. ISSN: 2366-0058. https://doi.org/10.1007/s00261-020-02882-z (2024).
132. Munro MG, Critchley HO, Fraser IS, Committee tFMD. The two FIGO systems for normal and abnormal uterine bleeding symptoms and classification of causes of abnormal uterine bleeding in the reproductive years: 2018 revisions. Int J Gynecol Obstetr. 2018;143:393–408. ISSN: 1879-3479. https://onlinelibrary.wiley.com/doi/abs/10.1002/ijgo.12666 (2024).
133. Holdsworth-Carson SJ. et al. Differences in the cellular composition of small versus large uterine fibroids. https://rep.bioscientifica.com/view/journals/rep/152/5/467.xml (2025).
134. Casey R, Rogers P, Vollenhoven B. An immunohistochemical analysis of fibroid vasculature. Hum Reprod. 2000;15:1469–1475. ISSN: 0268-1161. https://doi.org/10.1093/humrep/15.7.1469 (2025).
135. Sozen I, Senturk LM, Arici A. Effect of gonadotropin-releasing hormone agonists on monocyte chemotactic protein-1 production and macrophage infiltration in leiomyomatous uterus. Fertil Steril. 2001;76:792–796. ISSN: 0015-0282. https://www.sciencedirect.com/science/article/pii/S0015028201023780 (2025).
136. Goad J, et al. Single-cell sequencing reveals novel cellular heterogeneity in uterine leiomyomas. Hum Reprod. 2022;37:2334–49. ISSN: 0268-1161, 1460-2350. https://academic.oup.com/humrep/article/37/10/2334/6674607 (2025).
137. Corder RD, et al. Using rheology to quantify the effects of localized collagenase treatments on uterine fibroid digestion. Acta Biomater. 2021;134:443–52. ISSN: 1742-7061. https://www.sciencedirect.com/science/article/pii/S1742706121005237 (2024).
138. Wolańska M, Sobolewski K, Drozdzewicz M, Bańkowski E. Extracellular matrix components in uterine leiomyoma and their alteration during the tumour growth. Mol Cell Biochem. 1998;189:145–52. ISSN: 0300-8177.
139. Jamaluddin MFB, Nahar P, Tanwar PS. Proteomic characterization of the extracellular matrix of human uterine fibroids. Endocrinology. 2018;159:2656–69. ISSN: 1945-7170. https://academic.oup.com/endo/article/159/7/2656/4996506 (2025).
140. Jamaluddin MFB, et al. Proteomic profiling of human uterine fibroids reveals upregulation of the extracellular matrix protein periostin. Endocrinology 2018;159:1106–18. ISSN: 0013-7227. https://doi.org/10.1210/en.2017-03018 (2025).

141. Rossi M, et al. Mechanisms and pathogenesis of adenomyosis. Curr Obstetr Gynecol Rep. 2022;11:95–102. ISSN: 2161-3303. https://doi.org/10.1007/s13669-022-00326-7 (2025).
142. Bergeron C, Amant F, Ferenczy A. Pathology and physiopathology of adenomyosis. Best Pract Res Clin Obstetr Gynaecol. Adenomyosis. 2006;20:511–21. ISSN: 1521-6934. https://www.sciencedirect.com/science/article/pii/S1521693406000307 (2025).
143. Antero MF, Ayhan A, Segars J, Shih I-M. Pathology and pathogenesis of adenomyosis. Semin Reproduct Med. 2020;38:108–18. ISSN: 1526-8004. https://www.ncbi.nlm.nih.gov/pmc/articles/PMC7987203/ (2025).
144. Upson K, Missmer SA. Epidemiology of adenomyosis. Semin Reprod Med. 2020;38:89–107. ISSN: 1526-8004. https://www.ncbi.nlm.nih.gov/pmc/articles/PMC7927213/ (2025).
145. Peric H, Fraser IS. The symptomatology of adenomyosis. Best Pract Res Clin Obstetr Gynaecol. Adenomyosis. 2006;20:547–55. ISSN: 1521-6934. https://www.sciencedirect.com/science/article/pii/S1521693406000204 (2025).
146. Săsăran V, et al. Value of strain-ratio elastography in the diagnosis and differentiation of uterine fibroids and adenomyosis. J Personal Med. 2021;11:824. ISSN: 2075-4426. https://www.ncbi.nlm.nih.gov/pmc/articles/PMC8399978/ (2025).
147. Harmsen MJ, et al. Uterine junctional zone and adenomyosis: comparison of MRI, transvaginal ultrasound and histology. Ultrasound Obstetr Gynecol. 2023;62:42–60. ISSN: 1469-0705. https://onlinelibrary.wiley.com/doi/abs/10.1002/uog.26117 (2025).
148. Fusi L, Cloke B, Brosens JJ. The uterine junctional zone. Best Pract Res Clin Obstet Gynaecol Adenomyosis. 2006;20:479–91. ISSN: 1521-6934. https://www.sciencedirect.com/science/article/pii/S1521693406000356 (2025).
149. Ren Q, et al. Application of elastography to diagnose adenomyosis and evaluate the degree of dysmenorrhea: a prospective observational study. Reprod Biol Endocrinol. 2023;21:98. ISSN: 1477-7827. https://doi.org/10.1186/s12958-023-01145-y (2025).
150. Pongpunprut S, et al. A comparison of shear wave elastography between normal myometrium, uterine fibroids, and adenomyosis: a cross-sectional study. Int J Fertil Steril. 2022;16:49–54. ISSN: 2008-076X.
151. Acar S, Millar E, Mitkova M, Mitkov V. Value of ultrasound shear wave elastography in the diagnosis of adenomyosis. Ultrasound J Brit Medi Ultrasound Soc. 2016;24:205–13. ISSN: 1742-271X. https://www.ncbi.nlm.nih.gov/pmc/articles/PMC5098712/ (2025).
152. Frank ML, et al. Importance of transvaginal elastography in the diagnosis of uterine fibroids and adenomyosis. Ultraschall in Der Medizin (Stuttgart, Germany: 1980) 2016;37:373–8. ISSN: 1438-8782.
153. Stoelinga B, Hehenkamp WJK, Brölmann HaM, Huirne JaF. Real-time elastography for assessment of uterine disorders. Ultrasound Obstetr Gynecol. 2014;43:218–26. ISSN: 1469-0705. https://onlinelibrary.wiley.com/doi/abs/10.1002/uog.12519 (2025).
154. Görgülü FF, Okçu NT. Which imaging method is better for the differentiation of adenomyosis and uterine fibroids? J Gynecol Obstetr Hum Reprod. 2021;50:102002. ISSN: 2468-7847. https://www.sciencedirect.com/science/article/pii/S246878472030372X (2025).
155. Rees CO, et al. Quantitative ultrasound measurement of uterine contractility in adenomyotic vs. normal uteri: a multicenter prospective study. Fertil Steril. 2024;121:864–72. ISSN: 1556-5653.
156. Arena A, et al. Uterine peristalsis in women affected by adenomyosis: a step to-wards functional assessment. Int J Gynecol Obstetr. 2024;165:666–71. ISSN: 1879-3479. https://onlinelibrary.wiley.com/doi/abs/10.1002/ijgo.15299 (2025).
157. Ohuma EO, et al. National, regional, and global estimates of preterm birth in 2020, with trends from 2010: a systematic analysis. Lancet. 2023;402:1261–71. ISSN: 0140-6736, 1474-547X. https://www.thelancet.com/journals/lancet/article/PIIS0140-6736(23)00878-4/fulltext (2025).
158. Vink J, Myers K. Cervical alterations in pregnancy. London: Bailliere Tindall Ltd; 2018. ISSN: 15321932. https://www.ncbi.nlm.nih.gov/pmc/articles/PMC6282836/, pmc/articles/PMC6282836/?report=abstract%20.

159. Prediction and prevention of spontaneous preterm birth: ACOG practice bulletin, Number 234. Obstetr Gynecol. 2021;138(2):e65–90. https://doi.org/10.1097/AOG.0000000000004479
160. Waldorf et al. Uterine overdistention induces preterm labor mediated by inflammation: observations in pregnant women and nonhuman primates. Am J Obstetr Gynecol. 2015;213 (6):830.e1–19. https://doi.org/10.1016/j.ajog.2015.08.028
161. Bouvier D, et al. Risk factors and outcomes of preterm premature rupture of membranes in a cohort of 6968 pregnant women prospectively recruited. J Clin Med. 2019;8:1987. ISSN: 2077-0383. https://www.ncbi.nlm.nih.gov/pmc/articles/PMC6912547/ (2023).
162. Waldorf KM, et al. Uterine overdistention induces preterm labor mediated by inflammation: observations in pregnant women and nonhuman primates. Am J Obstetr Gynecol. 2015;213: 830.e1–19. ISSN: 10976868.
163. Thakur M, Mahajan K. StatPearls. Treasure Island: StatPearls Publishing; 2023. http://www.ncbi.nlm.nih.gov/books/NBK525954/.
164. Practice Bulletin No. 141: Management of Menopausal Symptoms. Obstetr Gynecol. 2014;123:202. ISSN: 0029-7844. https://journals.lww.com/greenjournal/fulltext/2014/01000/practice_bulletin_no__141__management_of.37.aspx (2025).
165. Stone J, House M. Measurement of cervical softness before cerclage placement with an aspiration-based device. Am J Obstetr Gynecol MFM 2023;5:100881. ISSN: 25899333. https://linkinghub.elsevier.com/retrieve/pii/S258993332300023X (2024).
166. Spontaneous preterm birth: Overview of risk factors and prognosis. 2024. https://www.uptodate.com/contents/spontaneous-preterm-birth-overview-of-risk-factors-and-prognosis (2024).
167. Galal M, Symonds I, Murray H, Petraglia F, Smith R. Postterm pregnancy. Facts Views Vis ObGyn 2012;4:175–87. ISSN: 2032-0418. https://www.ncbi.nlm.nih.gov/pmc/articles/PMC3991404/ (2024).
168. ACOG Practice Bulletin #55: management of postterm pregnancy. Obstetr Gynecol. 2004;104:639–46. ISSN: 0029-7844. http://journals.lww.com/00006250-200409000-00052 (2024).
169. Martin JA, et al. Births: final data for 2005. Natl Vital Stat Rep From Centers Dis Control Prevent Natl Center Health Stat Natl Vital Stat Syst. 2007;56:1–103. ISSN: 1551-8922.
170. Rath W, Kummer J, Königbauer JT, Hellmeyer L, Stelzl P. Synthetic osmotic dilators for pre-induction cervical ripening– an evidence-based review. Geburtshilfe und Frauenheilkunde 2023;83:1491–9. ISSN: 0016-5751. https://www.ncbi.nlm.nih.gov/pmc/articles/PMC10689108/ (2025).
171. Silver RM. Abnormal placentation: placenta previa, vasa previa, and placenta accreta. Obstetr Gynecol. 2015;126:654–68. ISSN: 0029-7844. https://journals.lww.com/greenjournal/Fulltext/2015/09000/Abnormal_Placentation__Placenta_Previa,_Vasa.30.aspx (2021).
172. Belfort MA. Placenta accreta. Am J Obstetr Gynecol. 2010;203:430–9. ISSN: 0002-9378. https://www.sciencedirect.com/science/article/pii/S0002937810011592 (2021).
173. Jauniaux E, Moffett A, Burton GJ. Placental implantation disorders. Obstetr Gynecol Clin North America. Hum Placenta Health Dis. 2020;47:117–32. ISSN: 0889-8545. https://www.sciencedirect.com/science/article/pii/S0889854519301111 (2021).
174. Jauniaux E, Jurkovic D, Hussein AM, Burton GJ. New insights into the etiopathology of placenta accreta spectrum. Am J Obstetr Gynecol. 2022;227:384–91. ISSN: 0002-9378. https://www.sciencedirect.com/science/article/pii/S0002937822001673 (2023).
175. Hull AD, Resnik R. Placenta accreta and postpartum hemorrhage. Clin Obstetr Gynecol. 2010;53:228–36. ISSN: 0009-9201. https://journals.lww.com/clinicalobgyn/Fulltext/2010/03000/Placenta_Accreta_and_Postpartum_Hemorrhage.23.aspx (2021).
176. Bartels HC, Postle JD, Downey P, Brennan DJ. Placenta accreta spectrum: a review of pathology, molecular biology, and biomarkers. Dis Markers. 2018;2018:e1507674. ISSN: 0278-0240. https://www.hindawi.com/journals/dm/2018/1507674/ (2021).

177. Boerma T, et al. Global epidemiology of use of and disparities in caesarean sections. Lancet 2018;392:1341–48. ISSN: 0140-6736. https://www.sciencedirect.com/science/article/pii/S0140673618319287 (2025).
178. Betran AP, Ye J, Moller A-B, Souza JP, Zhang J. Trends and projections of caesarean section rates: global and regional estimates. BMJ Global Health. 2021;6. ISSN: 2059-7908. https://gh.bmj.com/content/6/6/e005671 (2025).
179. Higgins MF, Monteith C, Foley M, O'Herlihy C. Real increasing incidence of hysterectomy for placenta accreta following previous caesarean section. Euro J Obstetr Gynecol Reprod Biol. 2013;171:54–6. ISSN: 1872-7654.
180. Paping A, et al. Uterine scars after caesarean delivery: from histology to the molecular and ultrastructural level. Wound Repair Regener. 2023;31:752–63. ISSN: 1067-1927, 1524-475X. https://onlinelibrary.wiley.com/doi/10.1111/wrr.13127 (2025).
181. Di Pasquo E, et al. Evaluation of the uterine scar stiffness in women with previous Cesarean section by ultrasound elastography: a cohort study. Clin Imaging. 2020;64:53–6. ISSN: 0899-7071. https://www.sciencedirect.com/science/article/pii/S0899707120300917 (2024).
182. Hofmeyr GJ, Say L, Gülmezoglu AM. WHO systematic review of maternal mortality and morbidity: the prevalence of uterine rupture. BJOG Int J Obstetr Gynaecol. 2005;112:1221–8. ISSN: 1470-0328.
183. Al-Zirqi I, Daltveit AK, Forsén L, Stray-Pedersen B, Vangen S. Risk factors for complete uterine rupture. Am J Obstetr Gynecol. 2017;216:165.e1–8. ISSN: 00029378. https://linkinghub.elsevier.com/retrieve/pii/S0002937816309127 (2025).
184. Rotas MA, Haberman S, Levgur M. Cesarean scar ectopic pregnancies: etiology, diagnosis, and management. Obstetr Gynecol. 2006;107:1373–81. ISSN: 0029-7844. http://journals.lww.com/00006250-200606000-00025 (2025).
185. Rozenberg P, et al. Evaluation of the usefulness of ultrasound measurement of the lower uterine segment before delivery of women with a prior cesarean delivery: a randomized trial. Am J Obstetr Gynecol. 2022;226:253.e1–9. ISSN: 00029378. https://linkinghub.elsevier.com/retrieve/pii/S000293782100870X (2025).
186. Lieberman E. Risk factors for uterine rupture during a trial of labor after cesarean. Clin Obstetr Gynecol. 2001;44:609. ISSN: 0009-9201. https://journals.lww.com/clinicalobgyn/fulltext/2001/09000/risk_factors_for_uterine_rupture_during_a_trial_of.18.aspx (2025).
187. Aboughalia H, et al. Imaging evaluation of uterine perforation and rupture. Abdominal Radiol. 2021;46:4946–66. ISSN: 2366-004X, 2366-0058. https://link.springer.com/10.1007/s00261-021-03171-z (2025).
188. Campo H, Santamaria X, Cervelló I, Simón C. In: Handbook of tissue engineering scaffolds: volume two. Amsterdam: Elsevier; 2019. p. 283–316. ISBN: 978-0-08-102561-1. https://linkinghub.elsevier.com/retrieve/pii/B9780081025611000117 (2025).
189. Koullali B, House MD. Handbook of tissue engineering scaffolds: volume two. Amsterdam: Elsevier; 2019, p. 333–43. ISBN: 978-0-08-102561-1. https://linkinghub.elsevier.com/retrieve/pii/B9780081025611000130 (2025).

Mechanobiology of the Uterus and Maternal Fetal Interface During Pregnancy

Cecelia E. Curtis, Jessica Terray, and Adrienne K. Scott

Abstract During pregnancy, the tissues of the female reproductive system dynamically remodel throughout gestation, at the onset of labor, and during postpartum involution. While hormones and biochemical signaling play an important role in the regulation of reproductive tissues, researchers are starting to uncover how the mechanical environment influences cells of the female reproductive system. During pregnancy, the extracellular matrix (ECM) is extremely dynamic. ECM remodeling results in changes in stiffness, anisotropy, and viscoelastic properties. Additionally, as the fetus grows, the stress and strain on tissues like the fetal membrane and the uterus increase. Mechanobiology, or the study of how cells respond to mechanical cues, is an emerging area of research in pregnancy. This chapter provides a brief overview of the mechanotransduction mechanisms that influence pregnancy from implantation to the onset of labor. Specifically, the chapter focuses on tissues that adapt, remodel, or support the increasing load of the fetus throughout pregnancy, including the fetal membranes, placenta, uterus, and cervix. Understanding how the biomechanical environment changes in pregnancy and regulates cell and tissue adaptations could elucidate important mechanisms of pregnancy, such as embryo implantation, dynamic tissue remodeling, rupture of the fetal membrane, the onset of labor, placental dysfunction, preterm birth, and more.

Keywords Mechanobiology · Pregnancy · Biomechanics · Mechanotransduction · Tissue remodeling · Uterus · Cervix · Placenta · Fetal membrane · In vitro models

---

Cecelia E. Curtis and Jessica Terray contributed equally with all other contributors.

C. E. Curtis · J. Terray · A. K. Scott (✉)
Aerospace and Mechanical Engineering, University of Notre Dame, Notre Dame, IN, USA

Bioengineering Program, University of Notre Dame, Notre Dame, IN, USA
e-mail: ccurtis6@nd.edu; jterray@nd.edu; ascott29@nd.edu

S. G. Zambuto, M. L. Oyen (eds.), *Biomaterials for Women's Health Engineering*,
https://doi.org/10.1007/978-3-032-10745-9_7

1 Mechanobiology

Mechanical forces have long been recognized to direct how tissues adapt, especially in the field of orthopedics. In 1638, Galileo reported that bone shape was related to mechanical loading. Later, the idea that bones adapt to mechanical stimuli, known as Wolff's law, was proposed by Julius Wolff in 1892 [1]. Since then, with the availability of advanced imaging and biomolecular techniques, researchers have been revealing the mechanisms of how cells adapt to mechanical forces. Cells sense mechanical cues, such as tensile, compressive, and shear stress, and adapt in response to these changes in mechanics. This change in behavior, or change in cell phenotype, occurs through various mechanisms including conformational changes of cell membrane proteins that result in activation of cellular pathways. Alternatively, force can be directly transferred to the nucleus and influence gene expression since the cytoskeleton and nucleus are connected through the LINC (linker of nucleoskeleton and cytoskeleton) complex. Mechanobiology is known to regulate many physiological processes like embryonic development, wound healing, adaptation of the cardiovascular system, and pregnancy. At the same time, aberrant mechanotransduction can contribute to disease states (e.g., fibrosis and cancer), but also may initiate or progress pregnancy complications [2].

1.1 Cell-Membrane Mechanosensors

Stretch-activated ion channels, focal adhesion complexes, and cell–cell junctions are all examples of sensors on the cell membrane that respond to mechanical force [2] (Fig. 1). For example, in response to stretch, certain ion channels like Piezo1 or Piezo2, transient receptor potential (TRP) channels, and TREK channels will allow the influx of ions, which initiates a cascade of cellular signaling pathways [3–5]. Focal adhesion complexes physically link the extracellular matrix (ECM) to the cytoskeleton via integrin receptors and are also mechanosensitive. Examples of force-sensitive focal adhesion proteins include talin, vinculin, and focal adhesion kinases (FAK) [6]. Talin proteins unfold under tension, bind to other focal adhesion proteins, such as vinculin and paxillin, and allow for adhesion growth and further cellular signaling [7, 8] (Fig. 1). FAKs sense ECM stiffness, initiating pathways that involve signaling molecules such as Rho/ROCK, PI3K/AKT, and MAPK, which ultimately activate transcription factors and lead to changes in gene expression [9]. Additionally, cell–cell junctions, such as cadherins, are known to control the growth and proliferation of cells through mechanical signals from neighboring cells [10] (Fig. 1).

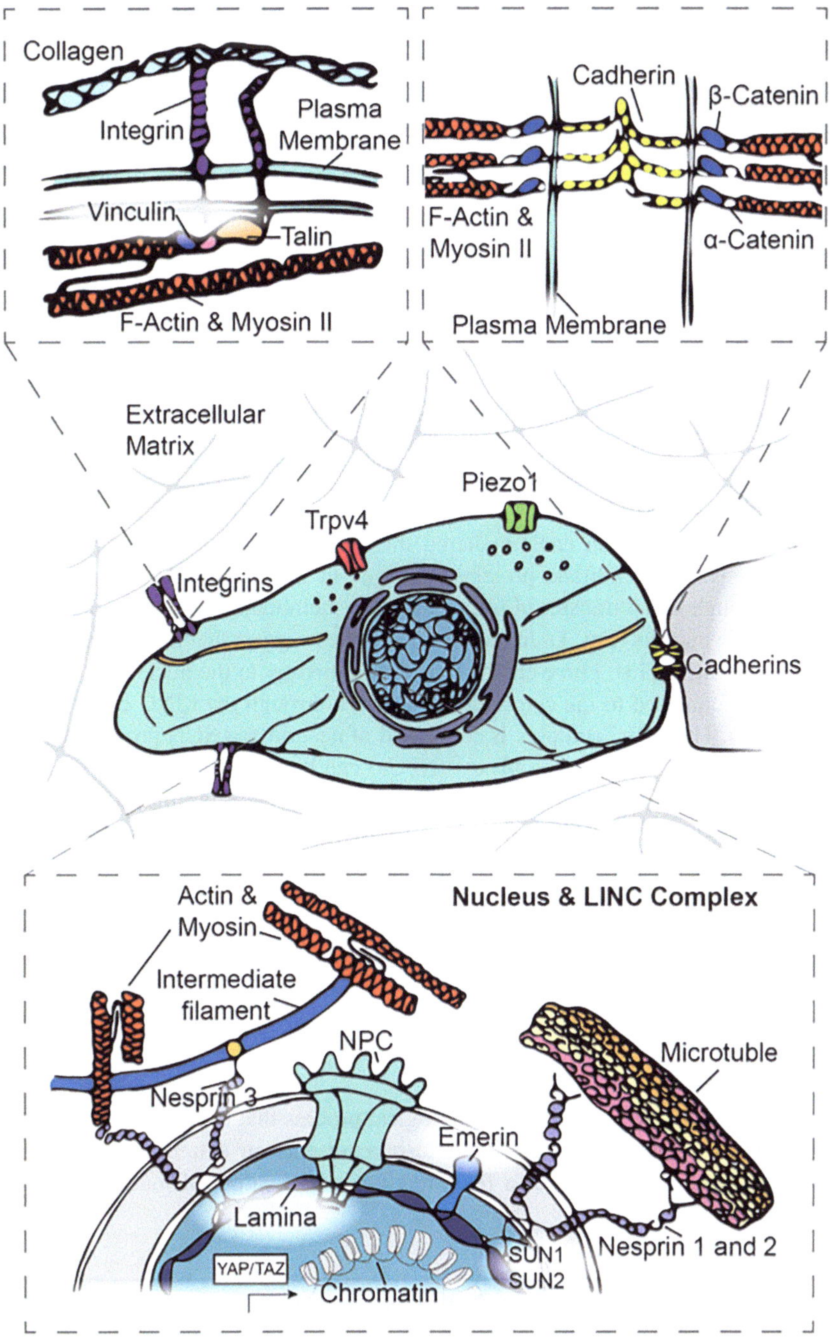

Fig. 1 The mechanical environment directs cellular phenotypes and cell fate. The cell contains various mechanosensitive proteins responsible for translating force into biochemical signals. Stretch-activated ion channels, integrins, and cadherins are proteins on the plasma membrane which respond to changes in the mechanical environments. Furthermore, the cytoskeleton,

1.2 The Cytoskeleton: A Network That Can Both Resist and Generate Forces

Cell membrane proteins not only influence molecular signaling cascades, but cell membrane responses can also alter the structure of the cytoskeleton network, which can lead to changes in gene expression [11]. The cytoskeleton is extremely dynamic, and the structure depends on the polarity of the actin fibers, microtubules, and intermediate filaments [9] (Fig. 1). Actomyosin networks can generate contractile forces, while intermediate filaments and microtubules maintain the cell structure and architecture inside the cell [12]. The active generation of force allows cells to exert traction on the surrounding ECM, migrate, and divide.

1.3 How the Nucleus Feels

While gene transcription can be altered through signaling pathways initiated by mechanosensitive membrane proteins, changes in gene transcription can also be altered through direct transfer of forces from the membrane to the cytoskeleton and finally to the nucleus (Fig. 1). In fact, recent studies suggest that the nucleus itself is mechanosensitive [13]. Force can be transferred directly to the nucleus because the nucleus is connected to the cytoskeleton network through the LINC complex [14–16] (Fig. 1). The LINC complex is composed of nesprin and SUN proteins (Fig. 1). Additionally, nuclear pore complexes (NPCs) can be opened in response to force, which can shuttle transcription factors and enzymes such as histone-modifying enzymes, myocardin-related transcription factor (MRTF-A), or Yes-associated protein/transcriptional coactivator with PDZ domain (YAP/TAZ) [17]. Structural proteins in the nuclear envelope, called lamins, also alter nuclear stiffness and have been shown to regulate gene transcription in mechanotransduction pathways [18].

2 Pregnancy Is Inherently a Biomechanical Process

Pregnancy is an extremely dynamic biological process that is not only governed by changes in biochemical signaling but also represents an extreme biomechanical transformation. The growth of a fetus requires coordination of multiple maternal

Fig. 1 (continued) including microtubules, filamentous actin, and intermediate filaments, can transmit force from the plasma membrane to the nucleus through the LINC (linker of nucleoskeleton and cytoskeleton) complex. Nuclear pore complexes (NPCs), emerin, and the nuclear lamina also mediate the transmission and integration of mechanical signals to the nucleus

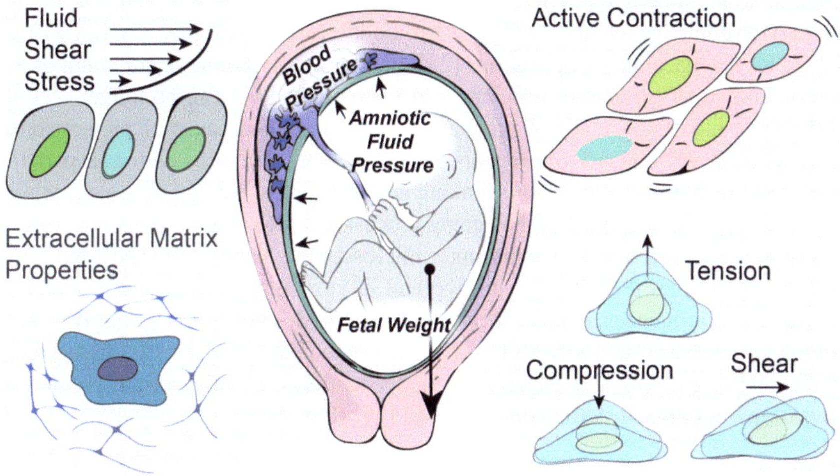

Fig. 2 Changes in biomechanics in pregnancy impact cellular behavior. Tissue remodeling, the growth of the fetus, and blood flow influence the mechanical environment experienced by cells during pregnancy. Increased shear stress due to blood flow in the placenta, decreasing stiffness of the cervix, and increased stretch of the uterus and fetal membrane are all mechanical cues that have been shown to influence cellular behavior. Additionally, smooth muscle cells in the myometrium and in the cervix also impact the pregnant mechanical environment through active contraction. Understanding the role of biomechanics and mechanobiology is critical to both understanding physiological pregnancy and preventing poor birth outcomes

tissues, including the uterus, cervix, and fetal-derived tissues, such as the placenta and fetal membranes (Fig. 2). The uterus expands from its prepregnancy state of about 10 milliliters in volume to the full-term pregnancy state of about 5 liters in volume [19]. As the uterus stretches, the cervix initially remains stiff and closed to accommodate the increasing load of the baby and force of baby movements. Similarly, the fetal membranes also remain intact, remodel, and stretch during pregnancy to act as a mechanical barrier to physical stress and infection. Additionally, the placenta vascular network grows and adapts to the oxygen and nutrient needs of the fetus. However, just prior to labor, the roles of these tissues reverse: the fetal membranes rupture; ECM remodeling of the cervix allows for softening, dilation, and birth; the uterus becomes contractile for labor; and the placenta detaches from the uterus and is delivered [20]. During the postpartum period, the maternal tissues are repaired and mostly return to the prepregnancy state, a process called postpartum involution [21]. Therefore, these tissues drastically remodel and adapt throughout the course of the 9-month human gestation [19]. Failure to adapt appropriately can lead to serious complications such as preterm labor, preeclampsia, uterine rupture, hemorrhage, or obstructed labor.

Although the mechanisms of how these tissues adapt in pregnancy are not fully understood, there are several tissue-scale observations that suggest that pregnancy and parturition are regulated by mechanical cues. Uterine overdistention, or increased stretch of the uterus due to multiple gestations (e.g., twins) or too much amniotic fluid, known as polyhydramnios, can increase the risk of preterm labor and premature rupture of membranes [22]. Chronic increased blood pressure is a serious risk factor for placental complications [23]. Premature shortening or softening of the cervix, known as cervical insufficiency, in which the cervix can no longer accommodate the increasing loads of pregnancy, is an identified cause of preterm birth [24]. Additionally, the risk of pregnancy complications increases with age, perhaps because of increased collagen crosslinking and resulting stiffening of tissues, which has been well characterized in the ageing process [25, 26].

Furthermore, research exploring microscopic length scales and the mechanobiology of these tissues in vivo and in vitro supports that the mechanical environment influences cellular behavior and ECM remodeling [27]. As such, pregnancy offers a powerful and understudied model of tissue-scale mechanobiology, with implications for understanding not only normal pregnancy physiology but also obstetric complications [28] (Fig. 2).

3 Fetal Membrane

The fetal membrane acts as a protective barrier during pregnancy to prevent infection and withstand the load of the growing fetus and the increased amniotic fluid pressure. The fetal membrane is a bilayer structure composed of the amnion and chorion [29] (Fig. 2). The amnion is avascular and is attached (after 14–16 weeks of gestation) to the thicker chorion layer, which has a higher cell density compared to the amnion. The main cell types in the fetal membrane include amnion epithelial cells, mesenchymal cells, fibroblasts, immune cells, and trophoblast cells [30]. The ECM of the chorioamnion is largely composed of collagen I, III, and IV, glycoproteins, fibronectin, and elastin [30, 31]. Since the amnion is stiffer and has a greater strength than the chorion, it predominantly supports the increasing loads throughout pregnancy [32]. The physical integrity of the chorioamnion is extremely important to be maintained until a term delivery. Prior to delivery, a biologically programmed weakening response allows the membranes to rupture [33]. This physiological weakening involves remodeling of the ECM, increases in matrix metalloproteinase (MMP) activity, and cellular apoptosis [34–36]. MMPs degrade ECM components, thereby altering the material properties of the ECM. The weak zone is often found above the cervix and is associated with an increase in MMP 9, a decrease in tissue inhibitor of metalloproteinase (TIMP) 3, and an increase in cell death through apoptosis [37–39]. Although this weakening response is necessary for birth, the mechanical integrity of the fetal membrane is not always maintained to term. Premature rupture of membranes (PPROM) occurs when the chorioaminion tissue fails, a tear develops, and the membranes detach from the uterine wall before 37 weeks of gestation [22].

Research into the mechanobiology of the fetal membrane has largely been driven by the aim of preventing PPROM (Table 1). The mechanical integrity of the chorioamnion tissues is largely attributed to the composition and organization of the ECM, in particular collagen [40, 41]. Therefore, understanding the

Table 1 Summary of mechanobiology studies of the fetal membrane

Involved tissue or cell	Model system	Driving change	Cellular or molecular response
Amniotic membrane	Human (ex vivo)	Cyclic stretch	Increased expression of mechanotransduction mediators Cx43 and AKT; Reduction in collagen and elastin content; Increased synthesis of glycosaminoglycans and inflammatory markers (MMP activity, PGE2 release) [22]
	Human (ex vivo)	Cyclic stretch	Increased collagen fiber polarization and gene expression of TGF-β1 and Cx43 [43]
	Human (ex vivo)	Uniaxial stretch	Orientation of collagen fibers in loading direction [44]
Amniotic and chorionic membranes and decidua	Human (ex vivo)	Static stretch	Increase in IL-8 [47]
Amnion epithelial cells	Human (in vitro)	Static stretch	Production of inflammatory markers (IL-1β, PGE2) [45, 46]
Amniocytes	Human (in vitro)	Static stretch	Elevated expression of IL-1β, IL-6, IL-8 [48]

biomechanical signaling that results in the remodeling and degradation of ECM is critical. For example, Barrett et al. found that a cyclic tensile strain increases the expression of mechanotransduction mediators connexin 43 (Cx43) and protein kinase B (AKT) [22, 42]. Additionally, cyclic tensile strain also influenced ECM remodeling through the increased synthesis of glycosaminoglycans, while inflammatory markers (MMP activity and prostaglandin E2, PGE2, release) also increased [22]. Similarly, Costa et al. reported that mechanical stimulation of preterm amniotic membranes increased collagen and gene expression of Cx43 and inflammatory marker TGF-β1 [43]. By inhibiting Cx43 and AKT, Barrett et al. found that strain-induced ECM changes associated with fetal membrane weakening could be prevented, indicating that Cx43 and AKT contribute to the mechanosensitivity of the fetal membrane and may be involved in the pathogenesis of PPROM [22]. Additionally, mechanical stretch not only causes cell mediated ECM remodeling, but also directly remodels the ECM through influencing fiber orientation and thus the overall mechanical properties. Perrini et al. observed progressive residual stretch and orientation of collagen fibers in the direction of uniaxial loading in term amniotic membranes, determining the resulting toughness of the membrane [44].

Other in vitro studies have demonstrated that the application of cyclic strain leads to the production of inflammatory markers (IL-1β, PGE2) through the activation of NF-kB in amnion epithelial cells [45, 46]. This observation is consistent with previous work that reported an increase in IL-8 in fetal membranes in response to mechanical stretch [47]. Furthermore, similar observations have been recorded in a nonhuman primate model of uterine overdistension in which the production of PGE2, IL-6, and IL-8 was elevated, suggesting that increased stretch of the fetal membrane due to uterine overdistension contributes to the production of these inflammatory biochemical markers [48].

4 Placenta

The placenta is a fetal-derived organ that develops from the trophoblast cells surrounding the fertilized blastocyst. The main function of the placenta is to provide an exchange surface to transfer oxygen, nutrients, and waste between the maternal and fetal circulatory systems. The predominant functional cell type of the placenta is the trophoblast cell, including syncytiotrophoblasts (STBs), cytotrophoblasts (CTBs), and extravillous trophoblasts (EVTs). Additionally, endothelial cells, fibroblasts, and immune cells are also found in the placenta. The ECM of the placenta primarily consists of collagens (I, III, IV, VI), non-collagenous glycoproteins (e.g., laminin, fibronectin, tenascin C), and proteoglycans (e.g., decorin) [49]. The tissue properties and blood flow surrounding cells in the placenta are extremely dynamic throughout pregnancy, and many placenta-related complications are associated with changes in this environment. Furthermore, the literature reports evidence of mechanosensitive molecules in both first-trimester and term placental tissue. Expression of TRPV6, Piezo1, and Polycystin-1 [50] proteins in the placenta suggest that mechanosensitive pathways play a role in the regulation of the trophoblast cell phenotype in vivo.

Changes in blood flow alter shear stresses that are exerted on cells from the movement of fluid (Fig. 2). The effects of shear stress on many cell types have been extensively explored in the mechanobiology literature (Table 2) [51]. In the placenta, shear stresses applied to vascular endothelial cells in the fetal capillaries are predicted to be low [52, 53] and shear stress from the maternal blood flow experienced by cells surrounding the villous tissue is estimated to be around 1 dyne/cm^2. However, the applied shear stress varies depending on location in the placenta and the shape of the villous tissue [50]. Throughout gestation, it is generally thought that fluid shear stress from the maternal blood decreases because arterial jetting is observed late first or early second trimester, which then subsides as the placenta grows [54]. Additionally, Doppler imaging of abnormal blood flow in the placenta is a well-known marker for placenta dysfunction [55]. For example, the measurement of resistance to blood flow of the spiral arteries is significantly higher in pregnancies with fetal growth restriction, preeclampsia, and gestational hypertension than in uncomplicated pregnancies [56]. The altered blood flow of the spiral arteries is particularly important since the spiral arteries are remodeled by extravillous trophoblast cells in early pregnancy to supply blood that contains nutrients and oxygen to the placenta. Trophoblast cell lines show mechanosensitive responses to fluid shear stress [50, 57, 58], including the production of growth factors [59], a change in metabolic activity [60], cell turnover [61], and motility [62]. Therefore, blood flow in contact with trophoblast cells in early pregnancy and throughout pregnancy may influence placenta development, cellular differentiation, and the development of particular pregnancy complications.

At the same time, elastography studies have demonstrated an increase in stiffness in placenta tissue in cases with fetal growth restriction [63], preeclampsia [64, 65], and gestational diabetes mellitus [66]. Placenta ECM stiffness also changes

Table 2 Summary of mechanobiology studies of the placenta

Involved tissue or cell	Model system	Driving change	Cellular or molecular response
Placenta	Mouse (in vivo)	Piezo1 knockout	Mechanosensitive ion channel Piezo1 is required for trophoblast fusion, and without this channel, the syncytiotrophoblast layer fails to form [77]
Syncytiotrophoblasts	Human (ex vivo)	Pregnancy and gestational age	Mechanosensitive pathways play a role in the regulation of the trophoblast cell phenotype, and applied shear stress varies depending on location in the placenta and the shape of the villous tissue [50]
	Human (in vitro)	Physical stresses applied via micropatterning	Stress patterns associated with budding morphogenesis enhance trophoblast fusion [73]
	Human (in vitro)	Fluid shear stress	Syncytiotrophoblasts under fluid shear stress increase production of growth factors [59]
Trophoblast cell line	Human (in vitro)	Fluid shear stress	Trophoblast cell lines show mechanosensitive responses including a change in metabolic activity [60]
	Human (in vitro)	Equibiaxial compressive, equibiaxial tensile, and uniaxial tensile stresses	Isometric compressive forces have been shown to enhance trophoblast fusion of 3D spheroid cultures [52]
	Human (in vitro)	Seeding on substrates with matrix rigidity gradients	Substrate stiffness altered trophoblast fusion. The percentage of cell fusion increased with a substrate with physiological stiffness (~1 kPa) compared to substrates with pathological (7 kPa) and supraphysiologically stiff environments (17 kPa and greater) [74]
	Human (in vitro)	Encapsulation in hydrogels with various gelatin bloom strengths	The outgrowth of spheroids composed of a trophoblast cell line decreased with increasing substrate stiffness [71]
Trophoblasts and HUVECs	Human (in vitro)	Fluid shear stress	Shear stress decreased apoptosis [61]

throughout gestation [67, 68] and the mechanical environment of the endometrium, where the blastocyst adheres during implantation, evolves during the different phases of the menstrual cycle [69]. In fact, recent studies suggest that the material properties of the microenvironment may influence trophoblast cells in the early stages of pregnancy (Table 2). After implantation, proliferative cytotrophoblasts, which differentiated from the cells making up the trophectoderm of the fertilized blastocyst, grow into columns that together form the cytotrophoblast shell. The cells in this layer give rise to extravillous trophoblast cells (EVTs), which invade the maternal decidua and remodel the maternal spiral arteries. Studies using a trophoblast cell line model (JAR) demonstrate that substrate stiffness influenced the number of focal adhesions and polymerization of F-actin cytoskeleton and these cells also migrated toward stiffer substrates [70]. Additionally, Zambuto et al. found that the outgrowth of spheroids composed of a trophoblast cell line decreased with increasing stiffness [71]. Therefore, the stiffness of the uterine microenvironment may regulate the success of implantation and the trajectory of placental development.

As the placenta develops and grows during pregnancy, one essential step in the development and maintenance of placenta function is the fusion of cytotrophoblast cells to form the multi-nucleated syncytiotrophoblast layer or the syncytium. The syncytium, composed of syncytiotrophoblast cells, encapsulates the chorionic villi, where the exchange of nutrients and waste occurs in the placenta. Dysregulated trophoblast fusion is associated with obstetric complications, since fusion is required for budding morphogenesis of the villi structures in the placenta [72]. While it is known that oxygen, cytokines, growth factors, and the general biochemical environment influence cytotrophoblast fusion, less is known about how the mechanical environment alters this critical process [73]. Recent work demonstrates that substrate stiffness altered trophoblast fusion. Specifically, the percentage of cell fusion increased with a substrate with physiological stiffness (~1 kPa) compared to substrates with pathological (7 kPa) and supraphysiologically stiff environments (17 kPa and greater) [74]. In addition to the elasticity of the microenvironment, stress patterns associated with budding morphogenesis enhance trophoblast fusion [73]. Furthermore, isometric compressive forces have been shown to also enhance trophoblast fusion of 3D spheroid cultures [52]. Interestingly, only an equibiaxial application of compressive stress to monolayer cultures, not uniaxial or equibiaxial tension, increased the expression of syndecan-1 and loss of E-cadherin associated with trophoblast fusion [52]. The application of controlled fluid shear stress and the mechanobiological response has also been explored in the context of trophoblast cell fusion. In fact, low shear stresses increased the rate of fusion of trophoblast stem cells [75].

Mechanisms of how trophoblast cells sense changes in fluid shear stress, compressive and tensile forces are in the process of being explored. That being said, literature reports an integral role of mechanotransduction in the formation of the placenta. Mechanosensitive transcriptional co-regulators, YAP and TAZ, are instrumental in early trophoblast differentiation [76]. Additionally, recent work suggests mechanosensitive ion channel Piezo1 is required for trophoblast fusion, and without this channel, the syncytiotrophoblast layer fails to form [77]. Elucidating the mechanisms of mechanotransduction in placenta pathophysiology could potentially lead to treatments for placenta-related complications such as preeclampsia or fetal growth restriction.

5 Uterus

The uterus is composed of three layers, including the endometrium, myometrium, and perimetrium. The endometrium and myometrium are known to be extremely dynamic tissues. The endometrium is the innermost tissue of the uterus and consists of a functional layer and a basal layer. The main cell types in the endometrium include luminal and glandular epithelial cells, stroma and stromal fibroblast cells, and immune cells [78]. Throughout the menstrual cycle, the collagenous matrix composition changes in response to hormone level cycling [49]. During pregnancy, the endometrium decidualizes, which is the process in which endometrial stromal cells differentiate into decidual cells that secrete ECM, such as collagen, fibronectin, and laminin. Measurements of the endometrium's mechanical properties indicate that the stiffness of the tissue increases during pregnancy [78]. While experimental data suggest that the stiffness of the myometrium does not change significantly with pregnancy, this muscular tissue also adapts to accommodate the growing fetus [78]. The expression of collagen II, fibrillin, elastin, and tenascin C increases during pregnancy in the myometrium, and the smooth muscle cells also undergo many adaptive phases [49]. First, the myocytes enter the proliferative phase, which is associated with an increase in the number of cells (hyperplasia). Next, in the synthetic phase, the uterine myocytes increase in size (hypertrophy). At the onset of labor, the myocytes become contractile, meaning that the previously unexcitable and uncoordinated muscle transitions to a muscle that is excitable and highly coordinated to allow for contractions to expel the fetus. The perimetrium, also known as the serosa, is the outermost layer of the uterus and is composed of epithelial cells embedded in a collagenous matrix. The perimetrium has been less well characterized, but recent work has demonstrated considerable remodeling with increased collagen deposition in pregnant tissues when compared to non-pregnant tissues [78].

Various in vitro studies have demonstrated that cells in the uterus are mechanosensitive (Table 3) [79]. During pregnancy in mice, the expression of mechanosensitive focal adhesion kinase (FAK)-related proteins increases, and this increase is reversed 1 day postpartum [79]. Recent studies have demonstrated that mechanosensitive ion channel, Piezo1, is also upregulated in both human and mouse uterine smooth muscle during pregnancy. Additionally, direct stimulation of the Piezo1 channel through a pharmacological treatment (Yoda1) resulted in increased contraction of uterine smooth muscle cells in vitro and a decreased pregnancy duration of mice in vivo. Inhibiting Piezo1 in mice with an intraperitoneal injection of Gsmtx4 extended the gestation of a common preterm labor mouse model induced through lipopolysaccharide (LPS) [80]. Additionally, stretch-sensing ion channel, TREK-1, may be involved in regulating the noncontractile and contractile state of the uterus. The TREK-1 channel becomes activated by stretch, stabilizes the membrane potential of cells, and reduces excitability. Evidence from the mouse uterus indicates that the expression of TREK-1 increases during pregnancy and then declines prior to the onset of labor [81]. Therefore, sensing stretch with TREK-1 may allow the uterus to be less excitable during pregnancy and promote the

Table 3 Summary of mechanobiology studies of the uterus

Involved tissue or cell	Model system	Driving change	Cellular or molecular response
Myometrial smooth muscle cells	Human and murine (ex vivo and in vitro)	Mechanical stretch	Upregulation of mechanosensitive Piezo1 channel. Piezo1 activation causes increased contraction and inhibition prolongs gestation in mice [80]
	Murine (ex vivo)	Mechanical stretch	Stretch-activated TREK-1 reduces excitability during pregnancy; downregulated before labor to promote contractions [81]
		Static stretch	Modulation of AP-1 transcription factors [86]
	Human (in vitro)	Mechanical stretch	Upregulation of transient reception potential canonical (TRPC) channels [85]
		Matrix stiffness variation	Increase in cell size, F-actin stress fibers, and focal adhesions with stiffness [87]
Uterine fibroids	Human (in vitro)	Matrix stiffness and hormonal stimuli	YAP/TAZ nuclear localization decreases on soft matrices and increases on stiff matrices with incorporation of estradiol and progesterone [89]
Leiomya cancer cells and myometrium tissue	Human (in vitro)	Cyclic stretch	Cell alignment along strain; upregulation of RhoA (increased cytoskeletal tension) [84]
Uterine horn	Murine (in vivo)	Artificial mechanical stretch in vivo	CASP3 activation [82]
Endometrial stromal cells	Human (in vitro)	Cyclic stretch	Upregulation of α-smooth muscle actin [90]
Uterine wall co-culture	Human (in vitro)	Fluid flow	Peristaltic intrauterine flow increases F-actin polymerization in mono- and co-cultures [91]

contractile state during labor. One research study actually isolated the effect of stretch by inserting a polymer balloon into the empty uterine horn of a unilateral pregnant rat (a rat with only fetuses in one uterine horn). These researchers observed that both the artificially mechanically stretched uterine horn and the pregnant uterine horn showed an activation of caspase 3 (CASP3), while the unstretched empty uterine horn did not [82]. While CASP3 is usually associated with apoptosis, it is thought that CASP3 plays a role in maintaining a quiescent, non-contractile state in pregnancy [82]. Overall, this in vivo mechanical stretching, along with studies that have simulated mechanical loading with the implantation of beads in the uterus, present powerful approaches to decouple mechanisms of stretch from pregnancy and demonstrate that stretch alone can activate cellular pathways in the uterus in vivo [82, 83].

Because labor involves frequent contraction, in vitro studies have focused on the uterine cell response to cyclic stretch (Table 3). In vitro studies demonstrate that in response to increased cyclic strain, myometrium cells align in the direction of strain and upregulate RhoA, which is a type of small Rho GTPase that generates cytoskeleton tension [84]. Myometrial smooth muscle cell expression of mechanosensitive ion channels, such as TWIK-related potassium channels and transient receptor potential canonical (TRPC) channels, increased with mechanical stretch [85]. In vitro studies have also explored the influence of static stretch, which constantly increases during pregnancy. With static stretch, the expression of activator protein-1 transcription factors (AP-1) is modulated [86]. The expression of these AP1 transcription factors is important because these molecules are responsible for the regulation of various ECM-related genes, including genes coding for collagen III, elastin, fibronectin, laminin, and MMPs [86]. Interestingly, when pretreating the cells with progesterone for 24 h, the magnitude of AP-1 gene expression decreased. Therefore, the integration of both mechanical cues and hormone signaling is essential to understand phenotypic shifts in the uterus [21].

Matrix stiffness has also been shown to influence the uterine smooth muscle cell phenotype; cells plated on stiff matrices increased in size, F-actin stress fibers, and focal adhesions [84, 87]. Additionally, myometrium smooth muscle cells display different calcium transient responses to oxytocin on stiff and soft substrates and with cell alignment on the corresponding substrates. Oxytocin is a primary regulator of myometrium contraction. Therefore, understanding how the stiffer and fibrous environments, such as fibrotic tissue that may arise from pathological tissue like fibroids, influence the myometrium will have critical implications for contractions during labor [88]. Moreover, the YAP/TAZ pathway may be involved in sensing changes in matrix stiffness in the uterine environment. Researchers have shown that softer environments decrease YAP/TAZ nuclear localization in both cells from the smooth muscle of the myometrium and uterine fibroids. Interestingly, the incorporation of estradiol and progesterone increased the nuclear localization of YAP/TAZ in response to stiff substrates, but only with cells isolated from the healthy myometrium and not with fibroids [89]. Therefore, cells in the smooth muscle of the myometrium may be more mechanosensitive in response to a change in hormone levels in the environment, while this may not be the case for cells in uterine fibroids.

While most of the research studying the mechanobiology of the uterus has focused on smooth muscle cells in the myometrium, cells in the endometrium have been shown to respond to mechanical stress as well. Cyclic mechanical strain increased the expression of alpha-smooth muscle actin which allowed for endometrial stromal cells to contract, suggesting that the endometrium can become contractile in response to stimulation from the myometrium [90]. Additionally, mechanical cues from peristaltic intrauterine flow can also impact the phenotype of endometrial cells; fluid flow has been shown to increase the polymerization of F-actin in mono-cell cultures and co-cultures [91, 92].

Outside of in vitro work and research conducted in mouse models, evidence from human pregnancy also suggests that mechanical forces regulate cell behavior in the uterus in pregnancy. For example, contractility of uterine smooth muscle cells from patients who gave birth to twins was higher than tissue from singleton pregnancies, suggesting that increased stretch is associated with smooth muscle contractility [93]. Additionally, birthweight correlated with cell contractility, further supporting this hypothesis [93].

6 Cervix

The cervix is a cylindrical extension of the distal end of the uterus and serves many functions in the nonpregnant and pregnant uterus. The cervix acts as a selective passageway that allows for menstrual fluids and sperm to pass, but also prevents pathogens from entering the uterus due to the secretion of mucus. The cervix remains closed most of pregnancy and supports the load of the growing fetus [24]. However, prior to birth, the ECM remodels, which allows for the softening, ripening, dilation, and the passage of the baby [24, 27, 94, 95]. The ECM of the cervix is primarily composed of water, fibrous collagen (type I and III), elastic fibers, proteoglycans, and glycosaminoglycans [96, 97]. Within the ECM, many cell types reside, including epithelial cells, smooth muscle cells, fibroblasts, immune cells, glandular cells, and vascular cells. Fibroblast cells in the cervix deposit and remodel the surrounding ECM and therefore can determine the physical properties of the cervix [98]. However, ECM remodeling is not the only mechanism of biophysical regulation of the cervix. Smooth muscle cells in the cervix are known to be contractile in nature which can modulate the capacity of the cervix to support the increasing load in pregnancy [99]. Specifically, smooth muscle cells form circumferential bundles around the internal os, or the opening of the cervix to the uterine cavity, which decrease in density toward the external os, or the opening of the cervix to the vaginal canal [99, 100]. In fact, it is hypothesized that the smooth muscle surrounding the internal os acts as a kind of sphincter in pregnancy. Understanding how ECM and active contraction regulation alter cervical remodeling is critical to understanding the progression to a term birth or early preterm labor (before 37 weeks of gestation).

Investigating how mechanical cues could direct ECM remodeling has been a key motivator in much of the cervix mechanobiology literature (Table 4). House et al. demonstrated that in response to dynamic loading, cervical fibroblasts embedded in a 3D matrix increased the production of collagen and sulfated glycosaminoglycans, which led to a stiffer matrix [101]. Similarly, when human cervical fibroblasts were exposed to cyclic stretch for 24, 36, and 48 h, there was an increase in the secretion of hyaluronic acid, a glycosaminoglycan that has been shown to increase throughout pregnancy [102, 103]. The specific mechanisms of mechanotransduction in the cervix have yet to be elucidated. However, researchers have observed an increase in expression of RNA and protein of cytoskeletal factors and associated signaling molecules throughout the course of the murine pregnancy, suggesting that the cytoskeleton may act as a mechanosensor in cervical cells throughout gestation [104]. Additionally, after birth, the expression of various cytoskeleton proteins, such as intermediate filaments and actin-binding proteins, drops after 48 h

Table 4 Summary of mechanobiology studies of the cervix

Involved tissue or cell	Model system	Driving change	Cellular or molecular response
Cervical fibroblasts	Primary human (ex vivo)	Dynamic mechanical loading in 3D culture	Increased collagen and sulfated glycosaminoglycan (sGAG) production leads to a stiffer matrix [101]
Cervical tissue	Murine (in vivo)	Pregnancy-related stretch	Increased RNA/protein expression of cytoskeletal and signaling molecules [104]
		Relaxation postpartum (↓ mechanical load)	Cytoskeletal protein expression (actin-binding, intermediate filaments) decreases within 48 hs [105]
Cervical smooth muscle cells	Primary human (in vitro)	Matrix stiffness variation	Cells on soft matrices show reduced contractility vs stiff matrices [100]

[105]. Taken together, these data suggest that mechanotransduction pathways are activated by the increased stretch of pregnancy and labor; however, direct experiments to test this hypothesis have not been completed.

In addition to exploring how mechanical cues alter cell ECM production and degradation, understanding the regulation of cell mechanics and active contraction is equally important. Researchers have investigated how force generation of cells changes in response to the biochemical environment. Specifically, Shukla et al. studied the effect of progesterone and proinflammatory cytokine, IL-1β, on cell adhesion and cell force generation by evaluating cell spreading and measuring traction forces through traction force microscopy (TFM) [106]. TFM is a technique that measures deformation of a substrate surrounding a cell to approximate the forces a cell is exerting on its environment. These studies showed that IL-1β decreased cell adhesion and cell force generation, while progesterone increased cell adhesion. Therefore, the external biochemical environments (e.g., inflammatory markers and hormones) influence cellular mechanics. In addition to the biochemical environment, the physical environment has also been shown to alter cellular mechanics in the cervix. Vink et al. demonstrated that cervical smooth muscle cells exhibited less contractility when exposed to soft matrices compared to stiff matrices [100]. While this is an observation seen in many different cell types, this experiment demonstrates that pregnant people with soft cervices may have less contractile smooth muscle, which could increase the risk for cervical insufficiency and preterm birth [107, 108].

7 Future Work at the Intersection of Mechanobiology, Pregnancy and Biomaterials

Despite the growing body of literature that explores the mechanobiology of pregnancy, critical gaps in our understanding remain. One of the greatest challenges of elucidating mechanisms of mechanobiology and studying pregnancy in general is the difficulty of accessing human reproductive tissues and cells longitudinally throughout gestation, given that pregnancy is a protected environment. Furthermore, pregnancy research is complicated by the fact that the anatomy and hormonal responses can vary drastically compared to humans. For example, mice have two uterine horns rather than one uterine cavity. Both the gross morphology and the degree of interdigitation of the fetal and maternal tissues in the placenta varies drastically in different animal species [109]. Progesterone is known to decrease throughout pregnancy in many animal models, but this process does not occur in human pregnancy [110]. To address the challenge of inadequate animal models, the progress of this field will depend on the integration and feedback of various in vitro, in silico, and in vivo experiments [111]. Several future directions of research have been outlined below to inform the design and execution of these computational and experimental studies.

- Full characterization of physiological and pathological tissue mechanical properties will be necessary to understand the cellular response to the pregnant mechanical environment. Developing mechanical models incorporating tissue heterogeneity, anisotropy, and time-dependent responses will provide the design criteria for engineering accurate in silico and in vitro models to study and predict the dynamics of pregnancy.
- Decoupling of tissue growth and remodeling from deformation will allow for an understanding of how much deformation cells experience and how the properties of reproductive tissues change in pregnancy.
- Pregnancy is governed by shifts in the endocrine and immune environment. Therefore, considering the interaction of hormones and the immune system when studying mechanobiology is critical.
- Cross talk between cells in different tissues cannot be ignored, as tissues in pregnancy are not isolated systems. Mechanically regulated pathways in cells in one tissue may influence the activation of cellular pathways in another.
- Characterizing and understanding mechanisms of postpartum involution raises questions of how and if tissues return to the prepregnant state. Additionally, questions of how obstetric history influences subsequent pregnancy need to be answered.
- While mechanisms of mechanotransduction in pregnancy and postpartum are being explored, further exploration is needed to start to develop drugs to interfere with discovered pathways that are mechanically regulated. Pharmaceutical treatments have the potential to override biomechanical signaling that may lead to obstetric complications.

With ethical and logistical limitations on obtaining ex vivo human samples, biomaterials provide a platform to study relevant mechanobiology of pregnancy by helping to recreate the dynamic and heterogeneous mechanical environments that cells experience in vivo. Because pregnancy involves continuous tissue remodeling and changes in stiffness, anisotropy, and viscoelasticity, biomaterial models that mimic these evolving extracellular matrix (ECM) properties can be used to investigate how mechanical cues regulate gene expression, cell phenotype, and tissue function. Throughout this review, engineered hydrogels, tunable substrates, and 3D culture systems have allowed researchers to decouple mechanical signals and have enabled precise control over parameters that help to drive the mechanobiology such as stiffness, flow, stretch, and strain. These biomaterial-based models therefore serve as essential tools to probe mechanotransduction pathways, explore how cells sense and respond to the pregnancy microenvironment, and ultimately improve our understanding of cell–tissue interactions that underlie healthy gestation and pregnancy-related pathologies.

A complete understanding of the complex mechanical environment that considers the change in hormonal and immune system responses, as well as the interaction between cell types, will allow for more physiologically relevant in vitro models to study the mechanobiology of pregnancy. Uncovering new mechanotransduction pathways could not only inform the development of therapeutics, but also in silico agent-based models that can predict the growth and remodeling of tissues [96, 112]. Comparing in vitro and in silico experiments to the in vivo environment will be essential for model validation and confidence. Ultimately, these potential advancements in the field of reproductive health will not only improve the understanding of normal physiology but also provide therapeutic and predictive tools to avoid or treat pregnancy complications rooted in mechanical dysfunction.

References

1. Willie B, Duda GN, Weinkamer R. Bone structural adaptation and Wolff's law. 2013. p. 17–45. https://doi.org/10.1039/9781849737555-00017.
2. Zuela-Sopilniak N, Lammerding J. Can't handle the stress? Mechanobiology and disease. Trends Mol Med. 2022;28:710–25. https://doi.org/10.1016/J.MOLMED.2022.05.010.
3. Jin P, Jan LY, Jan YN. Mechanosensitive ion channels: structural features relevant to mechanotransduction mechanisms. Annu Rev Neurosci. 2020;43:207–29. https://doi.org/10.1146/ANNUREV-NEURO-070918-050509/1.
4. Coste B, Mathur J, Schmidt M, Earley TJ, Ranade S, Petrus MJ, Dubin AE, Patapoutian A. Piezo1 and Piezo2 are essential components of distinct mechanically activated cation channels. Science (1979). 2010;330:55–60. https://doi.org/10.1126/SCIENCE.1193270/SUPPL_FILE/COSTE-SOM.PDF.
5. Sorum B, Docter T, Panico V, Rietmeijer RA, Brohawn SG. Tension activation of mechanosensitive two-pore domain K+ channels TRAAK, TREK-1, and TREK-2. Nat Commun. 2024;15(1):1–9. https://doi.org/10.1038/s41467-024-47208-5.
6. Kuo JC. Mechanotransduction at focal adhesions: integrating cytoskeletal mechanics in migrating cells. J Cell Mol Med. 2013;17:704. https://doi.org/10.1111/JCMM.12054.
7. Elosegui-Artola A, Oria R, Chen Y, Kosmalska A, Pérez-González C, Castro N, Zhu C, Trepat X, Roca-Cusachs P. Mechanical regulation of a molecular clutch defines force transmission and transduction in response to matrix rigidity. Nat Cell Biol. 2016;18(5):540–8. https://doi.org/10.1038/ncb3336.
8. Holland EN, Fernández-Yagüe MA, Zhou DW, O'Neill EB, Woodfolk AU, Mora-Boza A, Fu J, Schlaepfer DD, García AJ. FAK, vinculin, and talin control mechanosensitive YAP nuclear localization. Biomaterials. 2024;308:122542. https://doi.org/10.1016/J.BIOMATERIALS.2024.122542.

9. Martino F, Perestrelo AR, Vinarský V, Pagliari S, Forte G. Cellular mechanotransduction: from tension to function. Front Physiol. 2018;9:378185. https://doi.org/10.3389/FPHYS.2018.00824/XML/NLM.
10. Yap AS, Duszyc K, Viasnoff V. Mechanosensing and mechanotransduction at cell–cell junctions. Cold Spring Harb Perspect Biol. 2018;10:a028761. https://doi.org/10.1101/CSHPERSPECT.A028761.
11. Tamada M, Sheetz MP, Sawada Y. Activation of a signaling cascade by cytoskeleton stretch. Dev Cell. 2004;7:709–18. https://doi.org/10.1016/j.devcel.2004.08.021.
12. Fletcher DA, Mullins RD. Cell mechanics and the cytoskeleton. Nature. 2010;463(7280):485–92. https://doi.org/10.1038/nature08908.
13. Kirby TJ, Lammerding J. Emerging views of the nucleus as a cellular mechanosensor. Nat Cell Biol. 2018;20(4):373–81. https://doi.org/10.1038/s41556-018-0038-y.
14. Lombardi ML, Jaalouk DE, Shanahan CM, Burke B, Roux KJ, Lammerding J. The interaction between nesprins and sun proteins at the nuclear envelope is critical for force transmission between the nucleus and cytoskeleton. J Biol Chem. 2011;286:26743–53. https://doi.org/10.1074/jbc.M111.233700.
15. Lombardi ML, Lammerding J. Keeping the LINC: the importance of nucleocytoskeletal coupling in intracellular force transmission and cellular function. Biochem Soc Trans. 2011;39:1729–34. https://doi.org/10.1042/BST20110686.
16. Bouzid T, Kim E, Riehl BD, Esfahani AM, Rosenbohm J, Yang R, Duan B, Lim JY. The LINC complex, mechanotransduction, and mesenchymal stem cell function and fate. J Biol Eng. 2019;13:1–12. https://doi.org/10.1186/S13036-019-0197-9/FIGURES/8.
17. Elosegui-Artola A, Andreu I, Beedle AEM, Lezamiz A, Uroz M, Kosmalska AJ, Oria R, Kechagia JZ, Rico-Lastres P, Le Roux AL, Shanahan CM, Trepat X, Navajas D, Garcia-Manyes S, Roca-Cusachs P. Force triggers YAP nuclear entry by regulating transport across nuclear pores. Cell. 2017;171:1397–1410.e14. https://doi.org/10.1016/J.CELL.2017.10.008/ASSET/D5BB99B6-5F7D-4AD5-ACD4-B623284C925A/MAIN.ASSETS/GR7.JPG.
18. Cho S, Irianto J, Discher DE. Mechanosensing by the nucleus: from pathways to scaling relationships. J Cell Biol. 2017;216:305–15. https://doi.org/10.1083/JCB.201610042.
19. Louwagie EM, Russell SR, Hairston JC, Nottman C, Nhan-Chang C-L, Fuchs K, Gyamfi-Bannerman C, Booker W, Andrikopoulou M, Friedman AM, Zork N, Wapner R, Vink J, Mourad M, Feltovich HM, House MD, Myers KM. The biomechanical evolution of the uterus and cervix and fetal growth in human pregnancy. Npj Women's Health. 2024;2(1):1–9. https://doi.org/10.1038/s44294-024-00038-8.
20. Grimm MJ. Forces involved with labor and delivery—a biomechanical perspective. Ann Biomed Eng. 2021;49:1819–35. https://doi.org/10.1007/S10439-020-02718-3/TABLES/5.
21. Shynlova O, Tsui P, Jaffer S, Lye SJ. Integration of endocrine and mechanical signals in the regulation of myometrial functions during pregnancy and labour. Eur J Obstet Gynecol Reprod Biol. 2009;144:S2. https://doi.org/10.1016/j.ejogrb.2009.02.044.
22. Barrett DW, John RK, Thrasivoulou C, Mata A, Deprest JA, Becker DL, David AL, Chowdhury TT. Targeting mechanotransduction mechanisms and tissue weakening signals in the human amniotic membrane. Sci Rep. 2019;9(1):1–11. https://doi.org/10.1038/s41598-019-42379-4.
23. Chappell LC, Enye S, Seed P, Briley AL, Poston L, Shennan AH. Adverse perinatal outcomes and risk factors for preeclampsia in women with chronic hypertension. Hypertension. 2008;51:1002–9. https://doi.org/10.1161/HYPERTENSIONAHA.107.107565.
24. Myers KM, Feltovich H, Mazza E, Vink J, Bajka M, Wapner RJ, Hall TJ, House M. The mechanical role of the cervix in pregnancy. J Biomech. 2015;48:1511. https://doi.org/10.1016/J.JBIOMECH.2015.02.065.
25. Cavazos-Rehg PA, Krauss MJ, Spitznagel EL, Bommarito K, Madden T, Olsen MA, Subramaniam H, Peipert JF, Bierut LJ. Maternal age and risk of labor and delivery complications. Matern Child Health J. 2015;19:1202. https://doi.org/10.1007/S10995-014-1624-7.

26. Tang SY, Sharan AD, Vashishth D. Effects of collagen crosslinking on tissue fragility. Clin Biomech. 2008;23:122–3. https://doi.org/10.1016/j.clinbiomech.2007.08.010.
27. Jorge S, Chang S, Barzilai JJ, Leppert P, Segars JH. Mechanical signaling in reproductive tissues: mechanisms and importance. Reprod Sci. 2014;21(9):1093–107. https://doi.org/10.1177/1933719114542023.
28. Matsuzaki S. Mechanobiology of the female reproductive system, Reprod. Med Biol. 2021;20:371–401. https://doi.org/10.1002/RMB2.12404.
29. Joyce EM, Diaz P, Tamarkin S, Moore R, Strohl A, Stetzer B, Kumar D, Sacks MS, Moore JJ. In-vivo stretch of term human fetal membranes. Placenta. 2016;38:57–66. https://doi.org/10.1016/J.PLACENTA.2015.12.011.
30. Richardson L, Menon R. Fetal membrane at the feto-maternal interface: an underappreciated and understudied intrauterine tissue. Placenta Reprod Med. 2022;1:10.54844/prm.2022.0104. https://doi.org/10.54844/PRM.2022.0104.
31. Calvin SE, Oyen ML. Microstructure and mechanics of the chorioamnion membrane with an emphasis on fracture properties. Ann N Y Acad Sci. 2007;1101:166–85. https://doi.org/10.1196/ANNALS.1389.009.
32. Oyen ML, Cook RF, Calvin SE. Mechanical failure of human fetal membrane tissues. J Mater Sci Mater Med. 2004;15:651–8. https://doi.org/10.1023/B:JMSM.0000030205.62668.90.
33. Joyce EM, Moore JJ, Sacks MS. Biomechanics of the fetal membrane prior to mechanical failure: review and implications. Eur J Obstet Gynecol Reprod Biol. 2009;144:S121–7. https://doi.org/10.1016/j.ejogrb.2009.02.014.
34. McLaren J, Taylor DJ, Bell SC. Increased incidence of apoptosis in non-labour-affected cytotrophoblast cells in term fetal membranes overlying the cervix. Hum Reprod. 1999;14:2895–900. https://doi.org/10.1093/HUMREP/14.11.2895.
35. McLaren J, Taylor DJ, Bell SC. Increased concentration of pro-matrix metalloproteinase 9 in term fetal membranes overlying the cervix before labor: implications for membrane remodeling and rupture. Am J Obstet Gynecol. 2000;182:409–16. https://doi.org/10.1016/S0002-9378(00)70232-8.
36. Moore RM, Mansour JM, Redline RW, Mercer BM, Moore JJ. The physiology of fetal membrane rupture: insight gained from the determination of physical properties. Placenta. 2006;27:1037–51. https://doi.org/10.1016/J.PLACENTA.2006.01.002.
37. El Khwad M, Stetzer B, Moore RM, Kumar D, Mercer B, Arikat S, Redline RW, Mansour JM, Moore JJ. Term human fetal membranes have a weak zone overlying the lower uterine pole and cervix before onset of labor. Biol Reprod. 2005;72:720–6. https://doi.org/10.1095/BIOLREPROD.104.033647.
38. Menon R, Fortunato SJ. The role of matrix degrading enzymes and apoptosis in rupture of membranes. J Soc Gynecol Investig. 2004;11:427–37. https://doi.org/10.1016/J.JSGI.2004.04.001.
39. Lannon SMR, Vanderhoeven JP, Eschenbach DA, Gravett MG, Waldorf KMA. Synergy and interactions among biological pathways leading to preterm premature rupture of membranes. Reprod Sci. 2014;21:1215. https://doi.org/10.1177/1933719114534535.
40. Shilo D, Shalev E. New insights on the biomechanics of the fetal membrane. Front Biosci (Schol Ed). 2023;15:6. https://doi.org/10.31083/J.FBS1502006/6597BF3E717F7535350F1CC0C29B5354.PDF.
41. Strauss JF. Extracellular matrix dynamics and fetal membrane rupture. Reprod Sci. 2013;20:140. https://doi.org/10.1177/1933719111424454.
42. Chowdhury B, David AL, Thrasivoulou C, Becker DL, Bader DL, Chowdhury TT. Tensile strain increased COX-2 expression and PGE2 release leading to weakening of the human amniotic membrane. Placenta. 2014;35:1057–64. https://doi.org/10.1016/J.PLACENTA.2014.09.006.
43. Costa E, Thrasivoulou C, Becker DL, Deprest JA, David AL, Chowdhury TT. Cx43 regulates mechanotransduction mechanisms in human preterm amniotic membrane defects. Prenat Diagn. 2023;43:1284–95. https://doi.org/10.1002/PD.6429.

44. Perrini M, Mauri A, Ehret AE, Ochsenbein-Kölble N, Zimmermann R, Ehrbar M, Mazza E. Mechanical and microstructural investigation of the cyclic behavior of human amnion. J Biomech Eng. 2015;137:61010–1. https://doi.org/10.1115/1.4030054/444882.
45. Mohan AR, Sooranna SR, Lindstrom TM, Johnson MR, Bennett PR. The effect of mechanical stretch on cyclooxygenase type 2 expression and activator protein-1 and nuclear factor-kappaB activity in human amnion cells. Endocrinology. 2007;148:1850–7. https://doi.org/10.1210/EN.2006-1289.
46. Kanayama N, Fukamizu H. Mechanical stretching increases prostaglandin E2 in cultured human amnion cells. Gynecol Obstet Investig. 1989;28:123–6. https://doi.org/10.1159/000293546.
47. Maehara K, Kanayama N, El Maradny E, Uezato T, Fujita M, Terao T. Mechanical stretching induces interleukin-8 gene expression in fetal membranes: a possible role for the initiation of human parturition. Eur J Obstet Gynecol Reprod Biol. 1996;70:191–6. https://doi.org/10.1016/S0301-2115(95)02602-9.
48. Waldorf KMA, Singh N, Mohan AR, Young RC, Ngo L, Das A, Tsai J, Bansal A, Paolella L, Herbert BR, Sooranna SR, Gough GM, Astley C, Vogel K, Baldessari AE, Bammler TK, MacDonald J, Gravett MG, Rajagopal L, Johnson MR. Uterine overdistention induces preterm labor mediated by inflammation: observations in pregnant women and nonhuman primates. Am J Obstet Gynecol. 2015;213:830.e1–830.e19. https://doi.org/10.1016/J.AJOG.2015.08.028.
49. O'Connor BB, Pope BD, Peters MM, Ris-Stalpers C, Parker KK. The role of extracellular matrix in normal and pathological pregnancy: future applications of microphysiological systems in reproductive medicine. Exp Biol Med. 2020;245:1163. https://doi.org/10.1177/1535370220938741.
50. Lee TC, Moulvi A, James JL, Clark AR. Multi-scale modelling of shear stress on the syncytiotrophoblast: could maternal blood flow impact placental function across gestation? Ann Biomed Eng. 2023;51:1256. https://doi.org/10.1007/S10439-022-03129-2.
51. Lu D, Kassab GS. Role of shear stress and stretch in vascular mechanobiology. J R Soc Interface. 2011;8:1379–85. https://doi.org/10.1098/RSIF.2011.0177.
52. Parameshwar PK, Li C, Arnauts K, Jiang J, Rostami S, Campbell BE, Lu H, Rosenzweig DH, Vaillancourt C, Moraes C. Directed biomechanical compressive forces enhance fusion efficiency in model placental trophoblast cultures. Sci Rep. 2024;14(1):1–12. https://doi.org/10.1038/s41598-024-61747-3.
53. Tun WM, Yap CH, Saw SN, James JL, Clark AR. Differences in placental capillary shear stress in fetal growth restriction may affect endothelial cell function and vascular network formation. Sci Rep. 2019;9(1):1–10. https://doi.org/10.1038/s41598-019-46151-6.
54. Collins SL, Stevenson GN, Noble JA, Impey L. Developmental changes in spiral artery blood flow in the human placenta observed with colour Doppler ultrasonography. Placenta. 2012;33:782–7. https://doi.org/10.1016/J.PLACENTA.2012.07.005.
55. Papageorghiou AT, Yu CKH, Bindra R, Pandis G, Nicolaides KH. Multicenter screening for pre-eclampsia and fetal growth restriction by transvaginal uterine artery Doppler at 23 weeks of gestation. Ultrasound Obstet Gynecol. 2001;18:441–9. https://doi.org/10.1046/J.0960-7692.2001.00572.X.
56. Odibo AO, Kayisli U, Lu Y, Kayisli O, Schatz F, Odibo L, Chen H, Bronsteen R, Lockwood CJ. Longitudinal assessment of spiral artery and intravillous arteriole blood flow and adverse pregnancy outcome. Ultrasound Obstet Gynecol. 2022;59:350–7. https://doi.org/10.1002/UOG.23760.
57. Miura S, Sato K, Kato-Negishi M, Teshima T, Takeuchi S. Fluid shear triggers microvilli formation via mechanosensitive activation of TRPV6. Nat Commun. 2015;6(1):1–11. https://doi.org/10.1038/ncomms9871.
58. Brugger BA, Guettler J, Gauster M. Go with the flow—trophoblasts in flow culture. Int J Mol Sci. 2020;21:4666. https://doi.org/10.3390/IJMS21134666.

59. Lecarpentier E, Atallah A, Guibourdenche J, Hebert-Schuster M, Vieillefosse S, Chissey A, Haddad B, Pidoux G, Evain-Brion D, Barakat A, Fournier T, Tsatsaris V. Fluid shear stress promotes placental growth factor upregulation in human syncytiotrophoblast through the cAMP-PKA signaling pathway. Hypertension. 2016;68:1438–46. https://doi.org/10.1161/HYPERTENSIONAHA.116.07890/SUPPL_FILE/HYP_HYPE201607890_SUPP1.PDF.
60. Brugger BA, Neuper L, Guettler J, Forstner D, Wernitznig S, Kummer D, Lyssy F, Feichtinger J, Krappinger J, El-Heliebi A, Bonstingl L, Moser G, Rodriguez-Blanco G, Bachkönig OA, Gottschalk B, Gruber M, Nonn O, Herse F, Verlohren S, Frank HG, Barapatre N, Kampfer C, Fluhr H, Desoye G, Gauster M. Fluid shear stress induces a shift from glycolytic to amino acid pathway in human trophoblasts. Cell Biosci. 2023;13:1–21. https://doi.org/10.1186/S13578-023-01114-3/FIGURES/9.
61. James JL, Whitley GS, Cartwright JE. Shear stress and spiral artery remodelling: the effects of low shear stress on trophoblast-induced endothelial cell apoptosis. Cardiovasc Res. 2011;90:130–9. https://doi.org/10.1093/CVR/CVQ396.
62. Xie B, Wu H, Li J, Lv X, Zhou Y, Yu Q, Cui S, Zeng L, Li J, Huang X, Gao J, Luo S. Mechanical forces on trophoblast motility and its potential role in spiral artery remodeling during pregnancy. Placenta. 2022;123:46–53. https://doi.org/10.1016/J.PLACENTA.2022.03.013.
63. Arioz Habibi H, Alici Davutoglu E, Kandemirli SG, Aslan M, Ozel A, Kalyoncu Ucar A, Zeytun P, Madazli R, Adaletli I. In vivo assessment of placental elasticity in intrauterine growth restriction by shear-wave elastography. Eur J Radiol. 2017;97:16–20. https://doi.org/10.1016/J.EJRAD.2017.10.007.
64. Kılıç F, Kayadibi Y, Yüksel MA, Adaletli İ, Ustabaşıoğlu FE, Öncül M, Madazlı R, Yılmaz MH, Mihmanlı İ, Kantarcı F. Shear wave elastography of placenta: in vivo quantitation of placental elasticity in preeclampsia. Diagn Interv Radiol. 2015;21:202. https://doi.org/10.5152/DIR.2014.14338.
65. Cimsit C, Yoldemir T, Akpinar IN. Shear wave elastography in placental dysfunction: comparison of elasticity values in normal and preeclamptic pregnancies in the second trimester. J Ultrasound Med. 2015;34:151–9. https://doi.org/10.7863/ULTRA.34.1.151.
66. Yuksel MA, Kilic F, Kayadibi Y, Alici Davutoglu E, Imamoglu M, Bakan S, Mihmanli I, Kantarci F, Madazli R. Shear wave elastography of the placenta in patients with gestational diabetes mellitus. J Obstet Gynaecol (Lahore). 2016;36:585–8. https://doi.org/10.3109/01443615.2015.1110120.
67. Abbas Y, Carnicer-Lombarte A, Gardner L, Thomas J, Brosens JJ, Moffett A, Sharkey AM, Franze K, Burton GJ, Oyen ML. Tissue stiffness at the human maternal-fetal interface. Hum Reprod. 2019;34:1999–2008. https://doi.org/10.1093/HUMREP/DEZ139.
68. Scott AK, Fodera DM, Yang P, Arter A, Hines AM, Kolluru SS, Zambuto SG, Myers KM, Kamilov US, Odibo AO, Oyen ML. Bioengineering approaches for patient-specific analysis of placenta structure and function. Placenta. 2024. https://doi.org/10.1016/J.PLACENTA.2024.08.005.
69. Sternberg AK, Buck VU, Classen-Linke I, Leube RE. How mechanical forces change the human endometrium during the menstrual cycle in preparation for embryo implantation. Cells. 2021;10:2008. https://doi.org/10.3390/CELLS10082008.
70. Cao J, Li H, Tang H, Gu X, Wang Y, Guan D, Du J, Fan Y. Stiff extracellular matrix promotes invasive behaviors of trophoblast cells. Bioengineering. 2023;10:384. https://doi.org/10.3390/BIOENGINEERING10030384/S1.
71. Zambuto SG, Kolluru SS, Ferchichi E, Rudewick HF, Fodera DM, Myers KM, Zustiak SP, Oyen ML. Evaluation of gelatin bloom strength on gelatin methacryloyl hydrogel properties. J Mech Behav Biomed Mater. 2024;154:106509. https://doi.org/10.1016/J.JMBBM.2024.106509.
72. Langbein M, Strick R, Strissel PL, Vogt N, Parsch H, Beckmann MW, Schild RL. Impaired cytotrophoblast cell–cell fusion is associated with reduced Syncytin and increased apoptosis in

patients with placental dysfunction. Mol Reprod Dev. 2008;75:175–83. https://doi.org/10.1002/MRD.20729.

73. Ma Z, Sagrillo-Fagundes L, Tran R, Parameshwar PK, Kalashnikov N, Vaillancourt C, Moraes C. Biomimetic micropatterned adhesive surfaces to mechanobiologically regulate placental trophoblast fusion. ACS Appl Mater Interfaces. 2019;11:47810–21. https://doi.org/10.1021/ACSAMI.9B19906/SUPPL_FILE/AM9B19906_SI_001.PDF.
74. Ma Z, Sagrillo-Fagundes L, Mok S, Vaillancourt C, Moraes C. Mechanobiological regulation of placental trophoblast fusion and function through extracellular matrix rigidity. Sci Rep. 2020;10(1):1–12. https://doi.org/10.1038/s41598-020-62659-8.
75. Cao R, Wang Y, Liu J, Rong L, Qin J. Self-assembled human placental model from trophoblast stem cells in a dynamic organ-on-a-chip system. Cell Prolif. 2023;56:e13469. https://doi.org/10.1111/CPR.13469.
76. Nishioka N, ichi Inoue K, Adachi K, Kiyonari H, Ota M, Ralston A, Yabuta N, Hirahara S, Stephenson RO, Ogonuki N, Makita R, Kurihara H, Morin-Kensicki EM, Nojima H, Rossant J, Nakao K, Niwa H, Sasaki H. The Hippo signaling pathway components Lats and Yap pattern Tead4 activity to distinguish mouse trophectoderm from inner cell mass. Dev Cell. 2009;16:398–410. https://doi.org/10.1016/J.DEVCEL.2009.02.003/ATTACHMENT/B14B5D94-C679-478C-A2DA-A03FC380BBAE/MMC1.PDF.
77. Zhang Y, Shan KZ, Liang P, Lowry AJ, Feng L, Yang H. PIEZO1 drives trophoblast fusion and placental development. BioRxiv. 2025. 2025.03.25.645313. https://doi.org/10.1101/2025.03.25.645313.
78. Fodera DM, Russell SR, Jackson JLL, Fang S, Chen X, Vink J, Oyen ML, Myers KM. Material properties of nonpregnant and pregnant human uterine layers. J Mech Behav Biomed Mater. 2024;151:106348. https://doi.org/10.1016/J.JMBBM.2023.106348.
79. Wu X, Morgan KG, Jones CJ, Tribe RM, Taggart MJ. Myometrial mechanoadaptation during pregnancy: implications for smooth muscle plasticity and remodelling. J Cell Mol Med. 2008;12:1360. https://doi.org/10.1111/J.1582-4934.2008.00306.X.
80. Bi Y, Li H, Diao M, Liu Q, Huang L, Tao Y, Wan Y, Lin X. Piezo1 overexpression in the uterus contributes to myometrium contraction and inflammation-associated preterm birth. J Transl Med. 2024;22:1–15. https://doi.org/10.1186/S12967-024-05978-Y/FIGURES/7.
81. Monaghan K, Baker SA, Dwyer L, Hatton WC, Sik Park K, Sanders KM, Koh SD. The stretch-dependent potassium channel TREK-1 and its function in murine myometrium. J Physiol. 2011;589:1221. https://doi.org/10.1113/JPHYSIOL.2010.203869.
82. Shynlova O, Dorogin A, Lye SJ. Stretch-induced uterine myocyte differentiation during rat pregnancy: involvement of caspase activation. Biol Reprod. 2010;82:1248–55. https://doi.org/10.1095/BIOLREPROD.109.081158.
83. Rieger MM, Wong M, Burnett LA, Sesillo FB, Baynes BB, Alperin M. Mechanisms governing protective pregnancy-induced adaptations of the pelvic floor muscles in the rat preclinical model. Am J Obstet Gynecol. 2022;226:708.e1–708.e13. https://doi.org/10.1016/J.AJOG.2021.11.1353.
84. Norian JM, Owen CM, Taboas J, Korecki C, Tuan R, Malik M, Catherino WH, Segars JH. Characterization of tissue biomechanics and mechanical signaling in uterine leiomyoma. Matrix Biol. 2012;31:57–65. https://doi.org/10.1016/J.MATBIO.2011.09.001.
85. Dalrymple A, Mahn K, Poston L, Songu-Mize E, Tribe RM. Mechanical stretch regulates TRPC expression and calcium entry in human myometrial smooth muscle cells. Mol Hum Reprod. 2007;13:31–9. https://doi.org/10.1093/MOLEHR/GAL110.
86. Mitchell JA, Shynlova O, Langille BL, Lye SJ. Mechanical stretch and progesterone differentially regulate activator protein-1 transcription factors in primary rat myometrial smooth muscle cells. Am J Physiol Endocrinol Metab. 2004;287. https://doi.org/10.1152/AJPENDO.00275.2003/ASSET/IMAGES/LARGE/ZH10090417890006.JPEG.
87. Peyton SR, Raub CB, Keschrumrus VP, Putnam AJ. The use of poly(ethylene glycol) hydrogels to investigate the impact of ECM chemistry and mechanics on smooth muscle

cells. Biomaterials. 2006;27:4881–93. https://doi.org/10.1016/J.BIOMATERIALS.2006.05.012.
88. Maxey AP, Travis JM, McCain ML. Regulation of oxytocin-induced calcium transients and gene expression in engineered myometrial tissues by tissue architecture and matrix rigidity. Curr Res Physiol. 2023;6:100108. https://doi.org/10.1016/J.CRPHYS.2023.100108.
89. Purdy MKP, Ducharme M, Haak AJ, Ravix J, Tan Q, Sicard D, Prakash YS, Tschumperlin DJ, Stewart EA. YAP/TAZ are activated by mechanical and hormonal stimuli in myometrium and exhibit increased baseline activation in uterine fibroids. Reprod Sci. 2020;27:1074–85. https://doi.org/10.1007/S43032-019-00106-4/FIGURES/9.
90. Kim J, Ushida T, Montagne K, Hirota Y, Yoshino O, Hiraoka T, Osuga Y, Furuakwa KS. Acquired contractile ability in human endometrial stromal cells by passive loading of cyclic tensile stretch. Sci Rep. 2020;10(1):1–11. https://doi.org/10.1038/s41598-020-65884-3.
91. Elad D, Zaretsky U, Kuperman T, Gavriel M, Long M, Jaffa A, Grisaru D. Tissue engineered endometrial barrier exposed to peristaltic flow shear stresses. APL Bioeng. 2020;4:14. https://doi.org/10.1063/5.0001994/23045.
92. Shlomo Y, Gavriel M, Jaffa AJ, Grisaru D, Elad D. Arrangement into layers and mechanobiology of multi-cell co-culture models of the uterine wall. Hum Reprod. 2024;39:1767–77. https://doi.org/10.1093/HUMREP/DEAE130.
93. Turton P, Arrowsmith S, Prescott J, Ballard C, Bricker L, Neilson J, Wray S. A comparison of the contractile properties of myometrium from singleton and twin pregnancies. PLoS One. 2013;8:e63800. https://doi.org/10.1371/JOURNAL.PONE.0063800.
94. Colon-Caraballo M, Russell SR, Myers KM, Mahendroo M. Collagen turnover during cervical remodeling involves both intracellular and extracellular collagen degradation pathways. Biol Reprod. 2025;112:709–27. https://doi.org/10.1093/BIOLRE/IOAF012.
95. Barnum CE, Shetye SS, Fazelinia H, Garcia BA, Fang S, Alzamora M, Li H, Brown LM, Tang C, Myers K, Wapner R, Soslowsky LJ, Vink JY. The non-pregnant and pregnant human cervix: a systematic proteomic analysis. Reprod Sci. 2022;29:1542–59. https://doi.org/10.1007/S43032-022-00892-4/FIGURES/12.
96. Yoshida K. Bioengineering and the cervix: the past, current, and future for addressing preterm birth. Curr Res Physiol. 2023;6:100107. https://doi.org/10.1016/J.CRPHYS.2023.100107.
97. Yoshida K, Jayyosi C, Lee N, Mahendroo M, Myers KM. Mechanics of cervical remodelling: insights from rodent models of pregnancy. Interface Focus. 2019;9. https://doi.org/10.1098/RSFS.2019.0026.
98. Mahendroo M. Cervical remodeling in term and preterm birth: insights from an animal model. Reproduction. 2012;143:429–38. https://doi.org/10.1530/REP-11-0466.
99. Vink J, Mourad M. The pathophysiology of human premature cervical remodeling resulting in spontaneous preterm birth – where are we now? Semin Perinatol. 2017;41:427. https://doi.org/10.1053/J.SEMPERI.2017.07.014.
100. Vink J, Yu V, Dahal S, Lohner J, Stern-Asher C, Mourad M, Davis G, Xue Z, Wang S, Myers K, Kitajewski J, Chen X, Wapner RJ, Ananth CV, Sheetz M, Gallos G. Extracellular matrix rigidity modulates human cervical smooth muscle contractility-new insights into premature cervical failure and spontaneous preterm birth. Reprod Sci. 2021;28:237–51. https://doi.org/10.1007/S43032-020-00268-6.
101. House M, Sanchez CC, Rice WL, Socrate S, Kaplan DL. Cervical tissue engineering using silk scaffolds and human cervical cells. Tissue Eng Part A. 2010;16:2101–12. https://doi.org/10.1089/TEN.TEA.2009.0457/ASSET/IMAGES/LARGE/FIGURE7.JPEG.
102. Takemura M, Itoh H, Sagawa N, Yura S, Korita D, Kakui K, Kawamura M, Hirota N, Maeda H, Fujii S. Cyclic mechanical stretch augments hyaluronan production in cultured human uterine cervical fibroblast cells. Mol Hum Reprod. 2005;11:659–65. https://doi.org/10.1093/MOLEHR/GAH229.
103. Akgul Y, Holt R, Mummert M, Word A, Mahendroo M. Dynamic changes in cervical glycosaminoglycan composition during normal pregnancy and preterm birth. Endocrinology. 2012;153:3493–503. https://doi.org/10.1210/EN.2011-1950.

104. Gordon J, Mowa CN. Mechanobiology of mice cervix: expression profile of mechano-related molecules during pregnancy. Cell Tissue Res. 2019;376:443–56. https://doi.org/10.1007/S00441-018-02983-8/FIGURES/10.
105. Stanley RL, Ohashi T, Gordon J, Mowa CN. A proteomic profile of postpartum cervical repair in mice. J Mol Endocrinol. 2018;60:17–28. https://doi.org/10.1530/JME-17-0179.
106. Shukla V, Barnhouse V, Ackerman WE, Summerfield TL, Powell HM, Leight JL, Kniss DA, Ghadiali SN. Cellular mechanics of primary human cervical fibroblasts: influence of progesterone and a pro-inflammatory cytokine. Ann Biomed Eng. 2018;46:197–207. https://doi.org/10.1007/S10439-017-1935-0.
107. Lajiness JD, Conway SJ. The dynamic role of cardiac fibroblasts in development and disease. J Cardiovasc Transl Res. 2012;5. https://doi.org/10.1007/s12265-012-9394-3.
108. Conway CK, Varghese A, Mahendroo M, Miller KS. The role of biaxial loading on smooth muscle contractility in the nulliparous murine cervix. Ann Biomed Eng. 2021;49:1874–87. https://doi.org/10.1007/S10439-021-02778-Z/FIGURES/8.
109. Laundon D, Gostling NJ, Sengers BG, Chavatte-Palmer P, Lewis RM. Placental evolution from a three-dimensional and multiscale structural perspective. Evolution (N Y). 2024;78:13–25. https://doi.org/10.1093/EVOLUT/QPAD209.
110. Mitchell BF, Taggart MJ. Are animal models relevant to key aspects of human parturition? Am J Physiol Regul Integr Comp Physiol. 2009;297:525–45. https://doi.org/10.1152/AJPREGU.00153.2009/ASSET/IMAGES/LARGE/ZH60080968840005.JPEG.
111. Scott AK, Oyen ML. Virtual pregnancies: predicting and preventing pregnancy complications with digital twins. Lancet Digit Health. 2024;6:e436–7. https://doi.org/10.1016/S2589-7500(24)00086-4.
112. Clark AR, Yoshida K, Oyen ML. Computational modeling in pregnancy biomechanics research. J Mech Behav Biomed Mater. 2022;128:105099. https://doi.org/10.1016/J.JMBBM.2022.105099.

Myometrial Contractility and Uterine Peristalsis: Translating Biological Complexity into Bioengineered Systems

Karla I. Ortega Sandoval, Astha Lamichhane, Ritu Dave, Antonina I. Frolova, and Shreya A. Raghavan

Abstract The uterus is a multifunctional organ central to both reproductive and nonreproductive health. The contractility of its muscular wall, the myometrium, is a tightly regulated process, dynamically adapting across the menstrual cycle, pregnancy, labor, and postpartum periods. Dysfunctional myometrial contractility underlies significant clinical issues including dysmenorrhea, infertility, preterm birth, labor arrest, and postpartum hemorrhage. Understanding its function requires an appreciation for its intricate cellular and structural basis, multilayered regulation and nuanced contractile functions. This chapter discusses the central importance of myometrial contractility, providing biological context important for its investigation through bioengineering approaches. It also provides an overview of early and advanced bioengineering methods used to replicate or investigate myometrial contractility, identifying opportunities for future advancements in this field.

Keywords Myometrial contractility · Uterine peristalsis · Smooth muscle cells · Reproductive health

1 Introduction to Myometrial Contractility in the Uterus

The uterus is a hollow muscular organ in the pelvic cavity [1–3]. The organ is essential for menstruation, embryo implantation, placental development, pregnancy, and parturition. The uterine wall is composed of many distinct layers, including the innermost endometrium, the muscular myometrium, and the outermost serosa or perimetrium [3]. The myometrium, primarily composed of smooth muscle [4], is responsible for generating coordinated contractions that are central and essential to

K. I. Ortega Sandoval · A. Lamichhane · S. A. Raghavan (✉)
Department of Biomedical Engineering, Texas A&M University, College Station, TX, USA
e-mail: karla.ortegas@tamu.edu; alamichhane@tamu.edu; sraghavan@tamu.edu

R. Dave · A. I. Frolova
Department of Obstetrics and Gynecology, Center for Reproductive Health Sciences, Washington University School of Medicine, St. Louis, MO, USA
e-mail: ritudave@wustl.edu; frolovaa@wustl.edu

S. G. Zambuto, M. L. Oyen (eds.), *Biomaterials for Women's Health Engineering*,
https://doi.org/10.1007/978-3-032-10745-9_8

uterine function. Myometrial contractility is a core part of the mechanical competency of the uterus, and is a tightly regulated process that involves hormonal, neural, immune, and mechanical inputs that integrate into intracellular pathways.

Physiologically, myometrial contractility has diverse context-dependent roles that support the central function of the uterus in embryonic and fetal development, pregnancy, and parturition. To prepare for this function, the endometrium undergoes cyclic hormone-dependent remodeling. Guided by estrogen during the proliferative phase, endometrial growth and thickening occur. Following ovulation, progesterone secreted by the corpus luteum promotes endometrial transition into the secretory phase, preparing for potential embryo implantation. If fertilization does not occur, progesterone levels decline, leading to menstruation or shedding of the uterine lining [5, 6]. If fertilization occurs, myometrial contractile patterns transition to guide embryo implantation into the endometrial stroma and initiate placental development [7].

The myometrium facilitates physiologic functions of the nonpregnant uterus by varying its contractile patterns (waveform characteristics including amplitude, frequency, and direction) during the uterine menstrual cycle [8, 9]. During pregnancy, the myometrium maintains quiescence, allowing uterine expansion and stretch to accommodate a growing fetus heavily influenced by hormonal input from progesterone and human chorionic gonadotropin [2] and mechanical stretch [10]. Subsequently, during labor and delivery, the myometrium must transition to a highly contractile phenotype and expel the fetus. Leading up to parturition, a hormonal shift occurs in which estrogen predominates over progesterone. This estrogenic shift induces myometrial expression of contractile associated proteins such as the oxytocin receptor, which binds the peptide hormone oxytocin during labor to augment uterine contractions [11]. Postpartum, myometrial contractility is essential for placental separation and tamponade of the spiral arteries, preventing excessive bleeding, and returning the uterus toward a menstrual cycle.

Disruption of normal uterine function, particularly within the myometrium, can result in significant clinical sequelae both during and outside of pregnancy. Adenomyosis, a condition characterized by abnormal infiltration of endometrial tissue into the myometrium can cause debilitating pelvic pain and infertility [12, 13]. Leiomyomas (uterine fibroids), a common neoplasm in women, result from excessive proliferation of myometrial smooth muscle cells. Although benign, these can lead to abnormal uterine bleeding, pelvic discomfort, and infertility [14]. In addition to the structural abnormalities, altered myometrial peristalsis deeply impacts fertility. Hyperperistalsis (altered myometrial mechanical patterns) during in vitro fertilization has been associated with reduced embryo implantation, while insufficient peristalsis can impair sperm transport [15, 16]. Additionally, abnormal uterine peristaltic activity has been observed in women with adenomyosis and leiomyomas [17].

Myometrial dysfunction also has critical implications during pregnancy and parturition. Preterm birth, defined as delivery prior to 37 weeks of gestation, accounts for over a quarter of neonatal deaths and is characterized by premature transition of the myometrium to a contractile phenotype [18, 19]. Alternatively, inadequate myometrial contractility at term can result in prolonged gestation, labor dystocia, and cesarean delivery, all of which increase maternal and neonatal morbidity [20–25]. Failure of the uterus to adequately contract postdelivery, a process known as uterine atony, can lead to postpartum hemorrhage, a major cause of maternal morbidity and mortality [26, 27].

Having underscored the clinical significance of myometrial contractility, a reader may appreciate and recognize its central and fundamental importance to uterine function. The chapter first provides a structural basis for myometrial contractility, an overview of myometrial contractile patterns in physiology, and mechanisms of regulation across lifespan, physiology and pathophysiology. Subsequently, the later parts of the chapter explore the current state of bioengineering approaches used to investigate or replicate myometrial contractility, identifying scientific opportunities for future discovery.

2 Structural Basis of Myometrial Contractility

Understanding the anatomical and structural foundation of myometrial contractility is essential for unraveling the mechanisms governing uterine function in both health and disease. This section explores the myometrium's cellular architecture, offering insight into the generation and coordination of myometrial contractility.

2.1 Cell Types in the Myometrium

Single-cell atlases of the human myometrium highlight the rich diversity of cell types within this tissue [28–30]. Myometrial smooth muscle cells are the predominant population primarily responsible for generating contractions associated with uterine peristalsis and overall myometrial contractility. Other cell types within the myometrial microenvironment actively support this function, including stromal cells, endothelial cells and immune cells [30, 31]. Stromal cells like fibroblasts support myometrial structure through extracellular matrix maintenance, cell adhesion, and immune response mediation [30]. Endothelial cells support blood vessel morphogenesis and angiogenesis, and can also influence myometrial contractility through paracrine signaling to modulate myometrial tone [32]. Among the immune cell population, monocytes and macrophages are the most abundant and exhibit significant modulation in the setting of pregnancy and labor. Macrophages directly influence myometrial contractility by enhancing contractile protein expression in smooth muscle cells via secreted cytokines [33, 34]. Consequently, these cells play critical roles in initiating myometrial contractility during labor [35–37], while also contributing to uterine quiescence to prevent preterm birth [38]. Comparisons in single cell atlases between premenopausal, postpartum, perimenopausal and postmenopausal samples demonstrated significant changes in tissue composition, especially in the proportions of stromal, endothelial, and immune cells, underscoring the heterogeneity of the myometrium across the human lifespan [28].

Myometrial smooth muscle cells are primarily responsible for generating uterine contractions. Contraction itself arises from conserved mechanisms observed in smooth muscle cells throughout the body including vascular, gastrointestinal and airway smooth muscle. The key trigger for myometrial smooth muscle contractions is the electromechanical coupling initiated by a surge of calcium ions [4, 39]. A distinguishing feature of myometrial smooth muscle cells is a heightened sensitivity to oxytocin, which significantly modulates their excitability and contractility compared to other smooth muscle cell types [40, 41]. Through conserved pathways, intracellular calcium influx triggers actomyosin interaction, generating tension on the myometrial smooth muscle cell, ultimately resulting in contraction [42]. Therefore, the overall cellular coordination of myometrial contractility is governed not by unique molecular pathways, but by the functional integration of the layered arrangement of myometrial smooth muscle cells, and their cell–cell communication.

2.2 *Structural and Ultrastructural Organization of Myometrial Smooth Muscle Cells*

The macroscopic structural unit of the myometrium is the fasciculus, a collection of several cylindrical or sheetlike bundles of myometrial smooth muscle cells [43] with diameters in the millimeter scale. Early investigations used serial histological sectioning and trichrome staining to visualize myometrial architecture to reveal that each cylindrical bundle (~300 μm) housed similarly oriented smooth muscle cells with sheaths of connective tissue [44]. Originally, the myometrium was thought to have two layers, the inner circular layer and the outer longitudinal layer, with differing orientations of smooth muscle cells. However, with the advent of higher resolution imaging, tissue preparation methods and computational methods, a third mesh-like central layer was identified within the myometrium [45, 46]. Although the layers are less defined in the human myometrium compared to other species (Fig. 1) [4], they can still be classified based on the orientation of myometrial smooth muscle cells within the bundles into (i) the inner circular layer (sub-endometrial), where muscle cells are arranged concentrically around the longitudinal axis; (ii) middle mesh-like layer (stratum vasculare), where the bundle arrangement is diffuse and interconnected; and (iii) the outer longitudinal layer (subserosal) where muscle cells are primarily oriented along the longitudinal axis of the uterus. The fibers within the three layers often merge at the boundaries, allowing for functional integration and forceful, coordinated uterine contractions.

Within the fasciculi, smooth muscle cells are very densely packed, with most cells being contiguous. Gap junctions, located on the sarcolemma, enable direct cytoplasmic communication between adjacent cells, which is essential for ensuring coordinated contraction across the tissue. Connexin-43, the predominant gap junction

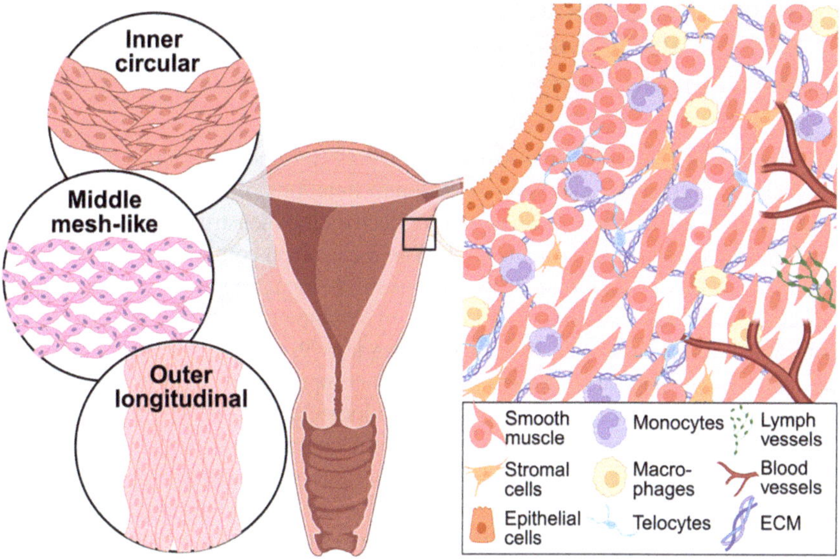

Fig. 1 The human myometrium is organized into three layers distinguished by the orientation of smooth muscle fibers. The innermost layer, located adjacent to the epithelial endometrium, features circularly arranged fibers. The middle layers consist of a mesh-like interwoven architecture. The outermost layer, adjacent to the serosa, contains fibers that run along the length of the uterus. The myometrium itself contains a diverse range of cells types. While smooth muscle makes up the majority of the tissue, other cell populations include stromal cells, telocytes, and immune cells such as monocytes and macrophages. Blood and lymphatic vessels are also embedded throughout supporting tissue function and communication

protein in the myometrium, forms low-resistance channels to facilitate electrical coupling between adjacent cells. This intercellular communication is essential for generating synchronous contractions across the uterus [4]. Connexin-43 expression increases in myometrial cells during labor to promote coordinated tissue-level contractility [47].

The overall structural and ultrastructural arrangement of myometrial smooth muscle cells directly dictates force production and myometrial contractility, ensuring that contractions are strong and coordinated enough to perform key reproductive functions, such as expelling menstrual debris or delivering a fetus during labor. Conversely, disruptions in this structural organization lead to dysfunctional myometrial contractility and associated reproductive disorders, as evidenced by structural alterations and adverse fertility outcomes in women with uterine fibroids [16] or endometriosis [48].

3 Myometrial Contractility and Uterine Peristalsis: Patterns and Significance in Physiology and Pathophysiology

The coordinated action of myometrial layers produces various patterns of myometrial contractility, determining different functions of the uterus. Myometrial contractions occur in several forms, varying across the menstrual cycle, pregnancy, labor, delivery, and post-partum (Fig. 2). The mechanical competency of the uterine myometrium was first identified by early methods including invasive intra-uterine pressure recordings, in vitro recordings of myometrial strips, and later with transvaginal ultrasound and MRI based imaging [9, 48–50]. A computationally inclined reader may also appreciate newer computational insights from high-resolution imaging corresponding to the biomechanics of the human uterus [51]. The insights demonstrate that myometrial contractility varies widely during the uterine menstrual cycle to perform different functions related to reproduction or menstruation. With an appreciation for the structural organization of the myometrium from the previous section, here we explore distinctions in macroscopic myometrial contractile patterns, their waveform characteristics, and their contribution to uterine function and physiology. Myometrial contractions occur in three primary forms: (i) uterine peristalsis; (ii) synchronized phasic; and (iii) tonic contractions, each with diverse functional implications. The regulation of these contractions occur at multiple levels, covered in the following section.

3.1 *Uterine Peristalsis*

Peristaltic contractions are slow, low magnitude, rhythmic, wavelike contractions that occur along the length of the uterus. They arise primarily from the sub-endometrial myometrium (or the inner circular layer) of the nonpregnant uterus. This functional localization was confirmed through imaging techniques including magnetic resonance imaging (MRI), transvaginal ultrasound, and video-vaginosonography, which showed peristaltic wave propagation confined to this inner myometrial layer [16]. Wave features differ by menstrual cycle phase. During the proliferative phase, under the influence of rising estrogen, peristaltic waves have high-frequency and high-amplitude contractions. Waves predominantly move from the cervix toward the fundus, producing intense displacement, guiding rapid transport of sperm [52]. During the secretory phase, opposing contractions, or waves that initiate simultaneously from both the cervix and fundus, are frequently observed. These bidirectional patterns are thought to stabilize the embryo within the uterine cavity, preventing expulsion through either the cervix or the fallopian tubes, while also supporting early embryo positioning and nutrient distribution during the implantation window [30, 53, 54]. Under continuing progesterone dominance, the myometrium enters a relatively quiescent state, marked by a reduction in both

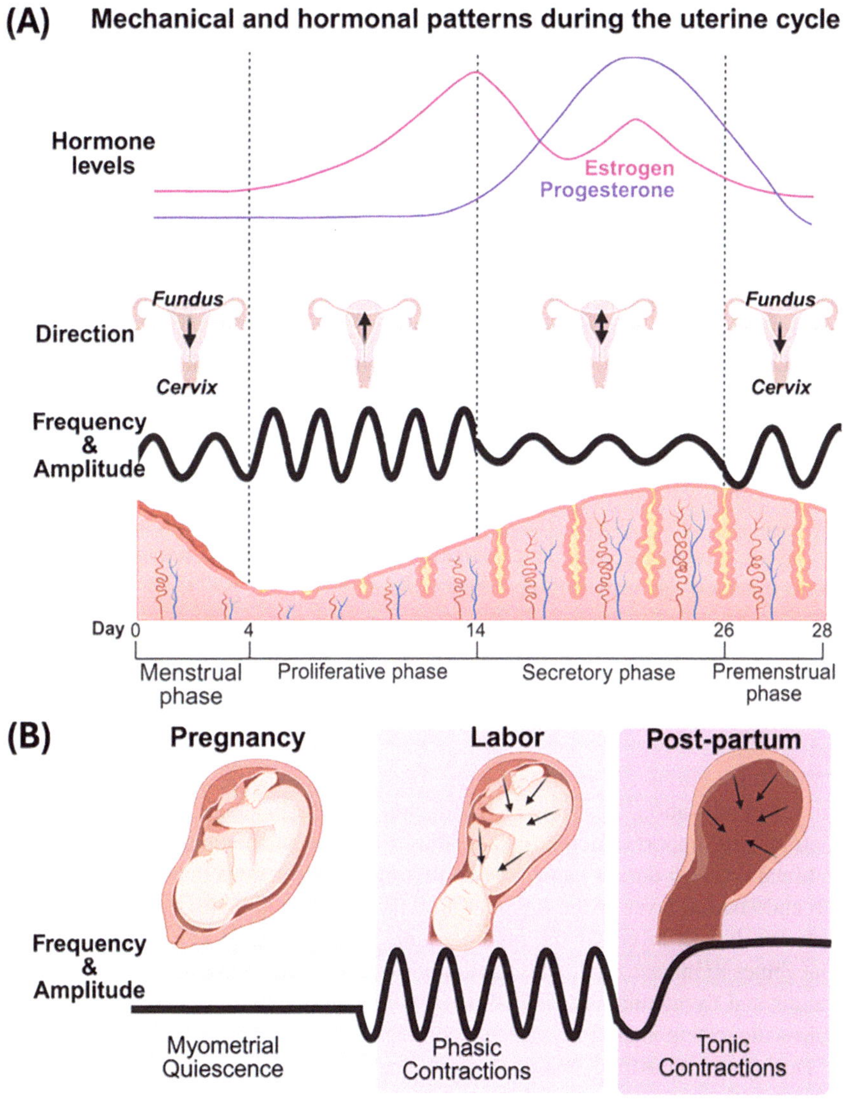

Fig. 2 (**a**) The pattern and direction of uterine peristalsis changes throughout the menstrual cycle, along with hormonal fluctuations. During menstruation, wave frequency and strength increase, with fundus-to-cervix contractions aiding endometrial and fluid expulsion. In the proliferative phase, estrogen promotes high-frequency, cervix-to-fundus waves that support sperm transport. The secretory phase is marked by slower, often bidirectional waves under progesterone dominance, promoting embryo implantation. As the cycle concludes, wave activity increases and directionality shifts again. (**b**) Uterine contractility across pregnancy, labor, and the postpartum period. During pregnancy, the myometrium remains largely quiescent, maintaining low activity to prevent premature contractions. Labor is characterized by strong, rhythmic phasic contractions involving all myometrial layers, which increase in frequency and amplitude to facilitate fetal expulsion. Postpartum, the uterus exhibits tonic contractions which promote uterine involution and help compress blood vessels at the placental site to prevent hemorrhage

contraction frequency and amplitude. This transition reflects the physiological shift toward uterine receptivity, optimizing the intrauterine environment for embryo implantation [54]. In the absence of embryo implantation, as the uterus proceeds toward menstruation, peristaltic waves increase in strength and frequency. The waves also shift direction, taking place from fundus to cervix to expel menstrual fluid.

Disruptions to patterns of uterine peristalsis in the form of altered waveforms (irregular frequency, higher amplitude, or lack of directionality) have dire consequences like infertility, implantation failure, and pain. Hyperperistalsis, characterized by increased frequency of peristaltic waves, has been strongly associated with conditions such as endometriosis and adenomyosis. This phenomenon was first identified using vaginal sonography in the mid-1990s, which also additionally revealed retrograde menstruation (from cervix to fundus instead of the opposite). Hyperperistalsis, therefore, is implicated in contributing to the development and dissemination of endometrial lesions outside the uterus in endometriosis [55]. Similarly, women with fibroids exhibit lower contraction amplitudes and frequencies. Although no direct causal relationships are established between endometriosis, fibroids, and other disorders and infertility, altered myometrial contractility impairs sperm transport and embryo implantation significantly [16, 31, 35] .

3.2 Phasic Contractions

Phasic contractions are strong, discrete bursts of contractile activity followed by periods of relaxation. Rhythmic, forceful, and periodic in nature, intermittent phasic contractions support endometrial shedding during menstruation, cervical dilation, and fetal delivery during labor. Unlike peristaltic contractions that only involve the sub-endometrial layer of the myometrium, the strong amplitudes of phasic contractions involve all layers of the myometrium. This transmural involvement directly contributes to intense contraction amplitudes, that are often implicated in menstrual cramps and dysmennorhea [56]. Women with fibroids often present with dysmenorrhea suggesting altered myometrial contractility as a potential cause [57].

During the menstrual phase, these contractions facilitate forward emptying of uterine content occurring fundus to cervix. Under the influence of oxytocin, phasic contractions of the myometrium during labor and delivery also aid in expelling the fetus. The frequency and amplitude of phasic contractions vary, occurring first at intervals of a few minutes during labor with increasing frequency as labor progresses. Amplitudes also increase during active labor, influenced by hormones and positive feedback from mechanical stretch (outlined in the following sections). Insufficient phasic contractions may contribute to labor dystocia or nonprogressive labor, often requiring uterotonics to augment contractions [58].

3.3 *Tonic Contractions*

Tonic contractions are prolonged, sustained contractions with minimal relaxation. Tone implies high-amplitude, long-duration contractions where the uterus maintains a heightened internal pressure while remaining firm and contracted [9]. These are typically associated with elevated levels of oxytocin following labor and delivery, or pathological states. Unlike normal rhythmic contractions, tonic contractions are continuous, contributing to a resting baseline tension. Basal tone in the uterus is required to maintain its shape and its readiness (to facilitate menstruation or pregnancy) [59]. In pathological nonpregnant states, excessive tonic contractions can lead to constant spasm [60]. However, in pregnancy and the postpartum period, myometrial tone is important to successful obstetric outcomes. Maintenance of uterine tone during pregnancy ensures quiescence, preventing premature contractility and preterm labor. Two of the most important functions of uterine tone occurs after fetal delivery. First, a strong basal tone is required for the uterus to shrink back to its prepregnancy size, a process known as involution, which returns the uterus to functional readiness to take on the menstrual cycle [59]. Secondly, a strong basal tone is required to compress the spiral arteries at the placental site. Loss of uterine tone (atony) consequently leads to severe postpartum hemorrhage [61].

3.4 *Ex Vivo and In Vitro Methods to Measure and Quantify Myometrial Contractility*

Organ Bath and Tissue Strip Measurements

The organ bath system remains a widely used ex vivo method for evaluating myometrial contractility. In this approach, strips or rings of myometrial tissue, derived from pregnant or nonpregnant uteri, are mounted between a fixed hook and an isometric force transducer. The tissues are preloaded and maintained within a temperature-controlled, oxygenated chamber containing physiological saline solution. Within this set up, pharmacological or physiological agents are administered to assess tissue responsiveness and contractility. This setup allows precise, real-time quantification of contractile parameters, including amplitude, frequency, duration, and basal tone, generated by the myometrial strips [62]. These metrics can reflect both spontaneous and stimulus-induced contractile activity and are crucial for characterizing normal and pathological uterine behavior [63]. For example, organ bath-based measurements were instrumental in characterizing how oxytocin and vasopressin increase contractile activity, and in supporting the use of antagonists such as atosiban to suppress preterm labor. Similarly, drugs like carbetocin and nifedipine were first screened for uterotonic and tocolytic effects in organ bath systems before entering clinical trials [64, 65].

Collagen-Based Contractility Assays
Three-dimensional (3D) collagen contractility assays provide a biophysically relevant platform for assessing cell-mediated contractile force. In this system, isolated myometrial cells are embedded in collagen lattices, which contract over time in response to cellular tension. As cells exert tractional forces, the gel contracts over time. The extent of contraction, measured by a reduction in gel area or volume, serves as a quantitative proxy for cellular contractile activity. Contraction is typically assessed using brightfield imaging followed by digital image analysis or by measuring dimensional changes with calipers or displacement [63, 66, 67]. This format supports mechanistic discovery, by allowing molecular perturbations like gene silencing, overexpression, and biochemical manipulation to dissect molecular pathways governing contractility [67]. However, collagen-based contractility assays do not decouple extracellular matrix remodeling and myometrial contractility, making the observed effects on area change an indirect readout of contractility.

4 Regulation of Myometrial Contractility and Peristalsis

The regulation of myometrial contractility and uterine peristalsis is a multifaceted process involving hormonal, neural, inflammatory, and mechanical signals that dynamically shape uterine behavior across reproductive cycle and pregnancy. This section will explore each of these regulatory mechanisms and how they collectively maintain the functional contractile dynamics of the uterus.

4.1 Hormonal Regulation

Myometrial contractility is tightly regulated by hormonal fluctuations throughout the menstrual cycle and pregnancy [68]. Oxytocin and prostaglandins are the primary uterotonic hormones, which directly augment myometrial contractility. Oxytocin is a pituitary hormone, which increases myometrial contraction frequency and amplitudes during labor by increasing calcium ion entry into myometrial smooth muscle cells. Oxytocin receptor expression is increased in the myometrium during labor [69]. In the nonpregnant uterus, oxytocin receptors are expressed at much lower levels. Consequently, while oxytocin still stimulates myometrial contractions, its effect is significantly less pronounced compared to labor [70]. In fact, elevated oxytocin receptor expression and even low serum concentrations of oxytocin are associated with painful menstruation and dysmennorhea [71]. Prostaglandins are synthesized locally within the uterus by several cell types, including decidual, myometrial and immune cells. Cyclooxygenase 2, one of the enzymes responsible for prostaglandin synthesis, is upregulated in the uterus at parturition and is one of the prototypical contractility-associated proteins. There are multiple prostaglandin subtypes, each with specific uterine effects. PGF2a and PGE2 are the main prostaglandins responsible for increased myometrial contractility.

The ovarian hormones progesterone and estrogen play crucial roles in regulating both the growth and contractility of the myometrium. Estrogens, mainly estradiol, enhance myometrial contractility and excitability, by increasing sensitivity to uterotonic hormones (prostaglandins and oxytocin), through upregulation of their receptors and synchronicity of contraction through the expression of connexin-43, the gap junction protein required for coordinated uterine contractions [52, 72, 73]. During the estrogen dominant proliferative phase of the uterine cycle, oxytocin and prostaglandin-induced increases in uterine peristalsis support sperm transport. A similar increase in phasic contractions induce endometrial shedding during menstruation [74]. Excessive stimulation of myometrial contractility during menses is associated with dysmenorrhea, which is why inhibitors of prostaglandin synthesis can be an effective treatment [75].

In contrast, progesterone promotes myometrial relaxation and quiescence [76] via multiple mechanisms. Progesterone suppresses myometrial smooth muscle cell expression of the oxytocin receptor [77, 78], inhibits prostaglandin synthesis, alters smooth muscle cell excitability [79], and inhibits the expression of connexin-43 [73]. Systemic levels of progesterone rise throughout pregnancy, maintaining myometrial quiescence. The onset of parturition is triggered by a decline in progesterone activity at the end of gestation, which in many species occurs through a systemic withdrawal, whether through lower synthesis or increased metabolism into inactive forms. However, in humans, circulating progesterone levels remain high until after delivery of the fetus and placenta. Instead, there is a functional withdrawal due to an altered balance in the expression of progesterone receptor isoforms in myometrial smooth muscle cells.

4.2 Neural Regulation

The uterus is innervated by sympathetic and parasympathetic fibers of the autonomic nervous system [80]. Cholinergic parasympathetic fibers stimulate myometrial contractions, by releasing acetylcholine that acts on muscarinic receptors on myometrial smooth muscle cells or noradrenaline [81]. Adrenergic sympathetic innervation is involved in myometrial contractility and endometrial secretory function [82]. α-adrenergic receptor activation leads to uterine contractions, whereas β-adrenergic receptors induce relaxation [83]. The entire sympathetic innervation of the uterus degenerates during pregnancy, and regenerates following parturition. While the functional significance for this plasticity is as yet unknown, it is thought to protect myometrial quiescence from potentially harmful overactivity of the sympathetic nervous system that may lead to premature labor [84]. In addition to the dramatic plasticity during pregnancy, innervation also varies with the uterine cycle along with cycling estrogen [85]. Although the myometrium is innervated, it is primarily a myogenic organ, meaning that its contractility is independent of neural activity with no motor neuronal synapses in the myometrium [86].

4.3 *Inflammatory Mediators and Cytokines in Myometrial Contractility and Peristalsis*

The transition of the myometrium from a quiescent to contractile state is driven by a shift from anti-inflammatory to pro-inflammatory signaling, primarily within myometrial smooth muscle cells and supported by infiltrating immune cells such as macrophages and neutrophils. This environment is characterized by elevated levels of pro-inflammatory cytokines (e.g., IL-1β, TNF-α), increased leukocyte infiltration, and upregulation of contraction associated proteins including connexin-43, and cyclooxygenase-2 (COX-2). Collectively, these changes promote myometrial contractility in preparation for labor or menstruation [87]. During menstruation, the withdrawal of progesterone leads to increased prostaglandin and inflammatory cytokines, such as IL-1β, TNF-α, and IL-6, contributing to myometrial contractions [88].

During pregnancy, the uterus remains in anti-inflammatory state until late gestation. Labor at term ends up leading to infiltration of inflammatory cells into the myometrium and cervix and increases production of pro-inflammatory cytokines (IL-1β, IL-6, TNF-α, and IL-8) [89]. This proinflammatory environment promotes myometrial contractility, expulsion of the fetus and placenta [89]. In the instance of infection, an activated inflammatory response state therefore may trigger preterm labor [89].

4.4 *Mechanical Factors*

Myometrial smooth muscle cells are highly mechanosensitive, and are regulated by many mechanical factors of the uterine microenvironment (Fig. 3). One of the primary mechanical regulatory mechanisms involves mechanical stretch, which occurs as the uterus expands. Especially in the context of pregnancy. Stretch activates mechanotransduction pathways, leading to an influx of sodium and calcium ions that alters myometrial smooth muscle cell excitability, and thereby its contractility [90]. Interestingly, myometrial smooth muscles adapt to passive stretch over time with extensive cytoskeletal remodeling, which ultimately results in enhanced contractility during the onset of labor [91]. In humans, myometrial strips from women who delivered twins exhibited greater contractile activity compared to those from singleton pregnancies [92]. However, excessive stretch, such as in cases of polyhydramnios can result in decreased myometrial contractile force [49]. Acute, rapid stretching also induces transient contractions driven by calcium ion influx [93, 94]. Following contraction, calcium levels return to baseline, allowing relaxation until the next activation cycle [60], allowing not just peristalsis but phasic contractile patterns. Before the onset of labor, mechanical stretch also increases oxytocin receptor expression, priming oxytocin responsiveness for labor and delivery [95]. Externally applying cyclic strain to myometrial smooth muscle

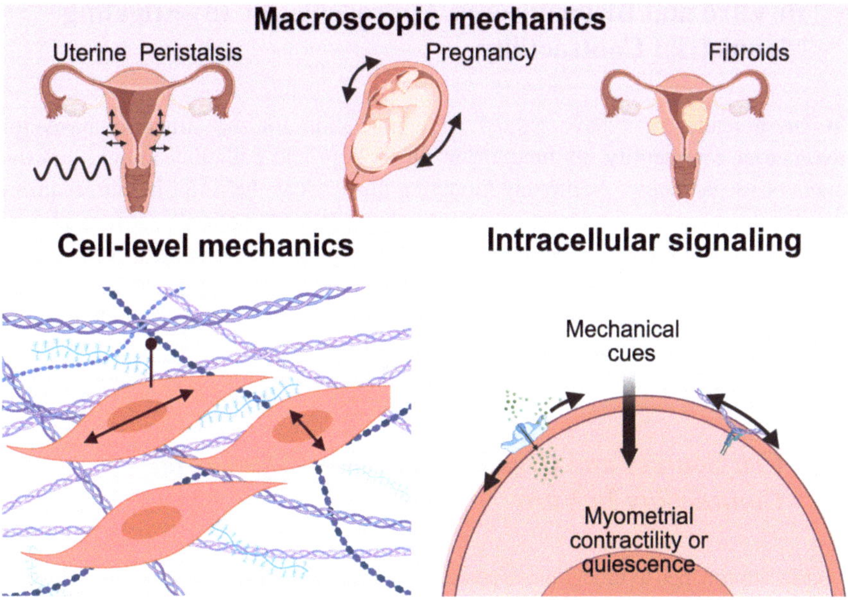

Fig. 3 Mechanical forces such as wave-like peristalsis, uterine stretch during pregnancy, external pressure from fibroids influence myometrial behavior. These external inputs are sensed through myometrial cell–ECM interactions involving integrins and mechanosensitive ion channels. Activation of mechanotransduction pathways leads to intracellular signaling events, including calcium influx and cytoskeletal remodeling, that modulate contractile activity. Depending on the mechanical context and hormonal environment, these signals can promote either increased contractility or support a quiescent state, allowing the uterus to adapt dynamically to physiological demands

cells (as those observed during low amplitude peristalsis), interestingly, results in altered elastin production, which further alters contractility by altering tissue material properties [96].

Another key mechanical variable in the uterus that impacts myometrial contractility is microenvironmental stiffness, reflecting the extracellular matrix and tissue material properties [97]. Physiologically, changes in stiffness occur through the uterine cycle during the proliferative, secretory and menstrual phases, as well as in pregnancy and postpartum remodeling. Pathological changes in stiffness also occur in uterine fibroids and adenomyosis [97–100]. In fact, stiffness is acutely related to the transformation of myometrial smooth muscle cells into a synthetic phenotype, connected to fibroid pathogenesis [101, 102]. Once placed in stiff or rigid microenvironments, myometrial smooth muscle cell responsiveness to calcium is altered, thereby altering oxytocin-induced contractility [103].

Interstitial and intrauterine fluid pressure also plays a role in regulating myometrial contractility, especially as it relates to coordination of global contractions. During labor, localized contractions elevate intrauterine pressure, increasing wall tension and recruiting additional contractile regions, thereby amplifying uterine responsiveness and coordination [104].

5 In Vitro and Bioengineered Approaches for Investigating Myometrial Contractility

So far, a reader may have gained an appreciation for the structural basis for myometrial contractility, its function in physiology and pathophysiology, and the layers of its regulation. Accurately modeling this intricate behavior in vitro requires the development of biomimetic systems that replicate both the structural and mechanical complexity of the native uterine myometrial environment for research and therapeutic applications. Here, we provide an overview of engineering methodologies used to tissue engineer the myometrium or the uterus, including some approaches that investigate myometrial contractility.

5.1 Cell Sources and Organoids to Assess Myometrial Contractility In Vitro

In vitro approaches to model the myometrium require stable cell sources as a starting point to combine with scaffolding or bioinks to create functionally bioengineered structures. Primary myometrial smooth muscle cells are the gold standard, typically isolated from human myometrial tissues during elective C-sections. Myometrial smooth muscle cells are isolated via enzymatic digestion (e.g., collagenase). Nutrient media composition is acutely important for the culture of smooth muscle cells to balance proliferation with the maintenance of the myometrial contractile phenotype [105, 106]. Primary human myometrial smooth muscle cells express many defining contractile markers including α-smooth muscle actin, caldesmon, the gap junction protein connexin-43, and the oxytocin receptor. For a limited number of passages, primary cells also remain responsive to both hormonal and inflammatory stimulation. Notably, cells isolated from different uterine regions exhibit distinct transcriptional and functional profiles, offering insight into spatial heterogeneity in contractile regulation [63]. Apart from limited passaging in vitro, another source of variability in primary tissues is the impact of donor variability and health status, inherent to all primary cells. In the context of the myometrium, this opens the interesting opportunity to study changes in myometrial contractility in cells derived from women with uterine fibroids [107], adenomyosis [108], or other underlying uterine disease. A standardized, and now commercially available, source of myometrial smooth muscle cells are telomerase-immortalized human myometrial smooth muscle cells [109, 110]. These immortalized cells offer reproducible behavior across many passages. Early in vitro studies for functional assessment of oxytocin used telomerase immortalized myometrial smooth muscle cells within collagen lattice gels, to assess myometrial contractility, similar to methods outlined in Sect. 3.4 [111]. Maintenance of key smooth muscle markers and basic contractile behavior, including responses to oxytocin [112] makes immortalized myometrial smooth muscle cells a robust starting point to study myometrial contractility and function.

Interestingly, myometrial stem cells have been identified in human myometrial samples based on the co-expression of CD44 and Stro-1 [113]. Encapsulating these cells into Matrigel resulted in the formation of a myometrial organoid, where stem cells differentiated and self-organized into mature myometrial smooth muscle cells and fibroblasts, producing extracellular matrix [114]. These organoids have been used widely in the study of uterine fibroid pathogenesis [114, 115], but not in investigations of myometrial contractility. Within the broader uterus ecosystem, organoids are better characterized for their use in investigating endometrial physiology and pathology, compared to myometrial contractility [116, 117]. Since myometrial contractility is influenced by many layers of regulation (outlined in Sect. 4), organoid systems may be particularly advantageous in gaining a nuanced understanding of how cell–cell communication influences contractility. However, the inaccessibility of luminal spaces in self-assembled organoids limits a direct measurement of contractility using organ bath based methods.

5.2 Engineered In Vitro Systems in Myometrial Contractility and Mechanobiology

The structure and arrangement of myometrial cells (the circular, mesh network and longitudinal alignment) is deeply related to its contractile ability. The ability for tissue engineering to enforce structure–function relationships by promoting cellular alignment render them inherently advantageous to investigate uterine physiology (summarized in Table 1). Early attempts at tissue engineering the myometrium used a variety of scaffold choices, including natural collagen and gel-like materials, decellularized extracellular matrices, and manufactured polymeric biomaterials [118]. Early work by Lü et al. [67] combined a custom molded collagen/Matrigel scaffold with static stretch to incorporate myometrial smooth muscle cells and endometrial cells. While contractility was not directly assayed, myometrial smooth muscle cells had the genotype and expressed contractile proteins at comparable levels to those observed in explant myometrial tissues. Decellularized extracellular matrices were popular sources of scaffolding material, preserving bioactivity and protein composition of the native uterus. While protocols for decellularization still continue to evolve, early work generated myometrial structures that were ~500 μm deep and demonstrated isometric, coordinated contractions in response to oxytocin stimulation [119]. Similar cultures of primary myometrial smooth muscle cells on polyglactin-910 mesh scaffolds also resulted in multicellular 3D structures that demonstrated contractility [66]. In recent years, as an appreciation for the mechanical competency of the myometrium grew, engineering approaches have also adapted to enable this important physiological functionality. Myometrial "ring" structures were generated using magnetic 3D bioprinting, where magnetized human myometrial cells (both primary and immortalized) were bioprinted into concentric ringlike structures, similar to the inner circular myometrium. Notably,

Table 1 A summary of methods and bioengineering studies investigating myometrial physiology

Reference	Model/innovation	Cell source	Approach/format	Major techniques	Key results and insights	Translational/clinical relevance
Young et al. [66]	3D polyglactin-910 (Vicryl) mesh scaffold for myometrial tissue culture	Primary human myometrial (term cesarean)	Cell seeding, mesh suspension	Live imaging, confocal, microelectrode, force measurement	Cells fill mesh, form 3D tissue with, bridge between meshes, generate measurable tension, and can produce coordinated contractions. First use of 3D scaffolds enabling physiological studies of human myometrium	Established a basis for interpreting physiological cell-to-cell interactions and mechanical behavior in human uterine tissue; useful for probing myometrial excitation and contractile dynamics
Fitzgibbon et al. [63]	Collagen gel contraction assay to study uterine SMC contractility	Primary human and immortalized myometrial SMCs	3D collagen lattice, embedded cells	SEM, fluorescence microscopy, RT-qPCR	TNFα and thrombin enhance contractility, indomethacin and Y-27632 reduce contraction; thrombin upregulates F2R gene	Functional assay for dissecting contractility regulation during inflammation and testing drugs for labor management
Lü et al. [67]	Multilayered uterine tissue constructs with smooth muscle via collagen/Matrigel	Human epithelial, stromal, smooth muscle + murine embryos	Layered scaffold, sequential cell seeding	Histology, immunostaining, SEM/TEM, embryo coculture	Constructs achieved tight junctions, desmosomes, pinopodes, embryo-supportive gene expression, enabled mouse embryo development ex vivo	Proof-of-principle for reconstruction of functional uterine wall; supports embryo implantation studies and fertility research
Young and Goloman [125]	Allo/xeno myometrial tissue reassembly using decellularized scaffolds	Human and rat myometrial cells	Recellularized, decellularized tissue scaffolds	Decellularization protocols, seeding, contractility measurements	Created functional "neo-myometrium": engineered tissues showed cell bundling, scaffold remodeling, coordinated contractions. Cross-species tissue engineering tested	Proved principles for constructing functional engineered myometrium for uterine repair and replacement; establishes importance of scaffold cellularization

Souza et al. [120]	Magnetically bioprinted human myometrial 3D cell rings (drug contractility assay)	Commercial and patient-derived myometrial SMCs	3D magnetic bioprinted rings	Nanoparticle labeling, image analysis, contractility monitoring	Rings contract spontaneously and show responses to indomethacin, nifedipine, and ibuprofen. Robustly detects dose-dependent contractility inhibition	Provides a high-throughput, scalable, and personalized platform for therapeutic testing of uterine contractility and pharmacological tocolytics
Elad et al. [123]	Dynamic endometrial barrier exposed to flow-generated shear	Human endometrial epithelial + myometrial cells	Flow chamber, 2D coculture	Peristaltic flow simulation, immunofluorescence, cytoskeleton quantification	Peristaltic shear increases F-actin mass and reorganizes cytoskeleton in both epithelial and myometrial layers, recapitulating physiological flow-induced changes	First in vitro system to mimic physical/mechanical environment of uterine wall, useful for mechanobiology and transport studies
Maxey et al. [103]	Micropatterned 2D/3D hydrogels for healthy vs. fibrotic myometrium	Human myometrial SMCs	Micropatterned hydrogels, variable stiffness/alignment	Calcium imaging, RNA sequencing, oxytocin/drug testing	Stiff isotropic architecture leads to shorter, lower Ca^{2+} transients. Soft, aligned matrices induce longer responses, gene profiling reveals TAS2R31 receptor downregulation and drug responses	Maps fibrotic remodeling's impact on contractility and gene expression with therapeutic screening relevance
Maxey et al. [126]	Engineered μMyometrium for contractility and inflammation studies	Human myometrial SMCs	3D microtissue	Traction force microscopy, cytokine stimulation	μMyometrium responds to PGF2α and cytokines (IL-6/IL-8) with increased contraction, PGE1/2 induces relaxation, explores how inflammation impacts contraction	Enables systematic study of myometrium regulation during preterm labor and inflammatory states. Scalable for screening mediators and pharmacological interventions

(continued)

Table 1 (continued)

Reference	Model/innovation	Cell source	Approach/format	Major techniques	Key results and insights	Translational/clinical relevance
Busch et al. [124]	Patient-derived 3D triculture myometrial/endometrial chip	Human endometrial stromal/epithelial + myometrial SMCs	Microfluidic microwell spheroid array	Live-cell tracing, hormone/cytokine exposure, ELISA, Ca^{2+} signaling	Triculture forms reproducible spheroids with epithelial periphery and stromal/myometrial core; responds to hormones and endothelin-1, expresses disease-relevant markers	Organotypic EMJ model for studies of placenta, adenomyosis, hormone response, and cellular invasion; platform for patient-specific disease modeling
Nietupski et al. [96]	Cyclic strain hydrogel-induced elastogenesis in engineered myometrium	Human myometrial SMCs	3D hydrogel constructs, cyclic bioreactor	Cyclic strain exposure, elastin quantification, gene expression	Cyclic strain increases elastin protein/mRNA (ELN/FBN1), promoting matrix assembly; hormone treatments do not significantly affect elastin	Demonstrates mechanical loading as a key driver of elastogenesis, guiding tissue engineering approaches for uterine repair

bioprinted hollow myometrial rings exhibited immediate contraction following printing, and exposure to clinically relevant tocolytics elicited a dose-dependent contractile response, validating the use of 3D bioprinted models for physiological relevance [120]. Microfabrication and micropatterning techniques have also been successfully applied to the myometrium. Precisely engineered rectangular microfeatures have directed the adhesion and alignment of primary human myometrial smooth muscle cells into three-dimensional structures. These myometrial constructs were contractile, generated forces in response to inflammatory mediators and contractile agonists like oxytocin, evaluated via traction force microscopy [121]. Interestingly, this bioengineering approach also revealed new insights into myometrial mechanobiology, where substrate stiffness altered myometrial contractile patterns, measured using transient calcium currents [103]. This is especially noteworthy because bioengineering approaches could hold the key in discovering an experimental link between the stiff uterine fibroid microenvironment and disruptions in myometrial contractility.

Myometrial cell mechanobiology is vastly understudied, despite our foundational understanding that mechanical factors regulate contractility. Here, microfluidic approaches and bioreactors have been particularly advantageous to investigate myometrial mechanobiology. Externally applied peristalsis bioreactor systems developed for broad smooth muscle structures could easily be adapted to study myometrial mechanobiology [122]. In recent times, there have also been more microfluidic approaches to model uterine peristalsis at the miniaturized scale. Endometrial and myometrial cells were cocultured in custom-designed microfluidic wells and exposed to rhythmic flow patterns generated by a custom 3D-printed belt mechanism. This time-controlled application of low-level shear stress induced cytoskeletal remodeling in both cell layers, effectively simulating the mechanical influence of natural uterine peristalsis on myometrial function [123]. Patterned microwell arrays were housed within a microfluidic channel network that allowed perfusion. A triculture model was established within the microwells with patient-derived endometrial, stromal and myometrial cells that self-assembled into the endometrial-myometrial junctional zone, producing calcium transients in response to endothelin, a surrogate measure of contractility [124].

6 Where Do We Go from Here?

Given the beautifully complex aspects of myometrial function, there is much to be leveraged from advanced bioengineering strategies (Fig. 4). Since structure is so closely aligned with function in the myometrium, biofabrication techniques that enable precise spatial deposition of multiple cell types from the myometrial microenvironment will be advantageous.

Beyond static structures, 4D bioprinting of structures that dynamically evolve over time in response to predetermined shape transformations [127], or those that alter the internal alignment of cells and their matrix [128] may better replicate the cyclic and changing uterine microenvironment under hormonal cycles. Integrating

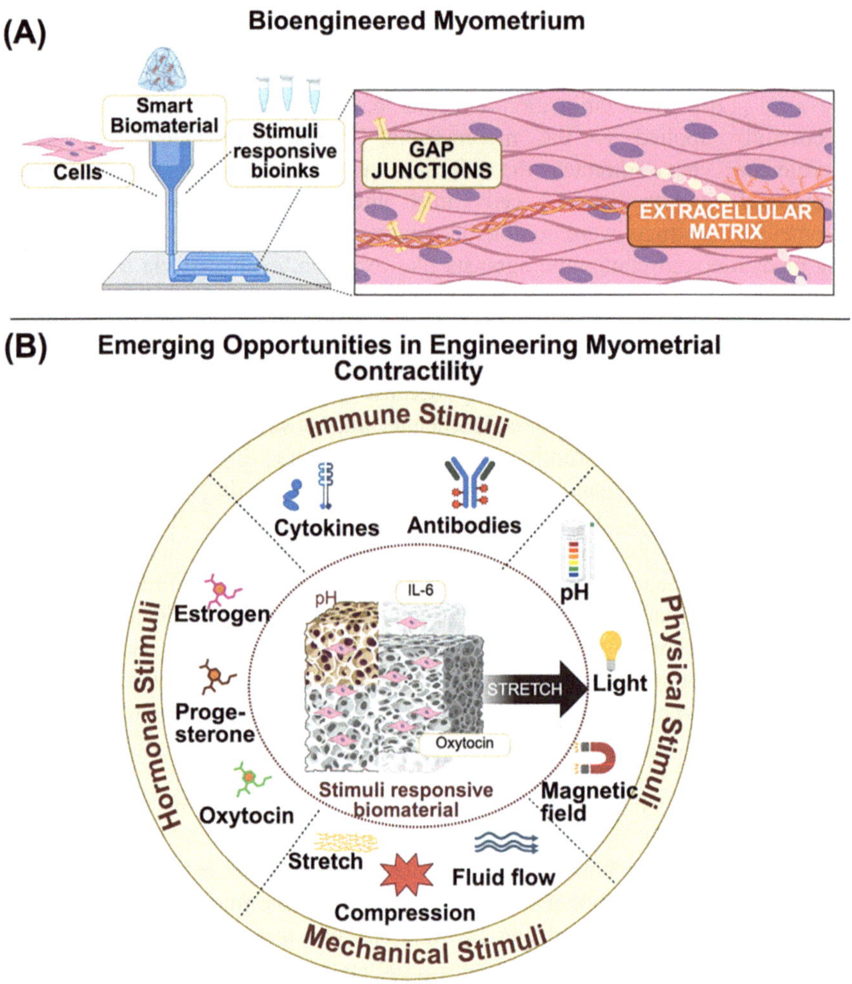

Fig. 4 Future opportunities in engineering the myometrium: (**a**) Bioprinted myometrial tissues with opportunities to mimic myocyte architecture, ECM components, and intracellular gap junctions, developed using smart biomaterials and bioinks. (**b**) Stimuli-responsive smart materials exhibiting shape-morphing and adaptive behaviors in response to physical, inflammatory, hormonal, and mechanical stimuli to accommodate a contractile myometrium

smart biomaterials into engineered systems are also vital for monitoring or modulating myometrial contractility. Models of the future may be fueled by recent advances in incorporating piezoelectric nanoparticles or conductive polymers into scaffolds to monitor mechanical strain in situ. Piezoelectric polymers and conductive hydrogels may enable real-time monitoring of myometrial contractility by transducing mechanical contractions into transmittable electrical signals [129]. The continued advancement of biomaterials and bioengineering methods will offer a transformative path toward engineering a mechanically competent myometrium, inspired by its inherent anatomic and physiological complexity.

Acknowledgments This work was supported by NIH NICHD R21HD118295 (SAR and AIF), and NSF CAREER Award BMMB-2440798 (SAR). The authors declare no competing conflicts of interest.

References

1. Ellis H. Anatomy of the uterus. Anaesth Intensive Care Med. 2005;6:74–5.
2. Louwagie EM, Russell SR, Hairston JC, et al. The biomechanical evolution of the uterus and cervix and fetal growth in human pregnancy. NPJ Womens Health. 2024;2:33.
3. Cunningham FG, Leveno KJ, Dashe JS, et al. Maternal physiology. In: Williams obstetrics, 26e. New York: McGraw Hill; 2022.
4. Malik M, Roh M, England SK. Uterine contractions in rodent models and humans. Acta Physiol (Oxf). 2021;231:e13607.
5. Jain V, Chodankar RR, Maybin JA, et al. Uterine bleeding: how understanding endometrial physiology underpins menstrual health. Nat Rev Endocrinol. 2022;18:290–308.
6. Dudley JS, Murphy CR, Thompson MB, et al. Uterine cellular changes during mammalian pregnancy and the evolution of placentation†. Biol Reprod. 2021;105:1381–400.
7. Taylor E, Gomel V. The uterus and fertility. Fertil Steril. 2008;89:1–16.
8. Kunz G, Leyendecker G. Uterine peristaltic activity during the menstrual cycle: characterization, regulation, function and dysfunction. Reprod Biomed Online. 2002;4(Suppl 3):5–9.
9. Bulletti C, de Ziegler D, Setti PL, et al. The patterns of uterine contractility in normal menstruating women: from physiology to pathology. Ann N Y Acad Sci. 2004;1034:64–83.
10. Yin Z, He W, Li Y, et al. Adaptive reduction of human myometrium contractile activity in response to prolonged uterine stretch during term and twin pregnancy. Role of TREK-1 channel. Biochem Pharmacol. 2018;152:252–63.
11. Uvnäs-Moberg K. The physiology and pharmacology of oxytocin in labor and in the peripartum period. Am J Obstet Gynecol. 2024;230:S740–s758.
12. Zondervan KT, Becker CM, Koga K, et al. Endometriosis. Nat Rev Dis Primers. 2018;4:9.
13. Moawad G, Fruscalzo A, Youssef Y, et al. Adenomyosis: an updated review on diagnosis and classification. J Clin Med. 2023;12:4828.
14. Yang Q, Ciebiera M, Bariani MV, et al. Comprehensive review of uterine fibroids: developmental origin, pathogenesis, and treatment. Endocr Rev. 2022;43:678–719.
15. Zhu L, Che HS, Xiao L, et al. Uterine peristalsis before embryo transfer affects the chance of clinical pregnancy in fresh and frozen-thawed embryo transfer cycles. Hum Reprod. 2014;29:1238–43.
16. Kuijsters NPM, Methorst WG, Kortenhorst MSQ, et al. Uterine peristalsis and fertility: current knowledge and future perspectives: a review and meta-analysis. Reprod Biomed Online. 2017;35:50–71.
17. de Boer A, Rees CO, Mischi M, et al. The influence of uterine abnormalities on uterine peristalsis in the non-pregnant uterus: a systematic review. J Endometr Uterine Disord. 2023;3:100038.
18. Zangeneh FZ, Hantoushzadeh S. The physiological basis with uterine myometrium contractions from electro-mechanical/hormonal myofibril function to the term and preterm labor. Heliyon. 2023;9:e22259.
19. Blencowe H, Cousens S, Chou D, et al. Born too soon: the global epidemiology of 15 million preterm births. Reprod Health. 2013;10(Suppl 1):S2.
20. Kissler K, Hurt KJ. The pathophysiology of labor dystocia: theme with variations. Reprod Sci. 2023;30:729–42.
21. Koutras A, Fasoulakis Z, Syllaios A, et al. Physiology and pathology of contractility of the myometrium. In Vivo. 2021;35:1401–8.

22. Bateman BT, Berman MF, Riley LE, et al. The epidemiology of postpartum hemorrhage in a large, nationwide sample of deliveries. Anesth Analg. 2010;110:1368–73.
23. Galal M, Symonds I, Murray H, et al. Postterm pregnancy. Facts Views Vis Obgyn. 2012;4: 175–87.
24. Olesen AW, Westergaard JG, Olsen J. Perinatal and maternal complications related to postterm delivery: a national register-based study, 1978-1993. Am J Obstet Gynecol. 2003;189:222–7.
25. Caughey AB, Stotland NE, Washington AE, et al. Maternal and obstetric complications of pregnancy are associated with increasing gestational age at term. Am J Obstet Gynecol. 2007;196:155.e1–6.
26. Mukherjee S, Arulkumaran S. Post-partum haemorrhage. Obstet Gynaecol Reprod Med. 2009;19:121–6.
27. Wang MJ, Oyelese Y. Postpartum hemorrhage. Matern Fetal Med. 2025;7:38–48.
28. Ulrich ND, Vargo A, Ma Q, et al. Cellular heterogeneity and dynamics of the human uterus in healthy premenopausal women. Proc Natl Acad Sci USA. 2024;121:e2404775121.
29. Punzon-Jimenez P, Machado-Lopez A, Perez-Moraga R, et al. Effect of aging on the human myometrium at single-cell resolution. Nat Commun. 2024;15:945.
30. Pique-Regi R, Romero R, Garcia-Flores V, et al. A single-cell atlas of the myometrium in human parturition. JCI Insight. 2022;7:e153921.
31. Ji K, Zhong J, Cui L, et al. Exploring myometrial microenvironment changes at the single-cell level from nonpregnant to term pregnant states. Physiol Genomics. 2024;56:32–47.
32. Ekerhovd E, Weidegard B, Brannstrom M, et al. Nitric oxide-mediated effects on myometrial contractility at term during prelabor and labor. Obstet Gynecol. 1999;93:987–94.
33. Boros-Rausch A, Dorogin A, Nadeem L, et al. A broad-spectrum chemokine inhibitor drives M2 macrophage polarization through modulation of the myometrial secretome. Cells. 2025;14:514.
34. Mackler AM, Ducsay TC, Ducsay CA, et al. Effects of endotoxin and macrophage-related cytokines on the contractile activity of the gravid murine uterus. Biol Reprod. 2003;69:1165–9.
35. Thomson AJ, Telfer JF, Young A, et al. Leukocytes infiltrate the myometrium during human parturition: further evidence that labour is an inflammatory process. Hum Reprod. 1999;14: 229–36.
36. Osman I, Young A, Ledingham MA, et al. Leukocyte density and pro-inflammatory cytokine expression in human fetal membranes, decidua, cervix and myometrium before and during labour at term. Mol Hum Reprod. 2003;9:41–5.
37. Rajagopal SP, Hutchinson JL, Dorward DA, et al. Crosstalk between monocytes and myometrial smooth muscle in culture generates synergistic pro-inflammatory cytokine production and enhances myocyte contraction, with effects opposed by progesterone. Mol Hum Reprod. 2015;21:672–86.
38. Gomez-Lopez N, Garcia-Flores V, Chin PY, et al. Macrophages exert homeostatic actions in pregnancy to protect against preterm birth and fetal inflammatory injury. JCI Insight. 2021;6: e146089.
39. Kajuluri LP, Li Y, Morgan KG. The uterine myocyte, contractile machinery and proteins of the myometrium and their relationship to the dynamic nature of myometrial function. Curr Opin Physio. 2020;13:14–9.
40. Shmygol A, Gullam J, Blanks A, et al. Multiple mechanisms involved in oxytocin-induced modulation of myometrial contractility. Acta Pharmacol Sin. 2006;27:827–32.
41. Ferreira JJ, Butler A, Stewart R, et al. Oxytocin can regulate myometrial smooth muscle excitability by inhibiting the Na(+) -activated K(+) channel, Slo2.1. J Physiol. 2019;597:137–49.
42. Aguilar HN, Mitchell BF. Physiological pathways and molecular mechanisms regulating uterine contractility. Hum Reprod Update. 2010;16:725–44.

43. Garfield R, Somlyo A. Structure of smooth muscle. In: Calcium and contractility: smooth muscle. Springer; 1985. p. 1–36.
44. Young RC, Hession RO. Three-dimensional structure of the smooth muscle in the term-pregnant human uterus. Obstet Gynecol. 1999;93:94–9.
45. Kagami K, Ono M, Iizuka T, et al. A novel third mesh-like myometrial layer connects the longitudinal and circular muscle fibers -a potential stratum to coordinate uterine contractions. Sci Rep. 2020;10:8274.
46. Lutton EJ, Lammers WJ, James S, et al. A computational method for three-dimensional reconstruction of the microarchitecture of myometrial smooth muscle from histological sections. PLoS One. 2017;12:e0173404.
47. Smith R, Imtiaz M, Banney D, et al. Why the heart is like an orchestra and the uterus is like a soccer crowd. Am J Obstet Gynecol. 2015;213:181–5.
48. Wang S, Anderson K, Pizzella S, et al. Noninvasive imaging of 4D electrical activation patterns of uterine peristalsis during normal menstrual cycles. NPJ Womens Health. 2024;2:1.
49. Caldeyro-Barcia R, Poseiro JJ. Physiology of the uterine contraction. Clin Obstet Gynecol. 1960;3:386–410.
50. Salerno JP. Observations on intrauterine pressure during first stage of labor. Am J Obstet Gynecol. 1938;36:294–302.
51. Myers KM, Elad D. Biomechanics of the human uterus. Wiley Interdiscip Rev Syst Biol Med. 2017;9:e1388.
52. Kunz G, Noe M, Herbertz M, et al. Uterine peristalsis during the follicular phase of the menstrual cycle: effects of oestrogen, antioestrogen and oxytocin. Hum Reprod Update. 1998;4:647–54.
53. Vidal A, Bora C, von Holzen J, et al. Cine-MRI for quantifying uterine peristalsis: a systematic review and meta-analysis. J Clin Med. 2025;14:1021.
54. Daido S, Kido A, Kataoka M, et al. MR imaging of uterine morphology and dynamic changes during lactation. J Magn Reson Imaging. 2017;45:617–23.
55. Kunz G, Beil D, Deininger H, et al. The dynamics of rapid sperm transport through the female genital tract: evidence from vaginal sonography of uterine peristalsis and hysterosalpingoscintigraphy. Hum Reprod. 1996;11:627–32.
56. de Ziegler D, Bulletti C, Fanchin R, et al. Contractility of the nonpregnant uterus: the follicular phase. Ann N Y Acad Sci. 2001;943:172–84.
57. Lethaby A, Vollenhoven B. Fibroids (uterine myomatosis, leiomyomas). BMJ Clin Evid. 2011;2011:0814.
58. Rosen H, Yogev Y. Assessment of uterine contractions in labor and delivery. Am J Obstet Gynecol. 2023;228:S1209–21.
59. Riemer RK, Heymann MA. Regulation of uterine smooth muscle function during gestation. Pediatr Res. 1998;44:615–27.
60. Pehlivanoğlu B, Bayrak S, Doğan M. A close look at the contraction and relaxation of the myometrium; the role of calcium. J Turk Ger Gynecol Assoc. 2013;14:230–4.
61. Driessen M, Bouvier-Colle MH, Dupont C, et al. Postpartum hemorrhage resulting from uterine atony after vaginal delivery: factors associated with severity. Obstet Gynecol. 2011;117:21–31.
62. Diao M, Zhou J, Tao Y, et al. RAC1 is involved in uterine myometrium contraction in the inflammation-associated preterm birth. Reproduction. 2022;164:169–81.
63. Fitzgibbon J, Morrison JJ, Smith TJ, et al. Modulation of human uterine smooth muscle cell collagen contractility by thrombin, Y-27632, TNF alpha and indomethacin. Reprod Biol Endocrinol. 2009;7:2.
64. Arrowsmith S. Human myometrial contractility assays. In: Werry EL, Reekie TA, Kassiou M, editors. Oxytocin: methods and protocols. New York: Springer US; 2022. p. 29–42.
65. Alotaibi MF. The response of rat and human uterus to oxytocin from different gestational stages in vitro. Gen Physiol Biophys. 2017;36:75–82.

66. Young RC, Schumann R, Zhang P. Three-dimensional culture of human uterine smooth muscle myocytes on a resorbable scaffolding. Tissue Eng. 2003;9:451–9.
67. Lü S-H, Wang H-B, Liu H, et al. Reconstruction of engineered uterine tissues containing smooth muscle layer in collagen/matrigel scaffold in vitro. Tissue Eng A. 2008;15:1611–8.
68. Hamburg-Shields E, Mesiano S. The hormonal control of parturition. Physiol Rev. 2024;104: 1121–45.
69. Blanks AM, Shmygol A, Thornton S. Regulation of oxytocin receptors and oxytocin receptor signaling. Semin Reprod Med. 2007;25:52–9.
70. Richter ON, Kubler K, Schmolling J, et al. Oxytocin receptor gene expression of estrogen-stimulated human myometrium in extracorporeally perfused non-pregnant uteri. Mol Hum Reprod. 2004;10:339–46.
71. Oladosu FA, Tu FF, Garfield LB, et al. Low serum oxytocin concentrations are associated with painful menstruation. Reprod Sci. 2020;27:668–74.
72. Clark K, Myatt L. Prostaglandins and the reproductive cycle. Glob Libr Womens Med. 2008: 17566-12.
73. Mesiano S, Welsh TN. Steroid hormone control of myometrial contractility and parturition. Semin Cell Dev Biol. 2007;18:321–31.
74. Richter ON, Bartz C, Dowaji J, et al. Contractile reactivity of human myometrium in isolated non-pregnant uteri. Hum Reprod. 2006;21:36–45.
75. Csapo A, Pulkkinen M, Henzl M. The effect of naproxen-sodium on the intrauterine pressure and menstrual pain of dysmenorrheic patients. Prostaglandins. 1977;13:193–9.
76. Mesiano S. Myometrial progesterone responsiveness and the control of human parturition. J Soc Gynecol Investig. 2004;11:193–202.
77. Soloff MS, Fernstrom MA, Periyasamy S, et al. Regulation of oxytocin receptor concentration in rat uterine explants by estrogen and progesterone. Can J Biochem Cell Biol. 1983;61:625–30.
78. Fuchs AR, Periyasamy S, Soloff MS. Systemic and local regulation of oxytocin receptors in the rat uterus, and their functional significance. Can J Biochem Cell Biol. 1983;61:615–24.
79. Young RC, Smith LH, McLaren MD. T-type and L-type calcium currents in freshly dispersed human uterine smooth muscle cells. Am J Obstet Gynecol. 1993;169:785–92.
80. Pinsard M, Mouchet N, Dion L, et al. Anatomic and functional mapping of human uterine innervation. Fertil Steril. 2022;117:1279–88.
81. Aleksandrovych V, Kurnik-Łucka M, Bereza T, et al. The autonomic innervation and uterine telocyte interplay in leiomyoma formation. Cell Transplant. 2019;28:619–29.
82. Wrobel KH, Kujat R. The bovine tubouterine junction: general innervation pattern and distribution of adrenergic, cholinergic, and peptidergic nerve fibers. Cell Tissue Res. 1993;274:493–501.
83. Bottari SP, Vokaer A, Kaivez E, et al. Differential regulation of alpha-adrenergic receptor subclasses by gonadal steroids in human myometrium. J Clin Endocrinol Metab. 1983;57: 937–41.
84. Brauer MM. Cellular and molecular mechanisms underlying plasticity in uterine sympathetic nerves. Auton Neurosci. 2008;140:1–16.
85. Monica Brauer M, Smith PG. Estrogen and female reproductive tract innervation: cellular and molecular mechanisms of autonomic neuroplasticity. Auton Neurosci. 2015;187:1–17.
86. Wray S, Prendergast C. The myometrium: from excitation to contractions and labour. In: Hashitani H, Lang RJ, editors. Smooth muscle spontaneous activity: physiological and pathological modulation. Singapore: Springer Singapore; 2019. p. 233–63.
87. Riaposova L, Kim SH, Hanyaloglu AC, et al. Prostaglandin F2α requires activation of calcium-dependent signalling to trigger inflammation in human myometrium. Front Endocrinol (Lausanne). 2023;14:1150125.
88. Maybin JA, Critchley HOD. Menstrual physiology: implications for endometrial pathology and beyond. Hum Reprod Update. 2015;21:748–61.

89. Mor G, Cardenas I, Abrahams V, et al. Inflammation and pregnancy: the role of the immune system at the implantation site. Ann N Y Acad Sci. 2011;1221:80–7.
90. Wray S, Burdyga T, Noble D, et al. Progress in understanding electro-mechanical signalling in the myometrium. Acta Physiol. 2015;213:417–31.
91. Wu X, Morgan KG, Jones CJ, et al. Myometrial mechanoadaptation during pregnancy: implications for smooth muscle plasticity and remodelling. J Cell Mol Med. 2008;12:1360–73.
92. Turton P, Arrowsmith S, Prescott J, et al. A comparison of the contractile properties of myometrium from singleton and twin pregnancies. PLoS One. 2013;8:e63800.
93. Moraitis AA, Cordeaux Y, Charnock-Jones DS, et al. The effect of an oxytocin receptor antagonist (Retosiban, GSK221149A) on the response of human myometrial explants to prolonged mechanical stretch. Endocrinology. 2015;156:3511–6.
94. Dalrymple A, Mahn K, Poston L, et al. Mechanical stretch regulates TRPC expression and calcium entry in human myometrial smooth muscle cells. Mol Hum Reprod. 2007;13:171–9.
95. Terzidou V, Sooranna SR, Kim LU, et al. Mechanical stretch up-regulates the human oxytocin receptor in primary human uterine myocytes. J Clin Endocrinol Metab. 2005;90:237–46.
96. Nietupski CA, Moset Zupan A, Schutte SC. Impact of cyclic strain on elastin synthesis in a 3D human myometrial culture model. Tissue Eng Part C Methods. 2024;30:279–88.
97. Fodera DM, Russell SR, Jackson JLL, et al. Material properties of nonpregnant and pregnant human uterine layers. J Mech Behav Biomed Mater. 2024;151:106348.
98. Leppert PC, Jayes FL, Segars JH. The extracellular matrix contributes to mechanotransduction in uterine fibroids. Obstet Gynecol Int. 2014;2014:783289.
99. Munro MG. Adenomyosis and uterine stiffness: what is the chicken? Which is the egg? Hum Reprod. 2023;38:527–8.
100. Sternberg AK, Buck VU, Classen-Linke I, et al. How mechanical forces change the human endometrium during the menstrual cycle in preparation for embryo implantation. Cells. 2021;10:2008.
101. Norian JM, Owen CM, Taboas J, et al. Characterization of tissue biomechanics and mechanical signaling in uterine leiomyoma. Matrix Biol. 2012;31:57–65.
102. Schutte SC, Ghosh D, Moset Zupan A, et al. Differential response to mechanical cues in uterine fibroid versus paired myometrial cells. Reprod Sci. 2023;30:3305–14.
103. Maxey AP, Travis JM, McCain ML. Regulation of oxytocin-induced calcium transients and gene expression in engineered myometrial tissues by tissue architecture and matrix rigidity. Curr Res Physiol. 2023;6:100108.
104. Young RC, Barendse P. Linking myometrial physiology to intrauterine pressure; how tissue-level contractions create uterine contractions of labor. PLoS Comput Biol. 2014;10:e1003850.
105. Mosher AA, Rainey KJ, Bolstad SS, et al. Development and validation of primary human myometrial cell culture models to study pregnancy and labour. BMC Pregnancy Childbirth. 2013;13:S7.
106. Palmberg L, Thyberg J. Uterine smooth muscle cells in primary culture. Alterations in fine structure, cytoskeletal organization and growth characteristics. Cell Tissue Res. 1986;246:253–62.
107. Bonazza C, Andrade SS, Sumikawa JT, et al. Primary human uterine leiomyoma cell culture quality control: some properties of myometrial cells cultured under serum deprivation conditions in the presence of ovarian steroids. PLoS One. 2016;11:e0158578.
108. Mehasseb MK, Taylor AH, Pringle JH, et al. Enhanced invasion of stromal cells from adenomyosis in a three-dimensional coculture model is augmented by the presence of myocytes from affected uteri. Fertil Steril. 2010;94:2547–51.
109. Soloff MS, Jeng YJ, Ilies M, et al. Immortalization and characterization of human myometrial cells from term-pregnant patients using a telomerase expression vector. Mol Hum Reprod. 2004;10:685–95.
110. Condon J, Yin S, Mayhew B, et al. Telomerase immortalization of human myometrial cells. Biol Reprod. 2002;67:506–14.

111. Devost D, Zingg HH. Novel in vitro system for functional assessment of oxytocin action. Am J Physiol Endocrinol Metab. 2007;292:E1–6.
112. Monga M, Ku CY, Dodge K, et al. Oxytocin-stimulated responses in a pregnant human immortalized myometrial cell line. Biol Reprod. 1996;55:427–32.
113. Mas A, Nair S, Laknaur A, et al. Stro-1/CD44 as putative human myometrial and fibroid stem cell markers. Fertil Steril. 2015;104:225–34 e3.
114. Banerjee S, Xu W, Chowdhury I, et al. Human myometrial and uterine fibroid stem cell-derived organoids for intervening the pathophysiology of uterine fibroid. Reprod Sci. 2022;29: 2607–19.
115. Omran MM, Vafaei S, Alkhrait S, et al. Utilising human myometrial and uterine fibroid stem cell-derived three dimentional organoids as a robust model system for understanding the pathophysiology of uterine fibroids. Cell Prolif. 2025;58:e70025.
116. Alzamil L, Nikolakopoulou K, Turco MY. Organoid systems to study the human female reproductive tract and pregnancy. Cell Death Differ. 2021;28:35–51.
117. Rawlings TM, Makwana K, Tryfonos M, et al. Organoids to model the endometrium: implantation and beyond. Reprod Fertil. 2021;2:R85–R101.
118. Almeida GHD, Iglesia RP, Araujo MS, et al. Uterine tissue engineering: where we stand and the challenges ahead. Tissue Eng Part B Rev. 2022;28:861–90.
119. Young RC, Goloman G. Allo- and xeno-reassembly of human and rat myometrium from cells and scaffolds. Tissue Eng Part A. 2013;19:2112–9.
120. Souza GR, Tseng H, Gage JA, et al. Magnetically bioprinted human myometrial 3D cell rings as a model for uterine contractility. Int J Mol Sci. 2017;18:683.
121. Maxey AP, Wheeler SJ, Travis JM, et al. Contractile responses of engineered human mumyometrium to prostaglandins and inflammatory cytokines. APL Bioeng. 2024;8:046115.
122. Clevenger AJ, Crawford LZ, Noltensmeyer D, et al. Rapid prototypable biomimetic peristalsis bioreactor capable of concurrent shear and multi-axial strain. Cells Tissues Organs. 2023;212: 96–110.
123. Elad D, Zaretsky U, Kuperman T, et al. Tissue engineered endometrial barrier exposed to peristaltic flow shear stresses. APL Bioeng. 2020;4:026107.
124. Busch C, Hill CJ, Paterson K, et al. Functional, patient-derived 3D tri-culture models of the uterine wall in a microfluidic array. Hum Reprod. 2024;39:2537–50.
125. Young RC, Goloman G. Allo- and xeno-reassembly of human and rat myometrium from cells and scaffolds. Tissue Eng A. 2013;19:2112–9.
126. Maxey AP, Wheeler SJ, Travis JM, et al. Contractile responses of engineered human μmyometrium to prostaglandins and inflammatory cytokines. APL Bioeng. 2024;8:046115.
127. Gao B, Yang Q, Zhao X, et al. 4D bioprinting for biomedical applications. Trends Biotechnol. 2016;34:746–56.
128. Pramanick A, Hayes T, Sergis V, et al. 4D bioprinting shape-morphing tissues in granular support hydrogels: sculpting structure and guiding maturation. Adv Funct Mater. 2025;35: 2414559.
129. Khan A, Joshi R, Sharma MK, et al. The potential of organic piezoelectric materials for next-generation implantable biomedical devices. Nano Trends. 2024;6:100032.

Biomaterial Tools for Modeling Endometriosis

Hannah S. Theriault and Brendan A. C. Harley

Abstract Endometriosis is a common gynecological disorder that can cause chronic pain and infertility. To better understand mechanisms of disease etiology and progression, researchers are increasingly turning to model systems. In vivo approaches have notable limitations, including limited ability to model human anatomy-related pathologies and poor translation of therapeutics developed in animal models. This chapter describes the current body of work surrounding the recent emergence of in vitro models of endometriosis. This work aims to describe methods by which researchers can consider specifying their work to stages of disease, lesion location, and interactions that could drive disease progression. This chapter defines a roadmap for the development of more robust and specific models of endometriosis with the goal of realizing translatable therapeutic strategies and noninvasive metrics of disease presence and progression.

Keywords Biomaterials · Endometriosis · In vitro · Tissue models · Therapeutics

H. S. Theriault
Department of Bioengineering, University of Illinois at Urbana-Champaign, Urbana, IL, USA

Carl R. Woese Institute for Genomic Biology, University of Illinois at Urbana-Champaign, Urbana, IL, USA
e-mail: hst4@illinois.edu

B. A. C. Harley (✉)
Carl R. Woese Institute for Genomic Biology, University of Illinois at Urbana-Champaign, Urbana, IL, USA

Department of Chemical and Biomolecular Engineering, University of Illinois at Urbana-Champaign, Urbana, IL, USA

Center for Gender and Sex in Health, University of Illinois at Urbana-Champaign, Urbana, IL, USA

Cancer Center at Illinois, University of Illinois at Urbana-Champaign, Urbana, IL, USA
e-mail: bharley@illinois.edu

S. G. Zambuto, M. L. Oyen (eds.), *Biomaterials for Women's Health Engineering*,
https://doi.org/10.1007/978-3-032-10745-9_9

1 Introduction

Endometriosis is a prevalent gynecologic pathology, affecting 10% of people who menstruate. Endometriosis can impact a spectrum of tissues, organs, and organ systems, with a large variety of subtypes and presentations. Generally, endometriosis is defined as a chronic inflammatory condition that primarily includes estrogen-dependent proliferation and metastasis of endometrial-like tissues throughout the pelvic cavity [1]. These ectopic tissues invade, to varying degrees, into pelvic tissues and organs, remodeling the underlying matrix, and results in pelvic adhesions and fibrotic tissue. Symptoms of the disease include, but are not limited to, dysmenorrhea, dyspareunia, menorrhagia, and infertility. Endometriosis is often co-diagnosed with a variety of other chronic inflammatory conditions [2].

1.1 Endometriosis Risk Factors

Endometriosis primarily occurs in people who menstruate (between menarche and menopause). It has been reported that race plays a role in disease risk; however, recent work has highlighted the potential selection biases by previous studies [3–6]. These prior studies and meta-analyses rarely considered socioeconomic status of patients (which determines access to care) and clinical biases against people of color (POC) seeking treatment for chronic pain conditions [7]. These inequalities in access to care, social stigma, or clinician biases toward populations likely heavily skew disease identification and patient outcomes. These biases are not something tissue engineers can easily recapitulate, but they must consider when reporting findings. Other risk factors for the development or exacerbation of endometriosis include a familial history of endometriosis, a familial history of immunological diseases, and exposure to environmental toxicants [8–12].

1.2 Categorical Division of Endometriosis

Endometriosis can be subdivided into categories of disease presentation based on lesion location or infiltration depth. Peritoneal, or superficial, endometriosis is described as lesions that do not invade far into pelvic tissues. Endometriotic lesions that extend beyond 5 mm under the surface of tissues are considered deep endometriosis [1]. Endometriosis presenting on the ovaries as invaginated or true cysts are described as endometriomas [7]. Although uncommon, endometriosis can occur in locations outside of the pelvis; this disease presentation is defined as extra-pelvic endometriosis. It is crucial to identify the type of endometriosis being studied, as disease type can influence clinical presentation, treatment options, methods for modeling disease, and potential origin (Fig. 1).

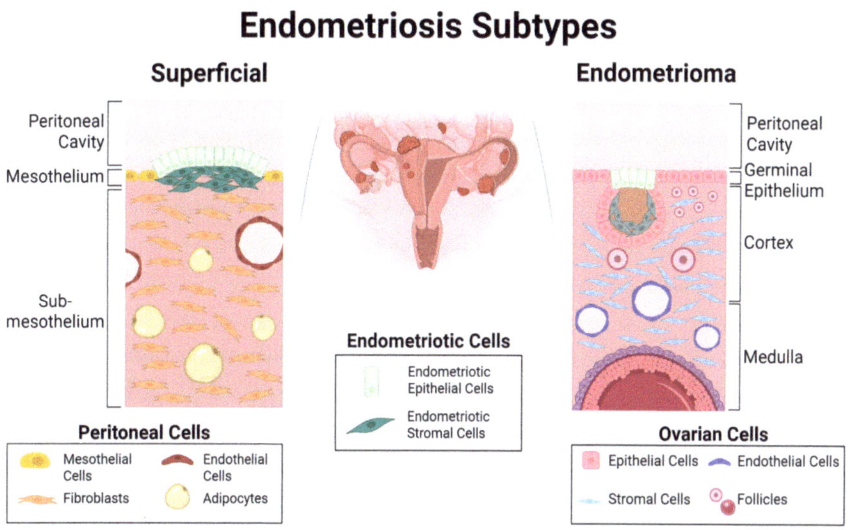

Fig. 1 Endometriosis subtype determines the structure of lesions. Superficial endometriotic lesions interact with the mesothelium of the peritoneum and often invade very minimally into the tissue. Endometriomas invade deeper into invaginations in the ovarian epithelium and can result in a fluid-filled center. (Figure made in BioRender)

1.3 Comparing the Endometrium and Endometriotic Tissues

Endometriotic tissue retains some intrinsic features of native, eutopic endometrial tissue including the presence of nuclear and cytosolic estrogen receptors (ERα, ERβ) [13]. The increased presence of these ERβs in endometriotic tissues results in increased proliferative capacity of these tissues and decreased progesterone receptors (PRs) [13, 14]. During the menstrual cycle, progesterone (P4) levels increase after ovulation to counteract the proliferative nature of estradiol (E2) and trigger the differentiation of native, eutopic endometrial stromal cells to a decidualized phenotype in preparation for pregnancy. Endometriotic tissues can develop a progesterone-resistant phenotype due to decreased PR expression [13, 14]. This cyclic interaction of ERs, lack of PRs, and local E2 levels in endometriotic tissue results in increased local inflammation and decreased apoptosis of ectopic cells (Table 1) [13, 14]. Clinicians often treat this altered hormonal state with gonadotropin-releasing hormone (GnRH) agonists/antagonists or progestins. The goal of these therapeutics is to suppress the hypothalamic–pituitary–gonadal (HPG) axis to decrease systemic estrogen levels or to block local estrogenic action with the synthetic progestins [15, 16]. These treatments typically only work in the short-term, and pose concerns about impacts on bone-density, inability to conceive naturally while on the medications, and mental health complications [17–19].

Table 1 Comparison of processes related to endometriosis as compared to native, healthy endometrium

Process	Endometriosis
Cellular components	(↓) Glandular epithelium [20]
	(↑) Stromal fibroblasts [20]
	(↓) Stem cells [21, 22]
	(=) Vascular cells; (↑) VEGF [23]
Receptors	(↓) ER [24, 25] (↓) PR [24, 25] (↑) ERβ/ERα ratio [26]
Estradiol levels	(↑) Local E2 near lesions [27]
Inflammation	(↑) Inflammation (ex. ↑ E2-mediated IL-1β) [27] (↑) Immune escape (sICAM1-mediated) [23]
Proliferation	(↑) Proliferation [27]
Apoptosis	(−) JNK [28] (↓) Apoptosis [28]

(↑) upregulated/increased, (↓) downregulated/decreased, (+) promoted, (−) inhibited, (=) equivalent, normal, or nonsignificant

1.4 Endometriosis Diagnosis and Treatment

The gold standard diagnostic for endometriosis includes laparoscopic surgery followed by histological examination of removed tissues. This diagnostic standard often results in delayed diagnosis because clinicians avoid invasive methods of diagnosis for as long as possible and undergoing laparoscopy can increase patient risk of surgical complications [29, 30]. Prior to surgery, patients often undergo various exclusion tests (transvaginal ultrasound, MRI, etc.) to rule out other conditions that can cause pelvic pain. Unfortunately, these imaging modalities have limitations in identifying lesions, especially deeper within the pelvic cavity [29, 30]. There are currently no commercially or clinically available noninvasive biomarker tests for identifying endometriosis in the United States [31–33]. During surgical identification of lesions, clinicians will employ an ablation or excision strategy to remove visible lesions and to improve fertility outcomes [34]. This treatment of endometriosis is largely palliative, with the goal of reducing patient pain levels and increasing quality of life. Resection outcomes are also tissue-dependent; resection of lesions on the ovaries can impact ovarian reserve and function [35]. Ablation techniques, primarily using CO_2, are often used for lesions that do not deeply infiltrate into tissues. Laparoscopic surgery is often followed by hormonal treatment. However, these types of treatments largely result in a tissue microenvironment significantly changed from pre-endometriosis lesion status via fibrosis and scar formation, complicating the prevention of lesion recurrence [36, 37]. This process of resection, especially related to endometriomas, can greatly negatively influence fertility outcomes [38].

1.5 *Modeling Disease*

To better understand underlying mechanisms of pathological etiology and progression, researchers aim to develop models of endometriosis. These models can be used for a range of studies from determining novel targets for therapeutics to high-throughput examination of personalized treatments for patients. Here, we describe the progression of endometriosis models, the importance of biomaterial models, the use of biomaterials in treatment of endometriosis, and the guiding principles researchers should consider when developing future work in this field.

2 Traditional In Vivo Models as the Gold Standard for Endometriosis Studies

2.1 *Small Animal Models of Endometriosis*

To understand the pathological mechanisms behind endometriosis initiation, researchers often use animal models. Rodent (mice, rats) and rabbit models of endometriosis are accessible animals for research purposes and can be used to investigate underlying mechanisms of disease. These systems utilize syngeneic transplantation of uterine tissue from one mouse into another to induce lesions [39–42] or will transplant human lesion tissue into an immunodeficient mouse model [43–47]. Researchers also identified significant increases (monocytic myeloid-derived suppressor cells, granulocytic myeloid-derived suppressor cells) and decreases (B-cells, macrophages) in peritoneal levels of early immune cell profiles in intraperitoneally induced endometriosis in C57BL/6 immunocompetent mice [42]. Notably, nude mice have been used to observe the impact of disrupted matrix metalloproteinase (MMP) regulation on endometriotic lesion development [46]. Although no model system can fully recapitulate human anatomy, rodent models lack a menstrual cycle (instead experiencing estrus cyclicity), possess dissimilar reproductive anatomy (closed reproductive system, bicornate uterus), and are phylogenetically distant from humans [48–51].

2.2 *Primate Models of Endometriosis*

To address the anatomical and phylogenetic differences, some researchers turn to the use of nonhuman primates (baboons, rhesus macaques) to study endometriosis. These animals share similar uterine anatomy (open reproductive system, simplex uterus), menstruate, and can develop spontaneous endometriosis [49, 52–54]. Baboon models have been used to identify the role of Th17 cells in the upregulation of increased levels of IL-17, which has been noted in the peritoneal fluid of humans with endometriosis [55]. Rhesus macaques have been used to study the interactive effects of polycystic ovarian syndrome (PCOS) on endometriosis progression [56].

2.3 Flaws of Animal Models for Endometriosis Studies

These in vivo models can investigate mechanistic interactions as well as provide valuable preclinical insights for novel therapeutics. However, the use of these animal models can experience substantial pushback from the public and governmental funding bodies due to ethical dilemmas surrounding animal-based research. Nonhuman primates in particular pose a significant financial burden and are not as accessible for wide use in research due to the need for special housing facilities (Fig. 2). With all animal models, there have been issues with translatability of findings to humans, pushing researchers toward the use of human cells in engineered in vitro model systems [57–59].

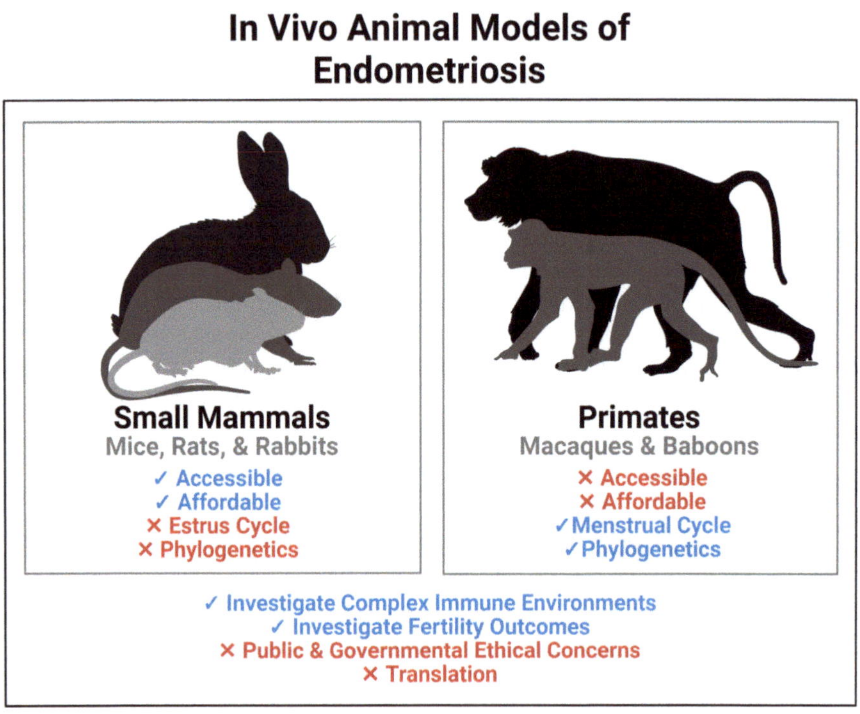

Fig. 2 Comparing small mammal in vitro models and primate models for endometriosis research. Here, we describe the overarching positive (blue) and negative (red) aspects of the use of these model systems. (Figure made in BioRender)

3 Cell Sources for Endometriosis Research

3.1 *Primary Components of Endometriosis Lesions*

To alleviate concerns about the use of animal models, but also with the goal of developing increasingly predictive models of human disease, investigators have started to consider in vitro models to investigate mechanisms of endometriosis initiation, progression, and recurrence. In vitro models can rely on the use of immortalized cell lines, induced pluripotent cells, or primary samples from patients. Immortalized cell lines are generally the most accessible cell source for researchers and constitute most early stage models. They are often commercially available or shared between research groups. These cell lines can be genetically stable and can be expanded many times without losing intrinsic morphological characteristics [60]. There is some debate over their use in model systems to generalize disease characteristics; however, they can behave differently than non-immortalized cells, often the patient-matched data is not reported, and there still can be passage-to-passage variability of transcriptomic and secreted factors [60, 61]. As the capacity increases, some investigators are increasingly opting for the use of primary cells. Primary cells are considered much more relevant in disease models; they conserve cell surface receptors in similar numbers (due to a lack of passaging), maintain similar signaling (due to a lack of culturing for extended periods on hard tissue culture plastic substrates), and can often be matched with patient data. The use of these tissues requires strict protocols to protect patient data (Institutional Review Board approval) and often necessitates a close relationship with clinicians. However, primary samples are often limited by low starting cell numbers, difficulties expanding sourced cells, and heterogeneous cell populations. Notably, while it may be an advantage to be able to connect a specific cell specimen with patient data, that also means that data analysis structures need to be built to consider the variability between patient specimens, patient lived-experiences, and experimental replicate to replicate. As a result, experiments must be meticulously planned to ensure the samples are used conservatively as once researchers deplete one patient biospecimen, they must procure a new sample from the same or a different patient. For endometriosis studies, this can also be particularly difficult, as endometriotic cells are retrieved during laparoscopic surgery and removed from the patients. Patients are often then placed on hormonal birth control to regulate the initiation of new lesions, so unless the patient ceases use of the medication, and elects to have new lesions removed, matched samples are often not possible.

As a result, researchers are increasingly considering alternative human cell sources. Potential noninvasive methods of cell sourcing includes the use of menstrual effluent from patients known to have endometriosis for the derivation of menstrual blood-derived stromal cells and stem cells (MenSCs) [62] as well as the potential to leverage patient-derived induced pluripotent stem cells (iPSCs). Although no current work reports the use of iPSCs for studying or modeling endometriosis, methods developed to differentiate cells to an "endometriotic state"

Table 2 Cell types used in endometriosis research. These include lesion-derived cells, endometrial cells, cancer cells, endothelial cells, immune cells, and stem cells [64–66]

Cell type	Cell name	Sample type	Citation
Endometriotic Epithelial	11z	F, PR, PT, NAR, NRR	[67, 68]
	12z	F, IM, PT, RA, NRR	[67, 68]
	49z	F, PR, PT, NAR, NRR	[67, 68]
	108z	F, PR, PT, NAR, NRR	[67, 68]
	EEC16	F, IM, OV, RA, NRR	[69]
	FbEM-1	F, IM, PT, RA, NRR	[70]
Endometriotic Stromal	iEC-ESC	F, IM, OV, RA, CC	[71, 72]
	22B	F, IM, PT, NAR, NRR	[67, 68]
Endometrial Adenocarcinoma	Ishikawa	F, IM, RA, AS	[73, 74]
Endometrial Stromal	T-hESC	F, IM, RA, NRR	[75]
	St-T1b	F, IM, RA, NRR	[76]
	iHUF	F, IM, V	[72]
Endometrial Epithelial	EECs	F, PR, RA, NRR	[77]
Stem cells	E-MSCs	F, PR, OV, RA, NRR	[78]
Endothelial cells	HUVECs	F, PR, V	[78]
Peritoneal surface epithelial cells	LP-9	F, PR, PT, RA, NRR	[72]
	HMrSV5	F, IM, PT, V	[79]
Ovarian surface Epithelial cells	OSEC10	F, PR, OV, NAR, NRR	[69]
	OSEC181	F, PR, OV, NAR, NRR	[69]
	OSEC11	F, PR, OV, NAR, NRR	[69]
Immune cells	U937	M, RA, CC	[79]
	PMs	F, PR, PT, NAR, NRR	[80]

F female, *M* male, *IM* immortalized, *PR* primary, *PT* peritoneal derived, *OV* ovarian derived, *RA* reproductive-aged, *NAR* no age reported, *CC* Caucasian, *AS* Asian, *NRR* no racial/ethnic data reported, *V* various age and race

could be reverse engineered to become a potential mechanism of disease treatment [63]. Table 2 details a range of cell types that are increasingly being used for endometriosis research.

3.2 Immune Cell Considerations

Dysregulation of immune cell infiltration into tissues is an important process by which the inflammatory environment surrounding endometriosis is hypothesized to be exacerbated [81, 82]. This dysregulation leads to modified activity of immune cell populations alongside an alteration of their secreted factors. In peritoneal fluid of patients with endometriosis, various cytokines implicated in angiogenesis and neutrophil recruitment are upregulated leading to increased incidence of these cells in the lesion microenvironment [83]. Neutrophils have also been shown to accumulate in ovarian endometriomas [84]. Natural killer cells (NKs) in endometriosis patients have been shown to have decreased cytotoxic functionality, resulting in the inability to properly recognize and clear ectopic cells that lead to lesions [84]. It has been found that during the proliferative phase, endometriosis patients had significantly increased numbers of macrophages present in their endometrium compared to healthy patients [85]. It has also been found that these endometrial macrophages tend to be more of the M1, pro-inflammatory, macrophage phenotype [86]. Th17 cells, a subtype of helper T cells, have been found to be of increased incidence in the endometrium and peritoneal fluid of endometriosis patients [84, 87]. Higher numbers of Th17 cells have been associated with more severe disease [84]. Table 3 outlines various immune cell populations that are integral to changes in the endometriosis lesion microenvironment that should be incorporated into in vitro investigations of the disease [88, 89].

3.3 Vascular Cell Considerations

Angiogenesis is another vital process in endometriosis by which new blood vessels are formed due to the recruitment of endothelial cells by endometriotic cells [102]. These cells form networks to provide nutrients and oxygen and are essential for the persistence and growth of endometriotic lesions in vivo. Clinicians often describe highly vascularized, new lesions as "red lesions" due to their bright red color from immense angiogenic processes [103, 104]. However, there are very few in vitro models of endometriotic cells and interactions with tissue-resident vascular cells, instead opting for the use of HUVECs, which are not tissue-specific [78].

Table 3 Immune cell dysregulation implicated in endometriosis disease

Cell name	Amount	Activity	Ability/secretion	Citation
Neutrophils	+	+	CXCL1$^+$, IL-8$^+$, IL-17α$^+$, VEGF$^+$	[83, 84, 90, 91]
Natural killers (NK)	±/=	−	Cytotoxicity$^-$	[84, 92–94]
Endometrial macrophages	+	=	CD163$^-$, IL-10$^+$, TGFβ$^+$, VEGF$^+$	[85, 86, 95, 96]
Peritoneal macrophages	+	=	Phagocytosis$^-$, IL-1β$^+$, IL-6$^+$, TNFα$^+$, VEGF$^+$	[95–97]
Treg (CD4+ T cell)	+/±	+	IL-10$^+$, TGFβ$^+$	[87, 98, 99]
Th17 (CD4+ T cell)	+	+	Endometriotic proliferation, IL-17α$^+$	[84, 87]
γδ (CD8+ T cell)	±/=	−	IL-17α$^+$	[100, 101]

(+) upregulated in endometriosis patients, (−) downregulated in endometriosis patients, (=) neutral, (±) conflicting literature, *CD163* cluster of differentiation 163, *CXCL1* human growth regulated protein alpha, *IL-1β* interleukin 1 beta, *IL-6* interleukin 6, *IL-8* interleukin 8, *IL-10* interleukin 10, *IL-17α* interleukin 17 alpha, *TGFβ* transforming growth factor beta, *TNFα* tumor necrosis factor alpha, *VEGF* vascular endothelial growth factor

3.4 Summary and Future Considerations for Cell Selection for Endometriosis Studies

It is important to note that studies utilizing various cell types do not always age-, sex-, disease-state, or lesion location-match their cells for experimentation. As described in Table 2, some studies employed the use of male-derived immune cells for endometriosis research. If available, researchers should attempt to sex-match all cell types used in their studies to ensure their results are not skewed by previous hormonal exposure. Researchers have shown that spheroids developed from various stages of disease and from various lesion locations can exhibit different cell signaling, invasive capacity, and cellular composition [20, 105]. More recently, researchers in the field have called the use of cells derived from healthy, native endometrium into question [106]. Some work uses these lines as a point of comparison; however, the intermixing of endometriotic lesion-derived cells and native endometrium-derived lines is ill-advised. Lesion-derived cells have been shown to display an enhanced capacity for invasion and migration [106, 107] while also displaying increased attachment [106, 108, 109]. The development of multicellular models of endometriosis should then aim to use endometriotic derived populations only and ideally use cells from the same lesion subtype. Thus, being selective with cell sourcing and being cautious about overgeneralizing conclusions to the whole of endometriosis is imperative for studies in this field.

4 Biomaterial Tools for Endometriosis Research

4.1 Bioinert Materials for In Vitro Endometriosis Studies

Biomaterial design is increasingly becoming a part of in vitro studies of endometriosis. Early generations of biomaterials were designed to interact with biological systems but not to elicit a cytotoxic biological response (bioinert) [110]. Early or simplified endometriosis studies often employ bioinert materials to understand basic mechanisms of endometriosis initiation and progression from an intracellular perspective (e.g., receptor activity, signaling cascades, transcriptomic analyses). The most ubiquitous bioinert materials fall under the umbrella of tissue culture plastics (TCPs). TCPs, such as polycarbonate, are used for scratch/wound-healing studies to investigate the invasive capacity of these cells, especially when treated with various cytokines, hormones, or therapeutics [74, 111, 112]. TCPs are also a primary component of transwell inserts, which are often used to quantify the migratory and chemotactic capacity of cells as well as to probe the effects of indirect coculture of other cell types with endometriotic cells [74, 78, 111, 113–115]. Other bioinert materials can be used to support the formation of endometriotic spheroids such as polyHEMA or alginate [69, 72]. Most immune-endometriosis studies to date have

Table 4 Bioinert materials used in endometriosis research

Material	Application	Investigation	Citation
Tissue culture plastic (TCP)	Transwell inserts	Migration, chemotaxis	[74, 111, 112]
	Scratch assay	Invasion, wound-healing	[74, 78, 111, 113–115]
	Low-adhesion properties	Spheroid formation	[69]
Alginate			[72]
Stainless steel			[75]

been conducted in 2D, in transwell assays, or without relevant ECM. Some of this work has elucidated the role of TNFα in enhancing endometriotic stromal cell proliferative capacity; however, this work was done in 2D on TCP [116]. Transwell inserts are useful for physically separating immune cells from endometriotic cells to investigate paracrine interactions. Table 4 describes three primary types of bioinert materials and their uses in endometriosis studies.

Studies that heavily rely on bioinert materials are often short-term, can only model simplistic multicellular interactions, and do not consider cell-matrix interactions. Further, it has been shown that experimenting on cells seeded on substrates of stiffnesses many magnitudes greater than many tissues can impact experimental results [117, 118]. These limitations require the use of more complex, physiologically relevant, bioactive, 3D biomaterials.

4.2 *Bioactive Materials for In Vitro Endometriosis Studies*

To model the complex tissue microenvironment of endometriotic lesions, researchers have turned to the use of bioactive materials. As opposed to bioinert materials, these are meant to explicitly interact with cells to elicit cellular responses. Often three-dimensional in nature, these materials can be engineered or selected to mimic distinct portions of the tissue(s) of interest including stiffness, porosity, degradability, adhesion sites, extracellular matrix (ECM) composition, etc. In endometriosis research, Matrigel is one of the most commonly used bioactive materials. It is derived from mouse sarcoma matrix and is used for invasion and tube formation studies [67, 72, 76, 78, 111, 112, 119, 120]. Matrigel retains cell binding motifs of natural tissues and readily supports cell cultured on top of or within the material. Matrigel, however, often reports batch-to-batch variability, and based on its derivation from mouse tumor stroma, it does not recapitulate the ECM composition of many human tissues.

Other naturally derived materials used in endometriosis research include collagens, gelatin, and fibrin [74, 76, 121–123]. Decellularized matrix also falls into the category of naturally derived biomaterials and has not yet been used in endometriosis research [124]. These materials, like Matrigel, maintain cell binding motifs and are naturally degradable by cells. These materials have less batch variability than Matrigel. They are difficult to tune to mimic specific tissue without incorporation of other compounds. Collagen I has been used to examine the directionality and invasive capacity of endometriotic multicellular spheroids, displaying the importance of ECM composition on in vitro modeling of endometriosis [76]. Fibrin gels have been used as a platform to culture primary endometriotic explants and investigate the effects of statins to inhibit endometriotic cell proliferation and endothelial network formation [122, 123].

Semisynthetic and synthetic materials can overcome the limitations of purely natural polymers and can be tuned to mimic specific tissues. Engineerable gelatin-based hydrogels, including those with light-based crosslinking moieties like methacrylamide functionalized gelatin (GelMA) as well as enzymatic-based crosslinking moieties like maleimide and thiol-functionalized gelatin (GelMAL, GelSH) allow for the retention of cell binding motifs and degradable sites as well as the ability to tightly control other parameters like mechanical properties and biotransport (e.g., diffusion). Derivatives of natural materials such as chitosan and elastin are described as semisynthetic due to additives that allow the resultant materials to be engineered more precisely [125]. Bioinert, synthetic polymers can be engineered to become bioactive. Commonly PEG or polyacrylamide can have proteins or peptides added to allow for cell degradation and attachment (e.g. VPM: protease-degradable; RGD: attachment sites) [125]. These materials have been used to mimic a variety of gynecological or pelvic tissues [126–128]. These bioactive materials can be applied to endometriosis research in a variety of ways including microfluidic devices, macrogels, microgels, and nanomaterials without even considering the multitude of methods cells can be incorporated into models with these materials (Table 5).

Table 5 Bioactive materials currently used or for proposed use in endometriosis research

Category	Material	Current or proposed	Citation
Natural materials	Matrigel	Current	[67, 72, 76, 78, 111, 112, 119, 120]
	Collagen	Current	[76, 121]
	Gelatin	Current	[74]
	Fibrin	Current	[122, 123]
	Decellularized matrix	Proposed	[124]
Semisynthetic materials	Gelatin derivatives (GelMA, GelMAL, GelSH)	Proposed	[127]
	Functionalized polyethylene glycol (PEG)	Proposed	[126]
	ECM-functionalized polyacrylamide	Current/proposed	[108]

4.3 Summary and Future Considerations for Biomaterials in Endometriosis Research

Researchers have many options for materials to use in endometriosis studies from the use of bioinert materials which has dominated the field to the novelty of biomaterials (Fig. 3). There is no one correct biomaterial for the study of endometriosis due to the heterogeneity of the disease. For tunability purposes and bioactivity, the use of semisynthetic materials is the most logical subcategory of biomaterials to implement in future studies. These materials can be tuned to mimic the stiffness of the tissue of interest (e.g., ovary, peritoneum, rectum), include relevant ECM though various chemical functionalization methods, and allow for degradation through various pathways. These methods can also capture changes that occur with age (changes in stiffness and composition), disease progression (fibrosis), etc. Researchers could also turn to the use of decellularized matrices from the tissues of interest; however, they may run into issues of replicability. Researchers must think critically about the materials they use, as work has shown that ECM composition plays a critical role in the ability of endometriosis cells to attach in vitro [108].

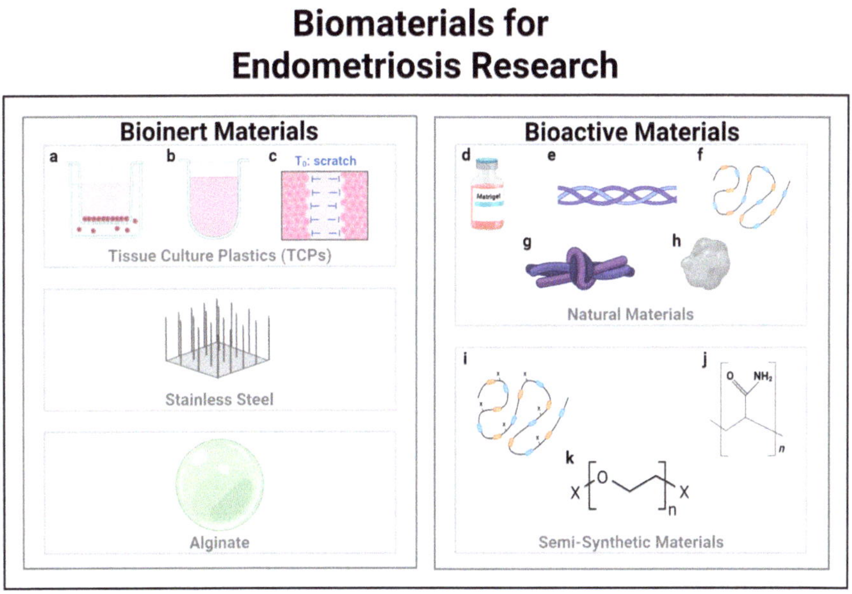

Fig. 3 Comparing types of biomaterials that are currently or could be used in endometriosis research. Under the TCP heading, there are (**a**) transwell inserts, (**b**) low-adhesion plates, and (**c**) well plates used for scratch-assays. Under naturally derived bioactive materials, there is (**d**) Matrigel, (**e**) collagen, (**f**) gelatin, (**g**) fibrin, and (**h**) decellularized matrix. Semisynthetic options for endometriosis research could include functionalized versions of (**i**) gelatin, (**j**) polyacrylamide, and (**k**) PEG. (Figure made in BioRender)

5 Signaling Considerations in Endometriosis Research

5.1 Developing Disease-Staged Models of Endometriosis

Once a material platform has been chosen, researchers decide how they will incorporate cell populations and various signals to mimic relevant stages of endometriosis development. This can be completed by seeding cell populations in a diffuse manner within the engineered hydrogels, seeding cells on top of a hydrogel substrate, forming spheroids then encapsulating them within or on top of the biomaterial, or some combination of these (Fig. 4). The methods by which investigators choose to incorporate cells can also be matched to potential stages of endometriosis based on theories of disease development.

For example, recent efforts have begun to use tissue engineering models targeted at specific stages of disease development (e.g., initiation, invasion, persistence/recurrence) [108]. This is particularly important in the design of in vitro model systems, as it is not possible to replicate all aspects of complexity of the lesion environment across a lifespan. Instead, models targeted to specific stages of disease development can provide researchers with insight about specific theories of disease

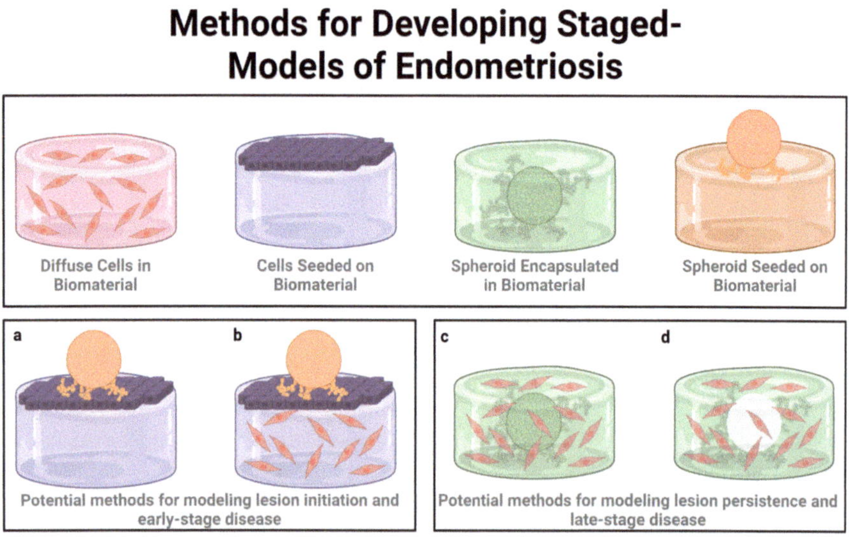

Fig. 4 Description of methods of incorporating cells with biomaterial tools to develop models that can recapitulate stages of disease development. Potential methods for modeling lesion initiation include (**a**) seeding a spheroid on top of a biomaterial that has previously had cells seeded on top (this could include tissue-specific epithelium) which could additionally include (**b**) vascular cells or support cells from the tissue of interest. Other methods for investigating lesion persistence could include (**c**) encapsulating a spheroid in a matrix with diffuse endothelial cells or other tissue-resident cells surrounding it. To investigate post-lesion recurrence, researchers could (**d**) "punch" the primary spheroid out of this system to investigate the capacity for further cell spread post "resection"

etiology and progression. It is also important to note the stage of disease being modeled to ensure the biomaterials being selected are relevant. For example, it has been hypothesized that early endometriotic cells would be interacting with otherwise healthy tissues that would be less fibrotic and more similar to stiffnesses of tissues reported in literature [129]. Disease status would also influence the extracellular matrix composition and alignment of the tissues [37]. Thus, when developing biomaterial tools to study early events of attachment, researchers would likely need to utilize softer biomaterials with less collagen content than later disease states which would require biomaterials with the inverse conditions.

5.2 Incorporating Immune Signals in Models of Endometriosis

The field has also become increasingly interested in the role of extracellular vesicles (EVs) on endometriosis development and progression. EVs can be immunosuppressive, facilitating immune evasion [130, 131]. Novel biomaterial tools aiming to investigate the immune–endometriosis axis should consider the inclusion of EVs in their studies. The immune system is vastly complex, and thus there are many ways in which researchers can integrate immune activity within 3D biomaterial models of endometriosis. What is important for investigators to consider is what stage of disease they are aiming to model, what tissue(s) they are aiming to model, and which immune cells/cytokines/EVs would be the most relevant to methodically investigate treating their endometriosis model system with.

5.3 Incorporating Angiogenic Signals in Models of Endometriosis

Investigators have shown that freshly isolated endometriotic cells (epithelial and stromal) cultured in hypoxic conditions increase VEGF secretions [132]. Angiogenesis is very closely linked to immune and endocrine activity through pathways related to IL-1β (estradiol increasing macrophage secretion of IL-1β which stimulates VEGF expression) [133, 134]. Beyond contributing data surrounding these processes, there is a novel interest in repurposing antiangiogenesis therapeutics used for cancer therapy for endometriosis treatment [135, 136]. By developing robust models of the interactions between endometriotic cells and their vascular microenvironment, preclinical evaluations of these therapeutics in a humanized model can be systematically tested.

5.4 *Incorporating Endocrine Signals in Models of Endometriosis*

Finally, hormones are critically important to the development and exacerbation of endometriosis progression through interactions with endometriotic cells directly, immune cell populations, and vascular cell recruitment. While some biomaterial models of that native endometrial microenvironment have begun to incorporate hormonal signals [137–140], there is significant opportunity to incorporate hormonal signals into models of endometriosis. For example, biomaterial models of endometriosis will likely require physiologically relevant concentrations of E2, but what concentrations constitute physiologically relevant across the menstrual cycle, with age, and as a function of anatomic localization (e.g., endometrioma lesions on the ovaries vs. endometriotic lesions on the peritoneal cavity) remain to be well-defined. This work could be conducted in more traditional hydrogel systems, or levels of E2 could be slowly altered in a microfluidic system to mimic the changes in E2 levels over the course of the menstrual cycle.

5.5 *Summary and Future Considerations for Signals in Endometriosis Research*

Here, we describe some of the most influential signaling processes in maintenance of an endometriotic disease state. Future work must consider the sequential investigation of these processes in 3D, physiologically relevant models. This progression should also consider the incorporation of epithelium, stroma, and/or endothelium from the specific tissue being studied. Organ-on-chip systems can readily incorporate various cellular and matrix components while studying the effect of paracrine and juxtracrine signaling. As the field develops increasingly complex models of these interactions, a shift to personalized investigation based on lived experiences (social stress, exposure to environmental toxicants, potential interactive effects caused by comorbid diseases, varied menstrual cyclicity, etc.) can perturb these base model systems and better understand how endometriosis can present differently in patients with different backgrounds.

6 Biomaterials for Endometriosis Diagnosis and Treatment

Beyond modeling disease pathology, biomaterials can also be considered for advancing endometriosis diagnosis and treatment. Biomaterials are often used to enhance drug or therapeutic efficacy by allowing for specific tracking to tissue targets or controlling the drug release kinetics [141–143]. In gene therapeutic development, researchers have been developing biomaterials that can suppress further endometriotic lesion formation by accumulating more acutely in lesions (hyaluronic acid-chitosan-polyetherimide conjugates) [144]. One example includes the use of poly lactic-co-glycolic acid (PLGA) encapsulated CTLA-4 antibodies to control the release and immune response to the therapeutic which showed promising halting of endometriosis progression in vivo [145]. Other biomaterial uses include the development of a PGLA-chitosan glue that targets endometriotic cells and causes apoptosis [146]. Biomaterial nanoparticles have been shown to decrease endometriotic cell viability in vitro [147] and decrease the presence of endometriotic glands and vascular density in vivo [148].

Early diagnosis of endometriosis is limited by the inability of current imaging modalities to identify differences in endometriotic and non-endometriotic tissues. Engineered nanoparticles have been shown to assist with noninvasive methods of endometriosis diagnosis. Researchers have found that hyaluronic acid modified iron oxide nanoparticles were able to create contrast during MRI imaging between endometriotic and non-endometriotic tissues [149].

Looking forward, biomaterials for the diagnosis and treatment of endometriosis will be integral to improving patient outcomes. The development of biomaterial tools for the early detection of endometriosis can utilize work done in the oncology space as a guide, using biomaterials to characterize lesions. Liquid biopsies, which circulating tumor cells can be extracted from, cultured in biomaterials can provide a patient-specific approach to cancer detection and treatment efficacy. This personalized approach to diagnosis could be applied to endometriosis studies by utilizing menstrual effluent with relevant biomaterial tools to determine the invasive capacity of cell populations and match with potential disease presence. The field of early cancer detection has also focused on overcoming limitations of current imaging modalities. Rarely is endometriosis identified through ultrasound or MRI techniques, especially early lesions. By identifying endometriosis-specific targets for that preferentially tracking of biomaterial-based imaging agents to endometriotic lesions, researchers could assist clinicians in early disease detection. As the field begins to better understand mechanisms of disease development and progression, the path to the development of materials for treatment will become clearer. Leveraging knowledge surrounding endometriosis–immune interactions could aid in the development of endometriosis immunotherapeutics. These immunomodulatory treatments could aid in immune clearance of endometriosis through increased production of phagocytic cells or tagging of endometriotic cells as foreign. Overall, the use of biomaterials for endometriosis treatment and identification has many avenues for growth. With more accurate detection methods, and precise control of therapeutics, clinicians will have the ability to better identify personalized treatments for endometriosis based on disease progression and subtype.

7 Concluding Challenges and the Future of Biomaterials in Endometriosis Studies

The use of tissue engineered models to investigate endometriosis lesion etiology, progression, and treatment is in its infancy. By critically choosing cells and biomaterials employed in endometriosis models, researchers are beginning to methodically investigate the mechanisms by which endometriosis initiates and progresses. Current limitations of applicability of findings using immortalized cell lines could be addressed by deriving primary samples from menstrual blood [62]. Because of the tunability of synthetic and semisynthetic biomaterials, their use in various stages of endometriosis research (composition, stiffness) is enticing as a path forward in studies that attempt to understand the influence of matrix environment on lesion activity. Investigators must also critically consider the method in which cells are interacting with the chosen materials, whether cells are seeded on or encapsulated within systems such as microgels, macrogels, or microfluidic chambers. Biomaterial models can recapitulate certain features of a living organism, especially using concise questions and careful planning of experimental approaches. As this field continues to grow, biomaterial models have huge potential to be used to evaluate therapeutic strategies with the hope that carefully designed systems will overcome translatability issues found in animal models. This imagined future is only possible via the interdisciplinary work of researchers from clinical, STEM, and humanities disciplines, who collectively have the ability to consider the mechanistic detail of endometriosis progression but also the skills to consider the role of social structure and the broader environment on disease etiology and progression. This path forward will require close collaboration between biologists, engineers, clinicians, social scientists, and patient advocates to ensure the models being developed will address pressing needs in the endometriosis clinical space.

Acknowledgments The authors would like to acknowledge funding sources, specifically the Eunice Kennedy Shriver National Institute of Child Health and Human Development of the National Institutes of Health under Award Numbers R01 HD118600 (BACH) and T32 HD108075 (HST). This content is solely the responsibility of the authors and does not necessarily represent the official views of the NIH. We acknowledge the use of BioRender to create figures.

References

1. International Working Group of AAGL, ESGE, ESHRE and WES, et al. An international terminology for endometriosis, 2021†,‡. Hum Reprod Open. 2021;2021(4):hoab029.
2. Shigesi N, et al. The association between endometriosis and autoimmune diseases: a systematic review and meta-analysis. Hum Reprod Update. 2019;25(4):486–503.
3. Bougie O, Nwosu I, Warshafsky C. Revisiting the impact of race/ethnicity in endometriosis. Reprod Fertil. 2022;3(2):R34–41.
4. Farland L, Horne A. Disparity in endometriosis diagnoses between racial/ethnic groups. BJOG: Int J Obstet Gynaecol. 2019;126(9):1115–6.

5. Katon JG, Plowden TC, Marsh EE. Racial disparities in uterine fibroids and endometriosis: a systematic review and application of social, structural, and political context. Fertil Steril. 2023;119(3):355–63.
6. Koninckx PR, et al. The epidemiology of endometriosis is poorly known as the pathophysiology and diagnosis are unclear. Best Pract Res Clin Obstet Gynaecol. 2021;71:14–26.
7. Bougie O, et al. Influence of race/ethnicity on prevalence and presentation of endometriosis: a systematic review and meta-analysis. BJOG: Int J Obstet Gynaecol. 2019;126(9):1104–15.
8. Missmer SA, et al. Incidence of laparoscopically confirmed endometriosis by demographic, anthropometric, and lifestyle factors. Am J Epidemiol. 2004;160(8):784–96.
9. Parazzini F, Vercellini P, Pelucchi C. Endometriosis: epidemiology, and etiological factors. In: Giudice LC, Evers JLH, Healy DL, editors. Endometriosis: Science and practice, Blackwell Publishing Ltd; 2011:19–26. https://doi.org/10.1002/9781444398519
10. Parazzini F, et al. Epidemiology of endometriosis and its comorbidities. Eur J Obstet Gynecol Reprod Biol. 2017;209:3–7.
11. Moen MH, Magnus P. The familial risk of endometriosis. Acta Obstet Gynecol Scand. 1993;72(7):560–4.
12. Lamb K, Hoffmann RG, Nichols TR. Family trait analysis: a case-control study of 43 women with endometriosis and their best friends. Am J Obstet Gynecol. 1986;154(3):596–601.
13. Kobayashi H, et al. Revisiting estrogen-dependent signaling pathways in endometriosis: potential targets for non-hormonal therapeutics. Eur J Obstet Gynecol Reprod Biol. 2021;258:103–10.
14. Pu H, et al. Regulation of progesterone receptor expression in endometriosis, endometrial cancer, and breast cancer by estrogen, polymorphisms, transcription factors, epigenetic alterations, and ubiquitin-proteasome system. J Steroid Biochem Mol Biol. 2023;227:106199.
15. Angioni S, et al. New trends of progestins treatment of endometriosis. Gynecol Endocrinol. 2014;30(11):769–73.
16. Brichant G, et al. New therapeutics in endometriosis: a review of hormonal, non-hormonal, and non-coding RNA treatments. Int J Mol Sci. 2021;22(19):10498.
17. Resta C, et al. Gonadotropin-releasing hormone (GnRH)/GnRH receptors and their role in the treatment of endometriosis. Cureus. 2023;15(4):e38136.
18. Yan H, et al. Oral gonadotropin-releasing hormone antagonists for treating endometriosis-associated pain: a systematic review and network meta-analysis. Fertil Steril. 2022;118(6):1102–16.
19. De Corte P, et al. Endometriosis and risk of depression among oral contraceptive users: a pooled analysis of cohort studies from 13 countries. Hum Reprod. 2025;40(3):479–86.
20. Tan Y, et al. Single-cell analysis of endometriosis reveals a coordinated transcriptional programme driving immunotolerance and angiogenesis across eutopic and ectopic tissues. Nat Cell Biol. 2022;24(8):1306–18.
21. Chan RW, Ng EH, Yeung WS. Identification of cells with colony-forming activity, self-renewal capacity, and multipotency in ovarian endometriosis. Am J Pathol. 2011;178(6):2832–44.
22. Cousins FL, Dorien FO, Gargett CE. Endometrial stem/progenitor cells and their role in the pathogenesis of endometriosis. Best Pract Res Clin Obstet Gynaecol. 2018;50:27–38.
23. Ulukus M, Cakmak H, Arici A. The role of endometrium in endometriosis. J Soc Gynecol Investig. 2006;13(7):467–76.
24. Bergqvist A, Fernö M. Endometriosis: oestrogen and progesterone receptors in endometriotic tissue and endometrium: comparison of different cycle phases and ages*. Hum Reprod. 1993;8(12):2211–7.
25. Jänne O, et al. Estrogen and progestin receptors in endometriosis lesions: comparison with endometrial tissue. Am J Obstet Gynecol. 1981;141(6):562–6.
26. Bulun SE, et al. Estrogen receptor-β, estrogen receptor-α, and progesterone resistance in endometriosis. Semin Reprod Med. 2010;28(01):036–43.
27. Chantalat E, et al. Estrogen receptors and endometriosis. Int J Mol Sci. 2020;21(8):2815.

28. Harada T, et al. Apoptosis in human endometrium and endometriosis. Hum Reprod Update. 2004;10(1):29–38.
29. Kinkel K, et al. Diagnosis of endometriosis with imaging: a review. Eur Radiol. 2006;16(2): 285–98.
30. Kido A, et al. MRI in the diagnosis of endometriosis and related diseases. Korean J Radiol. 2022;23(4):426–45.
31. Monnaka VU, et al. Overview of miRNAs for the non-invasive diagnosis of endometriosis: evidence, challenges and strategies. A systematic review. Einstein (São Paulo). 2021;19: eRW5704.
32. Moein Mahini S, et al. Non-invasive diagnosis of endometriosis: immunologic and genetic markers. Clin Chim Acta. 2023;538:70–86.
33. Scheck SM, et al. Non-invasive tests for endometriosis are here; how reliable are they, and what should we do with the results? Aust N Z J Obstet Gynaccol. 2024;64(2):168–70.
34. Kalaitzopoulos DR, et al. Treatment of endometriosis: a review with comparison of 8 guidelines. BMC Womens Health. 2021;21(1):397.
35. Koninckx PR, et al. Pathogenesis based diagnosis and treatment of endometriosis. Front Endocrinol. 2021;12:745548.
36. Vissers G, et al. The role of fibrosis in endometriosis: a systematic review. Hum Reprod Update. 2024;30(6):706–50.
37. Viganò P, et al. Cellular components contributing to fibrosis in endometriosis: a literature review. J Minim Invasive Gynecol. 2020;27(2):287–95.
38. Cranney R, Condous G, Reid S. An update on the diagnosis, surgical management, and fertility outcomes for women with endometrioma. Acta Obstet Gynecol Scand. 2017;96(6): 633–43.
39. Heard ME, et al. High-fat diet promotion of endometriosis in an immunocompetent mouse model is associated with altered peripheral and ectopic lesion redox and inflammatory status. Endocrinology. 2016;157(7):2870–82.
40. Li Y, et al. Progesterone alleviates endometriosis via inhibition of uterine cell proliferation, inflammation and angiogenesis in an immunocompetent mouse model. PLoS One. 2016;11 (10):e0165347.
41. Wieser F, et al. Retinoic acid suppresses growth of lesions, inhibits peritoneal cytokine secretion, and promotes macrophage differentiation in an immunocompetent mouse model of endometriosis. Fertil Steril. 2012;97(6):1430–7.
42. He Y, et al. Re-evaluation of mouse models of endometriosis for pathological and immunological research. Front Immunol. 2022;13:986202.
43. Wang N, et al. A red fluorescent nude mouse model of human endometriosis: advantages of a non-invasive imaging method. Eur J Obstet Gynecol Reprod Biol. 2014;176:25–30.
44. Perelló M, et al. Oral administration of pentoxifylline reduces endometriosis-like lesions in a nude mouse model. Reprod Sci. 2017;24(6):911–8.
45. Ma Y, He Y. Study of an antiangiogenesis gene therapy with endostatin on endometriosis in the nude mouse model. Clin Exp Obstet Gynecol. 2014;41(3):328–34.
46. Bruner-Tran KL, Osteen KG, Duleba AJ. Simvastatin protects against the development of endometriosis in a nude mouse model. J Clin Endocrinol Metabol. 2009;94(7):2489–94.
47. Nisolle M, Casanas-Roux F, Donnez J. Early-stage endometriosis: adhesion and growth of human menstrual endometrium in nude mice. Fertil Steril. 2000;74(2):306–12.
48. Taniguchi F, et al. Animal models for research on endometriosis. Front Biosci (Elite Ed). 2021;13(1):37–53.
49. Laganà AS, et al. Translational animal models for endometriosis research: a long and windy road. Ann Transl Med. 2018;6(22):431.
50. Tejada MA, et al. Rodent animal models of endometriosis-associated pain: unmet needs and resources available for improving translational research in endometriosis. Int J Mol Sci. 2023;24(3):2422.

51. Burns KA, et al. Endometriosis in the mouse: challenges and progress toward a 'best fit' murine model. Front Physiol. 2022;12:806574.
52. Nishimoto-Kakiuchi A, et al. Spontaneous endometriosis in cynomolgus monkeys as a clinically relevant experimental model. Hum Reprod. 2018;33(7):1228–36.
53. Harirchian P, et al. Lesion kinetics in a non-human primate model of endometriosis. Hum Reprod. 2012;27(8):2341–51.
54. Braundmeier AG, Fazleabas AT. The non-human primate model of endometriosis: research and implications for fecundity. Mol Hum Reprod. 2009;15(10):577–86.
55. Le N, et al. Effects of endometriosis on immunity and mucosal microbial community dynamics in female olive baboons. Sci Rep. 2022;12(1):1590.
56. Bishop CV, et al. The combined impact of testosterone and Western-style diet on endometriosis severity and progression in rhesus macaques†. Biol Reprod. 2022;108(1):72–80.
57. Fogg K, et al. Roadmap on biomaterials for women's health. J Phys Mater. 2023;6(1):012501.
58. Stejskalová A, et al. In vitro modelling of the physiological and diseased female reproductive system. Acta Biomater. 2021;132:288–312.
59. Rodrigues J, et al. 3D in vitro model (R)evolution: unveiling tumor-stroma interactions. Trends Cancer. 2021;7(3):249–64.
60. Irfan Maqsood M, et al. Immortality of cell lines: challenges and advantages of establishment. Cell Biol Int. 2013;37(10):1038–45.
61. Kolliopoulos V, et al. Donor sex and passage conditions influence MSC osteogenic response in mineralized collagen scaffolds. Adv Healthc Mater. 2024;13(27):2400039.
62. Nikoo S, et al. Menstrual blood-derived stromal stem cells from women with and without endometriosis reveal different phenotypic and functional characteristics. Mol Hum Reprod. 2014;20(9):905–18.
63. Miyazaki K, et al. Generation of progesterone-responsive endometrial stromal fibroblasts from human induced pluripotent stem cells: role of the WNT/CTNNB1 pathway. Stem Cell Rep. 2018;11(5):1136–55.
64. Gołąbek-Grenda A, Olejnik A. In vitro modeling of endometriosis and endometriotic microenvironment – challenges and recent advances. Cell Signal. 2022;97:110375.
65. Black V, et al. Modelling endometriosis using in vitro and in vivo systems. Int J Mol Sci. 2025;26(2):580.
66. Cheng Y-H, et al. A preliminary investigation of the roles of endometrial cells in endometriosis development via in vitro and in vivo analyses. Int J Mol Sci. 2024;25(7):3873.
67. Zeitvogel A, Baumann R, Starzinski-Powitz A. Identification of an invasive, N-cadherin-expressing epithelial cell type in endometriosis using a new cell culture model. Am J Pathol. 2001;159(5):1839–52.
68. Banu SK, et al. Gene expression profiles and functional characterization of human immortalized endometriotic epithelial and stromal cells. Fertil Steril. 2008;90(4):972–87.
69. Brueggmann D, et al. Novel three-dimensional in vitro models of ovarian endometriosis. J Ovarian Res. 2014;7(1):17.
70. de Joliniere J, et al. Human endometriosis-derived permanent cell line (FbEM-1): establishment and characterization. Hum Reprod Update. 1997;3(2):117–23.
71. Song Y, et al. Establishment of an immortalized endometriotic stromal cell line from human ovarian endometrioma. Reprod Sci. 2020;27(11):2082–91.
72. Song Y, et al. Spheroids as a model for endometriotic lesions. JCI Insight. 2023;8(11): e160815.
73. Guay S, Akoum A. Stable inhibition of interleukin 1 receptor type II in Ishikawa cells augments secretion of matrix metalloproteinases: possible role in endometriosis pathophysiology. Reproduction. 2007;134(3):525–34.
74. Zhao J, et al. Effect and mechanisms of kaempferol against endometriosis based on network pharmacology and in vitro experiments. BMC Complementary Med Ther. 2022;22(1):254.
75. Wendel JRH, et al. Three-dimensional biofabrication models of endometriosis and the endometriotic microenvironment. Biomedicines. 2020;8(11):525.

76. Stejskalová A, et al. Collagen I triggers directional migration, invasion and matrix remodeling of stroma cells in a 3D spheroid model of endometriosis. Sci Rep. 2021;11(1):4115.
77. Matsuzaki S, et al. Effects of matrix stiffness on epithelial to mesenchymal transition-like processes of endometrial epithelial cells: implications for the pathogenesis of endometriosis. Sci Rep. 2017;7(1):44616.
78. Canosa S, et al. Angiogenic properties of endometrial mesenchymal stromal cells in endothelial co-culture: an in vitro model of endometriosis. Mol Hum Reprod. 2017;23(3):187–98.
79. Králíčková M, et al. Altered immunity in endometriosis: what came first? Immunol Investig. 2018;47(6):569–82.
80. Loh F-H, et al. Effects of peritoneal macrophages from women with endometriosis on endometrial cellular proliferation in an in vitro coculture model. Fertil Steril. 1999;72(3):533–8.
81. Scheerer C, et al. Characterization of endometriosis-associated immune cell infiltrates (EMaICI). Arch Gynecol Obstet. 2016;294(3):657–64.
82. Chen S, Chai X, Wu X. Bioinformatical analysis of the key differentially expressed genes and associations with immune cell infiltration in development of endometriosis. BMC Genomic Data. 2022;23(1):20.
83. Wang X, et al. The abundance and function of neutrophils in the endometriosis systemic and pelvic microenvironment. Mediat Inflamm. 2023;2023(1):1481489.
84. Izumi G, et al. Involvement of immune cells in the pathogenesis of endometriosis. J Obstet Gynaecol Res. 2018;44(2):191–8.
85. Berbic M, et al. Macrophage expression in endometrium of women with and without endometriosis. Hum Reprod. 2008;24(2):325–32.
86. Takebayashi A, et al. Subpopulations of macrophages within eutopic endometrium of endometriosis patients. Am J Reprod Immunol. 2015;73(3):221–31.
87. Takamura M, et al. Simultaneous detection and evaluation of four subsets of CD4+ T lymphocyte in lesions and peripheral blood in endometriosis. Am J Reprod Immunol. 2015;74(6):480–6.
88. Seli E, Arici A. Endometriosis: interaction of immune and endocrine systems. Semin Reprod Med. 2003;21(02):135–44.
89. Abramiuk M, et al. The role of the immune system in the development of endometriosis. Cells. 2022;11(13):2028.
90. Milewski Ł, et al. Increased levels of human neutrophil peptides 1, 2, and 3 in peritoneal fluid of patients with endometriosis: association with neutrophils, T cells and IL-8. J Reprod Immunol. 2011;91(1):64–70.
91. Tabatabaei F, et al. Diagnostic significance of neutrophil to lymphocyte ratio in endometriosis: a systematic review and meta-analysis. BMC Womens Health. 2023;23(1):576.
92. Thiruchelvam U, Wingfield M, O'Farrelly C. Natural killer cells: key players in endometriosis. Am J Reprod Immunol. 2015;74(4):291–301.
93. Matsuoka S, et al. Expression of inhibitory-motif killer immunoglobulin-like receptor, KIR2DL1, is increased in natural killer cells from women with pelvic endometriosis. Am J Reprod Immunol. 2005;53(5):249–54.
94. Hoogstad-van Evert J, et al. The promises of natural killer cell therapy in endometriosis. Int J Mol Sci. 2022;23(10):5539.
95. Yang H-L, et al. The crosstalk between endometrial stromal cells and macrophages impairs cytotoxicity of NK cells in endometriosis by secreting IL-10 and TGF-β. Reproduction. 2017;154(6):815–25.
96. Hogg C, Horne AW, Greaves E. Endometriosis-associated macrophages: origin, phenotype, and function. Front Endocrinol. 2020;11:7.
97. Montagna P, et al. Peritoneal fluid macrophages in endometriosis: correlation between the expression of estrogen receptors and inflammation. Fertil Steril. 2008;90(1):156–64.

98. Li MQ, et al. CD4+Foxp3+ regulatory T cell differentiation mediated by endometrial stromal cell-derived TECK promotes the growth and invasion of endometriotic lesions. Cell Death Dis. 2014;5(10):e1436.
99. Podgaec S, et al. CD4+CD25highFoxp3+ cells increased in the peritoneal fluid of patients with endometriosis. Am J Reprod Immunol. 2012;68(4):301–8.
100. Hudecek R, et al. Blocking of EphA2 on endometrial tumor cells reduces susceptibility to Vδ1 gamma-delta T-cell-mediated killing. Front Immunol. 2021;12:752646.
101. Pawłowska A, et al. γδ T lymphocytes as a double-edged sword—state of the art in gynecological diseases. Int J Mol Sci. 2022;23(23):14797.
102. Laschke MW, Menger MD. Basic mechanisms of vascularization in endometriosis and their clinical implications. Hum Reprod Update. 2018;24(2):207–24.
103. Nisolle M, et al. Morphometric study of the stromal vascularization in peritoneal endometriosis **Supported in part by Fonds de la Recherche Scientifique Médicale, grant 3.4587.90, Brussels, Belgium. Fertil Steril. 1993;59(3):681–4.
104. Kuroda K, et al. Vascular density of peritoneal endometriosis using narrow-band imaging system and vascular analysis software. J Minim Invasive Gynecol. 2009;16(5):618–21.
105. Boretto M, et al. Patient-derived organoids from endometrial disease capture clinical heterogeneity and are amenable to drug screening. Nat Cell Biol. 2019;21(8):1041–51.
106. Gunther K, et al. Endometriosis is not the endometrium: reviewing the over-representation of eutopic endometrium in endometriosis research. Elife. 2025;14:e103825.
107. Kao A-P, et al. Comparative study of human eutopic and ectopic endometrial mesenchymal stem cells and the development of an in vivo endometriotic invasion model. Fertil Steril. 2011;95(4):1308–15.e1.
108. Theriault HS, et al. Matrix tropism influences endometriotic cell attachment patterns. Adv Funct Mater. 2025;35:02777.
109. Delbandi A-A, et al. Eutopic and ectopic stromal cells from patients with endometriosis exhibit differential invasive, adhesive, and proliferative behavior. Fertil Steril. 2013;100(3):761–9.
110. Zhao X. 1 – Introduction to bioactive materials in medicine. In: Zhao X, Courtney JM, Qian H, editors. Bioactive materials in medicine. Woodhead Publishing; 2011. p. 1–13.
111. Soni UK, et al. A high level of TGF-B1 promotes endometriosis development via cell migration, adhesiveness, colonization, and invasiveness†. Biol Reprod. 2018;100(4):917–38.
112. Liu H, et al. GLI1 is increased in ovarian endometriosis and regulates migration, invasion and proliferation of human endometrial stromal cells in endometriosis. Ann Transl Med. 2019;7(22):663.
113. Leiva MC, et al. Increased chemotactic activity of peritoneal fluid in patients with endometriosis. Am J Obstet Gynecol. 1993;168(2):592–8.
114. Witz CA, et al. An in vitro model to study the pathogenesis of the early endometriosis lesion. Ann N Y Acad Sci. 2002;955(1):296–307.
115. Fu X, et al. Osteopontin regulates endometrial stromal cell migration in endometriosis through the PI3K pathway. Reprod Sci. 2021;28(2):435–46.
116. Iwabe T, et al. Tumor necrosis factor-α promotes proliferation of endometriotic stromal cells by inducing interleukin-8 gene and protein expression. J Clin Endocrinol Metabol. 2000;85(2):824–9.
117. Wang N. Review of cellular mechanotransduction. J Phys D Appl Phys. 2017;50(23):233002.
118. Naqvi SM, McNamara LM. Stem cell mechanobiology and the role of biomaterials in governing mechanotransduction and matrix production for tissue regeneration. Front Bioeng Biotechnol. 2020;8:597661.
119. Kobayashi H. Invasive capacity of heterotopic endometrium. Gynecol Obstet Investig. 2000;50(Suppl. 1):26–32.
120. Qiu X-M, et al. IL-2 and IL-27 synergistically promote growth and invasion of endometriotic stromal cells by maintaining the balance of IFN-γ and IL-10 in endometriosis. Reproduction. 2020;159(3):251–60.
121. Gaetje R, et al. Invasiveness of endometriotic cells in vitro. Lancet. 1995;346(8988):1463–4.

122. Fasciani A, et al. Three-dimensional in vitro culture of endometrial explants mimics the early stages of endometriosis. Fertil Steril. 2003;80(5):1137–43.
123. Esfandiari N, et al. Effect of a statin on an in vitro model of endometriosis. Fertil Steril. 2007;87(2):257–62.
124. Francés-Herrero E, et al. Improved models of human endometrial organoids based on hydrogels from decellularized endometrium. J Pers Med. 2021;11(6):504.
125. Macchione MA, et al. Chapter 2 – Synthetic and semi-synthetic polymers for pharmaceutical applications. In: Nayak AK, et al., editors. Advances and challenges in pharmaceutical technology. Academic Press; 2021. p. 45–73.
126. Gnecco JS, et al. Organoid co-culture model of the human endometrium in a fully synthetic extracellular matrix enables the study of epithelial-stromal crosstalk. Med. 2023;4(8): 554–579.e9.
127. Zambuto SG, Clancy KBH, Harley BAC. A gelatin hydrogel to study endometrial angiogenesis and trophoblast invasion. Interface Focus. 2019;9(5):20190016.
128. Kim J, et al. Synthetic hydrogel supports the function and regeneration of artificial ovarian tissue in mice. NPJ Regen Med. 2016;1:16010.
129. Wynn TA. Cellular and molecular mechanisms of fibrosis. J Pathol. 2008;214(2):199–210.
130. Shomali N, et al. Exosomes: emerging biomarkers and targets in folliculogenesis and endometriosis. J Reprod Immunol. 2020;142:103181.
131. Freger S, Leonardi M, Foster W. Exosomes and their cargo are important regulators of cell function in endometriosis. Reprod Biomed Online. 2021;43(3):370–8.
132. Sharkey AM, et al. Vascular endothelial growth factor expression in human endometrium is regulated by hypoxia. J Clin Endocrinol Metab. 2000;85(1):402–9.
133. Lebovic DI, et al. Induction of an angiogenic phenotype in endometriotic stromal cell cultures by interleukin-1β. Mol Hum Reprod. 2000;6(3):269–75.
134. Akoum A, et al. Ectopic endometrial cells express high concentrations of interleukin (IL)-8 in vivo regardless of the menstrual cycle phase and respond to oestradiol by up-regulating IL-1-induced IL-8 expression in vitro. Mol Hum Reprod. 2001;7(9):859–66.
135. Chung MS, Han SJ. Endometriosis-associated angiogenesis and anti-angiogenic therapy for endometriosis. Front Glob Womens Health. 2022;3:856316.
136. Zheng W, et al. Anti-angiogenic alternative and complementary medicines for the treatment of endometriosis: a review of potential molecular mechanisms. Evid Based Complement Alternat Med. 2018;2018(1):4128984.
137. Zambuto SG, et al. Role of extracellular matrix biomolecules on endometrial epithelial cell attachment and cytokeratin 18 expression on gelatin hydrogels. ACS Biomater Sci Eng. 2022;8(9):3819–30.
138. Zambuto SG, et al. Response of neuroglia to hypoxia-induced oxidative stress using enzymatically crosslinked hydrogels. MRS Commun. 2020;10(1):83–90.
139. Zambuto SG, et al. Cell chirality of micropatterned endometrial microvascular endothelial cells. Adv Healthc Mater. 2024;13(12):e2303928.
140. Zambuto SG, et al. Endometrial decidualization status modulates endometrial microvascular complexity and trophoblast outgrowth in gelatin methacryloyl hydrogels. NPJ Womens Health. 2024;2(1):22.
141. Chen Q, et al. Emerging strategies for the treatment of endometriosis. Biomed Technol. 2024;7:46–62.
142. Yuxue J, et al. Applications of nanomaterials in endometriosis treatment. Front Bioeng Biotechnol. 2023;11:1184155.
143. Peng Y, et al. Emerging bioengineering breakthroughs in precision diagnosis and therapy for endometriosis and adenomyosis. J Mater Chem B. 2025;13(3):742–62.
144. Zhao M-D, et al. Hyaluronic acid reagent functional chitosan-PEI conjugate with AQP2-siRNA suppressed endometriotic lesion formation. Int J Nanomedicine. 2016;11:1323–36.

145. Liu Q, et al. Evaluation of PLGA containing anti-CTLA4 inhibited endometriosis progression by regulating CD4+CD25+Treg cells in peritoneal fluid of mouse endometriosis model. Eur J Pharm Sci. 2017;96:542–50.
146. Wang Y-C, et al. Polyglycolic acid/chitosan glue and apoptosis of endometriotic cells. Fertil Steril. 2005;84(1):75–81.
147. de Almeida Borges VR, et al. Development and pharmacological evaluation of in vitro nanocarriers composed of lamellar silicates containing copaiba oil-resin for treatment of endometriosis. Mater Sci Eng C. 2016;64:310–7.
148. Singh AK, Chakravarty B, Chaudhury K. Nanoparticle-assisted combinatorial therapy for effective treatment of endometriosis. J Biomed Nanotechnol. 2015;11(5):789–804.
149. Zhang H, et al. Hyaluronic acid-modified magnetic iron oxide nanoparticles for MR imaging of surgically induced endometriosis model in rats. PLoS One. 2014;9(4):e94718.

Ovary

Engineering Applications for In Vitro Ovarian Follicle Culture

Taylor Schissel, Emily E. Thomas, and Ariella Shikanov

Abstract This chapter reviews engineering strategies for developing bioengineered platforms to support in vitro ovarian follicle culture, a process vital for fertility preservation and reproductive biology research. Ovarian follicles are the functional units of the ovary, which serve as a source of both fertility and endocrine function. Follicles require a complex, dynamic microenvironment for proper development and hormone production, which can be challenging to replicate in vitro, leading to the need for novel biomaterials and engineering strategies. This chapter examines key engineering considerations, including matrix composition, stiffness, degradability, topography, bioactivity, and cell signaling within biomimetic hydrogels and scaffolds. It assesses natural, semisynthetic, and synthetic biomaterials for follicle encapsulation, highlighting their advantages and limitations. The importance of replicating the three-dimensional ovarian microenvironment, integrating paracrine and endocrine cues, and designing scalable, reproducible systems is emphasized. Advances such as 3D bioprinting and organ-on-a-chip technologies are discussed for their potential to improve clinical translation, high-throughput screening, and large-scale applications. Finally, barriers to translating advancements in follicle culture to the growth and maturation of early-stage human follicles are noted, and future directions are proposed for leveraging multi-omics techniques and advanced biomaterials to better model human ovarian biology and translate successful animal culture systems to human fertility preservation.

Keywords Biomimetic matrix · In vitro folliculogenesis · Follicle culture · Extracellular matrix · Natural and synthetic polymers

---

Taylor Schissel and Emily E. Thomas contributed equally with all other contributors.

T. Schissel · E. E. Thomas · A. Shikanov (✉)
University of Michigan, Ann Arbor, MI, USA
e-mail: tschisse@umich.edu; emilyet@umich.edu; shikanov@umich.edu

S. G. Zambuto, M. L. Oyen (eds.), *Biomaterials for Women's Health Engineering*,
https://doi.org/10.1007/978-3-032-10745-9_10

1 Introduction to Follicle Biology and Follicle Culture

The follicle is the structural and functional unit of the ovary that provides both reproductive and endocrine function. Each follicle is a multicellular structure with a single oocyte, or germ cell, that is surrounded by hormone-producing somatic cells, called granulosa and theca. At birth, all follicles are in a dormant state called the primordial stage, with a single layer of squamous granulosa cells surrounding the oocyte. The majority of these follicles will remain dormant throughout a person's life, with small cohorts of follicles periodically activating and entering the growing pool in a process called folliculogenesis (Fig. 1). Follicle activation is marked by the transition of granulosa cells to a cuboidal morphology, with subsequent proliferation in concentric layers around the oocyte as the follicle grows. At the later stages of folliculogenesis, theca cells, which produce estradiol precursor, androstenedione, are recruited to the growing structure, and granulosa cells differentiate into cumulus granulosa and mural granulosa cells. Folliculogenesis peaks with oocyte maturation and ovulation. In addition to nurturing the growing oocytes, follicles secrete a wealth

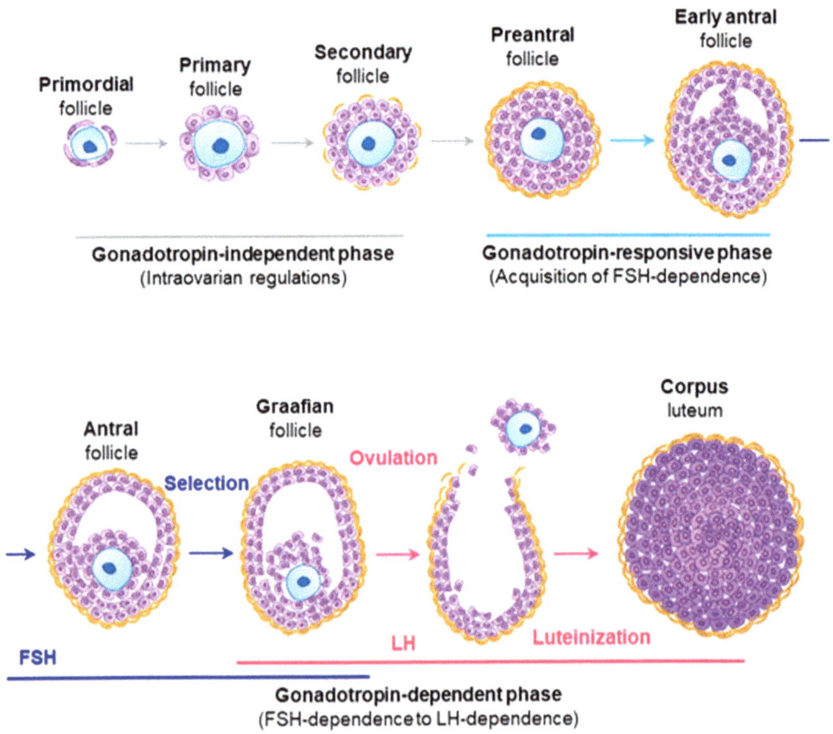

Fig. 1 The stages of folliculogenesis. Oocytes are represented in blue, granulosa cells in purple, and theca cells in yellow. FSH = follicle stimulating hormone. LH = luteinizing hormone. (Reproduced from Lee et al. [36], licensed under Creative Commons Attribution License (CC BY 4.0))

of steroid hormones, such as androstenedione, estradiol, and progesterone, as well as peptide hormones, including activins and inhibins, all of which play various roles in endocrine health.

In vitro culture platforms that can support follicle development from primordial follicle activation until ovulation could restore fertility in patients suffering from premature ovarian insufficiency. However, folliculogenesis is a complex and dynamic process that is not fully understood, thus hindering the development of a clinically translational culture system. Initially, these platforms were constructed in two-dimensions, but 2D cultures had limited success due to the lack of support for the three-dimensional structure of the follicle and poor mimicry of the native in vivo ovarian environment. The application of biomaterials to maintain the 3D structure of the follicle has proven to be a powerful tool to study questions related to basic ovarian biology, fertility preservation, the effects of environmental toxicants, nonhormonal contraceptive options, and pathologies like polycystic ovarian syndrome.

While significant advancements have been made in the development of bioengineered platforms for follicle culture, there is still ample room for innovation. Success in the culture of murine follicles has not been completely translated to the culture of human follicles. In this chapter, we will address the design criteria for engineering a platform for in vitro ovarian follicle development, with particular focus on hydrogels for follicle encapsulation. The use of biomaterials for in vivo applications is an extensive topic of its own, and we will direct the reader to chapter "Biomaterials to Facilitate Revascularization and Improve Outcomes of Ovarian Tissue Transplantation" to learn more.

2 Engineering Needs for Follicle Culture

Matrix composition (polymer selection), cell-driven biodegradation, sequestration of extracellular matrix (ECM) proteins, topography (spatial organization and geometry of the matrix), diffusion of cell-secreted growth factors and hormones, and scalability are considerations that must be addressed when engineering biomaterial platforms for ovarian follicle culture (Fig. 2).

For example, a dynamic, cell-responsive stiffness of the bioengineered matrix can match the unique composition of the human ovary, which consists of two structurally and functionally distinct compartments: the outer, denser layer called the cortex and the inner core called the medulla. Dormant follicles reside in the cortex, and as they activate and grow, they expand into the medulla, which is more permissive to large volumetric growth. Furthermore, there is constant crosstalk between the developing follicles and their environment, including other follicles, extra-follicular cells (endothelial cells, immune cells, pericytes, fibroblasts, etc.) and the extracellular matrix. When removing follicles from their native environment for in vitro culture, it is important to consider how these crucial elements can be reproduced in an engineered matrix that allows for diffusion of soluble factors and coexistence

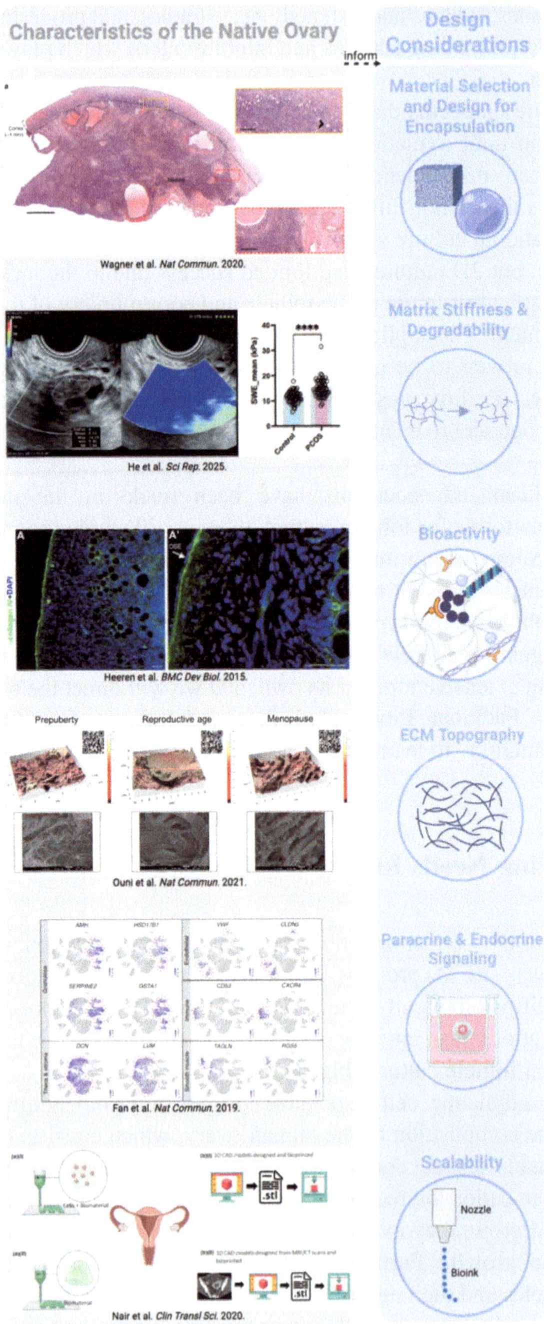

Fig. 2 Overview of design considerations for biomaterials for in vitro follicle culture. (**a**) As depicted in the H&E images, the native ovary contains diverse cell populations that reside in different microenvironments, which must be considered when choosing a biomaterial that will be used to encapsulate certain cell type(s) for culture. (**b**) Ovarian stiffness, shown in panel **b**, impacts folliculogenesis, which should be accounted for with the stiffness and degradability of the selected

of multiple cell types. Finally, reproducible, easily scaled-up designs can facilitate efficient, high-throughput follicle culture studies, particularly in toxicology, drug screening, and testing of new contraceptives.

2.1 *Ovarian Microenvironment*

The native ovarian extracellular matrix is a dynamic, fibrous network composed of extracellular matrix proteins including collagen, elastin, laminin, fibronectin, and proteoglycans, which surrounds and supports ovarian follicles and stromal cells. This matrix provides structural integrity, regulates cell signaling, and facilitates tissue remodeling during follicular development. Polymer scaffolds can be utilized to help recapitulate this ovarian microenvironment in vitro. To date, a wide variety of polymers have been used to create scaffolds for ovarian follicle culture. Both natural and synthetic materials have been used for follicle culture, and each has its own set of advantages and disadvantages. For example, natural materials may have inherent biodegradability leading to nontoxic by-products. Natural materials also possess intrinsic bioactivity, such as integrin binding and growth factor sequestration and presentation, leading to enhanced cell–matrix interaction. On the other hand, natural materials may vary in composition and quality, while synthetic materials provide greater batch-to-batch consistency. Synthetic materials often have enhanced tailorability, allowing researchers to more precisely control chemical and mechanical properties such as porosity, stiffness, and degradation rate. Additionally, synthetic materials may be more cost-effective as they can often be produced at scale at lower costs compared to some natural materials, making them more accessible for large-scale applications. Another class of biomaterials used for ovarian culture are semi-synthetic materials. This category includes naturally derived biomaterials that are chemically modified to enhance tunability. Semi-synthetics combine the benefits of both natural and synthetic materials as they can offer inherent bioactivity with

Fig. 2 (continued) biomaterial. (**c**) The native ovary contains a mosaic of ECM proteins, including collagen IV as shown, and material modifications can be made to an inert biomaterial to provide greater bioactivity and ECM remodeling. (**d**) Biomaterials can be designed to recapitulate the fibrous topography of the ovarian ECM, illustrated in the micrographs. (**e**) Folliculogenesis is dependent upon a complex milieu of paracrine and endocrine signals between the ovarian cell types, identified in panel **e**. Engineering strategies can be used to isolate these factors and analyze their effects on in vitro follicle development. (**f**) To be clinically effective for fertility preservation or drug screening, emerging technologies like 3D printing can be used to increase scalability. (All figures in the left column of this figure are reproduced under the Creative Commons Attribution License (CC BY 4.0) from the following sources: (**a**) Wagner et al. [66] (Fig. 1a). (**b**) He et al. [22]. Modifications made to the original figure (Fig. 3C, D). (**c**) Heeren et al. [23] (Fig. 7A, A'). (**d**) Ouni et al. [50] (Fig. 6A). (**e**) Fan et al. [14]. Modifications made to the original figure (Fig. 2e). (**f**) Nair et al. [46] (Fig. 4). Created in BioRender. Shikanov (2025) (https://BioRender.com/i92xu8d)

enhanced control of cross-linking and mechanical properties. Lastly, semisynthetic materials can easily be modified with additional bioactive cues through click chemistries. However, semisynthetics still often face the risk of batch-to-batch variability and may have reduced bioactivity compared to unmodified natural materials. A brief overview of natural, semisynthetic, and synthetic biomaterials commonly used for follicle culture is presented in Table 1.

2.2 *Follicle Growth and Expansion*

One of the first and most critical considerations in designing a follicle culture system is the stiffness of the material used to encapsulate the follicles. In the ovary, primordial follicles reside in the cortex, and they experience a less-permissive environment that contributes to maintaining quiescence [45]. On the other hand, growing follicles soften their surrounding matrix by secreting proteases, creating a more permissive environment to allow volumetric expansion (Fig. 3). This change in permissiveness highlights the importance of control over the initial stiffness surrounding the follicle, followed by cell-driven degradation and remodeling. Recently, studies using shear wave elastography have measured the stiffness of the adult, reproductive-age ovary, reporting values between 8 and 24 kPa, with values up to 30 kPa in older ovaries [22, 77, 80]. To mimic this range in vitro, hydrogel stiffness can be controlled by changing polymer concentration, cross-linker concentration, or other factors like cross-linking time or temperature that affect the degree of cross-linking. For example, the stiffness of alginate is easily controlled by its solid concentration ranging from 0.3% w/v used to create softer gels and >0.8% for stiffer gels. In lower-density alginates, murine and goat secondary and multilayer-stage follicles grew, developed antrums, secreted estradiol, and produced mature oocytes [4, 67, 71]. In contrast, primate primordial follicles cultured for 6 days retained their follicular structure only when encapsulated in higher density alginate hydrogels (2% compared to 0.5%) [25]. In addition to species-specific differences, this suggests that early-stage follicles may need a stiffer environment in vitro that recapitulates what those follicles would experience in the cortex in vivo, while follicles at secondary and later stages may need more permissive environments that do not hinder more accelerated cell proliferation. Building off this knowledge, several groups have investigated how to use a dynamic approach, where the stiffness of the material changes throughout culture to mimic the follicle's transition in vivo when expanding from the cortex to the medulla. One method utilized a two-step culture, encapsulating follicles in higher density and stiffer alginate hydrogels for the initial culture period followed with a second encapsulation in a lower-density hydrogel, or simply releasing the follicles into low-attachment plates for the latter culture phase [69, 81]. Alternatively, cell-driven degradation of the hydrogel can facilitate gradual softening of the follicular environment without additional, mid-experiment manipulation of the follicles [43, 58, 59]. In particular, the use of plasmin-degradable

Table 1 Summary of biomaterials used for in vitro follicle culture

Material	Alignment with engineering design criteria	Example usage
Natural polymers		
Alginate, a plant-derived polysaccharide	Offers highly tunable stiffness ranging from a few hundred to a few thousand Pascals but is not naturally degradable by mammalian cells; Is widely and easily produced enhancing scalability, but lacks biomimetic interactions with mammalian cells in general, and ovarian tissue specifically	[1, 4, 24, 30, 33, 51, 60, 72]
Cellulose, a polysaccharide derived from bacteria	Biocompatible with ovarian cell types but not mammalian-derived and not naturally degradable	[44]
Chitosan, a polysaccharide derived from shellfish	Biocompatible; biodegradable but degrades slowly, offering limited control; poor solubility at neutral pH required for ovarian follicle culture; high batch-to-batch variability	[20, 37]
Collagen, a human- or animal-derived protein	Abundant in the ovary; fibrous structure may mimic native ovarian topography and provide bioactive cues; offers tunable stiffness but with limited control over mechanical strength depending on the source and processing; is cell-degradable by matrix metalloproteinases (MMPs) produced by ovarian cell types; high batch-to-batch variability and can be expensive to produce at scale	[20, 37]
Decellularized ECM (dECM), a protein and polysaccharide mix; auto-, allo-, or xenogeneic	Closely mimics native ovary composition; May provide bioactive cues; however, required ECM processing may reduce bioactivity; limited control over degradation and stiffness; expensive to produce with high batch-to-batch variability	[8, 41, 52, 53]
Fibrin, a human- or animal-derived protein	Biocompatible and naturally derived; relatively rapid degradation with poor control making it incompatible with stability needed for long term ovarian follicle culture	[5, 7, 56, 58, 73]
Matrigel, a protein mix derived from cultured cancer cells	ECM rich and bioactive; contains proteins abundant in the native ovary including laminin; biodegradable; poor stiffness tunability; high batch-to-batch variation; may contain xenogenic contaminants	[19, 48, 49, 56, 78]

(continued)

Table 1 (continued)

Material	Alignment with engineering design criteria	Example usage
Wharton's Jelly, derived from human umbilical cord	ECM rich and bioactive; biodegradable; limited stiffness tunability; high batch-to-batch variation; derived from human umbilical cords, which limits accessibility	[79]
Semisynthetic polymers		
Dextran, polysaccharide derived from bacteria, as thiol-reactive dextran (SLO-dextran)	Biologically inert; highly tunable stiffness and mechanical properties; degradable by ovarian cell types when cross-linked with proteolytically degradable cross-linkers; compatible with electrospinning to introduce fibrous morphology to mimic the native structure of ovarian tissue; modification allows material to be conjugated to bioactive peptides using click chemistries	[40]
Gelatin, human- or animal-derived denatured protein, as gelatin-methacrylate (GelMA)	Derived from collagen which is abundant in the ovary; offers tunable stiffness and mechanical strength; proteolytically degradable by MMPs produced by ovarian cell types; high batch-to-batch variability and can be expensive to produce at scale; modification allows material to be conjugated to bioactive peptides using click chemistries	[68, 76]
Hyaluronic acid (HA), a naturally derived polysaccharide, as tyramine-modified HA	Abundant in the native ovary; biocompatible with mammalian cells; highly tunable stiffness and mechanical properties; degradable by hyaluronidase, which is secreted by follicles; batch-to-batch variability when produced at scale and relatively high cost; modification allows material to be conjugated to bioactive peptides using click chemistries	[9–11, 28]
Synthetic polymers		
Poly(caprolactone) (PCL)	Biologically inert; slow degradation by hydrolysis or enzymes; compatible with electrospinning to introduce fibrous morphology to mimic the native structure of ovarian tissue; limited batch-to-batch variation	[13]
Poly(ethylene glycol) (PEG)	Biologically inert; degradable by ovarian cell types when cross-linked with protease degradable cross-linkers; highly tunable stiffness; can be produced at scale with limited batch-to-batch variation	[27, 59]

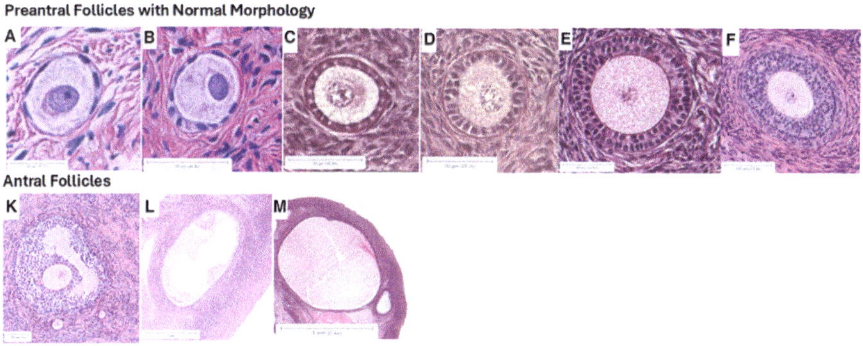

Fig. 3 Follicles undergo large-scale volumetric expansion during folliculogenesis, as shown with the primordial follicle ~25 μm in diameter (**a**), the growing preantral follicles (<50 μm up to ~200 μm) (**b–f**), early antrals reaching the milimeter range (**k–l**), and the late-stage antral follicle 6–9 mm in diameter (**m**). (Figure adapted from Yano Maher et al. [75] with permission from Elsevier. License number: 6130250319052)

cross-linkers is more conducive to human follicle culture, where the volumetric expansion from primordial follicle to ovulatory follicle is 10^5-fold, which would not be possible in a rigid, nondegradable system [59].

2.3 *Topography*

The surface topography, including both nanoscale and microscale features of the extracellular matrix, can have significant influences on cell behavior and function affecting adhesion, migration, proliferation, and differentiation [29]. When reconstructing the ovarian microenvironment in vitro, materials should incorporate topographic stimuli and instructive cues that may influence follicle development. For example, analysis of prepubertal, reproductive age, and menopausal ovarian tissue revealed differences in microscale biomechanics. In tissues from younger reproductive age individuals, intermediate collagen fibers were assembled into thicker bundles, and fiber orientation was significantly different when compared to tissue from older, nonreproductive age individuals [50]. Additionally, changes in ovarian topography often accompany ovarian diseases such as the increase in stiffness and fibrotic characteristics of polycystic ovarian syndrome (PCOS) [3, 57].

Inspired by the native topography of ovarian tissue, recent work has aimed to add micro- and nanoscale complexity to tissue-engineered constructs for ovarian follicle culture applications. Electrospun fibers were incorporated into hydrogel scaffolds, which more closely resemble the fibrous nature of native ECM [38]. Electrospun fibers decorated with ECM-sequestering peptides achieved more fibrillar retention of follicle-secreted ECM, mimicking the native ovarian environment and increasing the survival of isolated primordial follicles encapsulated in PEG hydrogels [47]. Beyond random incorporation of electrospun fibers, the controlled patterning of such fibers can further influence follicle culture outcomes, as seen with better survival and maturation rates in ovine follicles cultured on patterned PCL fibers compared to those cultured on randomly placed fibers [12]. Additionally, in 3D printed porous gelatin hydrogel scaffolds, the degree of contact with printed hydrogel struts influenced ovarian follicle survival. Constructs printed with strut patterns that created pores that facilitated increased scaffold interaction showed enhanced follicle survival as compared to pore geometries that led to reduced follicle-scaffold interaction [35]. Together, these studies illustrate the importance of controlling both the micro- and nanoscale topography of scaffolds for ovarian follicle culture.

2.4 *Bioactivity*

Beyond selection of the primary biomaterial for scaffold creation, additional modifications can be made to introduce biologically active signals to more closely mimic the native ovarian microenvironment. One approach is to encourage cell–matrix interactions through direct integrin binding. Modification of bulk dextran hydrogels with the fibronectin-derived, adhesion-promoting peptide RGD, which binds to cells' integrins, promoted antral follicle growth in culture of murine ovarian tissue and may play a role in theca cell differentiation [40]. A second approach is to encourage indirect cell–matrix interactions by sequestering follicle-secreted ECM to create a supportive niche for folliculogenesis. For example, modification of the bulk biomaterial scaffold with peptides that mimic cells' interactions with laminin, IKVAV and YIGSR, improved murine secondary stage follicle culture, resulting in oocyte meiotic competence [81]. Additionally, synthetic PEG hydrogels have been decorated with ECM-sequestering peptides (heparan-sulfate-binding peptide, AG73; basement membrane-binding peptide, BMB; and ECM-binding region of placental growth factor 2, RRR) to enhance retention of follicle-produced ECM, which increased both follicle growth and maturation in secondary-stage murine follicles [64].

2.5 *Cell Signaling*

The early stages of follicle activation and growth are mostly driven by local paracrine signals from neighboring cells and other follicles. At the later stages of folliculogenesis, follicles become sensitive to circulating gonadotropins, which are required for antral cavity formation, late-stage follicle growth, and dominant follicle selection. Thus, engineering a culture system capable of supporting follicle development from the paracrine-driven primordial stage to endocrine-driven antral stages will require methods that faithfully recapitulate these dynamic and complex cell signaling events in vitro.

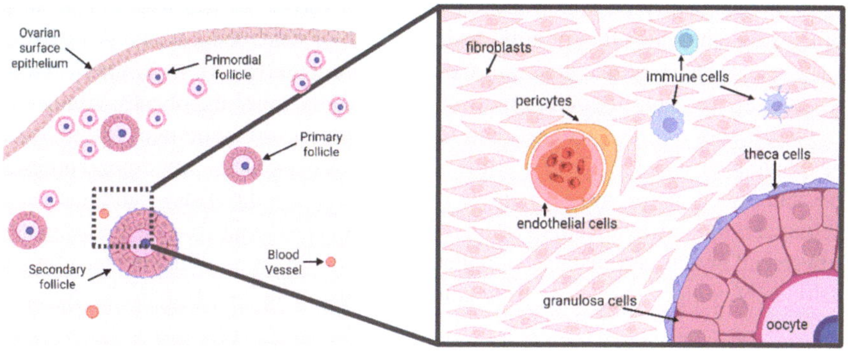

Fig. 4 The ovary contains a diverse population of cell types that contribute to folliculogenesis through paracrine signaling. (Created in BioRender. Thomas (2025) https://BioRender.com/wbv05w2)

Paracrine The ovary has a rich landscape of different cell types that contribute to follicle development (Fig. 4), and removing follicles from the ovary for culture disrupts that natural support system. Therefore, several groups have investigated multiple follicle culture or co-culture with feeder cells that supply critical factors for early follicle development in vitro. In mice, individually isolated and cultured primary follicles cannot survive in vitro, but they can be rescued by culturing them in groups of ten [26]. Smaller groups of five or fewer follicles survive, albeit with limited growth, while larger groups of ten follicles grow in a synergistic fashion, reaching optimal preovulatory sizes, secreting steroid hormones [82], and producing a greater number of meiotically competent oocytes compared to smaller groups [30]. In humans, group culture has also proven beneficial, with mature oocytes produced from group culture of 3–5 human follicles for 6 weeks [74]. Like culturing groups of follicles together, co-culture of follicles with feeder cells has also been shown to improve early-stage follicle development in vitro. Mouse ovarian stromal cells [62], mouse embryonic fibroblasts [60], mouse ovarian endothelial cells [32], and adipose-derived stem cells [16, 63] have all been shown to improve follicle outcomes, likely due to increased paracrine support for the follicle.

Endocrine Throughout folliculogenesis, growing follicles become increasingly dependent on endocrine hormones for growth and maturation. In vitro, this is achieved through media supplementation with follicle stimulating hormone, and later with luteinizing hormone or human chorionic gonadotropin to induce oocyte maturation. Most bulk hydrogels have nanoscale pores, allowing diffusion of nutrients and hormones to the encapsulated follicles. However, diffusion can be increased by modifying hydrogel porosity, which can be achieved via new technologies including 3D-printing matrices with defined porosity [35] or, as used with other in vitro culture models, microporous annealed particle hydrogels [17]. Under traditional culture systems, hydrogels are submerged in media in static conditions that do not recapitulate the dynamic flow experienced in the body. One area of emerging research is an ovary-on-a-chip approach, where ovarian cortical tissue or isolated follicles are cultured in microfluidic devices under constant media exchange [2]. Similarly, oocytes have been cultured in static, dynamic-passive (driven by gravity), and dynamic-active (pump) conditions, with significantly more meiotically competent oocytes, higher fertilization rates, and better blastocyst formation rates arising from the dynamic groups [55]. In 2017, this concept was expanded to multiple reproductive and endocrine organs in a single device, including the ovary, fallopian tube, uterus, cervix, and liver. This system, termed EVATAR, allowed media exchange between all organs and sustained circulating flow for 28 days, ultimately resulting in meiotically competent oocytes from cultured mouse follicles [70].

2.6 Scalability

In order to bring ovarian tissue engineering from the lab to clinical practice as a fertility preservation method, it is necessary to develop scalable methods that can be reproduced consistently for a large number of patients. Furthermore, increasing scalability will facilitate the use of tissue engineered products for large-scale studies designed for drug or environmental toxicants screening. Scalability is also an important consideration when seeking regulatory approval, as this process requires that the tissue engineering processes can be scaled up with minimal batch-to-batch variation, permitting reliable function without losing efficacy or safety. One method that offers promise for enhancing scalability of tissue-engineered constructs for ovarian follicle culture is 3D bioprinting. 3D bioprinting could permit automated and highly replicable construction of ovarian follicle culture scaffolds. For example, 3D bioprinting of a gelatin-based bioink permitted enhanced control over scaffold architecture for murine ovarian follicle culture, resulting in steroid hormone production and mature oocytes [35]. 3D bioprinting technology is actively being developed for use with many additional biomaterials commonly used in ovarian follicle culture [6]. Furthermore, microfluidic methods have been developed that may increase the ease and reliability of follicle encapsulation [21].

3 Current Challenges and Future Directions

Great strides have been made in the field of ovarian tissue engineering, particularly in the development of in vitro platforms for the culture of ovarian cortical tissue or isolated ovarian follicles. Currently, most work in the field is completed using animal models of folliculogenesis due to the scarcity of healthy, young human ovaries donated for research and due to sufficient similarity between human follicle development with other mammalian species, such as rodents, bovine, and nonhuman primates. For human follicle culture, several groups have developed multistep culture systems starting with the culture of pieces of intact ovarian tissue, followed by the dissection of growing follicles from the tissue and subsequent culture of these isolated follicles in low attachment plates [42, 61, 74]. The application of biomaterials for human follicle culture has been limited to the use of alginate to culture isolated secondary and multilayer stage follicles [69] or thin sections of ovarian cortex [34]. Only a few groups have been able to obtain mature oocytes from cultured human follicles [18, 42, 69, 74], with the most recent study proving that secondary-stage follicles from prepubertal patients can be cultured and oocytes matured, fertilized, and developed until the blastocyst stage [18]. To date, mature human oocytes have not been obtained by culturing primordial or primary follicles isolated from the tissue, nor from frozen-thawed ovarian tissue. Because early-stage follicles are the most abundant in the ovary and are also the most likely to survive cryopreservation, additional work must address these challenges in order to integrate in vitro follicle culture as a fertility preservation strategy that complements ovarian tissue cryopreservation. Future studies will be necessary to investigate if innovative platforms that have had success with animal models can be translated to human follicle culture, particularly for early-stage primordial and primary follicles isolated from the ovarian tissue. Excitingly, the recent surge in multi-omics approaches to studying the human ovary may aid in the translation of these platforms. Single-cell, bulk, and spatial RNA sequencing studies of the human ovary have provided a wealth of information about the ovarian transcriptome [15, 31, 39, 54, 66], which, when combined with insights from proteomic studies [65], can be leveraged to better inform follicle culture systems moving forward.

References

1. Amorim CA, Van Langendonckt A, David A, Dolmans M-M, Donnez J. Survival of human pre-antral follicles after cryopreservation of ovarian tissue, follicular isolation and in vitro culture in a calcium alginate matrix. Hum Reprod. 2009;24:92–9. https://doi.org/10.1093/humrep/den343.
2. Aziz AUR, Fu M, Deng J, Geng C, Luo Y, Lin B, Yu X, Liu B. A microfluidic device for culturing an encapsulated ovarian follicle. Micromachines. 2017;8:335. https://doi.org/10.3390/mi8110335.
3. Bonnans C, Chou J, Werb Z. Remodelling the extracellular matrix in development and disease. Nat Rev Mol Cell Biol. 2014;15:786–801. https://doi.org/10.1038/nrm3904.
4. Brito IR, Silva CMG, Duarte ABG, Lima IMT, Rodrigues GQ, Rossetto R, Sales AD, Lobo CH, Bernuci MP, Rosa-e-Silva ACJS, Campello CC, Xu M, Figueiredo JR. Alginate hydrogel matrix stiffness influences the in vitro development of caprine preantral follicles. Mol Reprod Dev. 2014;81:636–45. https://doi.org/10.1002/mrd.22330.
5. Brito I, Silva G, Sales A, Lobo C, Rodrigues G, Sousa R, Moura A, Calderón C, Bertolini M, Campello C, Smitz J, Figueiredo J. Fibrin–alginate hydrogel supports steroidogenesis, in vitro maturation of oocytes and parthenotes production from caprine preantral follicles cultured in group. Reprod Domest Anim. 2016;51:997–1009. https://doi.org/10.1111/rda.12779.
6. Chen S, Wang T, Chen J, Sui M, Wang L, Zhao X, Sun J, Lu Y. 3D bioprinting technology innovation in female reproductive system. Mater Today Bio. 2025;31:101551. https://doi.org/10.1016/j.mtbio.2025.101551.

7. Chiti MC, Dolmans M-M, Mortiaux L, Zhuge F, Ouni E, Shahri PAK, Van Ruymbeke E, Champagne S-D, Donnez J, Amorim CA. A novel fibrin-based artificial ovary prototype resembling human ovarian tissue in terms of architecture and rigidity. J Assist Reprod Genet. 2018;35:41–8. https://doi.org/10.1007/s10815-017-1091-3.
8. Chiti M-C, Vanacker J, Ouni E, Tatic N, Viswanath A, des Rieux A, Dolmans M-M, White LJ, Amorim CA. Ovarian extracellular matrix-based hydrogel for human ovarian follicle survival in vivo: a pilot work. J Biomed Mater Res B Appl Biomater. 2022;110:1012–22. https://doi.org/10.1002/jbm.b.34974.
9. Dahmardeh T, Ghanian MH, Ebrahimi B. A self-gelling hydrogel based on thiolated hyaluronic acid for three-dimensional culture of ovine preantral follicles. Int J Biol Macromol. 2023;253:127147. https://doi.org/10.1016/j.ijbiomac.2023.127147.
10. Desai N, Abdelhafez F, Calabro A, Falcone T. Three dimensional culture of fresh and vitrified mouse pre-antral follicles in a hyaluronan-based hydrogel: a preliminary investigation of a novel biomaterial for in vitro follicle maturation. Reprod Biol Endocrinol RBE. 2012;10:29. https://doi.org/10.1186/1477-7827-10-29.
11. Desai N, Spangler M, Nanavaty V, Gishto A, Brown A. New hyaluronan-based biomatrix for 3-D follicle culture yields functionally competent oocytes. Reprod Biol Endocrinol RBE. 2022;20:148. https://doi.org/10.1186/s12958-022-01019-9.
12. Di Berardino C, Liverani L, Peserico A, Capacchietti G, Russo V, Bernabò N, Tosi U, Boccaccini AR, Barboni B. When electrospun fiber support matters: in vitro ovine long-term folliculogenesis on poly (epsilon caprolactone) (PCL)-patterned fibers. Cells. 2022;11:1968. https://doi.org/10.3390/cells11121968.
13. Di Berardino C, Peserico A, Camerano Spelta Rapini C, Liverani L, Capacchietti G, Russo V, Berardinelli P, Unalan I, Damian-Buda A-I, Boccaccini AR, Barboni B. Bioengineered 3D ovarian model for long-term multiple development of preantral follicle: bridging the gap for poly(ε-caprolactone) (PCL)-based scaffold reproductive applications. Reprod Biol Endocrinol. 2024;22:95. https://doi.org/10.1186/s12958-024-01266-y.
14. Fan X, Bialecka M, Moustakas I, Lam E, Torrens-Juaneda V, Borggreven NV, Trouw L, Louwe LA, Pilgram GSK, Mei H, van der Westerlaken L, de Sousa C, Lopes SM. Single-cell reconstruction of follicular remodeling in the human adult ovary. Nat Commun. 2019;10 (3164):110–23. https://doi.org/10.1038/s41422-018-0125-4.
15. Fan X, Moustakas I, Bialecka M, del Valle JS, Overeem AW, Louwe LA, Pilgram GSK, van der Westerlaken LAJ, Mei H, Chuva de Sousa Lopes SM. Single-cell transcriptomics analysis of human small antral follicles. Int J Mol Sci. 2021;22:11955. https://doi.org/10.3390/ijms222111955.
16. Green LJ, Zhou H, Padmanabhan V, Shikanov A. Adipose-derived stem cells promote survival, growth, and maturation of early-stage murine follicles. Stem Cell Res Ther. 2019;10:102. https://doi.org/10.1186/s13287-019-1199-8.
17. Griffin DR, Weaver WM, Scumpia PO, Di Carlo D, Segura T. Accelerated wound healing by injectable microporous gel scaffolds assembled from annealed building blocks. Nat Mater. 2015;14:737–44. https://doi.org/10.1038/nmat4294.
18. Guo Y, Jia L, Zeng H, Sun P, Su W, Li T, Liang X, Fang C. Neurotrophin-4 promotes *in vitro* development and maturation of human secondary follicles yielding metaphase II oocytes and successful blastocyst formation. Hum Reprod Open. 2024;2024:hoae005. https://doi.org/10.1093/hropen/hoae005.
19. Guzel Y, Nur Şahin, Gizem, Sekeroglu, Mujde, Deniz A. Recombinant activin A enhances the growth and survival of isolated preantral follicles cultured three-dimensionally in extracellular basement matrix protein (matrigel) under serum-free conditions. Gynecol Endocrinol. 2014;30:388–91. https://doi.org/10.3109/09513590.2014.888411.
20. Hassani F, Ebrahimi B, Moini A, Ghiaseddin A, Bazrafkan M, Hassanzadeh G, Rezazadeh Valojerdi M. Chitosan hydrogel supports integrity of ovarian follicles during in vitro culture: a preliminary of a novel biomaterial for three dimensional culture of ovarian follicles. Cell J Yakhteh. 2020;21:479–93. https://doi.org/10.22074/cellj.2020.6393.

21. He X. Microfluidic encapsulation of ovarian follicles for 3D culture. Ann Biomed Eng. 2017;45:1676–84. https://doi.org/10.1007/s10439-017-1823-7.
22. He Y, Deng S, Wang Y, Wang X, Huang Q, Cheng J, Wang D, Lyu G. Evaluation of ovarian stiffness and its biological mechanism using shear wave elastography in polycystic ovary syndrome. Sci Rep. 2025;15:585. https://doi.org/10.1038/s41598-024-84338-8.
23. Heeren AM, van Iperen L, Klootwijk DB, de Melo Bernardo A, Roost MS, Gomes Fernandes MM, Louwe LA, Hilders CG, Helmerhorst FM, van der Westerlaken LAJ, Chuva de Sousa Lopes SM. Development of the follicular basement membrane during human gametogenesis and early folliculogenesis. BMC Dev Biol. 2015;15:4. https://doi.org/10.1186/s12861-015-0054-0.
24. Heise M, Koepsel R, Russell AJ, McGee EA. Calcium alginate microencapsulation of ovarian follicles impacts FSH delivery and follicle morphology. Reprod Biol Endocrinol RBE. 2005;3:47. https://doi.org/10.1186/1477-7827-3-47.
25. Hornick JE, Duncan FE, Shea LD, Woodruff TK. Multiple follicle culture supports primary follicle growth through paracrine-acting signals. Reproduction. 2013;145:19–32. https://doi.org/10.1530/REP-12-0233.
26. Hornick JE, Duncan FE, Shea LD, Woodruff TK. Isolated primate primordial follicles require a rigid physical environment to survive and grow in vitro. Hum Reprod. 2012;27:1801–10. https://doi.org/10.1093/humrep/der468.
27. Ihm JE, Lee ST, Han DK, Lim JM, Hubbell JA. Murine ovarian follicle culture in PEG-hydrogel: effects of mechanical properties and the hormones FSH and LH on development. Macromol Res. 2015;23:377–86. https://doi.org/10.1007/s13233-015-3045-x.
28. Jamalzaei P, Rezazadeh Valojerdi M, Montazeri L, Baharvand H. Applicability of hyaluronic acid-alginate hydrogel and ovarian cells for in vitro development of mouse preantral follicles. Cell J Yakhteh. 2020;22:49–60. https://doi.org/10.22074/cellj.2020.6925.
29. Janson IA, Putnam AJ. Extracellular matrix elasticity and topography: material-based cues that affect cell function via conserved mechanisms. J Biomed Mater Res A. 2015;103:1246–58. https://doi.org/10.1002/jbm.a.35254.
30. Jones A, Bernabé BP, Padmanabhan V, Li J, Shikanov A. Capitalizing on transcriptome profiling to optimize and identify targets for promoting early murine folliculogenesis in vitro. Sci Rep. 2021;111(11):1–14. https://doi.org/10.1038/s41598-021-92036-y.
31. Jones ASK, Hannum DF, Machlin JH, Tan A, Ma Q, Ulrich ND, Shen Y, Ciarelli M, Padmanabhan V, Marsh EE, Hammoud S, Li JZ, Shikanov A. Cellular atlas of the human ovary using morphologically guided spatial transcriptomics and single-cell sequencing. Sci Adv. 2024;10:eadm7506. https://doi.org/10.1126/sciadv.adm7506.
32. Kedem A, Aelion-Brauer A, Guo P, Wen D, Ding B-S, Lis R, Cheng D, Sandler VM, Rafii S, Rosenwaks Z. Activated ovarian endothelial cells promote early follicular development and survival. J Ovarian Res. 2017;10:64. https://doi.org/10.1186/s13048-017-0354-z.
33. Kreeger PK, Deck JW, Woodruff TK, Shea LD. The in vitro regulation of ovarian follicle development using alginate-extracellular matrix gels. Biomaterials. 2006;27:714–23. https://doi.org/10.1016/j.biomaterials.2005.06.016.
34. Laronda MM, Duncan FE, Hornick JE, Xu M, Pahnke JE, Whelan KA, Shea LD, Woodruff TK. Alginate encapsulation supports the growth and differentiation of human primordial follicles within ovarian cortical tissue. J Assist Reprod Genet. 2014;31:1013–28. https://doi.org/10.1007/s10815-014-0252-x.
35. Laronda MM, Rutz AL, Xiao S, Whelan KA, Duncan FE, Roth EW, Woodruff TK, Shah RN. A bioprosthetic ovary created using 3D printed microporous scaffolds restores ovarian function in sterilized mice. Nat Commun. 2017;8:15261. https://doi.org/10.1038/ncomms15261.
36. Lee EB, Chakravarthi VP, Wolfe WW, Rumi MAK. ERβ regulation of Gonadotropin responses during Folliculogenesis. Int J Mol Sci. 2021;22(19):10348. https://doi.org/10.3390/ijms221910348.

37. Liu C, Xia X, Miao W, Luan X, Sun L, Jin Y, Liu L. An ovarian cell microcapsule system simulating follicle structure for providing endogenous female hormones. Int J Pharm. 2013;455: 312–9. https://doi.org/10.1016/j.ijpharm.2013.07.004.
38. Liverani L, Raffel N, Fattahi A, Preis A, Hoffmann I, Boccaccini AR, Beckmann MW, Dittrich R. Electrospun patterned porous scaffolds for the support of ovarian follicles growth: a feasibility study. Sci Rep. 2019;9:1150. https://doi.org/10.1038/s41598-018-37640-1.
39. Man L, Lustgarten-Guahmich N, Kallinos E, Redhead-Laconte Z, Liu S, Schattman B, Redmond D, Hancock K, Zaninovic N, Schattman G, Rosenwaks Z, James D. Comparison of human antral follicles of xenograft versus ovarian origin reveals disparate molecular signatures. Cell Rep. 2020;32:108027. https://doi.org/10.1016/j.celrep.2020.108027.
40. Matsushige C, Kitazumi K, Beaman A, Miyagi M, Tallquist MD, Yamazaki Y. RGD peptide promotes follicle growth through integrins αvβ3/αvβ5 in three-dimensional culture. 2025. https://doi.org/10.1530/REP-24-0151.
41. McDowell HB, McElhinney KL, Tsui EL, Laronda MM. Generation of tailored extracellular matrix hydrogels for the study of in vitro folliculogenesis in response to matrisome-dependent biochemical cues. Bioengineering. 2024;11:543. https://doi.org/10.3390/bioengineering11060543.
42. McLaughlin M, Albertini DF, Wallace WHB, Anderson RA, Telfer EE. Metaphase II oocytes from human unilaminar follicles grown in a multi-step culture system. Mol Hum Reprod. 2018;24:135–42. https://doi.org/10.1093/molehr/gay002.
43. Mendez U, Zhou H, Shikanov A. Synthetic PEG hydrogel for engineering the environment of ovarian follicles. Methods Mol Biol Clifton NJ. 2018;1758:115–28. https://doi.org/10.1007/978-1-4939-7741-3_9.
44. Mihajlovic M, Pásztor-Jánoska DK, Cadenas J, Adrados CS, Andersen CY, Kristensen SG, Lind JU. 3D culture of ovarian follicles in granular and nanofibrillar hydrogels. Biomater Adv. 2024;164:213987. https://doi.org/10.1016/j.bioadv.2024.213987.
45. Nagamatsu G, Shimamoto S, Hamazaki N, Nishimura Y, Hayashi K. Mechanical stress accompanied with nuclear rotation is involved in the dormant state of mouse oocytes. Sci Adv. 2019;5:eaav9960. https://doi.org/10.1126/sciadv.aav9960.
46. Nair R, Kasturi M, Mathur V, Seetharam RN, S Vasanthan K. Strategies for developing 3D printed ovarian model for restoring fertility. Clin Transl Sci. 2024;17:e13863. https://doi.org/10.1111/cts.13863.
47. Nason-Tomaszewski CE, Thomas EE, Matera DL, Baker BM, Shikanov A. Extracellular matrix-templating fibrous hydrogels promote ovarian tissue remodeling and oocyte growth. Bioact Mater. 2024;32:292–303. https://doi.org/10.1016/j.bioactmat.2023.10.001.
48. Oktem O, Buyuk E, Oktay K. Preantral follicle growth is regulated by c-Jun-N-terminal kinase (JNK) pathway. Reprod Sci Thousand Oaks Calif. 2011;18:269–76. https://doi.org/10.1177/1933719110385709.
49. Oktem O, Oktay K. The role of extracellular matrix and activin-A in in vitro growth and survival of murine preantral follicles. Reprod Sci. 2007;14:358–66. https://doi.org/10.1177/1933719107303397.
50. Ouni E, Peaucelle A, Haas KT, Van Kerk O, Dolmans M-M, Tuuri T, Otala M, Amorim CA. A blueprint of the topology and mechanics of the human ovary for next-generation bioengineering and diagnosis. Nat Commun. 2021;12:5603. https://doi.org/10.1038/s41467-021-25934-4.
51. Pangas SA, Saudye H, Shea LD, Woodruff TK. Novel approach for the three-dimensional culture of granulosa cell-oocyte complexes. Tissue Eng. 2003;9:1013–21. https://doi.org/10.1089/107632703322495655.
52. Park EY, Park JH, Mai NTQ, Moon B-S, Choi JK. Control of the growth and development of murine preantral follicles in a biomimetic ovary using a decellularized porcine scaffold. Mater Today Bio. 2023;23:100824. https://doi.org/10.1016/j.mtbio.2023.100824.
53. Pors SE, Ramløse M, Nikiforov D, Lundsgaard K, Cheng J, Andersen CY, Kristensen SG. Initial steps in reconstruction of the human ovary: survival of pre-antral stage follicles in

a decellularized human ovarian scaffold. Hum Reprod Oxf Engl. 2019;34:1523–35. https://doi.org/10.1093/humrep/dez077.
54. Rooda I, Hassan J, Hao J, Wagner M, Moussaud-Lamodière E, Jääger K, Otala M, Knuus K, Lindskog C, Papaikonomou K, Gidlöf S, Langenskiöld C, Vogt H, Frisk P, Malmros J, Tuuri T, Salumets A, Jahnukainen K, Velthut-Meikas A, Damdimopoulou P. In-depth analysis of transcriptomes in ovarian cortical follicles from children and adults reveals interfollicular heterogeneity. Nat Commun. 2024;15:6989. https://doi.org/10.1038/s41467-024-51185-0.
55. Sadeghzadeh Oskouei B, Pashaiasl M, Heidari MH, Salehi M, Veladi H, Ghaderi Pakdel F, Shahabi P, Novin MG. Evaluation of mouse oocyte in vitro maturation developmental competency in dynamic culture systems by design and construction of a lab on a chip device and its comparison with conventional culture system. Cell J Yakhteh. 2016;18:205–13.
56. Sadr SZ, Fatehi R, Maroufizadeh S, Amorim CA, Ebrahimi B. Utilizing fibrin-alginate and matrigel-alginate for mouse follicle development in three-dimensional culture systems. Biopreserv Biobank. 2018;16:120–7. https://doi.org/10.1089/bio.2017.0087.
57. Shea LD, Woodruff TK, Shikanov A. Bioengineering the ovarian follicle microenvironment. Annu Rev Biomed Eng. 2014;16:29–52. https://doi.org/10.1146/annurev-bioeng-071813-105131.
58. Shikanov A, Smith RM, Xu M, Woodruff TK, Shea LD. Hydrogel network design using multifunctional macromers to coordinate tissue maturation in ovarian follicle culture. Biomaterials. 2011;32:2524–31. https://doi.org/10.1016/j.biomaterials.2010.12.027.
59. Shikanov A, Xu M, Woodruff TK, Shea LD. Interpenetrating fibrin-alginate matrices for in vitro ovarian follicle development. Biomaterials. 2009;30:5476–85. https://doi.org/10.1016/j.biomaterials.2009.06.054.
60. Tagler D, Tu T, Smith RM, Anderson NR, Tingen CM, Woodruff TK, Shea LD. Embryonic fibroblasts enable the culture of primary ovarian follicles within alginate hydrogels. Tissue Eng Part A. 2012;18:1229–38. https://doi.org/10.1089/ten.tea.2011.0418.
61. Telfer EE, McLaughlin M, Ding C, Thong KJ. A two-step serum-free culture system supports development of human oocytes from primordial follicles in the presence of activin. Hum Reprod Oxf Engl. 2008;23:1151–8. https://doi.org/10.1093/humrep/den070.
62. Tingen CM, Kiesewetter SE, Jozefik J, Thomas C, Tagler D, Shea L, Woodruff TK. A macrophage and theca cell-enriched stromal cell population influences growth and survival of immature murine follicles in vitro. Reprod Camb Engl. 2011;141:809–20. https://doi.org/10.1530/REP-10-0483.
63. Tomaszewski CE, Constance E, Lemke MM, Zhou H, Padmanabhan V, Arnold KB, Shikanov A. Adipose-derived stem cell-secreted factors promote early stage follicle development in a biomimetic matrix. Biomater Sci. 2019;7:571–80. https://doi.org/10.1039/c8bm01253a.
64. Tomaszewski CE, DiLillo KM, Baker BM, Arnold KB, Shikanov A. Sequestered cell-secreted extracellular matrix proteins improve murine folliculogenesis and oocyte maturation for fertility preservation. Acta Biomater. 2021;132:313–24. https://doi.org/10.1016/j.actbio.2021.03.041.
65. Virant-Klun I, Leicht S, Hughes C, Krijgsveld J. Identification of maturation-specific proteins by single-cell proteomics of human oocytes. Mol Cell Proteomics MCP. 2016;15:2616–27. https://doi.org/10.1074/mcp.M115.056887.
66. Wagner M, Yoshihara M, Douagi I, Damdimopoulos A, Panula S, Petropoulos S, Lu H, Pettersson K, Palm K, Katayama S, Hovatta O, Kere J, Lanner F, Damdimopoulou P. Single-cell analysis of human ovarian cortex identifies distinct cell populations but no oogonial stem cells. Nat Commun. 2020;11:1147. https://doi.org/10.1038/s41467-020-14936-3.
67. West ER, Xu M, Woodruff TK, Shea LD. Physical properties of alginate hydrogels and their effects on in vitro follicle development. Biomaterials. 2007;28:4439–48. https://doi.org/10.1016/j.biomaterials.2007.07.001.
68. Wu T, Gao YY, Su J, Tang XN, Chen Q, Ma LW, Zhang JJ, Wu JM, Wang SX. Three-dimensional bioprinting of artificial ovaries by an extrusion-based method using gelatin-methacryloyl bioink. Climacteric. 2022;25:170–8. https://doi.org/10.1080/13697137.2021.1921726.

69. Xiao S, Coppeta JR, Rogers HB, Isenberg BC, Zhu J, Olalekan SA, McKinnon KE, Dokic D, Rashedi AS, Haisenleder DJ, Malpani SS, Arnold-Murray CA, Chen K, Jiang M, Bai L, Nguyen CT, Zhang J, Laronda MM, Hope TJ, Maniar KP, Pavone ME, Avram MJ, Sefton EC, Getsios S, Burdette JE, Kim JJ, Borenstein JT, Woodruff TK. A microfluidic culture model of the human reproductive tract and 28-day menstrual cycle. Nat Commun. 2017;8:14584. https://doi.org/10.1038/ncomms14584.
70. Xiao S, Zhang J, Romero MM, Smith KN, Shea LD, Woodruff TK. In vitro follicle growth supports human oocyte meiotic maturation. Sci Rep. 2015;5:17323. https://doi.org/10.1038/srep17323.
71. Xu F, Lawson MS, Bean Y, Ting AY, Pejovic T, De Geest K, Moffitt M, Mitalipov SM, Xu J. Matrix-free 3D culture supports human follicular development from the unilaminar to the antral stage in vitro yielding morphologically normal metaphase II oocytes. Hum Reprod Oxf Engl. 2021;36:1326–38. https://doi.org/10.1093/humrep/deab003.
72. Xu J, Lawson MS, Yeoman RR, Molskness TA, Ting AY, Stouffer RL, Zelinski MB. Fibrin promotes development and function of macaque primary follicles during encapsulated three-dimensional culture. Hum Reprod. 2013;28:2187–200. https://doi.org/10.1093/humrep/det093.
73. Xu M, Banc A, Woodruff TK, Shea LD. Secondary follicle growth and oocyte maturation by culture in alginate hydrogel following cryopreservation of the ovary or individual follicles. Biotechnol Bioeng. 2009;103:378–86. https://doi.org/10.1002/bit.22250.
74. Xu M, West E, Shea LD, Woodruff TK. Identification of a stage-specific permissive in vitro culture environment for follicle growth and oocyte development. Biol Reprod. 2006;75:916–23. https://doi.org/10.1095/biolreprod.106.054833.
75. Yano Maher JC, Zelinski MB, Oktay KH, Duncan FE, Segars JH, Lujan ME, Lou H, Yun BH, Hanfling SN, Schwartz LE, Laronda MM, Halvorson LM, O'Neill KE, Gomez-Lobo V. Classification system of human ovarian follicle morphology: recommendations of the National Institute of Child Health and Human Development – sponsored ovarian nomenclature workshop. Fertil Steril. 2025;123:761–78. https://doi.org/10.1016/j.fertnstert.2024.11.016.
76. Ye M, Shan Y, Lu B, Luo H, Li B, Zhang Y, Wang Z, Guo Y, Ouyang L, Gu J, Xiong Z, Zhang T. Creating a semi-opened micro-cavity ovary through sacrificial microspheres as an in vitro model for discovering the potential effect of ovarian toxic agents. Bioact Mater. 2023;26:216–30. https://doi.org/10.1016/j.bioactmat.2023.02.029.
77. Yildirim M, Duran Kaymak S, Cayonu Kahraman N, Savran Ucok B, Engin-Ustun Y. Assessment of ovarian stiffness in women with polycystic ovary syndrome. J Ultrasound Med. 2025;44:1797–806. https://doi.org/10.1002/jum.16731.
78. Yoon JA, Lee K-A, Choi JK. A simplified 3D culture system for ovarian follicles utilizing a solid Matrigel drop to create an in vivo-like ovarian microenvironment. J Biomater Tissue Eng. 2019;9:558–61. https://doi.org/10.1166/jbt.2019.2018.
79. Zand E, Rajablou E, Siadat SF, Beiki B, Akbarinejad V, Amorim CA, Valojerdi MR, Tahaei LA, Fathi R. Successful 3D culture and transplantation of mouse isolated preantral follicles in hydrogel of bioengineered Wharton's jelly. PLoS One. 2023;18:e0290095. https://doi.org/10.1371/journal.pone.0290095.
80. Zaniker EJ, Zhang M, Hughes L, La Follette L, Atazhanova T, Trofimchuk A, Babayev E, Duncan FE. Shear wave elastography to assess stiffness of the human ovary and other reproductive tissues across the reproductive lifespan in health and disease†. Biol Reprod. 2024;110:1100–14. https://doi.org/10.1093/biolre/ioae050.
81. Zhao X, Zhang S, Gao S, Chang H-M, Leung PCK, Tan J. A novel three-dimensional follicle culture system decreases oxidative stress and promotes the prolonged culture of human granulosa cells. ACS Appl Mater Interfaces. 2023;15:15084–95. https://doi.org/10.1021/acsami.2c18734.
82. Zhou H, Decker JT, Lemke MM, Tomaszweski CE, Shea LD, Arnold KB, Shikanov A. Synergy of paracrine signaling during early-stage mouse ovarian follicle development in vitro. Cell Mol Bioeng. 2018;11:435–50. https://doi.org/10.1007/s12195-018-0545-8.

Biomaterials to Facilitate Revascularization and Improve Outcomes of Ovarian Tissue Transplantation

Despina I. Pavlidis and Ariella Shikanov

Abstract Primary ovarian insufficiency (POI) is a significant long-term consequence of gonadotoxic cancer treatments, which leads to infertility and systemic health concerns in survivors with ovaries. Ovarian tissue cryopreservation and transplantation (OTCT) is currently the only fertility preservation approach available to prepubertal patients or patients unable to delay cancer therapy, offering the potential to restore both fertility and physiological ovarian endocrine function. Despite promising outcomes, including up to 89% restoration of ovarian endocrine function and over 180 reported live births, OTCT remains limited by variable graft performance and functional longevity. A primary barrier to long-term OTCT success is massive primordial follicle loss following transplantation, driven largely by delayed graft revascularization and ensuing ischemic and reperfusion injuries. This chapter reviews the clinical background of OTCT, including tissue sources, transplantation sites, and current limitations. Special emphasis is placed on the mechanisms by which delayed revascularization induces ischemia, oxidative stress, follicle apoptosis, and abnormal follicle activation that collectively curtail graft function. The chapter then explores biomaterial strategies that enhance revascularization and follicle survival in preclinical human ovarian xenograft models, followed by emerging biomaterial systems from broader tissue engineering applications that inform the design and clinical translation of future OTCT approaches.

D. I. Pavlidis
Department of Biomedical Engineering, University of Michigan, Ann Arbor, MI, USA
e-mail: dpavlidi@umich.edu

A. Shikanov (✉)
Department of Biomedical Engineering, University of Michigan, Ann Arbor, MI, USA

Department of Obstetrics and Gynecology, University of Michigan, Ann Arbor, MI, USA

Macromolecular Science and Engineering, University of Michigan, Ann Arbor, MI, USA

Cellular and Molecular Biology Program, University of Michigan, Ann Arbor, MI, USA
e-mail: shikanov@umich.edu

S. G. Zambuto, M. L. Oyen (eds.), *Biomaterials for Women's Health Engineering*,
https://doi.org/10.1007/978-3-032-10745-9_11

Keywords Ovarian tissue transplantation · Graft revascularization · Ischemia · Reperfusion · Angiogenesis · Hydrogel scaffolds · Xenograft · Mesenchymal stem cells · Adipose tissue-derived stem cells · Endothelial cells · Growth factors · Granular hydrogels

1 Introduction

Improved cancer survival rates motivate the need to address the negative off-target effects of cancer treatments that persist long after remission and affect the quality of life of survivors. For cancer survivors with ovaries, one notable adverse effect is primary ovarian insufficiency (POI), a condition defined as the loss of ovarian activity before the age of 40 and characterized by irregular menstrual cycles with elevated gonadotropins and low estradiol [1]. Anticancer treatments such as chemotherapy and radiation are highly gonadotoxic and therefore prematurely deplete the nonrenewable ovarian follicle reserve, leading to infertility and POI [2, 3]. Consequently, POI and the associated loss of ovarian endocrine function can lead to systemic health issues, including cardiovascular disease, osteoporosis, mood disorders, and, in young patients, arrested puberty. Strategies to manage POI focus separately on: (1) establishing adequate gonadal hormone levels through hormone replacement therapy (HRT), and (2) preserving fertility through assistive reproductive technologies (ART) such as oocyte or embryo cryopreservation (Fig. 1). HRT, however, fails to replicate the dynamic hormone levels that arise from native feedback networks between organs and tissues of the endocrine system [4]. Furthermore, oocyte and embryo cryopreservation require hormone stimulation and time, making them unsuitable for pre- and peripubertal patients and patients who cannot delay anticancer treatment [5, 6]. For these patient populations, ovarian tissue cryopreservation and transplantation (OTCT) is the only option that offers the possibility of restoration of both fertility and physiological ovarian endocrine function (Fig. 1).

Ovarian tissue cryopreservation refers to the cryopreservation of a patient's ovarian tissue prior to anticancer treatment. Typically, only the ovarian cortex is cryopreserved as it houses the primordial follicles (PFs) that constitute the nonrenewable ovarian reserve (Fig. 2). Unlike oocyte or embryo cryopreservation, ovarian tissue cryopreservation does not require hormonal stimulation or reproductive maturity and can therefore be promptly performed without delaying anticancer treatments [5]. Once the patient is cancer-free, their cryopreserved tissue can be thawed and reimplanted in a process known as ovarian tissue transplantation. The ability of OTCT to offer both fertility preservation and restoration of ovarian endocrine function to a broad patient population largely depends on the number of PFs present in the tissue at the time of OTCT [8]. The effectiveness of OTCT, however, is hindered by ovarian tissue damage and significant loss of the PF pool upon tissue transplantation [5]. These obstacles are attributed to the avascular nature of the ovarian tissue transplantation procedure since direct vascular anastomosis of ovarian tissue is not possible, resulting in ischemic and reperfusion injuries to the transplanted tissue. Ovarian tissue and follicle apoptosis, as well as abnormal follicle

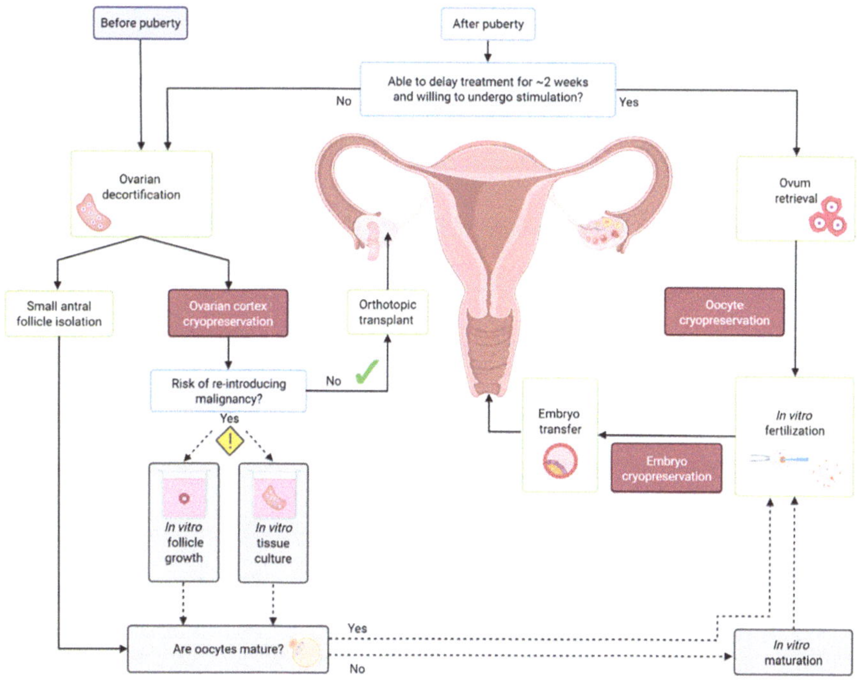

Fig. 1 Fertility preservation options for patients with ovaries undergoing cancer treatment. If the patient is postpubertal, able to delay cancer treatment, and willing to undergo hormonal stimulation, oocyte or embryo cryopreservation, followed by embryo transfer, can be performed. However, if the patient is prepubertal, or not able to delay treatment and undergo hormonal stimulation, OTCT is indicated. Procedures involving cryopreserved ovarian tissue in cases with potential malignancy risk (indicated as gray boxes following the yellow caution symbol) remain experimental and have not been translated to clinical practice. (Created in BioRender. Pavlidis (2025). https://BioRender.com/8i6gvo1)

activation, further hinder OTCT effectiveness; however, the specific factors causing these responses and strategies to mitigate these adverse effects remain under investigation.

This chapter provides an overview of the clinical background and limitations of OTCT with a focus on human ovarian tissue graft revascularization. A review of biomaterial strategies designed to enhance human ovarian tissue graft revascularization and emerging biomaterials with potential applications to OTCT is also provided.

2 Clinical Background

2.1 Ovarian Tissue Sources: Autograft Versus Allograft

OTCT typically involves the transplantation of a patient's previously cryopreserved ovarian tissue, also known as an "autograft." The history, clinical reports, successes,

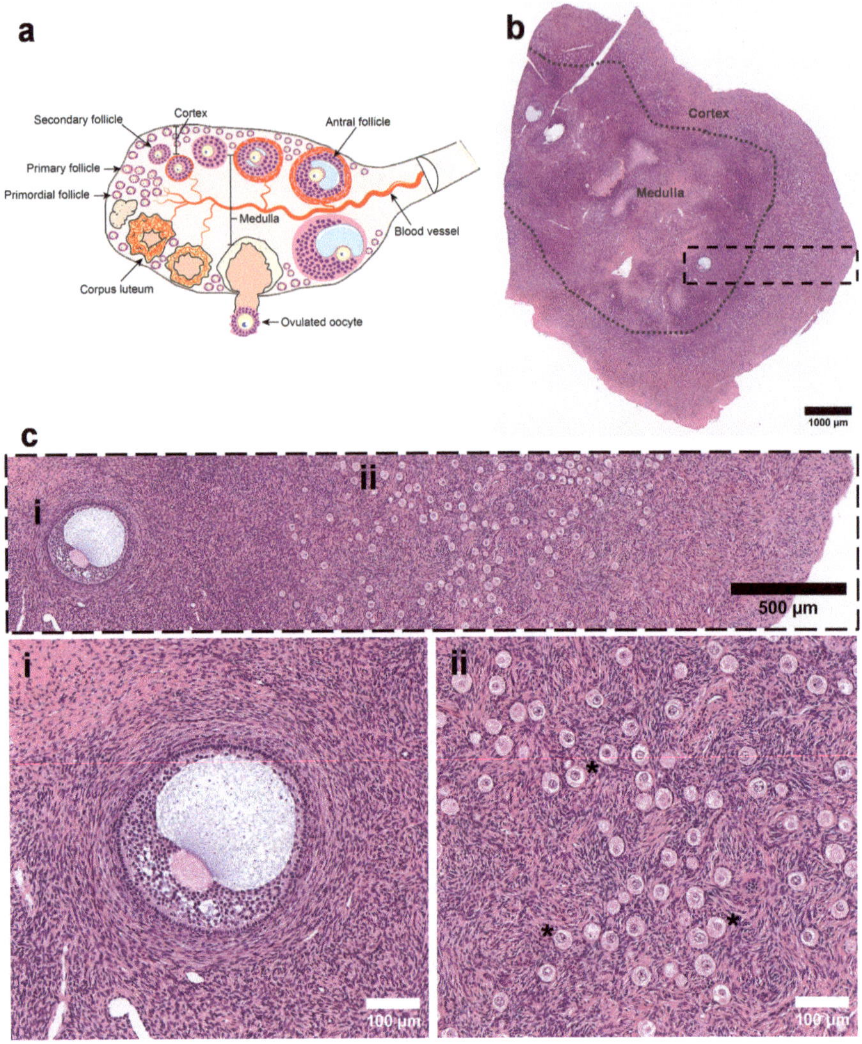

Fig. 2 Structure of the human ovary. (**a**) A schematic overview of human ovarian anatomy, highlighting the different developmental stages of follicles relative to the cortex and medulla. (Adapted from Zhang et al. [7], licensed under Creative Commons Attribution License (CC BY 4.0)). (**b**) Histological image of a human ovarian tissue sample showing the medulla and cortex. Scale bar = 1000 μm. (**c**) Magnified regions demonstrating (**i**) an antral follicle in the medulla and (**ii**) the primordial follicle ovarian reserve in the cortex. Examples of primordial follicles are indicated by asterisks (*). Scale bars = 500 μm (black), 100 μm (white)

and challenges associated with autotransplantation are described in detail in Sects. 2.3 and 3. There are instances, however, when a patient's ovarian tissue was not preemptively cryopreserved or when the patient's tissue is not suitable due to age or congenital conditions such as Turner syndrome [9]. In these instances, transplantation of donor ovarian tissue (i.e., an "allograft") can be used to restore fertility and ovarian endocrine function. To date, there have been a small number of ovarian allotransplantation cases recorded [9]. These have occurred between monozygotic twins or between genetically different but human leukocyte antigen (HLA)-compatible siblings who had previously undergone bone marrow transplantation with one sibling acting as donor to the other recipient sibling. In both scenarios, immunosuppression was not required for successful allotransplantation of ovarian tissue and restoration of ovarian endocrine function.

Recently, the first instance of a successful ovarian allotransplant utilizing immunosuppression was reported [10]. The allotransplant was performed between a donor and recipient sibling pair who were HLA-compatible but blood type incompatible, which required an immunosuppression protocol typically used for kidney transplantation to prevent rejection of the allograft. Ultimately, the recipient experienced restoration of ovarian endocrine function and had a live birth of a healthy infant. This case report is a promising advancement for patients who did not cryopreserve their ovarian tissue prior to undergoing gonadotoxic treatments. Nonetheless, allotransplantation with immunosuppression remains rare and experimental, and the current clinical practice recommends offering cancer patients the option to cryopreserve their own ovarian tissue.

2.2 *Transplantation Sites: Orthotopic Versus Heterotopic*

Orthotopic transplantation sites, either directly on the patient's remaining ovary or within the pelvic cavity near the ovary, are regarded as optimal environments for ovarian tissue health and follicle development since temperature, pressure, paracrine factors, and blood supply closely match the native microenvironment of the ovarian tissue [5]. The choice of transplantation site influences the outcomes of ovarian tissue transplantation, including graft revascularization [11]. Orthotopic transplantation sites also increase the probability of spontaneous pregnancy posttransplantation due to the tissue's proximity to the fallopian tubes.

In cases where restoration of ovarian endocrine function rather than pregnancy is the primary reason for ovarian tissue transplantation, minimally invasive heterotopic transplantation sites can be used, such as the subcutaneous forearm space or the abdominal wall [12]. Heterotopic transplantation sites provide easy access for ovarian tissue transplantation and tissue surveillance. Consequently, heterotopic sites are more appropriate for patients where orthotopic sites are not suitable due to tissue scarring or if there is a concern for disease recurrence upon ovarian tissue transplantation.

Despite these advantages, clinical studies suggest that heterotopic transplantation sites may not provide an optimal microenvironment for ovarian tissue health and follicle development [5]. In a 2001 study, Oktay et al. retrieved three oocytes from a patient with a graft transplanted to the subcutaneous forearm space [13]. Two of these oocytes were postmature, and one was matured in vitro but did not fertilize. In 2004, Oktay et al. noted that follicles in heterotopic grafts transplanted subcutaneously to the abdominal wall matured to smaller sizes (typically 10–11 mm) compared to 16–17 mm observed at orthotopic sites [14]. In this case study, 20 oocytes were obtained from one patient, 8 of which were candidates for in vitro fertilization. Of these candidates, three were already mature at retrieval and five were matured in vitro. None of the three mature oocytes fertilized, but two of the in vitro matured oocytes did, generating only one viable embryo for transfer to the patient's uterus.

These case study findings are also echoed in large clinical reviews. Among 285 patients across five European centers, only 5 underwent heterotopic ovarian tissue transplantation, with no pregnancies reported [8]. In contrast, of the 277 patients who underwent orthotopic ovarian tissue transplantation, 34% reported live birth. A meta-analysis of 12 studies spanning 201 patients found a 3% live birth rate for heterotopic ovarian tissue transplantation compared to 23% for orthotopic ovarian tissue transplantation [15]. In a direct comparison of patients treated by the same clinician, the number of viable embryos was significantly lower in the heterotopic group (1 vs. 8), and fertilization rates were similarly lower in the heterotopic group (26.5% vs. 97%) [16]. Collectively, these studies suggest that heterotopic sites, despite their advantages, are associated with suboptimal ovarian tissue health and follicle development, thereby leading to diminished oocyte and embryo quality as well as decreased chances of successful fertilization and pregnancy [17]. Orthotopic sites thus remain optimal environments for ovarian tissue health and follicle development.

2.3 OTCT Outcomes and Limitations

Since the first report of OTCT in 2000 [18], this procedure has demonstrated promising outcomes with at least 189 live births noted [19] and approximately 89% of patients having experienced restored ovarian endocrine function as soon as 4–5 months after ovarian tissue transplantation [8]. Despite these successful outcomes, the live birth rate remains low at just 28% (95% confidence interval: 24%–34%) and the duration of ovarian graft function varies widely from 0.7 to 5 years [19]. Several factors contribute to the limited success of OTCT.

First, follicle distribution in human ovarian tissue is heterogeneous and varies significantly between patients and even within the same ovary. Reliable nondestructive methods to evaluate the number of follicles in the tissue at the time of OTCT are not available. As such, there is limited ability to predict the lifespan of ovarian tissue grafts and the likelihood of pregnancy. Second, significant ovarian tissue damage and follicle loss occur shortly after ovarian tissue transplantation due to ischemia and reperfusion injuries. The combination of an unknown number of transplanted follicles and massive follicle loss after tissue transplantation results in shortened and variable functional longevity of the ovarian graft. One of the main obstacles to the long-term success of OTCT, which is described in the following section, continues to be poor ovarian tissue graft revascularization posttransplantation.

3 Human Ovarian Tissue Graft Revascularization

3.1 Ischemic Injury

The major determinants of OTCT effectiveness and graft longevity are the number of PFs present at the time of ovarian tissue cryopreservation and the number of PFs that survive the transplantation procedure. Xenotransplantation studies involving sheep and human ovarian tissue transplanted into immunodeficient mice have found that 50%–90% of PFs are lost shortly after tissue transplantation [20, 21]. It is hypothesized that this follicle loss occurs primarily due to tissue transplantation rather than tissue cryopreservation and thawing and, importantly, occurs before the tissue becomes revascularized [20]. Ovarian cortical tissue lacks large blood vessels amenable to surgical vascular anastomosis during ovarian tissue transplantation. Consequently, reestablishment of blood flow to the tissue depends solely on graft revascularization through angiogenesis and anastomosis with the host vasculature. Studies involving xenotransplantation of human ovarian tissue into immunodeficient mice have shown that the grafted tissue remains hypoxic for 3–5 days posttransplantation and that graft revascularization occurs within a 10-day window posttransplantation [22, 23] (Fig. 3). During this period, grafted ovarian tissue is subjected to insufficient blood flow (i.e., ischemia) and hypoxia. Consequently, hypoxia response elements produce inflammatory mediators that trigger the migration of neutrophils and macrophages into the tissue, causing tissue damage and fibrosis [11]. The limited effectiveness of OTCT is thus attributed to the avascular nature of the ovarian tissue transplantation procedure, which results in ischemic injury to the transplanted tissue (Fig. 4).

Within the native ovarian cortical microenvironment, PFs receive nutrients and oxygen via passive diffusion from nearby blood vessels [25]. Although PFs are naturally avascular and thus more resistant to ischemic injury than ovarian endothelial and stromal cells [11], ischemic damage to ovarian tissue likely contributes to the significant PF loss observed posttransplantation [26]. Ischemia-induced hypoxia also modulates cell proliferation and survival signaling pathways, such as PI3K/Akt, resulting in additional follicle loss through abnormal, premature follicle activation that may not be supported by the damaged ovarian stroma [26].

3.2 Reperfusion Injury

Paradoxically, revascularization of grafted tissue can lead to reperfusion injury, further exacerbating the preexisting ischemic injury [27]. Following prolonged ischemia, the influx of oxygen during reperfusion triggers a state of oxidative stress characterized by the overproduction of reactive oxygen species (ROS), such as superoxide anions (O_2^-), hydrogen peroxide (H_2O_2), and hydroxyl radicals ($OH^•$). ROS are by-products of physiological cellular metabolism that are regulated by

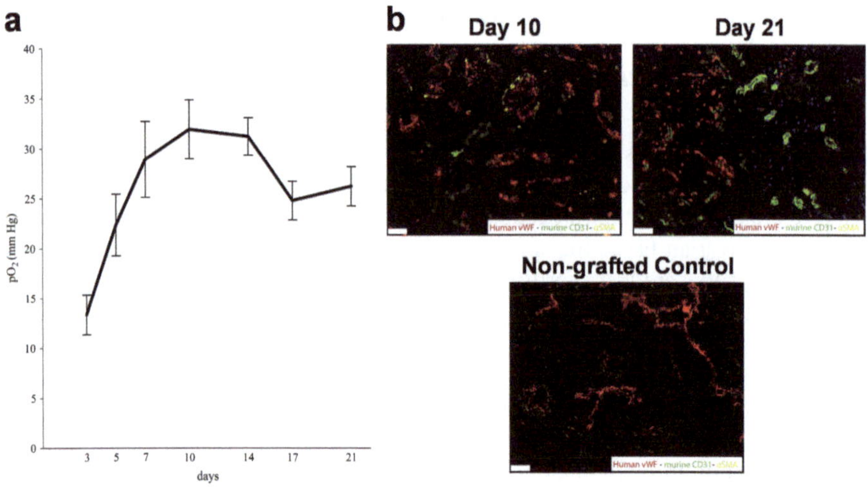

Fig. 3 Human ovarian xenograft reoxygenation and revascularization dynamics. (**a**) Oxygen partial pressure (pO_2) over time in human ovarian tissue grafts transplanted into immunodeficient mice. The x-axis indicates days post-tissue transplantation. (Adapted from Van Eyck et al. [22] with permission from Elsevier. License number: 6112080394522). (**b**) Revascularization of human ovarian tissue xenografts visualized by immunofluorescence staining of human (red) and mouse (green) vasculature 10 and 21 days posttransplantation. A non-grafted human ovarian tissue control is shown for comparison. Scale bars = 50 μm. (Adapted from Cacciottola et al. [23] with permission from Elsevier. License number: 6112080883161)

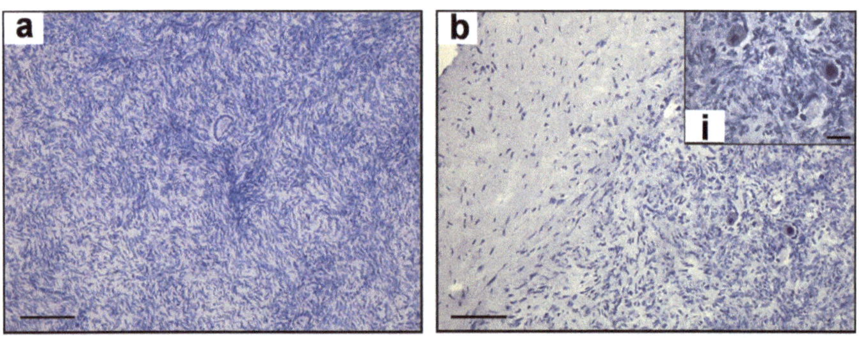

Fig. 4 Histologic evaluation of human ovarian tissue graft transplanted into immunodeficient mice. (**a**) Fresh ovarian tissue control showing healthy stroma with high cellular density. (**b**) Graft at 3 days posttransplantation demonstrates central necrosis surrounded by stroma with low cellular density. Inset (**i**) highlights abnormal follicles. Scale bars = 100 μm; inset scale bar = 25 μm. (Adapted from Van Eyck et al. [24] with permission from Elsevier. License number: 6112081141056)

antioxidant systems, including superoxide dismutase and catalase (enzymatic systems) and vitamins C and E (nonenzymatic systems) [28]. An imbalance between ROS production and antioxidant capacity, however, results in high ROS concentrations, which lead to oxidative damage of cellular components (e.g., DNA, lipids, proteins) and, consequently, cellular death [26]. While ischemia activates inflammatory pathways, reperfusion amplifies inflammation via cells such as neutrophils that release additional ROS and pro-inflammatory cytokines (e.g., TNF-α, IL-1, IL-6, IL-8) [27], further exacerbating cellular and extracellular matrix (ECM) damage following the initial ischemic injury [29].

A study focused on oxidative stress and ROS kinetics in human ovarian tissue xenotransplants found that ROS levels (measured as H_2O_2 concentrations via microdialysis) peaked 10 days after tissue transplantation, which matches the timepoint at which transplanted tissue typically becomes revascularized [23]. Notably, approximately 60% of the follicles were lost within the first 10 days of transplantation, prior to the ROS peak, and an additional ~20% of follicles were lost after the 10-day mark (Fig. 5). Analysis of human ovarian tissue xenotransplants at later time points (21 days posttransplantation) revealed modest increases in oxidative stress markers (Nrf2 and 8-hydroxy-deoxyguanosine) within the ovarian tissue and no evidence of such stress markers within follicles [30]. These studies suggest that both ischemic and reperfusion injuries contribute to the limited effectiveness of OTCT. Given that the severity of reperfusion injury is directly proportional to the duration of ischemia [31] (Fig. 6), developing tools that facilitate faster graft revascularization post-ovarian tissue transplantation are critical to improving the long-term effectiveness of OTCT.

4 Biomaterials for Human Ovarian Tissue Xenograft Revascularization

Facilitating faster graft revascularization post-ovarian tissue transplantation is one of the most commonly investigated approaches for mitigating ovarian tissue ischemia and reperfusion injuries and follicle loss [26]. Previously published reviews summarize various approaches for broadly improving ovarian tissue transplantation outcomes for tissue originating from human and nonhuman (rodent, ovine, bovine, nonhuman primate) sources [12, 26, 32]. These approaches include modulating transplanted tissue size as well as the use of growth factors, vitamins, antiapoptotic agents, antioxidants, and hormones. The following sections focus exclusively on biomaterial strategies for facilitating revascularization of human ovarian tissue xenografts (Table 1).

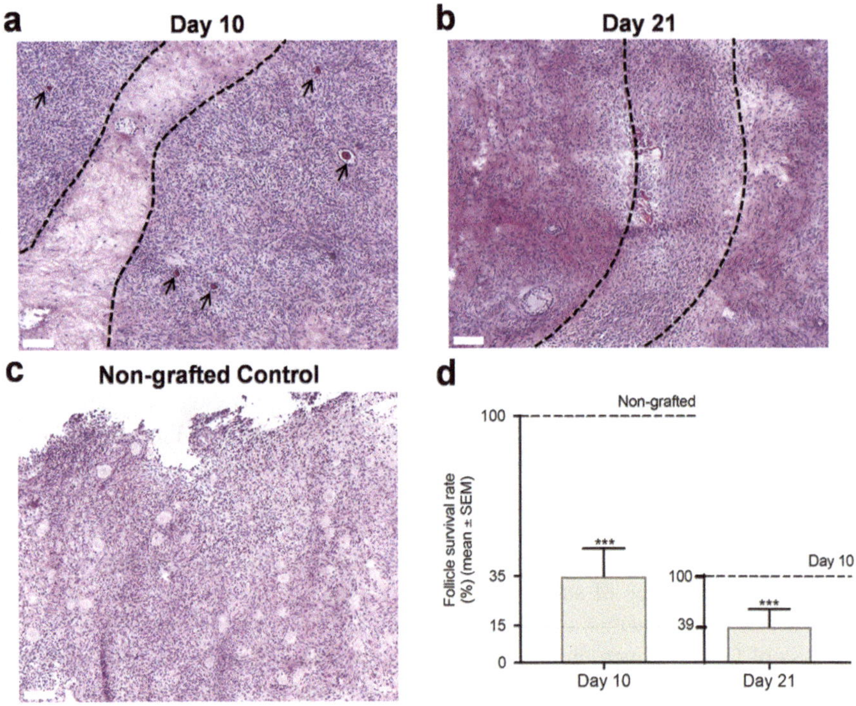

Fig. 5 Follicle loss in human ovarian xenografts. Histologic evaluation of human ovarian tissue grafts transplanted into immunodeficient mice for 10 (**a**) and 21 (**b**) days. Arrows indicate morphologically normal follicles. (**c**) Non-grafted ovarian tissue control shown for comparison. (**d**) Follicle survival rate in grafts retrieved 10 and 21 days posttransplantation (Adapted from Cacciottola et al. [23] with permission from Elsevier. License number: 6112080883161)

4.1 *Biomaterials as Scaffolds for Ovarian Tissue*

Biomaterials as scaffolds for transplanted ovarian tissue have shown promise for enhancing ovarian tissue revascularization and subsequently reducing ovarian tissue cell death. Reported materials include human recombinant type I collagen (CollPlant) [33], porcine small intestinal submucosa (SIS) [33], fibrin [34], and degradable gelatin hydrogels [35]. One study compared CollPlant and SIS by encapsulating and transplanting ovarian grafts into the back muscle of immunodeficient female mice [33]. At 21 days posttransplantation, CollPlant demonstrated better outcomes, including higher follicle numbers, fewer atretic follicles, and more proliferating granulosa cells compared to SIS. Both matrices, nonetheless, displayed similar graft revascularization patterns. Another study by the same group examined the effects of encapsulating ovarian tissue in fibrin, known to promote angiogenesis, alongside systemic treatment with simvastatin [34]. Simvastatin, a pharmaceutical agent for lowering cholesterol, has pleiotropic effects, including improving endothelial function, reducing inflammation, and promoting revascularization and

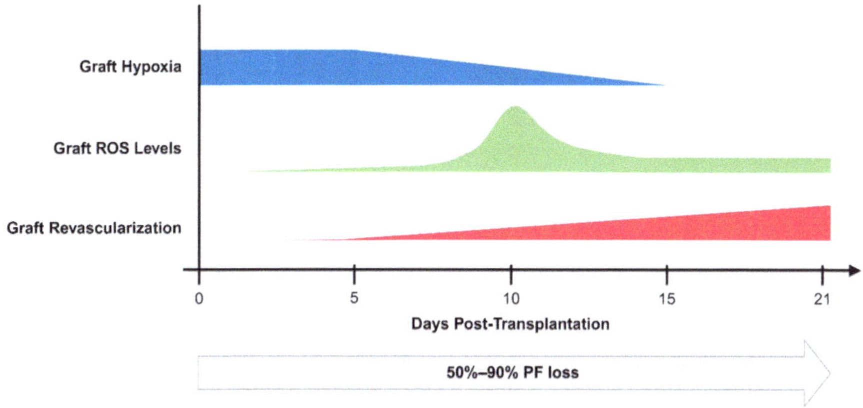

Fig. 6 Dynamics of hypoxia, ROS levels, and revascularization in human ovarian tissue grafts during the early posttransplantation period. Hypoxia due to slow revascularization primarily contributes to cell death and PF loss shortly after transplantation. ROS levels peak in grafts concurrently with increased graft revascularization, leading to reperfusion injury and augmenting the initial ischemic injury. (Created in BioRender. Pavlidis (2025). https://BioRender.com/fp4taln)

neovascularization in animal models. Similar to the CollPlant and SIS study, ovarian tissue was encapsulated in fibrin and transplanted into the back muscle of immunodeficient female mice. At 21 days posttransplantation, fibrin-encapsulated tissue displayed greater follicle proliferation compared to nonencapsulated tissue transplanted into non-treated hosts. In contrast, nonencapsulated tissue transplanted into simvastatin-treated hosts showed the highest level of follicle proliferation but also increased follicle atresia. Tissue revascularization was noted across all groups, with the highest levels identified in fibrin-encapsulated tissue transplanted into simvastatin-treated hosts. Mouse-specific vasculature was consistently more prominent than human-specific vasculature across all groups. Notably, only the fibrin-encapsulated tissue groups displayed large, organized vascular structures expressing both mouse and human markers. These tissues also retained more human vasculature than nonencapsulated tissues, indicating fibrin's positive role in tissue revascularization. Overall, the study demonstrated that fibrin encapsulation combined with simvastatin treatment synergistically improved posttransplantation outcomes for ovarian tissue grafts.

In contrast to systemic treatment with simvastatin, a local sustained delivery of basic fibroblast growth factor (bFGF) from degradable gelatin hydrogels encapsulating ovarian tissue has been explored [35]. bFGF is involved in various biological processes such as tissue repair, wound healing, and embryonic development and is known for its significant role in angiogenesis and in normal tissue maintenance. Analysis of the grafts transplanted into subcutaneous pockets on the backs of ovariectomized immunodeficient female mice after 6 weeks revealed that the bFGF gelatin hydrogel promoted angiogenesis in the ovarian grafts, leading to increased human and mouse blood vessel areas (human: 1.28% vs. 0.43%; mouse:

Table 1 Biomaterials used to enhance human ovarian tissue graft revascularization

Reference	Donor age (years)	Donor *n*	Tissue volume per implant	Implant location	Mouse strain	Mouse *n*	Duration	Material	Revascularization outcomes	Stroma outcomes	Follicle outcomes
Abir et al. [33]	9–22	9	5 × 5 mm	Heterotopic (back muscle)	nu/nu Balb/C	146	21 days	CollPlant, SIS	Similar revascularization patterns for CollPlant and SIS	CollPlant apoptosis > SIS apoptosis	CollPlant: ↑ total follicles, ↓ atretic follicles; SIS: ↑ total follicles, ↑ atretic follicles
Magen et al. [34]	10–23	6	5 × 5 mm	Heterotopic (back muscle)	nu/nu Balb/C	40	21 days	Fibrin	↑ Vascular density	Trend of ↓ apoptosis (ns)	↑ Follicle proliferation
Tanaka et al. [35]	29–34	4	5 × 10 × 1 mm	Heterotopic (subcutaneous back)	SCID	10	42 days	Gelatin (+bFGF)	↑ Vascular density	↑ Proliferation, ↓ fibrosis	↑ Primordial and primary follicles present
Xia et al. [36]	21	1	2.5 × 2.5 × 1 mm	Heterotopic (subcutaneous abdomen)	Athymic Balb/C	36	3, 7, 21 days	Matrigel (+MSCs)	↑ Vascular density, ↑ perfusion at 7 days	NR	↑ Primordial follicles present, ↓ primordial follicle apoptosis
Cheng et al. [37]	20–31	4	3 mm diameter	Heterotopic (renal capsule)	SCID	63	3, 7 days	Matrigel (+H-MSCs)	↑ Vascular density	↓ Apoptosis	↑ Total and primordial follicles present, ↓ atretic follicles, ↓ follicle apoptosis
Manavella et al. [38]	25–35	5	5 × 4 × 1 mm	Orthotopic (parietal peritoneum)	SCID	15	7 days	Fibrin (+ASCs)	↑ Vascular density, ↑ pO_2	Trend of ↓ fibrosis (ns)	↑ Total and primordial follicles present, ↓ follicle apoptosis
Manavella et al. [39]	25–35	5	5 × 4 × 1 mm	Orthotopic (parietal peritoneum)	SCID	10	7 days	Fibrin (+ASCs)	↑ Vascular density, ↑ VEGF expression and secretion	NR	NR

Cacciottola et al. [30]	20–35	5	6 × 4 × 1.5 mm	Orthotopic (parietal peritoneum)	Nu/nu Swiss	15	3, 10, 21 days	Fibrin (+ASCs)	Earlier vascularization	↑ Oxidative stress markers at 21 days	↓ HIF-1 in primordial follicles at 3 days, no presence of oxidative stress marker or DNA damage in follicles
Cacciottola et al. [40]	21–34	7	NR	Orthotopic (parietal peritoneum)	SCID	14	24 weeks	Fibrin (+ASCs)	NR	NR	↑ Total and primordial follicle present
Man et al. [41]	5–32	14	1 × 2 mm–6 × 3 mm	Heterotopic (fascia of gluteus maximus)	NSG	35	2–22 weeks	Fibrin (+ExECs, +AMH-ExECs)	Functional, perfused vessels	↓ Fibrosis	↑ Total follicles present, ↑ and larger antral follicles; AMH-ExECs: ↑ primordial follicles present

NR not reported, *SCID* severe combined immunodeficiency disease, *NSG* NOD (non-obese diabetic) SCID gamma, *SIS* small intestine submucosa, *bFGF* basic fibroblast growth factor, *ExECs* exogenous endothelial cells, *AMH-ExECs* exogenous endothelial cells expressing anti-Müllerian hormone, pO_2 partial pressure of oxygen, *VEGF* vascular endothelial growth factor, *HIF-1* hypoxia-inducible factor 1, a transcription factor involved in cellular response to hypoxia, *ns* no statistical significance

1.76% vs. 0.82%). It also contributed to greater numbers of primordial and primary follicles within the ovarian tissue, proliferative ovarian tissue stroma, and reduced fibrotic tissue area. Taken together, the sustained release of bFGF via a degradable hydrogel at the transplant site promoted ovarian tissue revascularization, maintaining a tissue environment that supported follicle survival.

The outcomes of these studies support the notion that implementing biomaterials can increase ovarian tissue revascularization in the early posttransplantation period, thereby improving follicle outcomes. This notion is further supported via the clinical use of AlloDerm—a commercial decellularized human extracellular tissue matrix (ECTM)—developed by Oktay et al. to transplant cryopreserved ovarian tissue into patients. Initial preclinical testing of AlloDerm for human ovarian tissue transplantation in a xenograft model showed good integration of AlloDerm into the ovarian stroma [42]. In a subsequent clinical study, seven patients underwent robot-assisted ovarian tissue transplantation with AlloDerm, which led to a longer mean graft longevity of 43.2 months compared to 29.2 months (derived from 79 transplant cases worldwide) [43]. When compared using age-matched samples, the AlloDerm grafts lasted 14 months longer compared to controls (47.4 vs. 33.7 months). Although the experimental design and limited sample size make it difficult to attribute the successful outcomes solely to the addition of the ECTM, these case studies highlight the promising role of biomaterial scaffolds for improving human OTCT outcomes.

4.2 Biomaterials as Scaffolds for Codelivery of Support Cells with Ovarian Grafts

Biomaterials have also been used to deliver support cells, such as mesenchymal stem cells (MSCs), to enhance ovarian tissue revascularization and reduce cell death due to their ability to differentiate into various cell lineages and secrete pro-angiogenic factors. One study investigated the use of Matrigel to co-transplant ovarian tissue and MSCs into the abdominal subcutaneous space of immunodeficient female mice for 3, 7, or 21 days [36]. The inclusion of MSCs increased graft revascularization at all time points. Notably, at 3 days posttransplantation, the microvascular density in the Matrigel/MSC group was double compared to the nonencapsulated group and the Matrigel-only group. From day 7 onward, MSCs also increased blood perfusion and reduced primordial follicle apoptosis in the ovarian tissue. Overall, co-transplantation of MSCs and ovarian tissue encapsulated in Matrigel demonstrated earlier graft revascularization and reperfusion along with reduced follicle apoptosis, which preserved the PF pool [36].

A separate study hypothesized that hypoxia could enhance MSC pro-angiogenic behavior and therefore examined the effect of hypoxia-preconditioned MSCs (H-MSCs) on ovarian tissue revascularization [37]. Ovarian tissue was co-transplanted with Matrigel-encapsulated H-MSCs under the renal capsule of ovariectomized immunodeficient female mice for 3 and 7 days. Results showed that H-MSCs increased revascularization levels as early as 3 days posttransplantation. At 3 days, tissue transplanted with H-MSCs had a vessel density of 107 vessels/mm^2 compared to transplanted tissue without MSCs (41 vessels/mm^2) or with normoxic MSCs (47 vessels/mm^2). The inclusion of H-MSCs also attenuated stroma cell and follicle apoptosis and decreased follicle atresia, leading to overall increased total and primordial follicle densities. Altogether, this study demonstrated that co-transplanting H-MSCs with ovarian tissue encapsulated in Matrigel enhanced early graft revascularization, correlating with reduced stroma and follicle apoptosis as well as PF pool preservation.

As an alternative to the typical one-step transplantation approach, a series of published studies have explored a two-step transplantation procedure involving adipose tissue-derived stem cells (ASCs) to support ovarian tissue revascularization. In these studies, a two-step transplantation procedure was utilized: 2 weeks prior to ovarian tissue transplantation, the graft site (parietal peritoneum) was seeded with ASCs encapsulated in fibrin. In the first study, ovarian tissue was transplanted into the prepared graft site for 7 days [38]. The ovarian tissue/ASC group demonstrated a greater by 8.4% graft vascular area compared to the fibrin-only group (4.03%) and tissue-only group (3.78%). Additionally, the ovarian tissue/ASC group had higher PF survival rates and lower apoptotic follicle percentages. This first study thus demonstrated that the angiogenic behavior of ASCs enhanced early graft revascularization, resulting in reduced follicle apoptosis rates and increased PF survival rates.

A follow-up study examined the mechanism by which ASCs enhance graft revascularization 7 days posttransplantation [39]. This study found that ASCs encapsulated in fibrin and transplanted into the graft site prior to ovarian tissue transplantation differentiated into human endothelial cell lineages as confirmed by positive staining for CD31 and CD34 markers. The encapsulated ASCs also showed increased expression and protein secretion of vascular endothelial growth factor (VEGF) soon after ovarian tissue transplantation. As such, ASCs facilitated revascularization in the early posttransplantation period by differentiating into endothelial-like cells and secreting pro-angiogenic cues.

An additional study, also utilizing the two-step transplantation procedure of fibrin-encapsulated ASCs followed with ovarian tissue transplantation, focused on hypoxia and oxidative stress throughout 21 days posttransplantation [30]. In this study, ROS levels peaked earlier (2 days posttransplantation) compared to the control tissue transplanted without fibrin or the two-step procedure (10 days posttransplantation). Since increases in ROS levels following ischemic injury are attributed to increases in oxygen levels via restoration of oxygen supply, these findings suggest that the two-step transplantation procedure contributed to earlier graft reperfusion and a shorter hypoxic period posttransplantation. Furthermore, only the ovarian tissue/ASC group displayed mouse blood vessels within the transplanted tissue as early as 3 days posttransplantation. Quantification of vascular components revealed that at 3, 10, and 21 days posttransplantation, human ovarian endothelial area in the ovarian tissue/ASC group remained similar to non-transplanted tissue controls. The sum of these results further supports the previous findings that graft site pretreatment with fibrin-encapsulated ASCs enhanced graft revascularization, reperfusion, and reoxygenation.

A long-term study spanning 24 weeks and using the same two-step transplantation procedure found that the transplanted ovarian tissue with ASCs contained greater follicle densities compared to a control group [40]. The non-transplanted tissue had 178 follicles/mm [3], and after 24 weeks, the follicle density for the ovarian tissue/ASC group was 92 follicles/mm^3, but only 69 follicles/mm^3 in the ovarian tissue-only group. Furthermore, in the ovarian tissue/ASC group, the follicles' stage distributions were similar to non-transplanted ovarian tissue, suggesting controlled follicle activation. In the non-transplanted tissue controls, PFs contributed to 76% of all follicles present in the tissue. After 24 weeks in vivo, PFs accounted for 63% of all follicles in the ovarian tissue/ASC group, while only 20% of all follicles in the ovarian-tissue-only group were still PFs. Collectively, this series of studies demonstrated that graft site pretreatment with fibrin-encapsulated ASCs facilitated ovarian tissue revascularization, thereby reducing tissue ischemic injury and supporting long-term preservation of the PF pool.

Finally, exogenous endothelial cells (ExECs) have been explored due to their potential to facilitate anastomosis to the host vasculature. Accordingly, ExECs were co-encapsulated in fibrin with ovarian tissue and subsequently transplanted under the fascia of the gluteus maximus of ovariectomized immunodeficient female mice [41]. Two weeks posttransplantation, this approach resulted in ExECs forming functional blood vessels at the interface of the graft and host tissue, which led to increased ovarian tissue graft viability and improved follicle outcomes. Specifically, reduced tissue fibrosis, increased total follicle counts, and the development of more and larger mature follicles were noted. ExECs engineered to express anti-Müllerian hormone (AMH) contributed to preservation of the PF pool, as evidenced by a ~2-fold increase in the percentage of PFs relative to non-AMH ExEC controls. Altogether, these studies highlight the effectiveness of utilizing support cells encapsulated in a biomaterial scaffold to facilitate ovarian tissue revascularization and improve follicle outcomes.

5 Broader Applications of Biomaterials for OTCT

The biomaterials reviewed thus far represent a small subset of the biomaterials broadly available in the fields of tissue engineering and regenerative medicine. The preceding sections reviewed published applications of biomaterials utilized for human ovarian tissue xenograft revascularization. Notably, these studies have exclusively used naturally derived biomaterials, which offer high biocompatibility and inherent bioactivity but are limited by batch-to-batch variability and lack orthogonal control over mechanical and biological functionalities—factors that can hinder clinical translation. In contrast, synthetic biomaterials offer increased control and modularity, enabling precise tailoring to specific biological applications The following sections therefore explore broader biomaterial strategies found in the literature that have not explicitly been applied to human ovarian tissue transplantation but hold potential for enhancing ovarian tissue graft revascularization.

5.1 Growth Factor Delivery via Biomaterials

Delivery of pro-angiogenic growth factors (GFs) from biomaterials can enhance graft revascularization by regulating endothelial cell migration and blood vessel formation and maturation. The clinical use of exogenous GFs, however, is limited by efficacy and safety concerns [44]. Due to their short half-life, free form GFs require frequent high-dose administrations to maintain effective local concentrations, resulting in undesirable off-target side effects [45]. Instead, incorporating GFs into biomaterials enables spatial and temporal regulation of GF delivery. For example, functionalization of poly(ethylene glycol) diacrylate (PEG-DA) hydrogels with VEGF resulted in sustained release in rat models, which increased vascular density and perfusion of the hydrogel grafts [46]. A different study utilized a dextran (DEX) and PEG-DA hydrogel formulation loaded with multiple GFs, including VEGF, angiopoietin-1 (Ang-1), insulin-like growth factor (IGF), and stromal cell-derived factor-1 (SDF-1) [47]. VEGF alone caused increased vascular density 1 week after implantation of the hydrogel graft in a rat model. The combination of multiple GFs, however, had a synergistic effect with VEGF, resulting in more and larger functional blood vessels within the hydrogel graft 3 weeks postimplantation, exemplifying the potential of biomaterial-based GF delivery to facilitate ovarian tissue graft revascularization.

5.2 Heparin Functionalization for Growth Factor Sequestration in Biomaterials

Hydrogels with increased affinity for GFs can enhance biomaterial strategies intended for graft revascularization [45]. Specifically, hydrogel platforms that replicate native ECM interactions provide an alternative to complex biomaterial chemistries needed for binding and controlled release of GFs. Within the native ECM, glycosaminoglycans such as heparin dynamically regulate GF activity by sequestering and releasing GFs. Accordingly, heparin is widely used in biomaterials to sequester GFs and extend their half-life, enabling control over GF spatial and temporal activity (Fig. 7).

At the simplest level, heparin can be incorporated into hydrogels merely to sequester endogenous GFs. Tissue injury and ischemia trigger the rapid upregulation of endogenous GFs such as VEGF and platelet-derived growth factor (PDGF) in order to induce angiogenesis [44]. Graft revascularization can therefore be increased

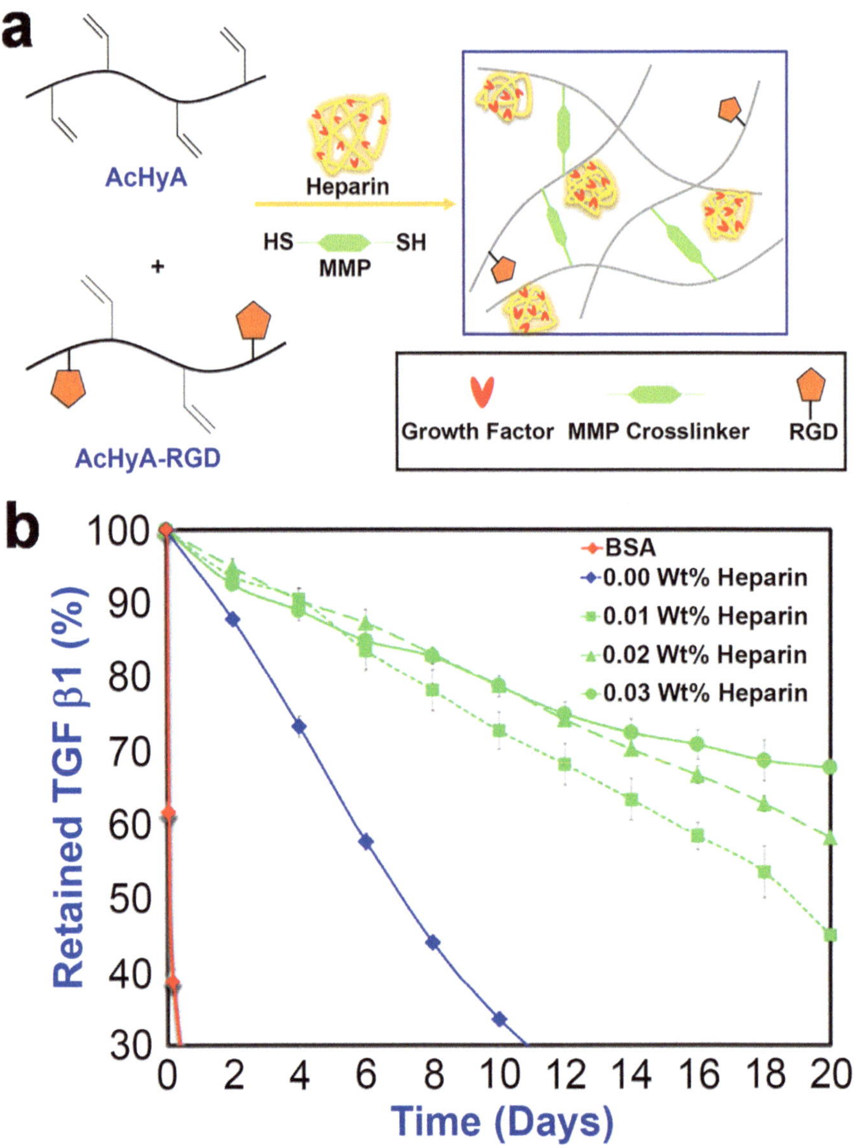

Fig. 7 Example of heparin incorporation into a biomaterial scaffold for growth factor sequestration. (**a**) Hyaluronic acid hydrogels containing an RGD peptide and heparin as a growth factor presenting agent. (**b**) Weight percentage of heparin included in the hydrogels influences growth factor (TGFβ-1) retention. (Adapted from Jha et al. [48] with permission from Elsevier. License number: 6112081357105)

by capitalizing on this innate tissue response through heparin sequestration of endogenous pro-angiogenic GFs within hydrogel scaffolds. For example, a hydrogel formed with Konjac glucomannan and heparin polysaccharides successfully sequestered locally produced endogenous GFs (VEGF, PDGF, bFGF) upon subcutaneous injection into mice [44]. The in situ sequestration of these pro-angiogenic GFs resulted in increased vascular density within the injected hydrogel.

Moreover, heparin can be used to sequester both exogenously delivered and endogenously produced GFs. For example, hyaluronic acid (HA) hydrogels were conjugated with heparin to sequester exogenous transforming growth factor beta-1 (TGFβ-1), which improved encapsulated stem cell function via heparin sequestration of endogenously produced pro-angiogenic GFs [48]. In vivo, the combination of heparin and sequestered TGFβ-1 promoted the formation of perfused vascular structures within the hydrogel graft. In a different example, porous scaffolds backfilled with a PEG hydrogel containing conjugated heparin improved in vivo revascularization of the scaffold [49]. The addition of exogenous VEGF to the scaffold via heparin sequestration resulted in a synergistic effect, further improving revascularization of the scaffold. Similarly, porous HA hydrogels loaded with VEGF through conjugated heparin resulted in increased vascular density within the HA grafts [50]. These examples highlight the synergistic potential of heparin-modified biomaterials for enhancing revascularization of ovarian tissue grafts.

5.3 *Granular Hydrogels*

Biomaterial architecture, such as porosity, is critical for efficient and unobstructed graft revascularization. Granular hydrogels—a class of "open-pore" hydrogel scaffolds composed of micron-scale hydrogels ("microgels")—have emerged as promising biomaterials for supporting endogenous tissue repair and enhancing graft revascularization (Fig. 8). Namely, microporous annealed particle (MAP) hydrogels feature secondary crosslinks between microgel subunits, which produce a uniform and interconnected cell-scale porous network that facilitates rapid cell infiltration and vascular ingrowth.

The first report of a PEG MAP hydrogel demonstrated increased vascular ingrowth and positive endothelial cell and pericyte (a capillary vessel support cell) staining in a mouse skin wound-healing model [52]. Notably, this was the first report of early (<7 days) pericyte migration into a synthetic or porous biomaterial without the use of exogenous GFs. Since then, multiple groups have investigated surgical approaches and hydrogel properties, such as microgel size and porosity, to further enhance graft revascularization. For instance, combining surgical micropuncture of host blood vessels with implants of MAP hydrogels revealed increased vascular network formation, particularly when "medium-sized" microgels (~80 μm diameter) were used as the MAP hydrogel subunits [53]. Alternatively, the use of porous

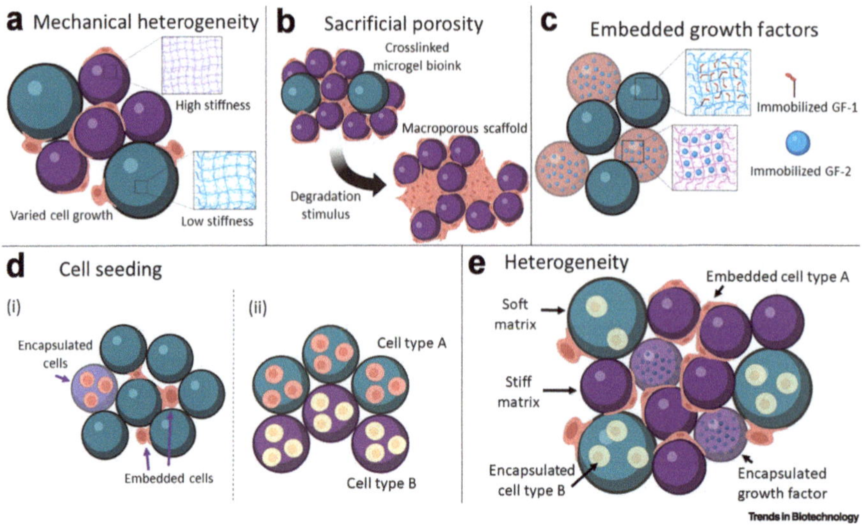

Fig. 8 Modular microgel compositions make granular hydrogels a versatile platform for graft revascularization. (**a**) Microgels with varying stiffnesses can be incorporated into a single granular hydrogel to modulate cell responses. (**b**) Sacrificial microgels can be included to increase porosity beyond the intrinsic porosity of granular hydrogels. (**c**) Microgels can be loaded with multiple bioactive factors to elicit specific cellular behaviors. (**d**) Multiple cell types can be encapsulated within individual microgels or the granular hydrogel scaffold. (**e**) The features illustrated in (**a**)–(**d**) can be combined to create complex matrices tailored to the target environment. (Adapted from Tuftee et al. [51] with permission from Elsevier. License number: 6132611085345)

microgels to introduce hierarchical porosity—created by combining the interstitial pores between MAP hydrogel microgels with additional pores within each microgel—resulted in increased endothelial cell recruitment compared to the nonporous microgel MAP scaffold, demonstrating that intraparticle porosity can further enhance graft revascularization [54].

The topographical benefits of granular hydrogels can also be combined with biofunctionalization to promote graft revascularization. Notably, the incorporation of heparin into a PEG MAP hydrogel demonstrated GF sequestration, resulting in extensive vascular ingrowth when applied in a mouse wound-healing model [55]. Additionally, a MAP hydrogel composed of PEG microgels loaded with heparin nanoparticles led to enhanced vessel formation and maturation when implanted in a mouse wound-healing model [56]. Overall, granular hydrogels can be designed to replicate ECM functions, offering both structural and biochemical cues that have the potential to enhance ovarian tissue graft revascularization.

5.4 *Oxygen-Modulating Biomaterials*

Acute hypoxia post-tissue injury initiates tissue repair mechanisms and can be utilized to drive tissue revascularization [57]. To leverage this, biomaterials that modulate oxygen to induce hypoxic conditions have been developed. For example, a hydrogel composed of gelatin and ferulic acid induced a hypoxic microenvironment in vivo, which promoted angiogenesis when injected subcutaneously into mice [58]. Similarly, gelatin microgels containing oxygen-modulating microcapsules promoted angiogenesis in a chick chorioallantoic membrane assay [59].

Alternatively, given the negative effects of prolonged ischemia and hypoxia on ovarian tissue transplantation outcomes, biomaterials can be designed to increase oxygen levels at the transplant site, thereby reducing ischemic injury. For instance, encapsulation of oxygen-releasing microspheres in a ROS-scavenging hydrogel resulted in increased vascular density in a mouse diabetic wound-healing model [60]. A different approach used ultrasound-responsive nanobubbles encapsulated in injectable microgels to deliver oxygen locally at specific times post-injury, which increased vascularization in a rat bone defect model [61]. These studies exemplify distinct but complementary oxygen-modulating biomaterial strategies that hold promise for enhancing revascularization of ovarian tissue grafts.

6 Conclusion and Future Directions

OTCT offers a life-changing advancement in treating infertility and loss of ovarian endocrine function in cancer survivors with POI. While many positive outcomes have been reported over the last two decades, OTCT continues to face limitations due to poor ovarian tissue graft revascularization and ensuing follicle loss. As discussed in this chapter, biomaterials have been employed as scaffolds for human ovarian tissue and support cells in an effort to enhance graft revascularization and mitigate follicle loss in human ovarian tissue xenograft models. These biomaterials, however, represent a small subset of the biomaterials broadly available in the fields of tissue engineering and regenerative medicine. In light of this, future biomaterial directions for human ovarian tissue transplantation could include controlled binding and release of signaling factors and hormones [44, 46–50, 62–64], granular hydrogels [52–56], and oxygen-modulating materials for spatiotemporal control of hypoxia [58–61]. These examples provide only a glimpse into the diverse biomaterial approaches available for tissue engineering and regenerative medicine, highlighting the many opportunities available to apply innovative biomaterials to OTCT (Fig. 9).

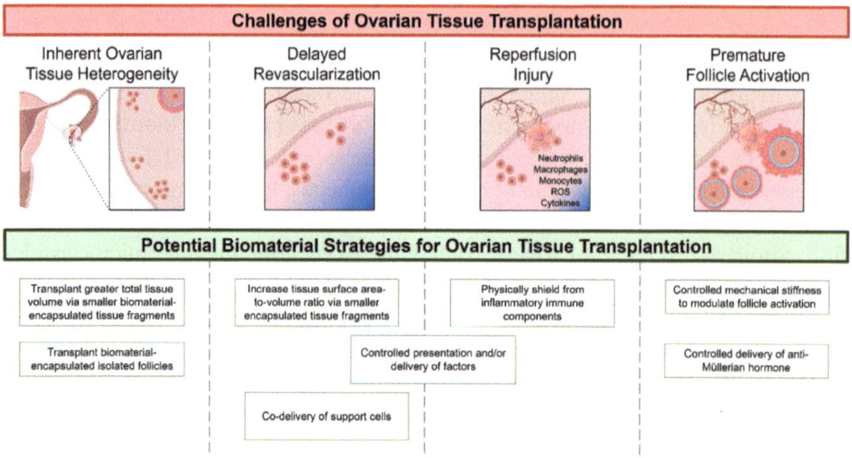

Fig. 9 Potential biomaterial strategies addressing the challenges associated with ovarian tissue transplantation. Ovarian tissue heterogeneity, particularly variations in follicle density, can be mitigated through biomaterial encapsulation. Increasing graft size may capture more follicles but exacerbates ischemic and reperfusion injury. Biomaterial encapsulation enables transplantation of greater total tissue volume as multiple smaller fragments, thereby increasing overall tissue surface area and the likelihood of implanting follicles. Alternatively, follicles isolated from ovarian tissue can be concentrated within a biomaterial scaffold to create an artificial ovary [65–68]. Delayed graft revascularization and associated ischemic injury can be further addressed by the same increase in tissue surface area and by co-delivery of support cells. Controlled presentation or delivery of pro-angiogenic, antioxidant, and immunomodulatory components can mitigate both ischemic and reperfusion injuries. Biomaterials can also shield ovarian tissue from inflammatory components during reperfusion. Finally, biomaterials can be used to prevent premature follicle activation by modulating scaffold mechanical stiffness and delivering anti-Müllerian hormone. (Created in BioRender. Pavlidis (2025). https://BioRender.com/6u4dhm8)

References

1. ESHRE, ASRM, CREWHIRL and IMS Guideline Group on POI, Panay N, Anderson RA, Bennie A, Cedars M, Davies M, Ee C, Gravholt CH, Kalantaridou S, Kallen A, Kim KQ, Misrahi M, Mousa A, Nappi RE, Rocca WA, Ruan X, Teede H, Vermeulen N, Vogt E, Vincent AJ. Evidence-based guideline: premature ovarian insufficiency. Fertil Steril. 2025;123:221–36.
2. Filippi F, Meazza C, Paffoni A, Raspagliesi F, Terenziani M, Somigliana E. Egg freezing in childhood and young adult cancer survivors. Pediatrics. 2016;138:e20160291.
3. Cattoni A, Parissone F, Porcari I, Molinari S, Masera N, Franchi M, Cesaro S, Gaudino R, Passoni P, Balduzzi A. Hormonal replacement therapy in adolescents and young women with chemo- or radio-induced premature ovarian insufficiency: practical recommendations. Blood Rev. 2021;45:100730.
4. Agarwal S, Alzahrani FA, Ahmed A. Hormone replacement therapy: would it be possible to replicate a functional ovary? Int J Mol Sci. 2018;19:3160.
5. Dolmans M-M, Manavella DD. Recent advances in fertility preservation. J Obstet Gynaecol Res. 2019;45:266–79.
6. Mercier A, Johnson J, Kallen AN. Prospective solutions to ovarian reserve damage during the ovarian tissue cryopreservation and transplantation procedure. Fertil Steril. 2024;122:565–73.

7. Zhang T, He M, Zhang J, Tong Y, Chen T, Wang C, Pan W, Xiao Z. Mechanisms of primordial follicle activation and new pregnancy opportunity for premature ovarian failure patients. Front Physiol. 2023;14:1113684.
8. Dolmans MM, von Wolff M, Poirot C, Diaz-Garcia C, Cacciottola L, Boissel N, Liebenthron J, Pellicer A, Donnez J, Andersen CY. Transplantation of cryopreserved ovarian tissue in a series of 285 women: a review of five leading European centers. Fertil Steril. 2021;115:1102–15.
9. Donnez J, Manavella DD, Dolmans M-M. Allotransplantation of human ovarian tissue. In: Donnez J, Kim SS, editors. Fertility preservation: principles and practice. Cambridge: Cambridge University Press; 2021. p. 410–9. https://doi.org/10.1017/9781108784368.037.
10. Silber SJ, Goldsmith S, Rubinoff B, Kelly E, Santos RD, Melo A, Brennan D. First successful ovarian cortex allotransplant to a turner syndrome patient requiring immunosuppression: wide implications. Fertil Steril. 2025;123:156–63.
11. Donfack NJ, Alves KA, Araújo VR, Cordova A, Figueiredo JR, Smitz J, Rodrigues APR. Expectations and limitations of ovarian tissue transplantation. Zygote. 2017;25:391–403.
12. Sönmezer M, Özkavukcu S. Chapter 14 – Surgical approach to orthotopic ovarian tissue transplantation. In: Oktay K, editor. Principles and practice of ovarian tissue cryopreservation and transplantation. Elsevier; 2022. p. 143–56. https://doi.org/10.1016/B978-0-12-823344-3.00001-7.
13. Oktay K, Economos K, Kan M, Rucinski J, Veeck L, Rosenwaks Z. Endocrine function and oocyte retrieval after autologous transplantation of ovarian cortical strips to the forearm. JAMA. 2001;286:1490–3.
14. Oktay K, Buyuk E, Veeck L, Zaninovic N, Xu K, Takeuchi T, Opsahl M, Rosenwaks Z. Embryo development after heterotopic transplantation of cryopreserved ovarian tissue. Lancet. 2004;363:837–40.
15. Xie B, Li J, Huang Y, Hang F, Hu Q, Yu J, Qin A. Assessing the impact of transplant site on ovarian tissue transplantation: a single-arm meta-analysis. Reprod Biol Endocrinol. 2023;21:120.
16. Oktay KH, Marin L. Comparison of orthotopic and heterotopic autologous ovarian tissue transplantation outcomes. Fertil Steril. 2024;121:72–9.
17. Oktay K, Babayev S. Chapter 18 – Approach to ovarian stimulation and in vitro fertilization in patients with transplanted ovarian tissue. In: Oktay K, editor. Principles and practice of ovarian tissue cryopreservation and transplantation. Elsevier; 2022. p. 185–92. https://doi.org/10.1016/B978-0-12-823344-3.00010-8.
18. Oktay K, Karlikaya G. Ovarian function after transplantation of frozen, banked autologous ovarian tissue. N Engl J Med. 2000;342:1919.
19. Khattak H, Malhas R, Craciunas L, Afifi Y, Amorim CA, Fishel S, Silber S, Gook D, Demeestere I, Bystrova O, Lisyanskaya A, Manikhas G, Lotz L, Dittrich R, Colmorn LB, Macklon KT, Hjorth IMD, Kristensen SG, Gallos I, Coomarasamy A. Fresh and cryopreserved ovarian tissue transplantation for preserving reproductive and endocrine function: a systematic review and individual patient data meta-analysis. Hum Reprod Update. 2022;28:400–16.
20. Baird DT, Webb R, Campbell BK, Harkness LM, Gosden RG. Long-term ovarian function in sheep after ovariectomy and transplantation of autografts stored at −196 C. Endocrinology. 1999;140:462–71.
21. Nisolle M, Casanas-Roux F, Qu J, Motta P, Donnez J. Histologic and ultrastructural evaluation of fresh and frozen-thawed human ovarian xenografts in nude mice. Fertil Steril. 2000;74:122–9.
22. Van Eyck AS, Jordan BF, Gallez B, Heilier JF, Van Langendonckt A, Donnez J. Electron paramagnetic resonance as a tool to evaluate human ovarian tissue reoxygenation after xenografting. Fertil Steril. 2009;92:374–81.
23. Cacciottola L, Manavella DD, Amorim CA, Donnez J, Dolmans MM. In vivo characterization of metabolic activity and oxidative stress in grafted human ovarian tissue using microdialysis. Fertil Steril. 2018;110:534–544.e3.

24. Van Eyck A-S, Bouzin C, Feron O, Romeu L, Van Langendonckt A, Donnez J, Dolmans M-M. Both host and graft vessels contribute to revascularization of xenografted human ovarian tissue in a murine model. Fertil Steril. 2010;93:1676–85.
25. So W, Dong R, Lee D, Abazarikia A, Hackfort BT, Cupp AS, Kim S-Y. Primordial follicle survival and changes in ovarian vasculature may be independently regulated during chemotherapy. Endocrinology. 2025;166:bqaf059.
26. Cacciottola L, Donnez J, Dolmans M-M. Ovarian tissue damage after grafting: systematic review of strategies to improve follicle outcomes. Reprod Biomed Online. 2021;43:351–69.
27. Cowled P, Fitridge R. Pathophysiology of reperfusion injury. In: Fitridge R, Thompson M, editors. Mechanisms of vascular disease: a reference book for vascular specialists. Adelaide: The University of Adelaide, Barr Smith Press; 2011. p. 331–50.
28. de Almeida AJPO, de Oliveira JCPL, da Silva Pontes LV, de Souza Júnior JF, Gonçalves TAF, Dantas SH, de Almeida Feitosa MS, Silva AO, de Medeiros IA. ROS: basic concepts, sources, cellular Signaling, and its implications in aging pathways. Oxidative Med Cell Longev. 2022;2022:1225578.
29. Zhang M, Liu Q, Meng H, Duan H, Liu X, Wu J, Gao F, Wang S, Tan R, Yuan J. Ischemia-reperfusion injury: molecular mechanisms and therapeutic targets. Signal Transduct Target Ther. 2024;9:12.
30. Cacciottola L, Nguyen TYT, Amorim CA, Donnez J, Dolmans M-M. Modulating hypoxia and oxidative stress in human xenografts using adipose tissue-derived stem cells. F S Sci. 2021;2: 141–52.
31. Ikhlas M, Atherton NS. Vascular reperfusion injury. Treasure Island: StatPearls Publishing; 2025.
32. Gadek LM, Joswiak C, Laronda MM. Thawing fertility: a view of ovarian tissue cryopreservation processes and review of ovarian transplant research. Fertil Steril. 2024;122:574–85.
33. Abir R, Stav D, Taieb Y, Gabbay-Benziv R, Kirshner M, Ben-Haroush A, Freud E, Ash S, Yaniv I, Herman-Edelstein M, Fisch B, Shufaro Y. Novel extra cellular-like matrices to improve human ovarian grafting. J Assist Reprod Genet. 2020;37:2105–17.
34. Magen R, Shufaro Y, Daykan Y, Oron G, Tararashkina E, Levenberg S, Anuka E, Ben-Haroush A, Fisch B, Abir R. Use of simvastatin, fibrin clots, and their combination to improve human ovarian tissue grafting for fertility restoration after anti-cancer therapy. Front Oncol. 2021;10:598026.
35. Tanaka A, Nakamura H, Tabata Y, Fujimori Y, Kumasawa K, Kimura T. Effect of sustained release of basic fibroblast growth factor using biodegradable gelatin hydrogels on frozen-thawed human ovarian tissue in a xenograft model. J Obstet Gynaecol Res. 2018;44:1947–55.
36. Xia X, Yin T, Yan J, Yan L, Jin C, Lu C, Wang T, Zhu X, Zhi X, Wang J, Tian L, Liu J, Li R, Qiao J. Mesenchymal stem cells enhance angiogenesis and follicle survival in human cryopreserved ovarian cortex transplantation. Cell Transplant. 2015;24:1999–2010.
37. Cheng J, Ruan X, Li Y, Du J, Jin F, Gu M, Zhou Q, Xu X, Yang Y, Wang H, Mueck AO. Effects of hypoxia-preconditioned HucMSCs on neovascularization and follicle survival in frozen/thawed human ovarian cortex transplanted to immunodeficient mice. Stem Cell Res Ther. 2022;13:474.
38. Manavella DD, Cacciottola L, Pommé S, Desmet CM, Jordan BF, Donnez J, Amorim CA, Dolmans MM. Two-step transplantation with adipose tissue-derived stem cells increases follicle survival by enhancing vascularization in xenografted frozen–thawed human ovarian tissue. Hum Reprod. 2018;33:1107–16.
39. Manavella DD, Cacciottola L, Payen VL, Amorim CA, Donnez J, Dolmans MM. Adipose tissue-derived stem cells boost vascularization in grafted ovarian tissue by growth factor secretion and differentiation into endothelial cell lineages. Mol Hum Reprod. 2019;25:184–93.
40. Cacciottola L, Nguyen TYT, Chiti MC, Camboni A, Amorim CA, Donnez J, Dolmans MM. Long-term advantages of ovarian reserve maintenance and follicle development using adipose tissue-derived stem cells in ovarian tissue transplantation. J Clin Med. 2020;9:1–18.

41. Man L, Park L, Bodine R, Ginsberg M, Zaninovic N, Man OA, Schattman G, Rosenwaks Z, James D. Engineered endothelium provides angiogenic and paracrine stimulus to grafted human ovarian tissue. Sci Rep. 2017;7:8203.
42. Oktay K, Bedoschi G, Pacheco F, Turan V, Emirdar V. First pregnancies, live birth, and in vitro fertilization outcomes after transplantation of frozen-banked ovarian tissue with a human extracellular matrix scaffold using robot-assisted minimally invasive surgery. Am J Obstet Gynecol. 2016;214(94):e1–94.e9.
43. Oktay K, Marin L, Bedoschi G, Pacheco F, Sugishita Y, Kawahara T, Taylan E, Acosta C, Bang H. Ovarian transplantation with robotic surgery and a neovascularizing human extracellular matrix scaffold: a case series in comparison to meta-analytic data. Fertil Steril. 2022;117:181–92.
44. Feng Y, Li Q, Wu D, Niu Y, Yang C, Dong L, Wang C. A macrophage-activating, injectable hydrogel to sequester endogenous growth factors for in situ angiogenesis. Biomaterials. 2017;134:128–42.
45. Teixeira SPB, Domingues RMA, Shevchuk M, Gomes ME, Peppas NA, Reis RL. Biomaterials for sequestration of growth factors and modulation of cell behavior. Adv Funct Mater. 2020;30: 1909011.
46. Phelps EA, Landázuri N, Thulé PM, Taylor WR, García AJ. Bioartificial matrices for therapeutic vascularization. Proc Natl Acad Sci. 2010;107:3323–8.
47. Sun G, Shen Y-I, Kusuma S, Fox-Talbot K, Steenbergen CJ, Gerecht S. Functional neovascularization of biodegradable dextran hydrogels with multiple angiogenic growth factors. Biomaterials. 2011;32:95–106.
48. Jha AK, Tharp KM, Ye J, Santiago-Ortiz JL, Jackson WM, Stahl A, Schaffer DV, Yeghiazarians Y, Healy KE. Enhanced survival and engraftment of transplanted stem cells using growth factor sequestering hydrogels. Biomaterials. 2015;47:1–12.
49. Janse van Rensburg A, Davies NH, Oosthuysen A, Chokoza C, Zilla P, Bezuidenhout D. Improved vascularization of porous scaffolds through growth factor delivery from heparinized polyethylene glycol hydrogels. Acta Biomater. 2017;49:89–100.
50. Lu D, Cai K, Zeng Z, Huang J, Ma N, Gao B, Yu S. VEGF loading heparinized hyaluronic acid macroporous hydrogels for enhanced 3D endothelial cell migration and vascularization. Biomater Adv. 2025;167:214094.
51. Tuftee C, Alsberg E, Ozbolat IT, Rizwan M. Emerging granular hydrogel bioinks to improve biological function in bioprinted constructs. Trends Biotechnol. 2024;42:339–52.
52. Griffin DR, Weaver WM, Scumpia PO, Di Carlo D, Segura T. Accelerated wound healing by injectable microporous gel scaffolds assembled from annealed building blocks. Nat Mater. 2015;14:737–44.
53. Ataie Z, Horchler S, Jaberi A, Koduru SV, El-Mallah JC, Sun M, Kheirabadi S, Kedzierski A, Risbud A, Silva ARAE, Ravnic DJ, Sheikhi A. Accelerating patterned vascularization using granular hydrogel scaffolds and surgical micropuncture. Small. 2024;20:2307928.
54. Kedzierski A, Kheirabadi S, Jaberi A, Ataie Z, Mojazza CL, Williamson ML, Hjaltason AM, Risbud A, Xiang Y, Sheikhi A. Engineering the hierarchical porosity of granular hydrogel scaffolds using porous microgels to improve cell recruitment and tissue integration. Adv Funct Mater. 2025;35:2417704.
55. Pruett LJ, Jenkins CH, Singh NS, Catallo KJ, Griffin DR. Heparin microislands in microporous annealed particle scaffolds for accelerated diabetic wound healing. Adv Funct Mater. 2021;31: 2104337.
56. Anderson AR, Caston ELP, Riley L, Nguyen L, Ntekoumes D, Gerecht S, Segura T. Engineering the microstructure and spatial bioactivity of MAP scaffolds instructs vasculogenesis in vitro and modifies vessel formation in vivo. Adv Funct Mater. 2025;35: 2400567.
57. Blatchley MR, Gerecht S. Acellular implantable and injectable hydrogels for vascular regeneration. Biomed Mater. 2015;10:034001.
58. Park KM, Gerecht S. Hypoxia-inducible hydrogels. Nat Commun. 2014;5:4075.

59. Molley TG, Jiang S, Ong L, Kopecky C, Ranaweera CD, Jalandhra GK, Milton L, Kardia E, Zhou Z, Rnjak-Kovacina J, Waters SA, Toh Y-C, Kilian KA. Gas-modulating microcapsules for spatiotemporal control of hypoxia. Proc Natl Acad Sci. 2023;120:e2217557120.
60. Guan Y, Niu H, Liu Z, Dang Y, Shen J, Zayed M, Ma L, Guan J. Sustained oxygenation accelerates diabetic wound healing by promoting epithelialization and angiogenesis and decreasing inflammation. Sci Adv. 2025;7:eabj0153.
61. Chen S, Han X, Cao Y, Yi W, Zhu Y, Ding X, Li K, Shen J, Cui W, Bai D. Spatiotemporalized hydrogel microspheres promote vascularized osteogenesis via ultrasound oxygen delivery. Adv Funct Mater. 2024;34:2308205.
62. Henry L, Labied S, Fransolet M, Kirschvink N, Blacher S, Noel A, Foidart J-M, Nisolle M, Munaut C. Isoform 165 of vascular endothelial growth factor in collagen matrix improves ovine cryopreserved ovarian tissue revascularisation after xenotransplantation in mice. Reprod Biol Endocrinol. 2015;13:12.
63. Fransolet M, Henry L, Labied S, Masereel M-C, Blacher S, Noël A, Foidart J-M, Nisolle M, Munaut C. Influence of mouse strain on ovarian tissue recovery after engraftment with angiogenic factor. J Ovarian Res. 2015;8:14.
64. Detti L, Fletcher NM, Saed GM, Sweatman TW, Uhlmann RA, Pappo A, Peregrin-Alvarez I. Xenotransplantation of pre-pubertal ovarian cortex and prevention of follicle depletion with anti-Müllerian hormone (AMH). J Assist Reprod Genet. 2018;35:1831–41.
65. Dolmans M-M, Martinez-Madrid B, Gadisseux E, Guiot Y, Yuan WY, Torre A, Camboni A, Van Langendonckt A, Donnez J. Short-term transplantation of isolated human ovarian follicles and cortical tissue into nude mice. Reproduction. 2007;134:253–62.
66. Dolmans M-M, Yuan WY, Camboni A, Torre A, Van Langendonckt A, Martinez-Madrid B, Donnez J. Development of antral follicles after xenografting of isolated small human preantral follicles. Reprod Biomed Online. 2008;16:705–11.
67. Paulini F, Vilela JMV, Chiti MC, Donnez J, Jadoul P, Dolmans M-M, Amorim CA. Survival and growth of human preantral follicles after cryopreservation of ovarian tissue, follicle isolation and short-term xenografting. Reprod Biomed Online. 2016;33:425–32.
68. Pors SE, Ramløse M, Nikiforov D, Lundsgaard K, Cheng J, Andersen CY, Kristensen SG. Initial steps in reconstruction of the human ovary: survival of pre-antral stage follicles in a decellularized human ovarian scaffold. Hum Reprod. 2019;34:1523–35.

Placenta

Biomaterials Related to the Placenta

Michelle L. Oyen

Abstract The placenta is the only human organ that is discarded when it is no longer needed. It is also the only organ that is grown from scratch for each new pregnancy, since it derives from the embryo, and is thus not genetically part of the mother's body. Its duty in providing nourishment for a growing fetus is highly specialized and short-lived. As an organ, the placenta is a key component of the interface between mother and fetus, regulating the transport of a range of atoms and molecules between two intrinsically distinct entities. Its primary role is to transport oxygen and nutrients from the mother's blood to her growing fetus and to filter waste products from the fetus's returning blood. While this intimacy enables fetal growth, it also means that undesirables in the maternal circulation may pass to the developing fetus, such as toxins or viruses. Because of its endocrine role in pregnancy, the placenta has an out-sized role in women's health in addition to being absolutely critical to the health of a developing fetus in utero. However, the human placenta remains a "black box" that is difficult to study, since there are no adequate animal models that fully capture the human placenta's structure and function and research involving pregnant women is limited. This gap in research methodologies requires the development of in vitro and in silico engineering approaches to model human placental function, utilizing engineering materials in both experimental and computational techniques. Here such biomaterials are considered in the context of organoids and tissue engineering, microphysiological systems, and for their role in computational modeling of placental function. This is a fast-growing and relatively recent field of research full of opportunities with potential to influence maternal and fetal outcomes.

Keywords Placenta · Trophoblast · Diffusion · Organoids · Microfluidics · Computational models

---

M. L. Oyen (✉)
Biomedical Engineering, Wayne State University, Detroit, MI, USA
e-mail: michelle.oyen@wayne.edu

S. G. Zambuto, M. L. Oyen (eds.), *Biomaterials for Women's Health Engineering*,
https://doi.org/10.1007/978-3-032-10745-9_12

1 Introduction

The placenta is a human's only truly disposable organ. It is treated as such an afterthought that it is normally only discussed as the "afterbirth"—the remnant tissue expelled from the body following a baby's birth. However, while the fetus is developing, the placenta performing the function of many fetal organs: while the lungs, liver, kidneys, and digestive system are all still under construction, the placenta does all of their jobs [1]. The placenta also functions as a supplement to the endocrine system of both mother and fetus and moderates immune interactions between the two. Because the placenta is fetal tissue, it is the same genetic sex as the fetus, and there are sex-related adaptations related to growth and development of both placenta and fetus that are only just beginning to be understood [2]. Overall, a successful pregnancy relies completely on the robust function of the placenta.

The placenta is responsible for transport of nutrients from mother to fetus, including oxygen, glucose, amino acids, fats, vitamins, and some immune molecules [1]. The reverse is also true, with the fetus returning carbon dioxide and urea back to the mother from the fetus. But not all nutrients that enter the placenta even reach the fetus: although estimates vary, around 50% of the oxygen and 30% of the glucose is consumed by the placenta itself, transmitting the balance to the fetus. The nutritional needs of the placenta are associated with its role as an endocrine producer, with large amounts of the steroid hormones progesterone and estrogen, as well as placental growth factor, human chorionic gonadotropin, and many others.

The placenta being a fetal tissue, it is fascinating that it creates hormones that circulate through the mother's body. Some problems in pregnancy are specifically placentally mediated, such as preeclampsia. In severe cases, induction or C-section is used prior to full-term gestation to save the life and health of the mother. Further, pregnancy has multigenerational effects, in that fetuses of either sex exposed to preeclampsia in pregnancy have greater risks of cardiovascular disease later in life [3]. For this reason, problems in pregnancy should be thought of as an issue of human health, not just female health specifically. Before we can consider the mature placenta's function and lack of function in later stages of pregnancy, we must first examine its origins and early development and examine how human placentation differs from that found in other mammals.

2 The Early Placenta

The placenta tissue itself is of embryonic origin. Following fertilization, the fertilized egg, or zygote (Fig. 1), begins to divide while remaining approximately the same size. Following the morula (16 to 32 cells) stage, the dividing embryo switches from a solid ball of cells to a hollow blastocyst (Fig. 1) and cell differentiation begins.

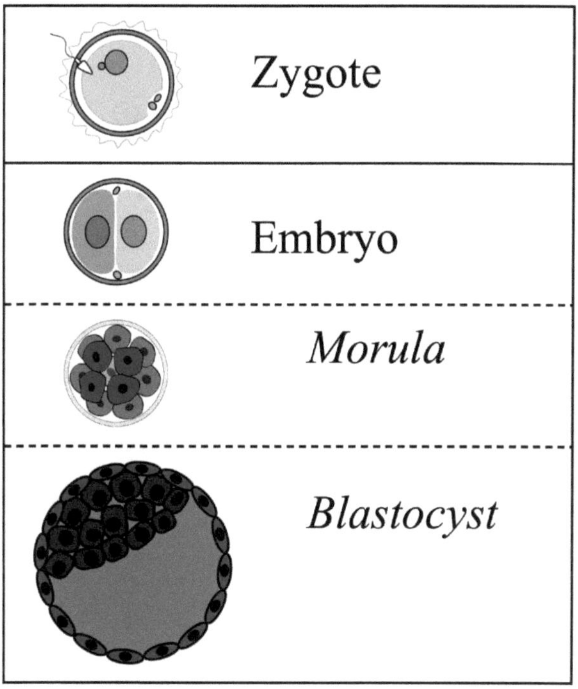

Fig. 1 A schematic illustration of a fertilized egg, or zygote, dividing into an embryo. There are many stages of embryonic development, including the morula (16 to 32 cells in a solid ball) and the hollow blastocyst, which hatches out of the zona pellucida prior to implantation

The placenta derives in part from the earliest differentiated cells at the blastocyst stage (5–6 days after fertilization), which separate into multiple cell types even prior to implantation (8–10 days after fertilization) (Fig. 2). The very first cell differentiation events in the blastocyst result in trophectoderm (future placenta) and inner cell mass (future fetus) (Fig. 2). The blastocyst is about 0.1 mm in diameter and only 100–200 individual cells at this stage.

As implantation occurs in three distinct stages (apposition, attachment, and invasion), cell differentiation continues. Figure 3 shows the postimplantation embryo. The decidual epithelium is closing back around the implanted embryo. The trophectoderm layer is differentiating into different trophoblast types, including the primitive syncytium and the invasive extravillus trophoblast.

During the first trimester of pregnancy, there is significantly more growth in the placenta than in the embryo. At the fourth month of pregnancy, (p.m.), the fetus overtakes the placenta in both linear dimension and weight [1], and for the remainder of pregnancy, the fetus's growth substantially outpaces that of the placenta. As the placenta continues to develop and grow, a complex network of vascular branches, known as villous trees, start to develop. The villous trees are characterized as mesenchymal, stem, intermediate, and terminal villi, where the mesenchymal villi give rise to the other three types as differentiation continues. Stem villi are like the tree trunks, intermediate villi resemble tree branches, and the terminal villi resemble the leaves at the tips of tree branches. The terminal villi are the critical component for

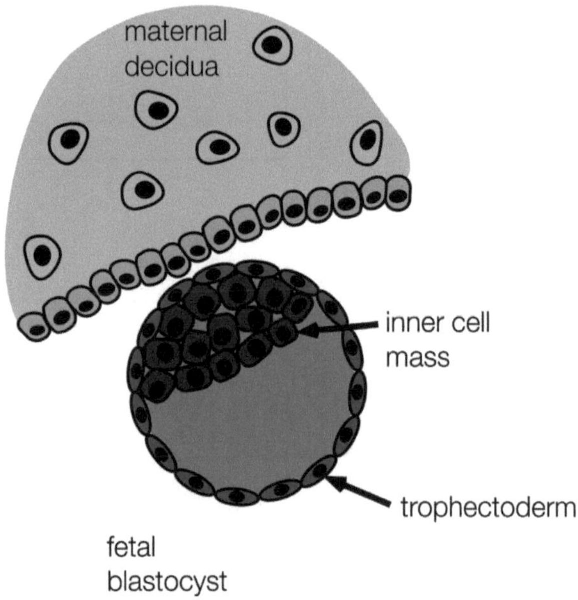

Fig. 2 A schematic illustration of a blastocyst immediately prior to implantation. The trophectoderm layer has differentiated from the inner cell mass, which will become the embryo proper and later the fetus. These first differentiation events have happened prior to implantation

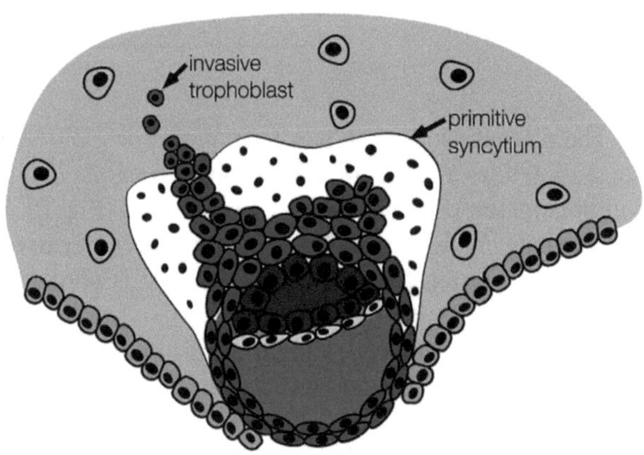

Fig. 3 A schematic illustration of a postimplantation blastocyst, with further differentiation of the trophoblastic cell lineages into the primitive syncytium and the invasive extravillus trophoblast

exchange of nutrients and waste between mother and embryo and are a complete and complex network by the third trimester of pregnancy.

3 The Mature Placenta

As the villous tree structures grow, the surface area available for gas and molecule exchange increases, while the distance between the maternal and fetal blood decreases [4]. The total length of fetal vasculature at term is over 500 km long and the total surface area for exchange is over 14 square meters, packed into a placenta with diameter about 20 cm and thickness about 5 cm [4]. The fetal circulation is closed, from the fetus via the umbilical cord and through the placental circulation. The maternal circulation is open, with blood emerging from the spiral arteries and taken back up by the uterine draining veins. This open-circuit maternal blood-flow arrangement is not found in most other animals and presents a particular risk to human women of hemorrhage at the maternal-placental interface either during pregnancy or following birth.

The normal third-trimester placenta has a fully formed and sophisticated interface between the open maternal circulation and the closed fetal circulation at the placental terminal villi (Fig. 4, inset). In these villi, oxygen and nutrients are transported from the maternal open circulation, which pools blood in the intervillous space (Fig. 4), to the fetus across the trophoblastic tissue layer. Placental oxygen transport occurs passively and can be described as a six-step process [5], in which the oxygen (1) dissociates from maternal red blood cells, (2) diffuses through maternal plasma, (3) diffuses across the trophoblastic epithelium, (4) diffuses across the basal lamina, villus stroma, and endothelium, (5) diffuses through fetal plasma, and finally (6) binds to the hemoglobin (Hb) of fetal erythrocytes. Steps (3) and (4) in this sequence are often combined and the composite tissue classed as the "villous membrane" [5] (Fig. 4).

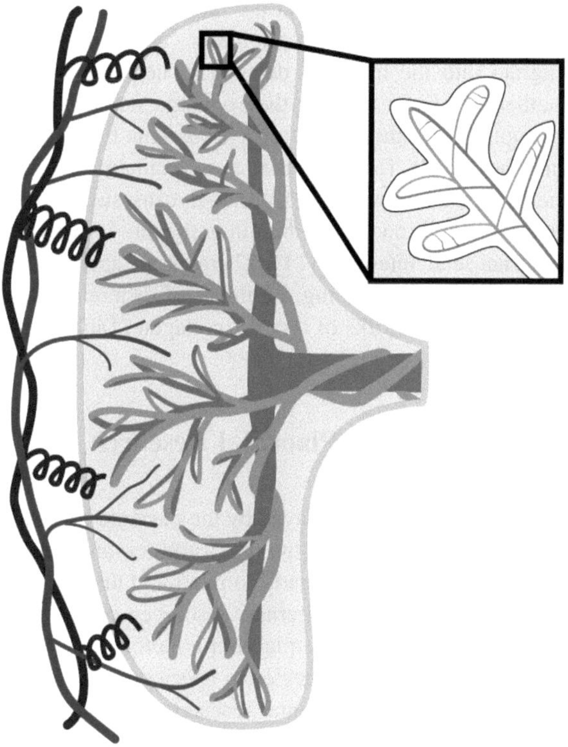

Fig. 4 A schematic illustration of a mature placenta, with open-loop maternal uterine vasculature (left), closed-loop fetal placental vasculature (center), and a zoomed-in view of a terminal villus tree (right)

Table 1 Extracellular matrix (ECM) collagen types I, III, IV, and VI molecules in the placenta and adjacent maternal uterine decidua (adapted from [12])

		Col I	Col III	Col IV	Col VI
Decidua basalis	Stroma	++	++	+++	++
(maternal)	Vessel wall	+	+	++	+
	Myometrium	+	+	+	+
Placenta	Villous core	+	+	+	+
(fetal)	Fetal vessel wall	+	+	+	+
	Basement membrane	–	–	+	+
	Cell column	–	–	+	–

Fetal hemoglobin is different from adult hemoglobin [6] and is produced during pregnancy and until a baby is a few months old—there is stronger binding of oxygen to the fetal hemoglobin than to the adult version, and that adds additionally to the transport of oxygen from maternal blood to fetal blood [7]. In contrast to oxygen transport, which is mostly passive and dominated by blood flow, transport of glucose and amino acids from mother to fetus relies on transporter proteins and is significantly affected by placental uptake of the nutrients [8]. Recent works have included computational models for more detailed placental transport kinetic studies of oxygen and solutes [9] and for quantifying the balance between transport and tissue metabolism [10].

The cells of the placenta are largely trophoblastic, including cytotrophoblasts, multinucleated syncytiotrophoblasts, and extra-villous trophoblasts. The latter migrate into the maternal decidua to help prepare the vascular structures of the mother's body for creating the exchange surface with the fetal placenta. In addition to trophoblasts, the placenta itself contains fibroblasts, immune cells, and vascular endothelial cells for lining the fetal vasculature. The extracellular matrix (ECM) of the placenta includes small proteoglycans such as decorin, with proteins such as laminin and fibronectin—laminin in the interior villi and fibronectin dominant at the maternal-fetal interface [11]. There is an abundance of collagen proteins in the placental ECM, including a number of different collagen types but notably three-dimensional networks of type IV collagen (Table 1, [12]).

4 Challenges in Placental Research

Despite the crucial role played by the placenta in pregnancy, much of the placenta's development in vivo is in the first trimester, and largely inaccessible to researchers. Our understanding of the early formation of the human placenta is extremely limited, and we have to locate alternative sources of information to understand placental development. The human placenta is notoriously difficult to study since placentas vary a great deal from species to species within mammals. There is thus no good "animal model" for placental research, and this is related to the wide variety of reproductive strategies found in mammals.

While all mammals share some physiological features in common, there are three distinct categories: monotremes, marsupials, and placental mammals. Only the placental mammals carry their offspring inside their bodies for the entirety of development. The fundamental function of the placenta requires the maternal blood supply to come close to the fetal blood to allow for exchange of gases, nutrients, and waste products between the mother and her progeny. Somewhat surprisingly, this identical function has not resulted in identical shapes and relative sizes of placentas across the placental mammals [13]. The placentas of different mammal species are surprisingly different in tissue distribution (one organ or many connected small ones) and geometry (a disc versus a belt when it is one organ, Fig. 5). Diffuse (horses and pigs) and cotyledonary (cows and sheep) placentation types have many different foci of exchange, or places where nutrients are passed, throughout the gestational sac, whereas the zonary (cats and dogs) and discoid (mice and humans) geometries are more concentrated in one location.

In addition to the placentas from different mammalian species being macroscopically different, the layers of tissue between the mother and fetus vary from species to

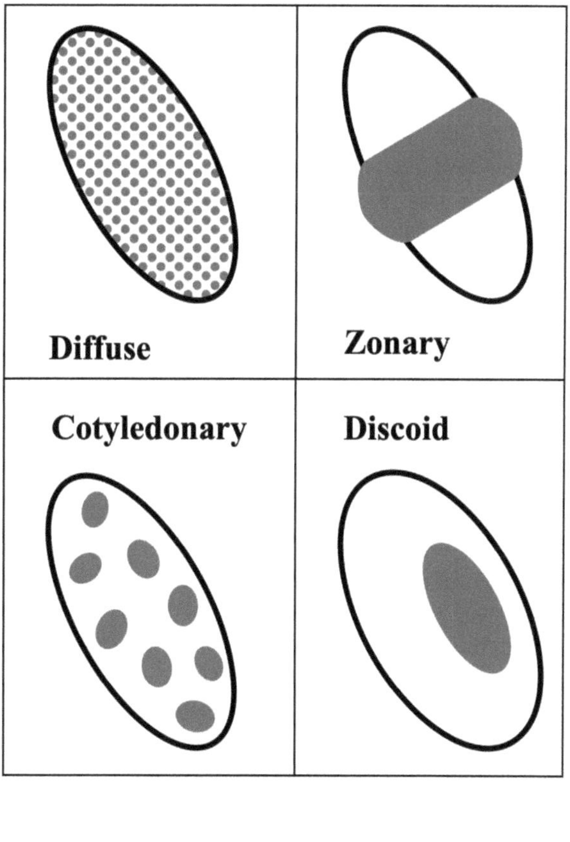

Fig. 5 A schematic illustration of the four primary macroscopic placenta shapes: diffuse, zonary, cotyledonary, and discoid

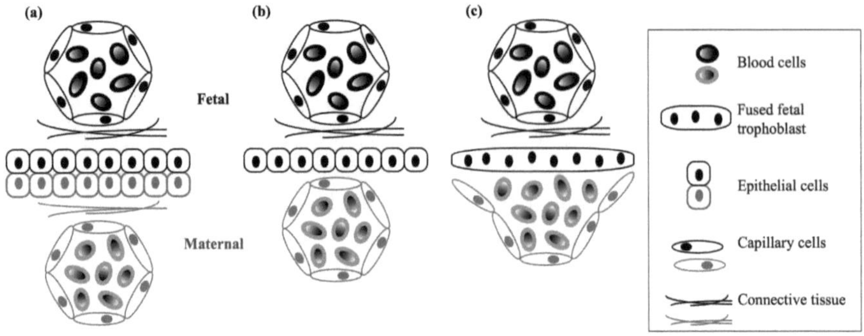

Fig. 6 A schematic illustration of (**a**) epitheliochorial, (**b**) endotheliochorial, and (**c**) hemochorial placentation

species [13]. Three different common examples of the many possible different arrangements are shown in Fig. 6, including for (Fig. 6a) epitheliochorial placentation, as in cows and pigs, and (Fig. 6b) endotheliochorial placentation, as in dogs and cats. Human placentation is hemochorial (Fig. 6c), the arrangement in which the fetal and maternal blood cells are in the closest proximity.

Figure 6c also demonstrates how the maternal circulation is open, in that blood cells are released from being contained within blood vessels. The surprising adaptation of open-loop blood circulation in the maternal uterus is pregnancy specific. The maternal circulation switches from closed in normal human physiology to open during the late first trimester of human pregnancy. The blood vessels near the placenta are remodeled by the fetal extravillous trophoblast cells, opening up their outlets into conical forms to increase flow to the placenta at decreased resistance. The blood leaves the arteries, pools on the fetal trophoblastic surface of the placenta, and is taken back up by maternal draining veins. The transport of oxygen from mother to fetus thus occurs from the maternal blood pool across the terminal villi of the placenta into the closed circulation of the fetal capillaries.

5 The Need for Placental Models

A significant fraction of preterm births is associated with pathologies of the placenta, as opposed to being of direct maternal or fetal origin [14]. In severe cases of maternal hypertension, medically indicated preterm births are initiated for the express purpose of removing the placenta to preserve the mother's life. Failures of early placentation are associated with the "great obstetrical syndromes" of preeclampsia (PE), fetal growth restriction (FGR), placental abruption, preterm labor, and stillbirth [15]. Although some knowledge exists about how insufficient trophoblast invasion in the first trimester leads to deficient spiral artery remodeling, the process of early human placental development in health and disease has been very difficult to study.

One method we have for understanding early pregnancy is to look at tissue samples from pregnant hysterectomies (surgical removal of the uterus), of which a large series of specimens was collected in the 1950s (and for which some images are available online [16]). These samples came about because the uterus was removed when no one was aware that the woman was pregnant, since simple pregnancy tests only arose in the 1960s. The hysterectomy images are excellent anatomical sources, but both rare and single-time glimpses of placental development.

This failure of trophoblast invasion has led to an interest in studying the process from a cellular biomechanics perspective [17]. The opposite case, of trophoblast invasion that is too deep instead of too shallow, is related to the trophoblastic cancer choriocarcinoma [18], which spreads easily from the uterus to the lungs. Although invasion of the uterus by trophoblast cells plays a critical role in reproductive outcome, limited understanding of the mechanisms controlling trophoblast invasion remains an obstacle to progress in pregnancy research.

The investigation of early-pregnancy development of the placenta was once limited by local governmental restrictions regarding the research use of embryonic stem cells. However, recent developments have led to multiple new approaches for placental research. Newer trophoblastic cell lines (Swan 71, ED27 and HTR-8/SVneo) have been developed from normal tissue, an improvement on earlier cell lines (JEG-3, JAR, BeWo) that were derived from choriocarcinomas. Both human-induced pluripotent stem cells (iPSCs) [19] and trophoblast stem cells [20] have now been leveraged to expand the cell sources available for placental research; further discussion of cell characteristics is beyond the scope of the current work since the focus here is on the enabling biomaterials that allow for three-dimensional cell studies in vitro.

Another enabling technology that has changed placental research in vitro has been the development of increasingly complex and tunable hydrogel materials. Hydrogels are known for their biological compatibility due to their large water content. Their fine structure can be tailored using chemical or physical chain entanglements in a variety of manners, some of which are shown schematically in Fig. 7. The schematic illustrations are for single-network-type hydrogels, but the addition of multiple chain types and different crosslinking mechanisms can make the hydrogels increasingly complex in underlying structure. This allows for incredible tuning of physical properties, such as pore size, and the corresponding properties of elasticity and viscosity and movement of fluid through the porous structure [21].

Despite the broad spectrum of clinical complications of pregnancy as presented above, the human placenta's early development remains something of an enigma. Bioengineering techniques for placental investigation are divided into three categories: (1) tissue engineering and organoids; (2) microfluidic devices; (3) computational modeling studies across length scales. Each of these will be considered specifically in the context of biomaterials as an enabling technology.

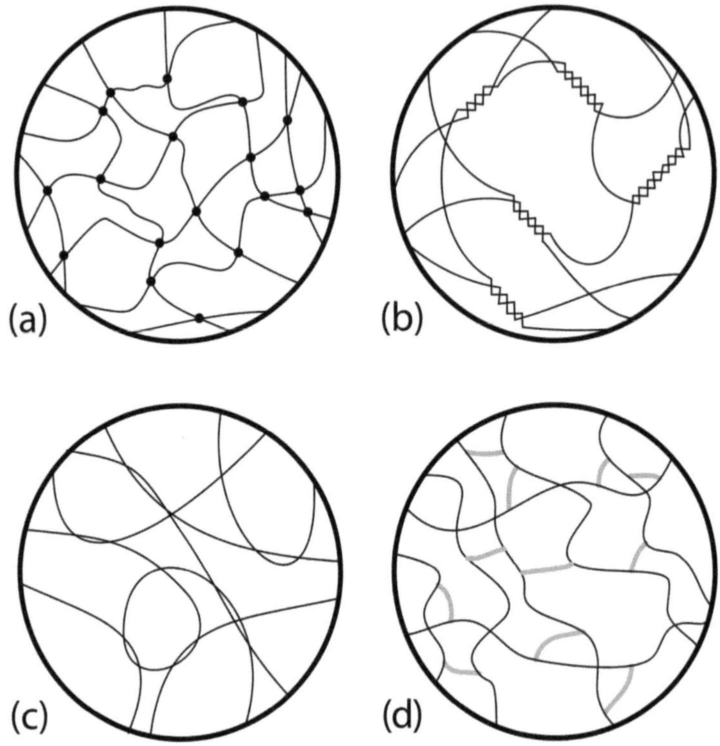

Fig. 7 A schematic illustration of (**a**) chemically point-crosslinked hydrogel, (**b**) gelatin hydrogel with helical crosslinks, (**c**) physically entangled hydrogel, and (**d**) methacrylated gelatin hydrogel

6 Organoids and Biomimetic Tissue Engineering

Organoids are used to try and replicate the stages of organogenesis in a dish. They typically are comprised of stem cells or stem-derived cells with some amount of artificial extracellular matrix in the form of a hydrogel. Many of these protocols have used the commercial hydrogel Matrigel (or its similar competitor Geltrex), derived from mouse tumor cells and recognized for its batch variability. Placental organoid models [22] have largely used Matrigel, which contains large amounts of collagen type IV, laminin, entactin, and heparan sulfate proteoglycan. This is useful for trophoblast studies, since placenta shares with this hydrogel formulation a large component of type IV collagen. However, since it is biologically derived, the lack of repeatability in the composition and physical properties [23] of Matrigel have limited the interpretability of results from such approaches.

Efforts to engineer a more controlled artificial ECM for placental (and other tissue) research have been plentiful in the last decade. Alternatives that have been used in reproductive research include synthetic polyethylene glycol(PEG)-based systems [24] and gelatin methacryloyl-based materials [25, 26]. However, there is much opportunity for optimizing a placenta-specific hydrogel matrix for tuning both chemical and mechanical cues to cells in a spatio-temporally controlled manner. The presence of collagen type IV could be important (Table 1) and related to the success of Matrigel and related biologically derived matrices to date. In addition to improving hydrogels for three-dimensional (3D) cell culture support, added complexity in placental organoids has been achieved through co-culture with different cell lineages, including those of the maternal uterine decidua for studying early development. However, careful consideration of the cell types is critical, since the older choriocarcinoma cell lines are poorly suited for generating functional organoids that truly mimic placental morphogenesis. There have also been challenges with placental organoids, in particular the fact that early versions using Matrigel were "inside out," with syncytiotrophoblast-like cells on the interior. New approaches have used collagen-coated beads in suspension culture to make a more realistic placenta-like architecture (Fig. 8) [27].

The repeatability of studies based on organoid, tissue engineering, or hybrid approaches using biomimicking hydrogels is an ongoing question that requires further research if these approaches are to substantially impact our understanding of the placenta. A consideration with hydrogel-based studies is the biomaterial's mechanical properties, including stiffness, time-dependent deformation, and physical pore size, and how these properties compare with the native placental tissue. Such properties of placenta have not been measured much in the past, although recent approaches using placental nanoindentation have shown promise [28]. Abbas et al. [23] examined Matrigel and quantified its batch-to-batch stiffness variability also using nanoindentation and found its variation consistent with its having a non-reproducible composition. Ideally, a trophoblast hydrogel biomaterial growth environment would include both the necessary chemical and biomechanical cues for cell differentiation and villus formation. Overall, the biomechanical properties of the uterus [29] and placenta [28] have been studied very little compared with other

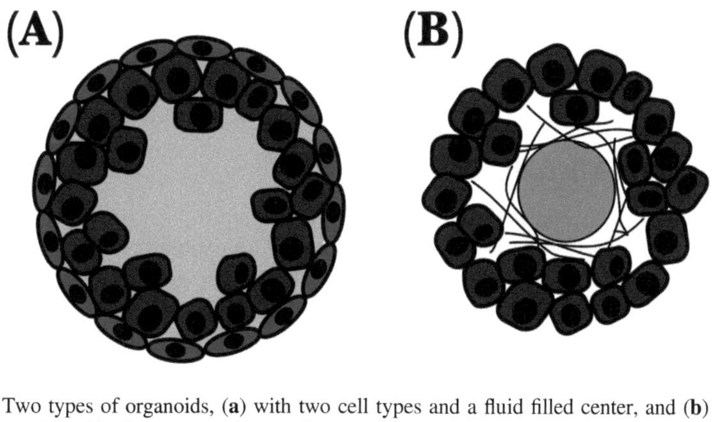

Fig. 8 Two types of organoids, (**a**) with two cell types and a fluid filled center, and (**b**) with an ECM-coated bead in the center and one cell type. After [27]

human tissues, and this presents another research opportunity that will enhance the use of in vitro approaches for placental biomaterials research.

In addition to considerations of homogeneous hydrogels, recent efforts have examined structured biomaterials with relevance to the placenta. Trophoblast fusion was interrogated using micro-patterned surfaces [30]. Three-dimensional bioprinting has recently been used to generate biomimetic methacrylated gelatin membranes designed to improve this technique with a more cell-friendly environment for creating placental-type barriers [31]. Bioprinting has been increasingly popular for making placenta models [32–34]. Similar gelatin-based materials and 3D printing techniques have been used to develop a trophoblast invasion assay based on concentric rings of cell- and growth-factor chemoattractant loaded hydrogel in a truly 3D system without a membrane barrier [35]. Comparisons have been made between bioprinted PEG materials and Matrigel with differences in trophoblast differentiation depending on the matrix [34], demonstrating how important the selection of biomaterials is in this field.

Tissue engineering approaches tend to focus more on the ECM components and their structure and organization as well as physical properties relevant to organ function. Tissue engineering of the placenta is quite sensibly more focused on improved development of in vitro models and not yet in developing an artificial placenta for organ replacement in vivo. In fact, many studies related to tissue engineering of the placenta use decellularization and dehydration of the tissue to produce a naturally derived ECM for use in other applications [36, 37], since the placenta itself is frequently discarded and therefore available for other uses post-birth. Some quite complex materials have been produced for bioprinting that were composites of silk, gelatin, and placental extracts [38].

That said, Gargus et al. [39] presented a thorough review of tissue engineering approaches for both male and female reproductive tissues, including uterus and placenta. The primary focus was on tissue transplantation, with some discussion of drug delivery and even the fetus's futuristic ex vivo development. This demonstrates the potential for future tissue engineering approaches that go well beyond what is currently being done in research with nearer-term goals. That said, the recapitulation of functional placental tissue has also been popular in the domain of microfluidics approaches and will be discussed in the next section below.

7 Placental Microfluidic Devices

Recently, several approaches have been considered for examining the placenta in the context of a "placenta-on-a-chip" framework. The chip devices, increasingly known as microphysiological systems, allow for physiological fluid flow, clearly relevant in a placenta context. While polydimethylsiloxane (PDMS) is the most commonly used material in microfluidic devices [40], other polymers or hydrogels [41] could also serve as functional materials. The excitement about a potential placenta-on-a-chip is related not just to the placenta's research importance but also to the lack of existing in vitro models for studying its functions. Because of the complexities of obtaining and culturing relevant cell types, microfluidic devices are favored as they allow for experiments using small cell numbers.

The mechanics of trophoblast migration have been investigated in a PDMS chip with a central hydrogel chamber [17]. The assay was adapted from a common approach to study cancer metastasis [42]. Cells were seeded in a central hydrogel-filled channel and exposed to a chemical gradient established across the hydrogel, and trophoblast migration (outside the ultrasound (US), using primary cells) was assessed in response to a gradient of the uterine chemoattractant granulocyte-macrophage colony-stimulating factor (GM-CSF, Fig. 9). This is important as there are questions surrounding whether the invasive nature of the many different trophoblast-like cell lines is diminished relative to primary cells.

Microfluidic approaches have also shown potential in devices that consider the placenta's critical barrier function between mother and fetus [43]. These types of studies have been focused on drug transport or environmental contaminants that can be transmitted across the placental barrier. Such approaches have been reviewed [44], and it is clear that there are substantial advantage for these in vitro strategies for testing pharmaceutical agents and microorganisms and their transport across the placental barrier to the fetus, given the limitations of animal models in human pregnancy

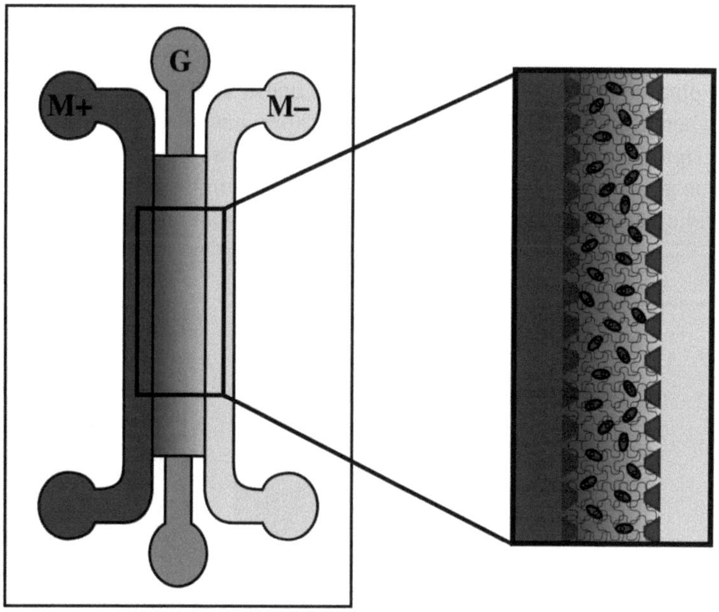

Fig. 9 A trophoblast invasion assay where primary cells were placed in Matrigel in the central chamber (G, zoom), and media was flowed on each side channel with (M+) and without (M−) a chemoattractant molecule of interest, here GM-CSF [17]

All of the in vitro models considered here have advanced placental research dramatically in just the last five years. However, in parallel, there has been significant growth in the study of computational models of the placenta in silico, taking research out of the wet lab and into the bioengineering modeling domain.

8 Computational Placenta Models

Pregnancy is an excellent case for the use of computational modeling in cases where experiments are challenging [45], or in combination with experiments. The placenta has been the focus of recent biomechanical models across a wide range of length scales, demonstrating the potential for computational modeling in understanding placental pathology and placenta-related clinical conditions. The development of new computational approaches for investigations of the placenta's fundamental functions, such as blood flow, shear stress, and oxygen diffusion, have been the subject of recent scientific meetings [46] and review papers [47–49]. In addition to baseline models of normal placental function, recent works have used computer-generated models to examine altered placental structure and oxygen transport in clinical conditions such as FGR [50]. Recent approaches to collecting geometrical representations of placentas for modeling purposes have included two-dimensional placental cross-section scans [51], 3D confocal laser scanning image stacks [52, 53], 3D micro-computed tomography (microCT) images utilizing polymer casts [54], optical coherence tomography (OCT) [28], and even synchotron imaging [55].

However, a significant challenge associated with all of these geometrically accurate placental computational models is the question of experimental validation. This is where a combined computational and experimental approach with biomaterials has significant potential. For example, Fig. 10 shows a schematic simulation of a diffusion gradient across three different hydrogels as in the central chamber of the microfluidic device shown above in Fig. 7. (Real simulations appear in [17].) The

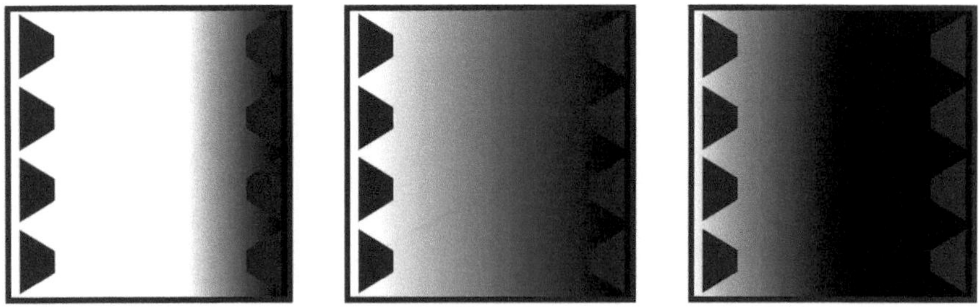

Fig. 10 A schematic simulation of three different hydrogels from the center channel of the device in Fig. 7, where the diffusion gradient established in the hydrogel chamber depends on the pore size and hydraulic permeability of three different hydrogel formulations. Inspired by Abbas et al. [17]

difference in hydrogel parameters, such as pore size and hydraulic permeability, would give rise to three different diffusion gradients, which may be expected to affect trophoblast cell migration differently. Another approach is to 3D print upscaled models of experimental geometries and match the Reynolds numbers to allow for macroscopic experiments associated with microscopic computational models, as was done by Plitman Mayo et al. for examining placental capillary blood flow [53]. Either way, the combination of experiments and simulations, enhanced with knowledge of relevant biomaterials, provides a new direction for placental research that should expand the capabilities of modeling or experiments on their own independently.

9 Conclusion

Biomaterials approaches to the study of the placenta are a relatively new field, with most of the work discussed herein happening within the last decade. All three primary fields here, organoids and tissue engineering, microfluidic devices, and computational models, involve a significant element of biomaterials research and development opportunity. As discussed in the review of placental development and structure, the organ is critical to pregnancy but not static, as it grows and develops from even before implantation through to the end of pregnancy. In humans, it is largely available to study easily only in its final form immediately following birth, and by that time it is a very different entity than in its formative stages. Animal experimentation is essentially useless when it comes to the human placenta, since its structure and relationship with the mother are completely different than in other mammals. Deepening our understanding of the earliest stages of pregnancy can thus only be accomplished through alternative and creative methods that include biomaterials and other bioengineering techniques. Given the large scale of the challenges with having a successful pregnancy—high rates of pregnancy loss including miscarriage and stillbirth and also significant morbidity and mortality associated with high rates of preterm birth—there is much to be gained and learned here through scientific and engineering examination of the human placenta via biomaterials.

Conflicts of Interest There are no conflicts of interest to declare.

References

1. Baergen RN, Burton GJ, Kaplan CG. editors. Benirschke's pathology of the human placenta. 7th ed. Cham: Springer; 2022. 939 pp.
2. Meakin AS, Cuffe JSM, Darby JRT, Morrison JL, Clifton VL. Int J Mol Sci. 2021;22:6386.

3. Paramsothy A, Hegvik T-A, Engeland A, Bjørge T, Egeland GM, Klungsøyr K. Hypertension. 2023;80. https://doi.org/10.1161/hypertensionaha.122.20682.
4. Gonzalez-Ortiz M. Advances in maternal-fetal biomedicine, cellular and molecular mechanisms of pregnancy pathologies. 1st ed. Advances in experimental medicine and biology series, vol. 1428. Description based on publisher supplied metadata and other sources. Cham: Springer International Publishing AG; 2023. 1315 pp.
5. Mayhew T. Ann Anat Anatomis Anzeiger. 2014;196:34–40.
6. Khandros E, Blobel GA. Blood. 2024;144:845–52.
7. Houben NAM, Lopriore E. Pediatr Res. 2024;97:1767–8.
8. Bell A, Hay W, Ehrhardt R. Bioscient Proc. 1999;54:401–10.
9. Erlich A, Pearce P, Mayo R, Jensen, O, Chernyavsky I. Sci Adv. 2019;5:6326.
10. Lewis R, Cleal J, Sengers B. Placenta. 2020;93:43–8.
11. Natale BV, Kotadia R, Gustin K, Harihara A, Min S, Kreisman MJ, Breen KM, Natale DR. Stem Cells Develop. 2023;32:622–37.
12. Oefner C, Sharkey A, Gardner L, Critchley H, Oyen M, Moffett A. Placenta. 2015;36:59–68.
13. Moffett A, Loke C. Nat Rev Immunol. 2006;6:584–94.
14. Villar J, Papageorghiou A, Knight H, Gravett M, Iams J, Waller S, Kramer M, Culhane J, Barros F, Conde-Agudelo A, Bhutta Z, Goldenberg R. Am J Obstetr Gynecol. 2012;206:119–23.
15. Brosens I, Pijnenborg R, Vercruysse L, Romero R. Am J Obstetr Gynecol. 2011;204:193–201.
16. http://www.trophoblast.cam.ac.uk/Resources/boyd-collection
17. Abbas Y, Oefner C, Polacheck W, Gardner L, Farrell L, Sharkey A, Kamm R, Moffett A, Oyen M. J R Soc Inter. 2017;14:20170131.
18. Jiao L, Ghorani E, Sebire N, Seckl M. Gynecol Oncol. 2016;141:624–31.
19. Dong C, Theunissen TW. In: Human Naïve Pluripotent Stem Cells. Berlin: Springer US; 2021. p. 91–104.
20. Okae H, Toh H, Sato T, Hiura H, Takahashi S, Shirane K, Kabayama Y, Suyama M, Sasaki H, Arima T. Cell Stem Cell. 2018;22:50–63.e6.
21. Oyen ML. Int Mater Rev. 2013;59:44–59.
22. Turco M, et al. Nature. 2018;564:263–7.
23. Abbas Y, Carnicer-Lombarte A, Gardner L, Thomas J, Brosens J, Moffett A, Sharkey A, Franze K, Burton G, Oyen M. Hum Reprod. 1999;34:1999–2008.
24. Slaby EM, Plaisier SB, Brady SR, Hiremath SC, Weaver JD. Biomater Sci. 2024;12:933–48.
25. Zambuto S, Clancy K, Harley B. Interf Focus. 2019;9. https://doi.org/10.1101/548024.
26. Zambuto SG, Kolluru SS, Harley BA, Oyen ML. Placenta. 2024;157:67–75.
27. Zhou J, Sheridan M, Tian Y, Dahlgren K, Messler M, Peng T, Zhao A, Ezashi T, Schulz L, Ulery B, Roberts R, Schust D. iScience. 2025;28:112099.
28. Scott AK, Fodera DM, Yang P, Arter A, Hines AM, Kolluru SS, Zambuto SG, Myers KM, Kamilov US, Odibo AO, Oyen ML. Placenta. 2025;166:154–63.
29. Fodera DM, Russell SR, Jackson JL, Fang S, Chen X, Vink J, Oyen ML, Myers KM. J Mech Behav Biomed Mater. 2024;151:106348.
30. Ma Z, Sagrillo-Fagundes L, Tran R, Parameshwar P, Kalashnikov N, Vaillancourt C, Moraes C. ACS Appl Mater Interf. 2020. https://doi.org/10.1021/acsami.9b.19906.
31. Kreuder A-E, Bolanos-Rosales A, Palmer C, Thomas A, Geiger M-A, Lam T, Amler A-K, Markert U, Lauster R, Kloke L. Scient Rep. 2020;10:15606.
32. Kuo C-Y, Eranki A, Placone J, Rhodes K, Aranda-Espinoza H, Fernandes R, Fisher J, Kim P. ACS Biomater Sci Eng. 2016;2:1817–26.
33. Kuo C-y, Guo T, Cabrera-luque J, Arumugasaamy N, Bracaglia L, Garcia-vivas A, Santoro M, Baker H, Fisher J, Kim P. J Biomed Mater Res Part A. 2018;106:1476–87.
34. Richards C, Chen H, O'Rourke M, Bannister, A, Owen G, Volkerling A, Ghosh A, Gorrie, CA, Gallego-Ortega D, Bottomley AL, Padula MP, McGrath KC, Cole L, Hansbro PM, McClements L. Nat Commun. 2025;16. https://doi.org/10.1038/s41467-025-62996-0.
35. Ding H, Illsley N, Chang R. Scient Rep. 2019;9:18854.

36. Rameshbabu A, Ghosh P, Subramani E, Bankoti K, Kapat K, Datta S, Maity P, Subramanian B, Roy S, Chaudhury K, Dhara S. J Mater Chem B. 2016;4:613–25.
37. Roy A, Mantay M, Brannan C, Griffiths S. BioMed Res Int. 2022;2022. https://doi.org/10.1155/2022/6751456.
38. Schneider KH, et al. Biomater Res. 2023;27. https://doi.org/10.1186/s40824-023-00431-5.
39. Gargus E, Rogers H, Mckinnon K, Edmonds M, Woodruff T. Nat Biomed Eng. 2020;4:574.
40. Sackmann E, Fulton A, Beebe D. Nature. 2014;507:181–9.
41. Berendsen J, Kruit S, Atak N, Willink E, Segerink L. Anal Chem. 2020;92:3302–6.
42. Xu H, Liu X, Le W. TrAC Trends Anal Chem. 2018;105:1–6.
43. Arumugasaamy N, Rock K, Kuo C-Y, Bale T, Fisher J. Adv Drug Delivery Rev. 2020;161–162:161–175.
44. Pemathilaka R, Reynolds D, Hashemi N. Interf Focus. 2019;9:20190031.
45. Scott AK, Oyen ML. Lancet Digit Health. 2024;6:e436–7.
46. Acharya G, et al. Placenta. 2018;64:S4–8.
47. Clark A, Lee T, James J. WIREs Mechan Dis. 2020;13. https://doi.org/10.1002/wsbm.1502.
48. Mayo PR. Comput Struct Biol J. 2018;16:298–306.
49. Wheeler ML, Oyen ML. Ann Biomed Eng. 2021;49:1805–18.
50. Sun C, Groom K, Oyston C, Charley L, Clark A, James J. In: The placenta in fetal growth restriction: what is going wrong? Placenta; 2020. p. 10–18.
51. Lecarpentier E, Bhatt M, Bertin G, Deloison B, Salomon L, Deloron P, Fournier T, Barakat A, Tsatsaris V. PLOS ONE. 2016;11:e0147262.
52. Mayo PR, Charnock-Jones D, Burton G, Oyen M. Placenta. 2016;43:54–60.
53. Mayo PR, Olsthoorn J, Charnock-Jones D, Burton G, Oyen M. J Biomech. 2016;49:3780–7.
54. Bappoo N, Kelsey L, Parker L, Crough T, Moran C, Thomson A, Holmes M, Wyrwoll C, Doyle B. Biomech Model Mechanobiol. 2017;16:1361–72.
55. Tun WM, Poologasundarampillai G, Bischof H, Nye G, King, ONF, Basham M, Tokudome Y, Lewis RM, Johnstone ED, Brownbill P, Darrow M, Chernyavsky IL. J R Soc Interf. 2021;18:20210140.

The Placenta as a Biomaterial

Renata Dos Reis Marques and Marley J. Dewey

Abstract The placenta is often considered a "waste" material after birth, yet it contains a variety of factors important for regenerative medicine, many of which have been used as biomaterials to support wound repair. Herein, we discuss the placenta structure and components, processing the placenta for regenerative medicine approaches, biomaterials applications of the placenta, placenta-derived stem cells and factors in biomaterials, and clinical applications of placentas. Specifically, we focus on the amniotic membrane, chorionic membrane, and placental disc layers in our chapter. This chapter aims to discuss similarities and differences between placental layers used in biomaterial applications, and current methods for using the placenta as a biomaterial for wound repair. We contrast the placenta layer biological components, mechanical properties, cell types, processing procedures, and differences in wound healing outcomes. Universally, the placenta provides an immunomodulatory material rich in factors that can prevent chronic inflammation. We also examine factors of the placenta, such as soluble factors, cells, and extracellular vesicles, which can be used separately from biomaterials as factors for repair. Finally, we discuss companies and biomaterial products made from the placenta, which are used clinically for wound healing applications. This chapter highlights the recent advances in biomaterials made from the placenta and the importance of which layer of the placenta is used for repair.

Keywords Placenta · Amnion · Chorion · Placental disc · Biomaterials · Stem cells · Regenerative medicine · Wound repair

R. Dos Reis Marques · M. J. Dewey (✉)
Department of Bioengineering, University of California Santa Barbara, Santa Barbara, CA, USA
e-mail: rdosreismarques@ucsb.edu; marleydewey@ucsb.edu

S. G. Zambuto, M. L. Oyen (eds.), *Biomaterials for Women's Health Engineering*,
https://doi.org/10.1007/978-3-032-10745-9_13

1 Introduction

Tissue engineering and regenerative medicine are fields dedicated to designing therapies that can regrow damaged or diseased tissues. Most research in these fields has focused on the development of materials or molecules, such as synthetic or organic polymers and growth factors, to aid the body in accelerating normal healing. One material that has received recent attention is the placenta, a temporary organ formed during pregnancy that connects the fetus to the mother. The placenta is composed of multiple layers, mainly the placental disc, amniotic membrane, and chorionic membrane (see Sect. 2). The placenta is often considered a "waste product" after birth; however, there is a breadth of research that has demonstrated the potential for placentas to be used as a natural material for wound repair due to their anti-scarring, anti-inflammation, and anti-infection properties. To date, thousands of research articles have been published investigating the beneficial and pro-regenerative properties of the placenta, which we discuss herein.

A brief search on September 25, 2025, of research articles and clinical trials using various elements of the placenta as biomaterials for tissue engineering or regenerative medicine was conducted to examine how various components were used in research and the clinic (Table 1). Most research and clinical trials have been performed on the amniotic membrane and placenta-derived cells. Compared to a similar published article in 2017, this trend remains, as more research and clinical trials were performed using the amniotic membrane and cells derived from the placenta (mesenchymal stem cells, cord blood cells) than the other components of the placenta [1].

Within this chapter, we will examine the structure of the placenta, the properties and components of each layer, how the placenta is processed for biomaterial and medical applications, and how the placenta is used as a biomaterial in the clinic. As a medical waste product, the placenta represents a rich and potentially sustainable source for highly regenerative wound therapies.

2 Placenta Structure and Components

The placenta is composed of an umbilical cord, an amniotic membrane, an intermediate layer, a chorionic membrane, and a placental disc (Fig. 1). The *umbilical cord* connects from the fetus to the chorion and includes typically one artery and one vein to transport nutrients and waste [2, 3]. The *amniotic membrane* (or amnion) is closest to the fetus. The amniotic tissue microenvironment is characterized by a single epithelial layer, a basement membrane, a compact layer, and an avascular stroma [4]. There are primarily two populations of stem cells that populate the amniotic membrane: amniotic epithelial cells, which reside in the epithelial monolayer, and amniotic mesenchymal stromal cells, which are found in the stromal layer. The extracellular matrix of the amniotic membrane is largely enriched for fibronectin,

Table 1 Number of research articles published and clinical trials (ongoing or completed) involving the placenta as a biomaterial, for tissue engineering, or regenerative medicine as of 2025

Placenta component	Search terms	Research articles published (pubmed.ncbi.nlm.nih.gov)	Clinical trials (clinicaltrials.gov)
Placental disc	(((placental disc) OR (placenta disc)) AND ((biomaterial) OR (tissue engineering) OR (regenerative medicine)))	6	0
Amniotic membrane	(((amniotic membrane) OR (amnion)) AND ((biomaterial) OR (tissue engineering) OR (regenerative medicine)))	1620	9
Chorionic membrane	(((chorionic membrane) OR (chorion)) AND ((biomaterial) OR (tissue engineering) OR (regenerative medicine)))	540	1
Placenta extract	(((placenta extract) OR (placenta solution)) AND ((biomaterial) OR (tissue engineering) OR (regenerative medicine)))	167	0
Placenta cells	(((placenta cells) OR (placenta derived cells) OR (placenta stem cells)) AND ((biomaterial) OR (tissue engineering) OR (regenerative medicine)))	1600	2
Placenta extracellular vesicles	(((placenta extracellular vesicles) OR (placenta exosomes) OR (placenta vesicles)) AND ((biomaterial) OR (tissue engineering) OR (regenerative medicine)))	107	0
Placenta growth factors	(((placenta growth factors) OR (placental growth factors)) AND ((biomaterial) OR (tissue engineering) OR (regenerative medicine)))	482	0

Search terms were typed into the database of either PubMed or clinicaltrials.gov (intervention/treatment), and the number of hits was reported. Search was conducted on September 25, 2025

laminin, various collagens (I, III, IV, V, VI), and proteoglycans [5]. The structural integrity and mechanical properties of the amnion are largely afforded by collagens III, IV, and V present in the basement membrane [6]. In fact, the amniotic membrane represents one of the thickest basement membranes in the body (0.2–0.5 mm) and is devoid of blood vessels, nerves, and lymphatic vessels [7]. The amniotic membrane serves as a barrier as well as a layer to protect the mechanical integrity of the placenta as a whole [8].

Between the amniotic and the chorionic membranes lies an *intermediate layer*, often termed a "spongy layer," which may be acellular or contain relatively scarce cells (fibroblasts) and mainly collagens (I, III and IV), proteoglycans, and glycoproteins (hyaluronic acid and heparan sulfate) [9]. The umbilical cord attaches to the *chorion*, and within the chorion, villous "trees" spread into the placental disc. The maternal blood circulates through these villous spaces to exchange nutrients, gas, and waste with the fetus. The chorion comprises three layers: a trophoblast layer, a

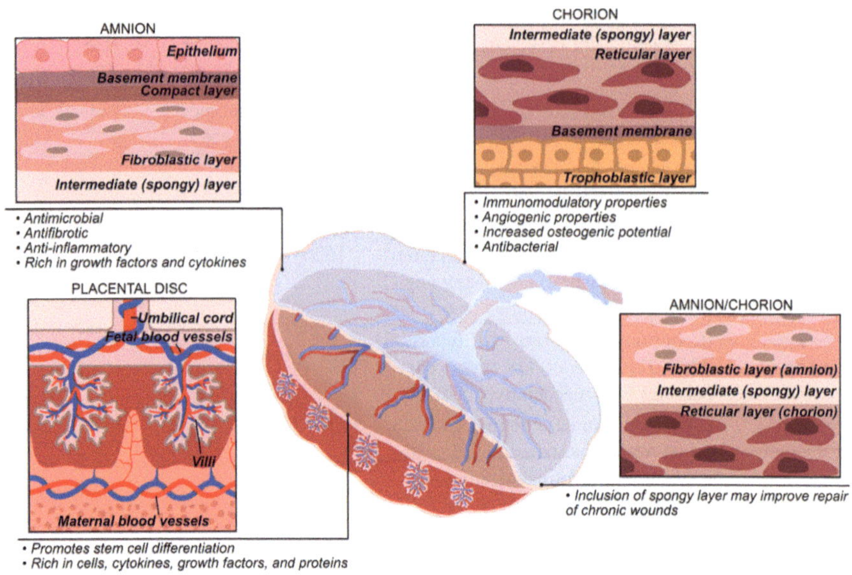

Fig. 1 Placenta tissue structure and properties

basement membrane, and reticular layer (also known as the extraembryonic mesoderm), the latter of which is in contact with the amniotic membrane and intermediate layer. The chorion is composed of a variety of densely-packed collagens (types I, III, IV, V, and VI) and infiltrated by fibroblasts and macrophages [10, 11]. Interestingly, hematopoietic stem cells have been found within the chorion during fetal development, but cease to exist at term [12]. Laminin and fibronectin are commonly found within the chorion, and one of the key defining features of the chorion from the amniotic membrane is villi within the chorion, which act as channels for transporting blood and nutrients and waste between the mother and the fetus [9]. Interestingly, a proteomic characterization of the human chorion revealed that there are more signaling molecules (proteins) per square centimeter of tissue than in the amniotic membrane. Of these signals, the chorion is enriched in aminopeptidase-N (APN), angiopoietin-2 (ANG-2), basic fibroblast growth factor (b-FGF), endocrine gland vascular endothelial growth factor (EG-VEGF), hepatocyte growth factor (HGF), insulin-like growth factor 1 (IGF-1), platelet-derived growth factor AA and BB (PDGF-AA, PDGF-BB), tissue inhibitor of metalloproteinases 2 and 4 (TIMP-2, TIMP-4), while the amnion is enriched in Gelctin-7 (GAL-7), transforming growth factor β1 (TGF-β1), and interleukin-1F [13]. Within canine chorionic membranes, other proteins were observed, such as proteins related to ECM remodeling (matrix metalloproteinase 2 and tissue inhibitor of metalloproteinases 3) and vascularization (vascular endothelial growth factor and relaxin), and tissue decellularization impacted protein enrichment [14].

The *placental disc* connects to the maternal endometrium and provides blood supply to the fetus. Due to this, the placental disc is highly vascularized and contains various collagens (I, III, IV, VI) as well as glycoproteins and proteoglycans (fibronectin, fibrillin I, laminin, thrombospondin, tenascin C, decorin, Heparan sulfate, elastin) [15, 16]. Within the placental disc, there are also a plethora of different cell types, including mesenchymal stem cells, immune cells, fibroblasts, trophoblasts, endothelial cells, and vascular smooth muscle cells, as well as a variety of cytokines and other nutrients [17]. A variety of cytokines have also been identified in commercially available placenta products (amnion–chorion), including angiogenin, ANG-2, bFGF, placental growth factor (PGF), vascular endothelial growth factor (VEGF), epidermal growth factor (EGF), and keratinocyte growth factor (FGF-7) [18, 19]. Tissue sampling across the different layers of the placenta (basal plate, chorionic plate, and the middle part connecting the two surfaces of the placenta) demonstrated differences in protein content between these layers. Specifically, there were 14, 8, and 21 distinct proteins in the three layers, and functionally, the basal plate region had increased endothelial cell activity and increased cell-cycle arrest (senescence) [20].

Mechanically, the chorion membrane provides elasticity to the placenta. It has a stiffness (Young's modulus) of approximately 2.3 MPa, whereas the amnion is much stiffer with a Young's modulus of 21 MPa [21, 22]. This trend is similarly reflected in the maximum principal stress of the amnion, which is 4 MPa [23], chorion 168 kPa [24], and placental disc 900 kPa [25]. Interestingly, the amnion supports much of the mechanical robustness of the placenta; if the amnion fails, the entire placenta fails, whereas if the chorion fails (mechanically), the amnion may stay intact [21]. This is intriguing considering the thickness of the different layers, as the placenta as a whole roughly measures 3 cm thick in the center, with the placental disc providing the greatest volume compared to the amnion (44 μm) and chorion (188 μm) [3, 22].

3 Placenta Biomaterial Processing

Like many tissue-derived materials, the placenta is often decellularized before use (Fig. 2). This process involves washing steps to remove blood, decellularization steps commonly using chemicals, drying steps, and sterilization steps. Common decellularization techniques include mechanical force, enzymes (Trypsin–EDTA, dispase, thermolysin), detergents (SDS, Triton-X, CHAPS), chelating agents (EDTA), and hypotonic and hypertonic solutions [26–30]. In general, decellularization methods can include any combination of physical, chemical, or biological treatments, but these require a careful balance between the sufficient removal of immunogenic components (i.e., cells) and maintenance of tissue structure (i.e., extracellular matrix) that gives rise to the tissue's bioactivity. Typically, any layer of the placenta is first washed in water or PBS, then most often decellularized using a low concentration of SDS (2–0.1%). Sometimes low concentrations of

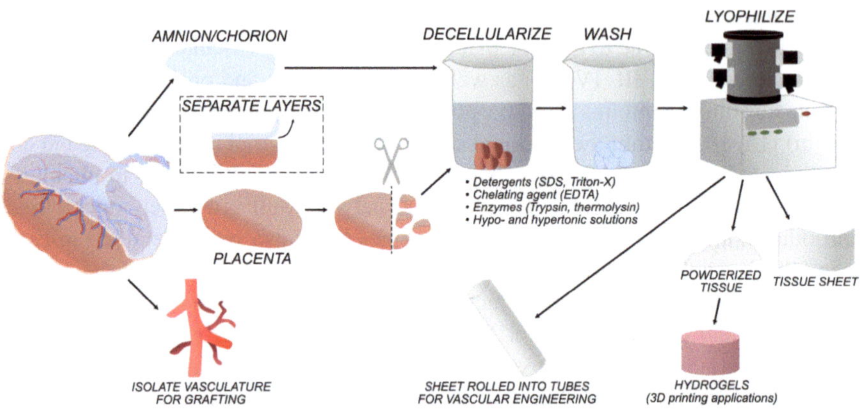

Fig. 2 Processing of placental tissues for biomaterial applications. Placenta processing typically begins with layer separation. Following this process, parts of the placenta are decellularized, lyophilized, and then processed into powder, sheets, tubes, or hydrogels. Finally, placenta biomaterials will be sterilized prior to wound application

EDTA (1–0.05%) or low concentrations of Triton-X (0.5–1%) are also used. Some researchers will treat the placenta with 0.2–0.016% DNase and/or RNase to promote further removal of foreign nucleic acids. Often layers of the placenta are frozen (−80 °C) after decellularization and subsequently freeze-dried to remove water. Of note, processing of the placental disc is often slightly different due to the thickness of this material. To decellularize the placental disc, processing typically starts with homogenizing, blending, or cutting up the placenta into pieces and then centrifuging these pieces in distilled water to remove blood. Subsequent centrifugation steps may also be used to remove washing solutions as well. To avoid cutting up placental disc fragments to effectively decellularize this whole tissue, the human placenta can be perfused through the umbilical cord with decellularization detergents. For the amnion and chorion, due to the thin nature of these materials, they can be processed without cutting and kept in a sheet form. Interestingly, the majority of clinical and laboratory applications utilizing the placenta do not include the spongy layer; however, recent studies investigating this layer have found that it can provide improved wound repair of nonhealing wounds such as ulcers, trauma, or surgical wounds [31].

As with any tissue, there are optimal decellularization solutions to achieve proper decellularization without damaging biological or mechanical components. Unfortunately, while several decellularization methods have been proposed and contrasted in literature, there remains a lack of procedural standardization in the field. For instance, one comparative study has concluded that a hypertonic solution-based decellularization method increases amniotic membrane porosity, mesenchymal stem cell activity (attachment, proliferation), and in vivo skin remodeling compared to treatment with 0.25% Trypsin–EDTA [32]. A different study has shown that the use of thermolysin enhances preservation of basement membrane structure and composition compared to EDTA- and dispase-based methods [27]. In contrast, a study examined various concentrations of SDS and Triton-X 100 and various wash times of the placenta and found that 0.5% SDS and Triton-X for 30 min showed optimal decellularization with minimal negative effects on placental tissue [33]. However, each decellularization method possesses its own drawbacks, namely, detergents disrupt cell membranes and denature proteins, while freeze–thaw cycles can fracture the extracellular matrix due to ice crystal formation. Effective decellularization is usually then confirmed with Hematoxylin and Eosin staining for nuclei and structural impacts, and a dsDNA quantification assay after digestion in Proteinase K (commonly PicoGreen assay) and achieving <50 ng/mg dry tissue [34]. In addition to decellularization, cryopreservation and lyophilization of placenta tissues are commonly utilized to promote prolonged storage before implantation. For instance, one study proposed a treatment of the amniotic membrane with nonionic surfactants to remove cellular material, followed by trehalose treatment to promote protein retention after lyophilization (i.e., lyopreservation). This combination successfully retained collagen and sulfated glycosaminoglycans with an increase in tissue tensile strength and hydrophilicity [35]. After decellularization, the placenta can also be sterilized using gamma irradiation or other methods such as 0.1% peracetic acid or 70% ethanol. However, a study examined how placenta processing can impact placenta hydrogel formation, and gamma irradiation resulted in unstable hydrogels [36].

After decellularization, layers of the placenta have been used as sheets, particles, or digested into a hydrogel. The placenta can also be used as a whole and decellularized, even from small animals, such as mice, for small-scale placenta applications, while maintaining the ability for cells to naturally attach and proliferate [37]. The placenta has been used as a sponge in various applications by combining decellularized placenta particles with other biomaterials, such as alginate, gelatin, or synthetic polymers, and then lyophilizing [38]. Likewise, in particle form, the amnion and chorion can be directly incorporated into collagen sponges during fabrication [39, 40], or soaked to release soluble factors, which can be added to biomaterials after fabrication [41]. To note, fabrication of sponges and other lyophilized 3D structures using the placental disc usually encounters challenges with good mechanical stability. To overcome this, researchers have investigated three different crosslinking methods with glutaraldehyde (soak, fumigation, slurry) and found that the fumigation method had better mechanical and biological (biocompatibility) properties than the other methods [42]. Hydrogels are often created by digesting particles in pepsin to form a gel, which can then be used to coat graft materials to enhance reendothelialization [43], or to use as a scaffold itself for tissue regeneration approaches [44]. Freezing and cryomilling can also be used to create placental particles, and after digestion, it can be combined with other materials such as gelatin and silk fibroin for FRESH 3D printing applications of placenta hydrogels [45]. It is important to note that when extracting ECM components or digesting the placenta tissue, the reagents used (pepsin, Tris, serum) can impact the isolation of collagens and bioactive elements [46]. While most commonly the layers of the placenta are used as a sheet or particles, sheets of the placenta can also be rolled into a tube for vascular graft applications [47]. It is also important to note that if using in sheet form, the orientation of the chorion, or other layers, after isolation may be important to consider, as the trophoblast side and mesoderm side have different properties, although both are biocompatible with endothelial cells and fibroblasts [48].

4 Placenta Biomaterial Applications

4.1 Placental Disc

The placental disc has been used for a variety of different regenerative medicine applications, including skin, bone, and stem cell differentiation, among other applications; however, there are some missing details in some applications using the placenta, including whether this is the disc only or a combination of multiple layers (disc, amnion, and chorion). Generally, as shown in Table 1, there is a strikingly lower amount of research and clinical applications of the placental disc, even though there is a much greater amount of this tissue harvestable from the placenta than the amnion and chorion. For skin applications, the placental disc is often combined with another biomaterial. After removing the umbilical cord, amniotic membrane, and chorionic membrane layers, the placenta can be decellularized and combined with alginate (50:50) to create a biomaterial for skin repair. This combination results in mechanical properties matching native skin and promotes angiogenesis, epithelization, and granulation tissue formation in full-thickness skin repair rat models [38]. The placenta has also been combined with sericin (silk cocoon protein) to create an angiogenic scaffold capable of significantly reducing the wound size of excisional wounds in rats compared to a saline control [49]. Similarly, decellularized placentas have been combined with silk fibroin, and higher amounts of placenta increased the viability of adipose-derived mesenchymal stem cells [50]. Extracellular matrix derived from the placenta has been combined with gelatin and alginate to create 3D-printable hydrogels, and the addition of the placenta resulted in no signs of an immunological response and increased granulation tissue formation, angiogenesis, and reepithelialization of full-thickness cutaneous wounds in mice compared to biomaterials without placental ECM [51]. Decellularized placenta particles have been likewise combined with synthetic polymers, such as PEG-based polymers, to create hydrogels that are 3D-printable, and the addition of the placenta to PEG hydrogels allowed for greater skin and macrophage cell adherence and proliferation than PEG alone [52].

The placenta has also been fabricated as a sponge for bone repair applications. Adipose-derived stem cells and macrophages were cocultured on a placenta sponge and demonstrated an upregulation of four different osteogenic genes and greater mineralization than scaffolds without the placenta [53]. The placenta could also serve as a hydrogel for human-induced pluripotent stem cell (iPSC) differentiation, as decellularized placental hydrogels could differentiate iPSC spinal cord organoids into neurons in comparison to traditionally used Matrigel [54]. The placenta can serve as a substrate for neonatal mouse spermatogonial cells proliferation and differentiation, and after 35 days of culture on placental extracellular matrix and 2D well plates, the percentage of Prm1-positive cells (differentiation marker) in the placental group (36.4%) significantly surpassed that of the 2D group (10.96%) [55]. An overview of various articles published on uses of the placenta as a biomaterial can be seen in Table 2.

4.2 Amnion

The amniotic membrane was first used as a skin graft as early as 1910 [56]. Since then, the amnion and its extracts have been used in various additional tissue engineering applications, including musculoskeletal, vascular, ocular, nerve, and urothelial regeneration, among many others. While the amnion presents a distinct tissue microenvironment, it is rich in growth factors and cytokines that promote cell adhesion, proliferation, differentiation, and immune modulation, all critical biological processes in the wound healing cascade. In addition, the amniotic membrane exhibits antimicrobial, antifibrotic, and anti-inflammatory properties [57–60]. These characteristics make the amnion an attractive biomaterial for tissue repair. Typically, the amniotic membrane is placed on a wound and secured by sutures, glue, or bandages. When decellularized, the amniotic membrane can be used as a natural, biocompatible material; however, poor tissue mechanical properties, rapid degradation, and difficulty in handling pose significant drawbacks in its clinical use. Modifications to the amniotic membrane have been proposed to address these challenges. Crosslinking agents, such as transglutaminase [61], glutaraldehyde [62, 63], methacrylic anhydride [64], and carbodiimides [63, 65, 66], can improve tissue mechanical properties but may reduce tissue bioactivity and biocompatibility. Amniotic membrane extracts (i.e., isolated through lyophilization and/or incorporated into composite materials) retain some regenerative properties, yet the extracellular matrix is destroyed without guaranteed improvements to mechanical properties. One study has suggested the fabrication of a composite hydrogel consisting of methacrylated decellularized amnion and methacrylated gelatin to address limited tissue mechanical integrity and promote skin wound healing. The combination of methacrylated amnion and gelatin exhibited significantly increased tensile strength compared to decellularized amnion, methacrylated amnion, and methacrylated gelatin alone without a loss of fibroblast viability. An evaluation of in vivo performance of the composite methacrylated amnion–gelatin hydrogel demonstrated enhanced skin thickness, angiogenesis, and wound healing in a rabbit model [64]. Powderized amnion has also been successfully incorporated into a 3D-printed, bilayered methacrylated gelatin–gelatin composite scaffold to promote angiogenesis in a coculture model including keratinocytes, fibroblasts, and endothelial cells for skin tissue engineering [67]. Interestingly, intact amniotic membrane has also been combined with flexible electrodes to stimulate the release of epidermal growth factor (EGF) from amniotic mesenchymal interstitial cells, thus increasing bioactivity to outpace rapid degradation of the amnion that typically limits its clinical applicability

Table 2 Summary of placental disc biomaterials literature

References	Placental processing	Biomaterial fabrication	Wound repair application	Outcome
Alizadeh et al. [38]	Umbilical cord, amnion, and chorion were removed and placental disc was decellularized with SDS and triton-X	Placenta was combined with sodium alginate and freeze-dried	Full-thickness skin wound repair	50:50 alginate to placenta was superior at repairing wounds and matching mechanical properties to skin
Bhoopathy et al. [49]	Amnion was removed, remaining placenta was decellularized with SDS and DNase/RNase	Sericin (silk) was combined with placenta and freeze-dried	Open excision wound healing	Greater wound closure with treatment group compared to untreated control
Mehrabi et al. [50]	Amnion was removed, remaining placenta was decellularized with SDS and triton-X	Combined placenta and silk fibroin into a hydrogel	Breast tissue engineering	Higher placental ratio hydrogels exhibited greater adipose-derived stem cell expansion
Bashiri et al. [51]	Placenta was decellularized with SDS and triton-X	Combined placenta with gelatin and alginate into a hydrogel bio-ink	Full-thickness skin wound repair	5% placenta hydrogel supported the best tissue repair
Fan et al. [52]	Placenta was decellularized with SDS, DNase, and PAA	Combined placenta with PEG-based hydrogels	Skin and immune cell attachment	Macrophage and fibroblast cells adhered and proliferated on gels
Khosrowpour et al. [53]	Placenta was decellularized with SDS and triton-X	Placenta was freeze-dried	Osteogenic differentiation of stem cells	Improved osteogenic gene expression and mineralization with groups containing the placenta
Wang et al. [54]	Placenta was decellularized with tris–HCl, DNase, RNase, and triton-X	Placenta was solubilized to create hydrogel	Spinal cord organoids	Differentiated iPSCs into neurons, accelerating spinal cord organoid formation compared to Matrigel
Asgari et al. [55]	Umbilical cord, amnion, and chorion were removed and placental disc was decellularized with SDS	Placenta was freeze-dried	In vitro spermatogenesis	Improves sperm cell proliferation and differentiation

To note, many articles do not include information on what parts of the placenta remained or were removed in skin repair [68]. Electrospun polycaprolactone has also been used to reinforce the amnion in a composite membrane for full-thickness skin grafting. Compared to the amnion alone, this polycaprolactone–amnion composite material exhibited improved stability, mechanical properties, and degradation rates, thereby promoting accelerated wound closure and epidermal and dermal regeneration [69].

In addition to skin tissue engineering, the amniotic membrane has been used as a biomaterial for guided musculoskeletal tissue regeneration, including tissues such as bone [39, 70, 71], tendon [72, 73], and cartilage [74, 75]. For instance, the amnion is commonly combined with hydroxyapatite, a naturally occurring form of calcium phosphate mineral that is native to bone tissue, to guide osteogenesis. After decellularization, biomineralization of the amnion can be accomplished by immersion of the tissue in simulated body fluid to initiate hydroxyapatite nucleation within the matrix [71]. The amniotic membrane can also be ground or powderized and incorporated into a mineralized composite biomaterial during fabrication [39, 70]. The addition of amnion into mineralized scaffolds for bone repair can be beneficial owing to its anti-inflammatory properties; in fact, mineralized collagen–amnion scaffolds have been shown to increase osteogenesis of adipose mesenchymal stem cells in the presence of interleukin-1β, a pro-inflammatory cytokine secreted by macrophages during the inflammation stage of wound healing [39]. A similar study combined amniotic membrane matrix with an anisotropic collagen–glycosaminoglycan scaffold to improve material mechanical properties and immune modulation in tendon repair. In this case, the amnion was either directly incorporated into the material as a powder or used as a sheet wrapped around the scaffold to mimic commercially available tendon wraps. Soluble factors released from amniotic membrane sheets included anti-inflammatory factors (interleukin-10, interleukin-1RA, TIMP-1/2), as well as pro-inflammatory factors (interleukin-1β, interleukin-8, tumor necrosis factor-α). While the addition of amniotic membrane to collagen–glycosaminoglycan scaffolds did not significantly improve material strength, this study further corroborated that the amnion is able to mitigate highly inflammatory conditions that typically hinder tissue regeneration [40]. Using a different approach, others have leveraged the amniotic membrane as a strategy to control spatiotemporal release of exogenous bone morphogenic protein 2 (BMP-2) from a collagen sponge and, in turn, mitigate heterotopic ossification in bone repair. Interestingly, the amnion surrounding the collagen sponge was able to sequester more BMP-2 compared to synthetic poly(ε-caprolactone), effectively reducing heterotopic ossification; however, osteogenesis was delayed in earlier stages of regeneration. The amnion's enhanced sequestration of BMP-2 is likely due to its extracellular matrix structure (glycosaminoglycans, adhesion ligands, proteins), immunomodulatory properties, and unique capacity to bind growth factors [76]. The amniotic membrane and its extracts have also been leveraged toward repair of musculoskeletal tissue junctions, such as osteochondral [77, 78] and rotator cuff tendon–bone interfaces [79].

Amniotic membrane grafts have been used for ocular surface reconstruction in cases of chemical burn [80], Stevens–Johnson syndrome [81], pterygium excision [82], conjunctival surface reconstruction [83], corneal ulceration [84], and many others. The amnion is reported to repair the ocular surface by promoting epithelialization [80], reducing inflammation [85], inhibiting fibrosis [80], and suppressing corneal neovascularization [86]. In clinical applications, the amniotic tissue may serve as a surgical patch, a scaffold for tissue replacement, or both. Additionally, the amnion can be grafted in the stromal layer of the cornea (inlay transplantation), closer to the corneal surface (onlay transplantation), or a combination of the two. Notably, the amniotic basement membrane is enriched for collagens IV and VII, much like the corneal epithelial basement membrane [87]. One comparative study investigated the effect of amniotic membrane sidedness (i.e., cell layer) and tissue processing methods on corneal epithelial cell behavior and inflammatory response. Of the three commercially available amniotic membrane grafts interrogated in this study (Biovance 3L Ocular, Ambio2, AmnioGraft), in vitro epithelial cell activity was reported to be maximized on the stromal layer of Biovance 3L Ocular, including an increased initial response to inflammatory challenge [88]. In addition to amniotic tissue grafts, amnion extracts have also been leveraged for enhanced corneal repair strategies, including chitosan–dextran nanoparticles loaded with amnion extract [89] and hydrogel platforms for amniotic protein extract delivery [90]. A summary of select studies utilizing the amniotic membrane and its extracts in biomaterials for repair of diverse tissues can be seen in Table 3.

4.3 Chorion

The chorionic membrane has been used for a variety of wound repair applications, including dental (periodontal surgeries), to aid in implant surgeries, and bone repair, among others [91]. Intriguingly, in many of these studies, there were no inflammatory or infectious complications or rejection of the implant, which is often seen in many other biomaterial approaches to repair wounds. This is likely due to the chorionic membrane's propensity for immune modulation. Incorporating chorionic membrane particles or soluble factors derived from the chorion into a mineralized collagen sponge results in increased immunomodulatory gene expression in mesenchymal stem cells, mainly CCL2, HGF, and IL6, and osteogenic gene expression remained unaffected [41]. In a study of skin wound repair, the chorion was also incorporated as nanoparticles into a biomaterial, and the chorion nanoparticles were thought to achieve anti-inflammatory impacts [92]. The chorion can also be used as a hydrogel, and when injected into rat hearts post myocardial infarction, could reduce scar volume, maintain normal electrical activity, and reduce immune cells and inflammation at the site of injury [44]. The chorion can also be used as an angiogenic material, both by deriving bioactive components from the chorion and by using the native mechanical structure of the chorion. When compared to the amnion, the native artery and vascularized nature of the chorion can be leveraged for vascular grafting with success [93], whereas the amnion lacks this structure. Arteries can be isolated manually from the chorion (<1 mm diameter), decellularized, and applied in a rat arteriovenous loop model, which demonstrated no immunological response and

Table 3 Summary of amniotic membrane biomaterials literature

References	Placental processing	Biomaterial fabrication	Wound repair application	Outcome
Zhang et al. [64]	Chorion was removed, amnion was decellularized with EDTA and mechanical scraping	Methacrylated amnion combined with methacrylated gelatin to form a photocrosslinkable hydrogel	Skin defect healing	Improved tensile strength significantly; promoted fibroblast proliferation in vitro and collagen deposition and angiogenesis in vivo
Pazhouhnia et al. [67]	Amnion was frozen, crushed into powder, washed, and dissolved in PBS	Amniotic extract dissolved in PBS added to methacrylated gelatin/gelatin hydrogel	Skin tissue engineering	Increased viability of endothelial cells
Wang et al. [68]	Amnion was separated from chorion and soaked in serum-free medium	Metal Mg/Fe electrodes were electrosputtered on poly(lactic-*co*-glycolic acid) film and layered onto amnion	Full-skin defect healing	Promoted epithelialization and neovascularization in vivo
Pinky et al. [69]	Amnion was separated from chorion and decellularized using EDTA, trypsin, and mechanical scraping	Wet decellularized amnion was "sandwiched" onto electrospun polycaprolactone and lyophilized	Full-thickness skin excision wound healing	Improved stability and delayed degradation; promoted epidermis and dermis formation
Firouzeh et al. [71]	Amnion was separated from chorion, decellularized using urea, and freeze-dried	Decellularized amnion was mineralized by immersion in simulated body fluid	Bone tissue engineering	Supported mesenchymal stem cell viability and osteogenic differentiation
Dewey et al. [39]	Amniotic membrane was separated from placenta and decellularized with thermolysin	Amnion was ground to fine particles, added to mineralized collagen suspension, then lyophilized	Craniofacial bone defects	Osteogenesis increased under inflammatory challenge
Hortensius et al. [40]	Amniotic membrane was separated from placenta, decellularized with thermolysin, and lyophilized	Lyophilized amnion was homogenized into particles and combined with collagen; dry amnion sheets were wrapped around collagen scaffolds	Tendon repair	Pro-inflammatory cytokines downregulated
Priddy et al. [76]	Dehydrated amnion/chorion (AmnioFix) was used	Collagen sponge surrounded by amniotic membrane	Large bone defects	Decreased heterotopic ossification in vivo

(continued)

Table 3 (continued)

References	Placental processing	Biomaterial fabrication	Wound repair application	Outcome
Jun et al. [77]	Amnion was isolated from placenta and decellularized with trypsin and by mechanical scraping	Rabbit cartilage fragments added to decellularized amnion scaffolds	Osteochondral defects	Improved subchondral bone regeneration and integration with cartilage
Wang et al. [79]	Amnion was detached from placenta, decellularized with triton-X 100 and trypsin–EDTA, and lyophilized	Decellularized amniotic membrane used as biomaterial	Rotator cuff repair	Promoted healing and improved mechanical properties; decreased in quality compared to normal rotator cuff
Shimazaki et al. [80]	Amniotic membrane with chorion was cryopreserved with dimethyl sulfoxide	N/A	Ocular surface reconstruction after chemical/thermal burns	Promoted conjunctival epithelialization and suppressed fibrosis
Tsubota et al. [81]	Amniotic membrane was frozen for 2 weeks	N/A	Advanced ocular cicatricial pemphigoid and stevens–Johnson syndrome	Ocular reconstruction was achieved in most cases
Prabhasawat et al. [82]	Amnion was separated from chorion, flattened onto nitrocellulose paper, cut, and cryopreserved in culture medium and glycerol	N/A	Ptegyrium excision	Low recurrence rate of pterygia
Tseng et al. [83]	Amnion was separated from chorion, flattened onto nitrocellulose paper, cut, and cryopreserved in culture medium and glycerol	N/A	Reconstruction of conjunctival defects after surgical removal or symblepharon lysis	Some patients showed successful surface reconstruction, though others experienced adverse effects
Lee et al. [84]	Amnion was separated from chorion, flattened onto nitrocellulose paper, cut, and cryopreserved in culture medium and glycerol	N/A	Persistent epithelial defects with ulceration	All but one patient healed in 4 weeks without recurrence

Bakhshandeh et al. [89]	Amnion was cryogenically frozen and pulverized	Amniotic extract encapsulated into dextran sulfate–chitosan nanoparticles, then incorporated into poly(ε-caprolactone) scaffold	Corneal transplantation	Enhanced anti-angiogenic property of scaffold
Basasoro et al. [90]	Amnion was detached from chorion, rinsed, cryopreserved, and homogenized in phenylmethanesulfonyl fluoride and PBS	Amnion proteins were incorporated into a hyaluronic acid-based hydrogel or a hydrogel composed of various polymers	Corneal repair	Wound closure improved compared to untreated controls with limitations

reendothelialization of the graft surface [94]. Similarly, vascular grafts have been harvested and effectively decellularized from the chorion of bovine placentas [95]. The chorion has also been chemically modified with methacryloyl groups to develop a hydrogel with high mechanical properties (kPa) and promoted endothelial cell tube formation without the addition of other angiogenic factors [96]. The amnion and chorion (separately) have also been combined with methacrylated hyaluronic acid to create 3D-printable structures, and despite these different layers having different ECM and growth factor contents, both supported endothelial cell vasculogenesis equally [97].

The chorion has demonstrated differences in osteogenesis when compared to the amnion, as extracts from the chorion could induce greater MG-63 mineralization than extracts from the amnion [98]. This was due to differences in enriched growth factors, such as osteopontin, osteomodulin, bFGF, TGF-β1, Thy-1, netrin 4, retinol-binding protein, and DJ-1, and was achieved through the noncanonical Wnt-mediated CXCL signaling-dependent pathway [98]. The chorion also has potentially greater antibacterial properties than the amnion, as there were more bacterial growth inhibition zones around chorionic membranes than amniotic membranes [99]. Finally, human mesenchymal stem cells may be able to adhere, engraft, and proliferate on decellularized chorion better than on decellularized amnion [100]. Thus, many important mechanical and biological considerations may influence researchers' use of the amnion or chorion for wound repair. An overview of various articles published on uses of the placenta as a biomaterial can be seen in Table 4.

4.4 *Amnion–Chorion*

While the amnion and chorion membranes have been used separately for repair, these can be isolated together as a joint amnion–chorion therapy. The amnion and chorion combined have been used for a variety of different regenerative medicine applications, including bone, dental, and skin, among others. For bone repair applications, digested amnion and chorion were incorporated into a chitosan and nanohydroxyapatite hydrogel, and improved the hydrogel's mechanical properties, such as swelling, degradation, mechanical strength, and SAOS-2 cell attachment, differentiation, and mineralization for improved bone repair applications [101]. The amnion–chorion has been used for dental repair applications, such as dental pulp regeneration, as a dressing to improve the viability and differentiation of root canal stem cells, due to the membrane's ability to promote an anti-inflammatory response, which prevents tissue necrosis [102]. For skin applications, the amnion and chorion can be carefully processed together without separation of the layers. Subcutaneous implantation of a decellularized amnion–chorion graft into mice resulted in host-cell infiltration, angiogenesis, tissue remodeling, and structural layer retention for up to 10 weeks [103]. An overview of various articles published on uses of the placenta as a biomaterial can be seen in Table 5.

Table 4 Summary of chorion biomaterials literature

References	Placental processing	Biomaterial fabrication	Wound repair application	Outcome
Kolliopoulos et al. [41]	Amnion and chorion separated, snap-frozen in liquid nitrogen, freeze-dried, and powderized	Chorion and amnion particles were lyophilized with mineralized collagen to fabricate sponges or scaffolds were soaked in soluble extracts	Bone repair	Mineralized collagen–chorion scaffolds upregulated immunomodulatory genes while amnion scaffolds osteogenic, angiogenic, and immunomodulatory genes
Francis et al. [44]	Chorion was decellularized with N-lauryl sarcosine	Placenta was solubilized to create hydrogel	Myocardial infarction	Injections of chorion repaired myocardium
Mahheidari et al. [92]	Chorion was freeze-thawed and decellularized with SDS, triton-X, and DNase	Chorion was milled into nanoparticles and incorporated into a alginate/ carboxymethyl cellulose hydrogel	Full-thickness skin repair	Wound area size was reduced with hydrogel
Schneider et al. [93]	Arteries were isolated from the chorion and decellularized using triton-X and EDTA or SDS and EDTA, and then PAA	Heparin was crosslinked onto grafts	Vascular replacement	SDS altered the matrix of grafts but both grafts were functionally remodeled
Falkner et al. [94]	Arteries were isolated from the chorion and decellularized using triton-X, EDTA, DNase, and PAA	Heparin was crosslinked onto grafts	Vascular replacement	Grafts had no immunological responses and host cells infiltrated the graft
Oliveira et al. [95]	Chorion was decellularized with SDS and triton-X, then the entire vascular system was isolated	Vascular grafts were re-cellularized with canine yolk sav cells	Vascular replacement	Vessels were viable and cytocompatible
Martins et al. [96]	Chorionic membrane was detached from amnion and chorionic plate and umbilical cord and	Chorion was methacrylated to create a hydrogel	Vascular replacement and repair	Hydrogels were mechanically tunable and prolonged culture of endothelial cells

(continued)

Table 4 (continued)

References	Placental processing	Biomaterial fabrication	Wound repair application	Outcome
	decellularized with SDS, triton-X, and nuclease treatments			
Comperat et al. [97]	Chorion was decellularized using tris/EDTA, CHAPS, NaOH, EDTA, and NaCl	Chorion was solubilized to create hydrogel bio-inks	Vascular replacement and repair	Both amnion and chorion bioinks supported endothelial cell health
Zare-Bidaki et al. [99]	Chorion and amnion were mechanically separated	Membranes were used without washing or freezing	Antibacterial effects	Chorion membranes had superior antibacterial effects compared to the amnion
Lakkireddy et al. [100]	Chorion and amnion were separated and decellularized with SDS, triton-X, and NaOH and sterilized with UV radiation	Cells were seeded directly onto decellularized membranes	Stem cell compatibility	Human mesenchymal stem cells adhered and proliferated on chorion membranes better than amnion

Table 5 Summary of amnion–chorion biomaterials literature

References	Placental processing	Biomaterial fabrication	Wound repair application	Outcome
Khazaei et al. [101]	Placental cotyledons were detached from the chorion–amnion and then the chorion–amnion was decellularized with SDS and EDTA	Chorion–amnion was combined with nanohydroxyapatite and chitosan to make a hydrogel	Bone tissue engineering	Amnion and chorion increased SAOS-2 cell proliferation and osteogenic differentiation and calcium deposition
Wetzell et al. [103]	Amnion and chorion were not separated during decellularization, preserving a trophoblast layer	Chorion–amnion used as a sheet (biopsies)	Wound repair	Supports fibroblast cell proliferation and cell infiltration and tissue remodeling

4.5 Placenta-Derived Cells and Factors in Biomaterials

The placenta is an organ rich in cells and growth factors. There are several distinct types in the placenta, including trophoblasts, stromal/mesenchymal cells, Hofbauer (macrophage) cells, epithelial cells, vascular smooth muscle cells, pericytes, and endothelial cells. Placenta-derived stem cells are the most widely reported cell type in tissue repair applications. Importantly, placenta-derived stem cells can vary in biological characteristics (activity, differentiation ability, others) depending on their location within the tissue [104]. Some studies isolate these cells in a nonspecific manner, suggesting a heterogeneous stem cell population in culture. In general, the placenta offers a relatively noninvasive and abundant source of stem cells compared to other tissues, such as bone marrow. Additionally, placenta-derived stem cells lack ethical concerns and tumorigenicity typically associated with embryonic stem cells [105]. Within the amniotic membrane specifically, it is widely accepted that two distinct types of stem cells exist: amniotic mesenchymal stem cells and amniotic epithelial stem cells. Intriguingly, amniotic epithelial cells express pluripotent stem cell markers (octamer-binding transcription factor 4, SRY-box 2, Nanog) and can differentiate into any of the three germ layers [105, 106]. Similarly, amniotic and chorionic mesenchymal stem cells are multipotent and can undergo "classical" trilineage differentiation (osteogenic, chondrogenic, and adipogenic), though other lineages have been reported for amniotic mesenchymal stem cells (skeletal muscle [107], cardiomyocytes [108], and others) [109]. Likewise, amniotic fluid and chorion have been identified as sources of mesenchymal stem cells. Notably, one study further classifies placenta-derived mesenchymal stem cells by location within the placenta tissue: amniotic membrane, chorionic membrane, chorionic plate, and chorionic villi. These cells have been shown to possess biological activity unique to their origin; for instance, chorionic villi stem cells favored chondrogenic and osteogenic lineages, whereas their amniotic membrane-derived counterparts tended toward osteogenic and neurogenic differentiation [104]. Given previous evidence of distinct, location-dependent stem cell characteristics within placental tissues, it is possible that enrichment of specific cell subpopulations could further optimize biomaterial systems toward their intended application. Both amniotic membrane and chorionic mesenchymal stem cells can be isolated in the first, second, and third trimester mesoderm of the amniotic and chorionic membranes, respectively. The isolation of mesenchymal stem cells from the placenta is relatively easy to accomplish. The amniotic membrane must be first separated from the whole placenta, at which point the tissue is minced, incubated in trypsin to remove epithelial cells, and enzymatically digested to release mesenchymal stem cells [109]. Amniotic fluid mesenchymal stem cells can be isolated by aspiration of amniotic fluid during the second and third trimesters of pregnancy (amniocentesis) or during Caesarean section [110–112]. On the other hand, the trophoblastic layer of the chorion must first be mechanically and enzymatically removed prior to tissue digestion for cell isolation [109].

Because of their many benefits, placenta-derived mesenchymal stem cells have attracted significant interest in the tissue engineering space. Both natural and synthetic material compositions can be compatible with these cells, regardless of placental tissue or extract incorporation within the material. Various biomaterial applications of amniotic mesenchymal stem cells have been reported in literature, including electrospun polylactic acid-*co*-polycaprolactone vascular grafts [113], photo-crosslinked gelatin–collagen composite hydrogel for intrauterine adhesion prevention [114], gradient collagen–hydroxyapatite scaffolds to promote tendon–bone interface repair [115], and placenta extracellular matrix/silk fibroin sponges to accelerate bone regeneration [116]. On the other hand, the pluripotent nature of amniotic epithelial stem cells coupled with their immunomodulatory properties offer a unique advantage in regenerative medicine [117]. For instance, multiple studies have combined amniotic epithelial stem cells with biomaterials for tendon regeneration [118, 119]. In addition to effective tenogenesis, researchers have shown that amniotic epithelial stem cells cultured on poly(lactic-*co*-glycolic) acid 3D scaffolds exhibited an increase in secreted immunomodulatory factors into conditioned culture medium compared to those cultured on tissue culture-treated plastic. Further functional studies modeling paracrine signaling demonstrated that conditioned medium secreted by cells on 3D scaffolds significantly increased interleukin-6 secretion by macrophages, a pro-inflammatory cytokine that plays a critical role in tendon regeneration [119]. Other applications of amniotic epithelial stem cells include a nanochitosan–polypyrrole–alginate composite material for spinal cord injury repair [120] and a polyurethane cardiac patch for myocardial infarction treatment [121]. Amniotic fluid mesenchymal stem cells likewise present a possible candidate cell population for tissue repair. For example, though bone marrow mesenchymal stem cells are commonly utilized in bone biomimetic materials, their amniotic fluid-derived counterparts have been shown to exhibit a five-fold increased mineralized matrix deposition in a poly-ε-caprolactone scaffold after 15 weeks of culture. It is important to note, however, that osteogenic differentiation of amniotic fluid stem cells was relatively delayed [122]. These results highlight the importance of accounting for source-specific stem cell bioactivity and application-specific requirements in the development of biomaterials-based therapies.

Extracellular vesicles (EVs), or lipid bilayer-bound nanoparticles encapsulating signaling molecules (proteins, RNAs, lipids, others) secreted naturally by cells, can be isolated from placenta cells and the placenta itself as factors for repair. EVs can be isolated from placenta-derived cells, placental tissue, and amniotic fluid. These EVs retain some regenerative qualities of the placenta, offering a potential alternative to cell-based therapies for wound repair. Typically, EVs are harvested from cells by first the in vitro culture of stem cells and the collection of conditioned medium, and then subsequent isolation of EVs from this conditioned medium. For example, amniotic mesenchymal stem cells secrete EVs exhibiting angiogenic properties, including increased proliferation, migration, and vessel formation of endothelial cells (HUVEC) [123]. These effects on HUVEC activity have been shown to persist in high-glucose environments modeling diabetic wound healing [124]. In addition to applications in diabetic skin wounds, amniotic mesenchymal stem cell EVs have been shown to repair dystrophic skeletal muscle [125] and mitigate retinal degeneration induced by oxidative stress [126]. EVs isolated from amniotic epithelial cells similarly possess therapeutic properties. For example, one study has shown that these extracellular vesicles facilitate reepithelialization, reduce fibrosis, and promote transparency of the cornea after chemical burn [127]. In general, EVs can be directly injected into the body or incorporated into biomaterials for controlled delivery. Intriguingly, EVs isolated from placenta-derived mesenchymal stem cells in culture have been combined with an amniotic membrane hydrogel for repair of diabetic wounds. In addition to common markers of regeneration, including accelerated wound closure, increased angiogenesis, and increased collagen density, an increase in antioxidative factors (glutathione, catalase, and superoxide dismutase) was also observed in rat skin samples treated with this hydrogel [128]. Others have proposed a different therapeutic strategy in which chorionic plate mesenchymal stem cell-derived EVs are loaded with ellagic acid, a small molecule drug, and embedded within a methacrylated gelatin hydrogel for diabetic skin wound healing [129]. However, while several studies have reported the therapeutic capacity of placenta stem cell-derived EVs, relatively few have explored the incorporation of these as a stimulus in biomaterials for tissue repair. Importantly, EVs were recently found to reside within the extracellular matrix of soft tissues [130], revealing a novel mechanism of cell–environment interactions that could be leveraged in biomaterials design for wound healing. These tissue-resident EVs have been isolated from the placenta tissue itself and encapsulated in a fibrin hydrogel for peripheral nerve regeneration in a murine model. The EV-laden hydrogel did not significantly enhance sciatic function compared to the fibrin-only hydrogels, though the authors discussed that this could be due to low concentrations of bioactive factors (growth factors, EVs) or material properties [131].

Beyond cells and EVs, the placenta is also rich in growth factors and cytokines (see Sect. 2 for specific components). Extracts are typically produced by lysing full-term placentas, which result in a noncellular fluid rich in biological factors [1]. Interestingly, full-term placenta extracts resulted in improved hematopoietic stem cell activity compared to placenta extracts at earlier gestational terms [132]. One study found that placental extracts contain various antioxidants, and 15% of this antioxidant activity could be attributed to collagen peptides [133]. Another study found that placenta extracts promoted keratinocyte activity, and these extracts had distinct activities from growth factors alone (EGF) and other serums (cord serum, maternal serum, others) [134]. Extracts from placental villi have been injected into full thickness skin defects in mice and shown an increase in wound closure compared to a control, likely attributed to early-stage transforming growth factor-beta (TGF-β) expression in the wound site and VEGF in the late stage [135]. Placenta extracts have also been used to treat dry skin cosmetically, and a double-blind patient trial found that ingesting porcine placenta extracts resulted in an improvement in skin dryness after 4 weeks [136]. In terms of biomaterial applications, placenta extracts have been combined with 3D-printed gelatin hydroxyapatite hydrogels to improve bone regeneration in vitro and in vivo compared to hydrogels without placenta extract [137]. Extracts have also been encapsulated into alginate microbeads to release anti-oxidative and anti-inflammatory factors [138]. Additionally, soaking mineralized collagen sponges in soluble extracts isolated from the amnion and chorion resulted in greater stem cell activity compared to incorporation of the matrix itself into the sponges; however, both matrix particles and soluble extracts resulted in osteogenesis and improved angiogenesis and immunomodulation [41]. Overall, there are limited studies examining placenta extracts and soluble factors combined with biomaterials for wound repair, and most extract studies focus on cosmetic-related applications. Select studies incorporating placenta-derived factors in biomaterials for tissue repair are summarized in Table 6.

5 Clinical Applications of Placental Biomaterials

As the placenta is often considered a "waste" material or "disposable organ," use of the placenta as a biomaterial can be thought of as a potentially sustainable resource for tissue engineering. Potential limitations include patient heterogeneity and the quality of the harvested material due to patient-derived preexisting conditions or incidents during pregnancy. While donor variability may be an issue for many regenerative medicine applications, a study comparing decellularized amnion–chorion membranes from three different pig breeds demonstrated minimal differences in structural, biochemical, and mechanical characteristics [139]. Most clinical studies use either the amniotic membrane or a combination of the amnion and chorion for wound repair applications and sometimes refer to this combination as the "placenta." Few companies use the chorion alone as a membrane for repair, which is intriguing considering the differences in repair noted in Sect. 4.3 between the amnion and chorion, as well as the mechanical and compositional properties noted in Sect. 2. Of these companies that have clinical products, only Interfyl (Celularity) was reported to comprise just the chorion (Table 7). Similarly, Axiofill (Mimedx) was the only product comprised of just the placental disc.

In a comparative study of clinically available ECM products comparing ovine forestomach, porcine placenta, porcine peritoneal, and porcine small intestinal submucosa, the performance of these for dermal reconstruction based on pathological scores found that the placenta was similar to peritoneal ECM, but the forestomach ECM outperformed all groups [140]. A company's processing of placenta products may also play a large role in bioactivity. In a study comparing three different companies' placenta-derived products, Interfyl (Cellularity) interacted more favorably with human tenocytes in vitro, such as greater tenocyte proliferation and maintenance of tenocyte differentiation [141]. In a systematic review, it was found that placental-derived factors (amniotic fluid, amniotic sac, umbilical cord, and mixtures) had 6.24 times greater chronic diabetic ulcer closure than conventional treatments, indicating a dramatic potential for the use of the placenta in clinical wound repair applications [142]. Various studies have cited the use of placenta extracts in research and obtained their extracts through companies; however, details of these methods and research to back applications are limited.

Table 6 Summary of placenta-derived factors used in biomaterials literature

References	Placental processing	Biomaterial fabrication	Wound repair application	Outcome
Varyani et al. [128]	Human placenta/amniotic sacs were decellularized with trypsin–EDTA, triton, and sodium deoxycholic acid, then freeze-dried	Placenta mesenchymal stem cell-derived EVs were immobilized into a decellularized amnion hydrogel	Diabetic wound healing	EV-containing hydrogels demonstrate greatest regenerative capacity compared to hydrogel-only and control groups
Tian et al. [129]	N/A	Ellagic acid was encapsulated in chorionic plate mesenchymal stem cell-derived EVs and added to methacrylated gelatin hydrogels	Diabetic wound healing	Improved reepithelialization, collagen deposition, and EGFR expression
Kobayashi et al. [131]	Amnion was decellularized under high hydrostatic pressure and digested with liberase to release EVs	Amnion–derived EVs encapsulated in fibrin hydrogel	Peripheral nerve regeneration	Sciatic function index was not significantly different between EV-fibrin hydrogels and fibrin-only hydrogels
Lee et al. [137]	Not reported	Gelatin–hydroxyapatite scaffolds were immersed in placental extract	Bone tissue engineering	Adipose stem cell proliferation and osteogenic marker expression increased with placental extract
Taweechaipaisankul et al. [138]	Placentas were cryogenically frozen or freeze-dried, ground, dissolved in buffer, then pasteurized	Placenta extracts were encapsulated in alginate microbeads	N/A	Placental extract release delayed in microbeads; antioxidative and anti-inflammatory effects
Go et al. [98]	Chorion and amnion were frozen in liquid nitrogen and finely ground	Ground particles were soaked and extracts collected	Bone formation	Chorion extracts enhanced osteogenic differentiation of MG-63 cells compared to amnion

Table 7 Summary of clinical placenta products to date

Product name	Company	Description	Application(s)	References
Placenta				
InnovaMatrix	ConvaTek	Porcine placenta	Ulcers, partial and full-thickness wounds, burns	Ragsdale et al. [143], Fife et al. [144]
Grafix	Osiris Therapeutics	Human placenta containing cells, growth factors, and ECM	Acute or chronic wounds	Gibbons [145], Du et al. [146]
Axiofill	Mimedx	Acellular human placental disc	Replacement or supplementation of damaged tissue (tissue defects)	Ganesh et al. [147]
Dermavest	AediCell	Human placental disc (majority), amnion, chorion, and umbilical cord	Replacement or supplementation of damaged tissue (tissue defects)	Ganesh et al. [147]
Plurivest	AediCell	Human placental disc, amnion, chorion, and umbilical cord	Replacement or supplementation of damaged tissue (tissue defects)	Ganesh et al. [147]
Revita	StimLabs	Human placenta will all layers	Acute or chronic wound covering	Wilmas et al. [148]
NuShield	Organogenesis Inc	Dehydrated placenta allograft with all layers	Wound site protection	McQuilling et al. [149]
Amnion				
Dermacyte	Merakris	Human amniotic membrane with preserved basement membrane and fibroblast layer	Protective covering for partial and full-thickness wounds and surgical sites	Ditmars et al. [150]
Omnigen	NuVision biotherapies	Dehydrated amniotic membrane affixed by a bandage contact lens	Dry eye disease	Travé-Huarte and Wolffsohn [151]
AmnioGraft	BioTissue	Cryopreserved amniotic membrane graft	Improved patient outcomes after ocular surface reconstruction	Mao et al. [88], Huang et al. [152], Chuck et al. [153]
Biovance 3L ocular	Celularity	Decellularized and dehydrated amniotic membrane	Corneal and conjunctival disorders, pterygium repair, fornix reconstruction	Mao et al. [88]

(continued)

Table 7 (continued)

Product name	Company	Description	Application(s)	References
Ambio2	IOP Ophthalmics	Processed, dehydrated amniotic membrane allograft	Protective covering in surgical applications, including pterygium excision, conjunctival chalasis, and corneal ulcers	Mao et al. [88], Miyakoshi et al. [154]
Ambio5	IOP Ophthalmics	Processed, dehydrated, and multilayered amniotic membrane allograft	Protective covering in surgical applications, including fornix reconstruction, symblepharon, and stevens–Johnson syndrome	Naxer et al. [155]
AmbioDisk	IOP Ophthalmics	Processed, sutureless amniotic membrane allograft	Treatment of ocular surface diseases/defects (e.g., corneal erosions, acute burns, epithelial defects, etc.)	Choi and Jeon [156]
AmnioGen	HCT regenerative	Dehydrated amniotic tissue	Wound healing, ophthalmology	Huang et al. [152]
ProKera	BioTissue	Cryopreserved amniotic membrane	Keratitis, corneal scars, chemical burns, corneal defects, and partial limbal stem cells deficiency	Morkin and Hamrah [157]
Affinity	Organogenesis	Fresh amniotic tissue-derived allograft	Protective covering for acute and chronic wound healing	McQuilling et al. [149], Harmon et al. [158]
AmnioBioGraft	Alamo biologics	Patch tissue-derived from amniotic membrane	Chronic and nonhealing skin wounds, cutaneous wounds, ocular injuries, burns	
PalinGen Hydromembrane	Amnio technology	Processed amniotic tissue allograft stored in saline	Physical and biological support for wound healing; full and partial thickness, acute and chronic wounds	

(continued)

Table 7 (continued)

Product name	Company	Description	Application(s)	References
PalinGen membrane	Amnio technology	Processed, air-dried amniotic tissue allograft	Physical and biological support for wound healing; full and partial thickness, acute and chronic wounds	
PalinGen XPlus membrane	Amnio technology	Similar to PalinGen membrane, crosslinked with glutaraldehyde	Physical and biological support for wound healing; full and partial thickness, acute and chronic wounds	
AmnioExcel	Integra	Processed, dehydrated amniotic membrane	Protective wound covering	Snyder et al. [159], Lintzeris et al. [160], Barr [161], Abdo [162], Rosenblum [163], Thompson et al. [164], Boyar and Galiczewski [165]
AmnioDerm	Biohealing	Processed amniotic membrane	Wound covering, vascularization, scar reduction, anti-inflammation, epithelialization; venous leg ulcers, arterial and neuropathic skin ulcers, lymphedema ulcers	
Chorion				
Interfyl	Celularity	Human decellularized chorionic plate	Replacement or supplementation of damaged tissue (tissue defects)	Ganesh et al. [147]
Amnion–chorion				
Epifix	Mimedx	Human amnion–chorion	Acute or chronic wounds, ulcers	Du et al. [146], Bianchi et al. [166]
AmnioBand	Mtf biologics	Minimally processed human amnion–chorion	Acute or chronic wounds	Du et al. [146], Glat et al. [167]

(continued)

Table 7 (continued)

Product name	Company	Description	Application(s)	References
PelloGraft	Surgenex	Amnion–chorion	Chronic ulcers	
Vendaje AC	BioStem technologies	Dehydrated human amnion–chorion	Protective covering (surgery, wounds, burns)	Sabol et al. [168]
AmnioGain	Surgical Esthetics	Dehydrated human amnion–chorion	Dental surgeries	
Neomem Xac	Cytagenix	Amnion–chorion	Dental applications	
AmnioExcel plus	Integra	Amnion–chorion–amnion layered sheet (tri-layer)	Protective barrier for soft tissue repair	Holder [169]
ACApatch	Extremity care	Dehydrated amnion–chorion–amnion (including spongy layer)	Protective barrier for wound repair	
Matrion	LifeNet health	Amnion and chorion and trophoblast layer	Protective barrier for soft tissue wound repair	Wetzell et al. [103]
AmnioExcite	Salvin	Amnion and chorion and trophoblast layer	Amnion and chorion and trophoblast layer	Wetzell et al. [103]
WoundFix	Skye biologics	Amnion and chorion and trophoblast layer	Acute or chronic wounds	
WoundEx 200	Skye biologics	Dehydrated amnion–chorion membrane	Acute or chronic wounds	
AmnioShield	Atec spine	Double-sided amniotic and chorionic tissue membrane	Wound covering, scar reduction	
Placenta-derived factors and cells				
Human placenta extract	Melsmon pharmaceutical	Liquid ampule form of 100 mg placenta villi (placenta extract)	Illness, surgery, aging, cancer	Hong et al. [135]
PLx	Snowden	Hydrolyzed human placenta powder extract (placenta extract)	Cosmetics, diet	Togashi et al. [133]
Amniomatrix	Integra	Cryopreserved liquid suspension allograft derived from amniotic membrane and amniotic fluid	Tissue repair of tunneling and deep wounds	

(continued)

Table 7 (continued)

Product name	Company	Description	Application(s)	References
NuCel	Organogenesis	Cryopreserved amniotic suspension including extracellular matrix proteins, amniotic fluid cells, anti-inflammatory cytokines, and growth factors	Bone fusion, tendon repair, limb salvage, wounds, and burns	
Clarix Flo	Amniox medical	Injectable particulate amniotic membrane and umbilical cord	Promote wound healing, reduce scarring and inflammation	
AmnioELITE	Surgilogix	Nonsurgical, liquid treatment containing amniotic tissue and fluid components (collagens, growth factors, amino acids, cytokines, etc.)	Repair of chronic wounds	
Allogen	Vivex biologics	Frozen, liquid allograft derived from amniotic fluid	Tissue repair; orthopedics, neurosurgery, spinal surgery, and general surgery	

6 Conclusion

The placenta represents a potentially sustainable and highly bioactive material and source of factors for regenerative medicine applications. Layers of the placenta have been used in multiple clinical trials to date and have unique properties and components, such as anti-inflammatory, antimicrobial, and angiogenic. Of notable interest, most research and clinical applications have focused on cells derived from the placenta and the use of the amniotic membrane alone; however, the placental disc and chorion can offer different biological factors and potential differences in healing outcomes. Specifically, the unique vasculature of the chorion and the ability to harvest arteries from this layer make it valuable for vascular applications. Based on our review, researchers should better define what parts of the placenta they are using, and how they are isolating extracts, as some articles mention using the placenta but are missing whether this is the placental disc only or all layers of the placenta (amnion, chorion, and placental disc). We also recommend examining multiple patient placenta samples to better understand donor variability concerns.

Future promising applications include more studies examining the placental disc and examining extracellular vesicles and placenta extracts within biomaterials as cell-free alternatives to repair.

Acknowledgments The authors would like to thank the National Institutes of Health T32 Fellowship funding 1T32GM141846 (R.D.M.). This work was also partially supported by the National Science Foundation through the Materials Research Science and Engineering Center (MRSEC) at UC Santa Barbara: NSF DMR-2308708 (Seed, M.J.D.), the Connie Frank Foundation Fellowship (R.D.M.), and the University of California-Santa Barbara Regents in Bioengineering Fellowship (R.D.M.).

References

1. Pogozhykh O, Prokopyuk V, Figueiredo C, Pogozhykh D. Placenta and placental derivatives in regenerative therapies: experimental studies, history, and prospects. Stem Cells Int. 2018;2018:4837930. https://doi.org/10.1155/2018/4837930.
2. Benirschke K, Burton GJ, Baergen RN. Anatomy and pathology of the umbilical cord. In: Benirschke K, Burton GJ, Baergen RN, editors. Pathology of the human placenta. Berlin, Heidelberg: Springer; 2012. p. 309–75. https://doi.org/10.1007/978-3-642-23941-0_12.
3. Burton GJ, Sibley CP, Jauniaux ERM. Chapter 1 – Placental anatomy and physiology. In: Gabbe SG, Niebyl JR, Simpson JL, Landon MB, Galan HL, Jauniaux ERM, Driscoll DA, Berghella V, Grobman WA, editors. Obstetrics: normal and problem pregnancies (seventh edition). Philadelphia: Elsevier; 2017. p. 2–25. https://doi.org/10.1016/B978-0-323-32108-2.00001-9.
4. Van Herendael BJ, Oberti C, Brosens I. Microanatomy of the human amniotic membranes. Am J Obstet Gynecol. 1978;131:872–80. https://doi.org/10.1016/S0002-9378(16)33135-0.
5. Department of Nanomedicine and Tissue Engineering, Shaheed Beheshti Medical University, Tehran, Iran, Niknejad H, Peirovi H, Jorjani M, Ahmadiani A, Ghanavi J, Seifalian A. Properties of the amniotic membrane for potential use in tissue engineering. Eur Cell Mater. 2008;7:88–99. https://doi.org/10.22203/eCM.v015a07.
6. Arrizabalaga JH, Nollert MU. Human amniotic membrane: a versatile scaffold for tissue engineering. ACS Biomater Sci Eng. 2018;4:2226–36. https://doi.org/10.1021/acsbiomaterials.8b00015.
7. Danforth DN, Hull RW. The microscopic anatomy of the fetal membranes with particular reference to the detailed structure of the amnion. Am J Obstet Gynecol. 1958;75:536–50. https://doi.org/10.1016/0002-9378(58)90610-0.
8. Moreno S, Massee M, Campbell S, Bara H, Koob TJ, Harper JR. PURION® processed human amnion chorion membrane allografts retain material and biological properties supportive of soft tissue repair. J Biomater Appl. 2024;39:24–39. https://journals.sagepub.com/doi/full/10.1177/08853282241246034. Accessed 9 Apr 2025.
9. Benirschke K, Burton GJ, Baergen RN. Anatomy and pathology of the placental membranes. In: Benirschke K, Burton GJ, Baergen RN, editors. Pathology of the human placenta. Berlin, Heidelberg: Springer; 2012. p. 249–307. https://doi.org/10.1007/978-3-642-23941-0_11.
10. Malak TM, Ockleford CD, Bell SC, Dalgleish R, Bright N, Macvicar J. Confocal immunofluorescence localization of collagen types I, III, IV, V and VI and their ultrastructural organization in term human fetal membranes. Placenta. 1993;14:385–406. https://doi.org/10.1016/S0143-4004(05)80460-6.
11. Roy A, Mantay M, Brannan C, Griffiths S. Placental tissues as biomaterials in regenerative medicine. Biomed Res Int. 2022;2022:6751456. https://doi.org/10.1155/2022/6751456.

12. Muench MO, Kapidzic M, Gormley M, Gutierrez AG, Ponder KL, Fomin ME, Beyer AI, Stolp H, Qi Z, Fisher SJ, Bárcena A. The human chorion contains definitive hematopoietic stem cells from the fifteenth week of gestation. Development. 2017;144:1399–411. https://doi.org/10.1242/dev.138438.
13. McQuilling JP, Vines JB, Kimmerling KA, Mowry KC. Proteomic comparison of amnion and chorion and evaluation of the effects of processing on placental membranes. Wounds. 2017;29:E36–40.
14. de Sá Schiavo Matias G, da Silva Nunes Barreto R, Carreira ACO, Junior MYN, Fratini P, Ferreira CR, Miglino MA. Proteomic profile of extracellular matrix from native and decellularized chorionic canine placenta. J Proteome. 2022;256:104497. https://doi.org/10.1016/j.jprot.2022.104497.
15. Chen CP, Aplin JD. Placental extracellular matrix: gene expression, deposition by placental fibroblasts and the effect of oxygen. Placenta. 2003;24:316–25. https://doi.org/10.1053/plac.2002.0904.
16. Protzman NM, Mao Y, Long D, Sivalenka R, Gosiewska A, Hariri RJ, Brigido SA. Placental-derived biomaterials and their application to wound healing: a review. Bioengineering. 2023;10:829. https://doi.org/10.3390/bioengineering10070829.
17. Lim JJ, Koob TJ. Placental cells and tissues: the transformative rise in advanced wound care. In: Worldwide wound healing – innovation in natural and conventional methods. IntechOpen; 2016. https://www.intechopen.com/chapters/53065. Accessed 9 Apr 2025.
18. Chen J, Lopez CD, Girard AO, Abousy M, Redett RJ, Groves M, Yang R. Dehydrated human amnion/chorion membrane allografts for myelomeningocele and wound reconstruction. Childs Nerv Syst. 2021;37:3721–31. https://doi.org/10.1007/s00381-021-05352-z.
19. Koob TJ, Lim JJ, Massee M, Zabek N, Denozière G. Properties of dehydrated human amnion/chorion composite grafts: implications for wound repair and soft tissue regeneration. J Biomed Mater Res B Appl Biomater. 2014;102:1353–62. https://doi.org/10.1002/jbm.b.33141.
20. Manna S, Scheel J, Noone A, McElwain CJ, Scaife C, Gupta S, English J, McCarthy C, McCarthy FP. A proteomic profile of the healthy human placenta. Clin Proteomics. 2023;20:1. https://doi.org/10.1186/s12014-022-09388-4.
21. Verbruggen SW, Oyen ML, Phillips ATM, Nowlan NC. Function and failure of the fetal membrane: modelling the mechanics of the chorion and amnion. PLoS One. 2017;12:e0171588. https://doi.org/10.1371/journal.pone.0171588.
22. Helmig R, Oxlund H, Petersen LK, Uldbjerg N. Different biomechanical properties of human fetal membranes obtained before and after delivery. Eur J Obstet Gynecol Reprod Biol. 1993;48:183–9. https://doi.org/10.1016/0028-2243(93)90086-R.
23. Oyen ML, Cook RF, Calvin SE. Mechanical failure of human fetal membrane tissues. J Mater Sci Mater Med. 2004;15:651–8. https://doi.org/10.1023/B:JMSM.0000030205.62668.90.
24. Manoogian SJ, Bisplinghoff JA, McNally C, Kemper AR, Santago AC, Duma SM. Dynamic tensile properties of human placenta. J Biomech. 2008;41:3436–40. https://doi.org/10.1016/j.jbiomech.2008.09.020.
25. Chua WK, Oyen ML. Do we know the strength of the chorioamnion?: a critical review and analysis. Eur J Obstet Gynecol Reprod Biol. 2009;144:S128–33. https://doi.org/10.1016/j.ejogrb.2009.02.029.
26. Wilshaw S-P, Kearney J, Fisher J, Ingham E. Biocompatibility and potential of acellular human amniotic membrane to support the attachment and proliferation of allogeneic cells. Tissue Eng A. 2008;14:463–72. https://doi.org/10.1089/tea.2007.0145.
27. Hopkinson A, Shanmuganathan VA, Gray T, Yeung AM, Lowe J, James DK, Dua HS. Optimization of amniotic membrane (AM) denuding for tissue engineering, tissue engineering part C. Methods. 2008;14:371–81. https://doi.org/10.1089/ten.tec.2008.0315.
28. Wilshaw S-P, Kearney JN, Fisher J, Ingham E. Production of an acellular amniotic membrane matrix for use in tissue engineering. Tissue Eng. 2006;12:2117–29. https://doi.org/10.1089/ten.2006.12.2117.

29. Zhang Z, Lu B, Zou L, Huang X, Yang F, Lv H. Decellularized human amniotic membrane scaffolds: influence on the biological behavior of dental pulp stem cells. BMC Oral Health. 2024;24:394. https://doi.org/10.1186/s12903-024-04130-y.
30. Khosravimelal S, Momeni M, Gholipur M, Kundu SC, Gholipourmalekabadi M. Protocols for decellularization of human amniotic membrane. In: Methods in cell biology. Elsevier; 2020. p. 37–47. https://doi.org/10.1016/bs.mcb.2019.11.004.
31. Psathas E, Egger B, Mayer D. Dehydrated human amnion/chorion membrane allograft with spongy layer to significantly improve the outcome of chronic non-healing wounds. Int Wound J. 2024;21:e14356. https://doi.org/10.1111/iwj.14356.
32. Tauseef H, Ahmed K, Chaudhary F, Salim A, Mohiuddin OA. The impact of decellularization method on the cytocompatibility and wound healing capability of human amniotic membrane. Adv Biol. 2025;9:2400509. https://doi.org/10.1002/adbi.202400509.
33. Asgari F, Asgari HR, Najafi M, Eftekhari BS, Vardiani M, Gholipourmalekabadi M, Koruji M. Optimization of decellularized human placental macroporous scaffolds for spermatogonial stem cells homing. J Mater Sci Mater Med. 2021;32:47. https://doi.org/10.1007/s10856-021-06517-7.
34. Crapo PM, Gilbert TW, Badylak SF. An overview of tissue and whole organ decellularization processes. Biomaterials. 2011;32:3233–43. https://doi.org/10.1016/j.biomaterials.2011.01.057.
35. Sarkar S, Rajput JH, Poundarik AA. Lyopreservation and nonionic decellularization of human amnion scaffolds for enhancing regeneration in chronic nonhealing ulcers. ACS Appl Bio Mater. 2025;8:2151–66. https://doi.org/10.1021/acsabm.4c01711.
36. Gujjar S, Tyagi A, Sainger S, Bharti P, Nain V, Sood P, Jayabal P, Sharma JC, Sharma P, Rajput S, Pandey AK, Pandey AK, Abnave P, Mathapati S. Biocompatible human placental extracellular matrix derived hydrogels. Adv Biol. 2024;8:2300349. https://doi.org/10.1002/adbi.202300349.
37. Barreto RS, Romagnolli P, Fratini P, Mess AM, Miglino MA. Mouse placental scaffolds: a three-dimensional environment model for recellularization. J Tissue Eng. 2019;10:2041731419867962. https://doi.org/10.1177/2041731419867962.
38. Alizadeh S, Nasiri M, Saraei M, Zahiri M, Khosrowpour Z, Sineh Sepehr K, Nouri M, Zarrabi M, Kalantari N, Shafikhani SH, Gholipourmalekabadi M. Optimization of an affordable and efficient skin allograft composite with excellent biomechanical and biological properties suitable for the regeneration of deep skin wounds: a preclinical study. ACS Appl Bio Mater. 2024;7:7378–90. https://doi.org/10.1021/acsabm.4c01016.
39. Dewey MJ, Johnson EM, Slater ST, Milner DJ, Wheeler MB, Harley BAC. Mineralized collagen scaffolds fabricated with amniotic membrane matrix increase osteogenesis under inflammatory conditions, regenerative. Biomaterials. 2020;7:247–58. https://doi.org/10.1093/rb/rbaa005.
40. Hortensius RA, Ebens JH, Dewey MJ, Harley BAC. Incorporation of the amniotic membrane as an immunomodulatory design element in collagen scaffolds for tendon repair. ACS Biomater Sci Eng. 2018;4:4367–77. https://doi.org/10.1021/acsbiomaterials.8b01154.
41. Kolliopoulos V, Dewey MJ, Polanek M, Xu H, Harley BAC. Amnion and chorion matrix maintain hMSC osteogenic response and enhance immunomodulatory and angiogenic potential in a mineralized collagen scaffold. Front Bioeng Biotechnol. 2022;10:1034701. https://www.frontiersin.org/articles/10.3389/fbioe.2022.1034701. Accessed 3 Oct 2023.
42. Zhan T, Niu W, Zang C, Liu X, Cheng L, Xu Y. Study of glutaraldehyde-treated crosslinking protocols for placental decellularized matrix sponges. Biomater Adv. 2024;165:214003. https://doi.org/10.1016/j.bioadv.2024.214003.
43. Rohringer S, Schneider KH, Eder G, Hager P, Enayati M, Kapeller B, Kiss H, Windberger U, Podesser BK, Bergmeister H. Chorion-derived extracellular matrix hydrogel and fibronectin surface coatings show similar beneficial effects on endothelialization of expanded polytetrafluorethylene vascular grafts. Mater Today Bio. 2022;14:100262. https://doi.org/10.1016/j.mtbio.2022.100262.

44. Francis MP, Breathwaite E, Bulysheva AA, Varghese F, Rodriguez RU, Dutta S, Semenov I, Ogle R, Huber A, Tichy A-M, Chen S, Zemlin C. Human placenta hydrogel reduces scarring in a rat model of cardiac ischemia and enhances cardiomyocyte and stem cell cultures. Acta Biomater. 2017;52:92–104. https://doi.org/10.1016/j.actbio.2016.12.027.
45. Schneider KH, Goldberg BJ, Hasturk O, Mu X, Dötzlhofer M, Eder G, Theodossiou S, Pichelkastner L, Riess P, Rohringer S, Kiss H, Teuschl-Woller AH, Fitzpatrick V, Enayati M, Podesser BK, Bergmeister H, Kaplan DL. Silk fibroin, gelatin, and human placenta extracellular matrix-based composite hydrogels for 3D bioprinting and soft tissue engineering. Biomater Res. 2023;27:117. https://doi.org/10.1186/s40824-023-00431-5.
46. Hackethal J, Dungel P, Teuschl AH. Frequently used strategies to isolate extracellular matrix proteins from human placenta and adipose tissue, tissue engineering part C. Methods. 2021;27: 649–60. https://doi.org/10.1089/ten.tec.2021.0150.
47. Frazão LP, Fernandes AM, Oliveira C, Martins A, Silva TH, de Castro JV, Nogueira-Silva C, Neves NM. New vascular graft using the decellularized human chorion membrane. ACS Biomater Sci Eng. 2021;7:3423–33. https://doi.org/10.1021/acsbiomaterials.1c00293.
48. Frazão LP, Vieira de Castro J, Nogueira-Silva C, Neves NM. Decellularized human chorion membrane as a novel biomaterial for tissue regeneration. Biomolecules. 2020;10:1208. https://doi.org/10.3390/biom10091208.
49. Bhoopathy J, Dharmalingam S, Sathyaraj WV, Rajendran S, Rymbai S, Senthil R, Atchudan R. Sericin/human placenta-derived extracellular matrix scaffolds for cutaneous wound treatment—preparation, characterization, *in vitro* and *in vivo* analyses. Pharmaceutics. 2023;15: 362. https://doi.org/10.3390/pharmaceutics15020362.
50. Mehrabi A, Mousazadeh S, Mollafilabi A, Nafissi N, Milan PB. Synthesis and characterization of a silk fibroin/placenta matrix hydrogel for breast reconstruction. Life Sci. 2023;334:122236. https://doi.org/10.1016/j.lfs.2023.122236.
51. Bashiri Z, Rajabi Fomeshi M, Ghasemi Hamidabadi H, Jafari D, Alizadeh S, Nazm Bojnordi M, Orive G, Dolatshahi-Pirouz A, Zahiri M, Reis RL, Kundu SC, Gholipourmalekabadi M. 3D-printed placental-derived bioinks for skin tissue regeneration with improved angiogenesis and wound healing properties. Mater Today Bio. 2023;20: 100666. https://doi.org/10.1016/j.mtbio.2023.100666.
52. Fan Y, Lüchow M, Badria A, Hutchinson DJ, Malkoch M. Placenta powder-infused thiol-Ene PEG hydrogels as potential tissue engineering scaffolds. Biomacromolecules. 2023;24:1617–26. https://doi.org/10.1021/acs.biomac.2c01355.
53. Khosrowpour Z, et al. Coculture of adipose-derived mesenchymal stem cells/macrophages on decellularized placental sponge promotes differentiation into the osteogenic lineage. Artif Organs. 2023;47:47–61. https://onlinelibrary.wiley.com/doi/10.1111/aor.14394. Accessed 9 Apr 2025.
54. Wang Z, Liu R, Liu Y, Zhao Y, Wang Y, Lu B, Li H, Ju C, Wu W, Gao X, Xu H, Cheng S, Cao Y, Jia S, Hu C, Zhu L, Hao D. Human placenta decellularized extracellular matrix hydrogel promotes the generation of human spinal cord organoids with dorsoventral organization from human induced pluripotent stem cells. ACS Biomater Sci Eng. 2024;10:3218–31. https://doi.org/10.1021/acsbiomaterials.4c00067.
55. Asgari F, Asgari H, Najafi M, Hajiaghalou S, Pirhajati-Mahabadi V, Mohammadi A, Gholipourmalekabadi M, Koruji M. In vitro proliferation and differentiation of mouse spermatogonial stem cells in decellularized human placenta matrix. J Biomed Mater Res B Appl Biomater. 2024;112:e35414. https://doi.org/10.1002/jbm.b.35414.
56. Davis JS II. Skin grafting at the Johns Hopkins Hospital. Ann Surg. 1909;50:542–9. https://doi.org/10.1097/00000658-190909000-00002.
57. Hortensius RA, Harley BA. Naturally derived biomaterials for addressing inflammation in tissue regeneration. Exp Biol Med (Maywood). 2016;241:1015–24. https://doi.org/10.1177/1535370216648022.

58. Inge E, Talmi YP, Sigler L, Finkelstein Y, Zohar Y. Antibacterial properties of human amniotic membranes. Placenta. 1991;12:285–8. https://doi.org/10.1016/0143-4004(91)90010-D.
59. Kjaergaard N, Hein M, Hyttel L, Helmig RB, Schønheyder HC, Uldbjerg N, Madsen H. Antibacterial properties of human amnion and chorion in vitro. Eur J Obstet Gynecol Reprod Biol. 2001;94:224–9. https://doi.org/10.1016/S0301-2115(00)00345-6.
60. Ricci E, Vanosi G, Lindenmair A, Hennerbichler S, Peterbauer-Scherb A, Wolbank S, Cargnoni A, Signoroni PB, Campagnol M, Gabriel C, Redl H, Parolini O. Anti-fibrotic effects of fresh and cryopreserved human amniotic membrane in a rat liver fibrosis model. Cell Tissue Bank. 2013;14:475–88. https://doi.org/10.1007/s10561-012-9337-x.
61. Chau DYS, Brown SV, Mather ML, Hutter V, Tint NL, Dua HS, Rose FRAJ, Ghaemmaghami AM. Tissue transglutaminase (TG-2) modified amniotic membrane: a novel scaffold for biomedical applications. Biomed Mater. 2012;7:045011. https://doi.org/10.1088/1748-6041/7/4/045011.
62. Spoerl E, Wollensak G, Reber F, Pillunat L. Cross-linking of human amniotic membrane by glutaraldehyde. Ophthalmic Res. 2004;36:71–7. https://doi.org/10.1159/000076884.
63. Alibabaei-Omran F, Zabihi E, Seifalian AM, Javanmehr N, Samadikuchaksaraei A, Gholipourmalekabadi M, Asghari MH, Nouri HR, Pourbagher R, Bouzari Z, Seyedmajidi S. Bilateral crosslinking with glutaraldehyde and 1-Ethyl-3-(3-dimethylaminopropyl) carbodiimide: an optimization strategy for the application of decellularized human amniotic membrane in tissue engineering. J Tissue Eng Regen Med. 2024;2024:1–14. https://doi.org/10.1155/2024/8525930.
64. Zhang Q, Chang C, Qian C, Xiao W, Zhu H, Guo J, Meng Z, Cui W, Ge Z. Photo-crosslinkable amniotic membrane hydrogel for skin defect healing. Acta Biomater. 2021;125:197–207. https://doi.org/10.1016/j.actbio.2021.02.043.
65. Skopinska-Wisniewska J, Michalak M, Tworkiewicz J, Tyloch D, Tuszynska M, Bajek A. Modification of the human amniotic membrane using different cross-linking agents as a promising tool for regenerative medicine. Materials. 2023;16:6726. https://doi.org/10.3390/ma16206726.
66. Lai J-Y. Carbodiimide cross-linking of amniotic membranes in the presence of amino acid bridges. Mater Sci Eng C. 2015;51:28–36. https://doi.org/10.1016/j.msec.2015.02.021.
67. Pazhouhnia Z, Noori A, Farzin A, Khoshmaram K, Hoseinpour M, Ai J, Ebrahimi M, Lotfibakhshaiesh N. 3D-bioprinted GelMA/gelatin/amniotic membrane extract (AME) scaffold loaded with keratinocytes, fibroblasts, and endothelial cells for skin tissue engineering. Sci Rep. 2024;14:12670. https://doi.org/10.1038/s41598-024-62926-y.
68. Wang Y, Wu H, Xiao A, Zhu J, Qiu J, Yang K, Liu Q, Hao S, Hui L, Zhou X, Hou Q, Su H, Meng Z, Chang L. Combined amniotic membrane and self-powered electrical stimulator bioelectronic dress promotes wound healing. ACS Appl Mater Interfaces. 2024;16:15809–18. https://doi.org/10.1021/acsami.3c18547.
69. Pinky A, Sharma V, Arora EP, Rao S, Arava AK, Agrawal M, Jassal S. Mohanty, modulating the hAM/PCL biocomposite for expedited wound healing: a chemical-free approach for boosting regenerative potential. ACS Biomater Sci Eng. 2024;10:3842–54. https://doi.org/10.1021/acsbiomaterials.3c01740.
70. Jia Z, Ma H, Liu J, Yan X, Liu T, Cheng YY, Li X, Wu S, Zhang J, Song K. Preparation and characterization of polylactic acid/Nano hydroxyapatite/Nano hydroxyapatite/human acellular amniotic membrane (PLA/nHAp/HAAM) hybrid scaffold for bone tissue defect repair. Materials. 2023;16:1937. https://doi.org/10.3390/ma16051937.
71. Firouzeh A, Shabani I, Karimi-Soflou R, Shabani A. Osteogenic potential of adipose stem cells on hydroxyapatite-functionalized decellularized amniotic membrane. Colloids Surf B: Biointerfaces. 2024;240:113974. https://doi.org/10.1016/j.colsurfb.2024.113974.
72. Mao X, Wang Y, Zhang X, Yao Z, Yuan Z, Yao L, Wang L, Mao H. Decellularised amniotic membrane-TDSCs composite promotes Achilles tendon healing. Sci Rep. 2025;15:15556. https://doi.org/10.1038/s41598-025-00596-0.

73. Liu C, Zhang X, Zhao L, Hui L, Liu D. Multilayer amnion-PCL nanofibrous membrane loaded with celecoxib exerts a therapeutic effect against tendon adhesion by improving the inflammatory microenvironment. Heliyon. 2023;9:e23214. https://doi.org/10.1016/j.heliyon.2023.e23214.
74. Abd Halim NFA, Ab Aziz A, Tan S-L, Selvaratnam V, Kamarul T. A systematic review of human amnion enhanced cartilage regeneration in full-thickness cartilage defects. Biomimetics (Basel). 2024;9:383. https://doi.org/10.3390/biomimetics9070383.
75. Jin CZ, Park SR, Choi BH, Lee K-Y, Kang CK, Min B-H. Human amniotic membrane as a delivery matrix for articular cartilage repair. Tissue Eng. 2007;13:693–702. https://doi.org/10.1089/ten.2006.0184.
76. Priddy LB, Krishnan L, Hettiaratchi MH, Karthikeyakannan S, Gupte N, Guldberg RE. Amniotic membrane attenuates heterotopic ossification following high-dose bone morphogenetic protein-2 treatment of segmental bone defects. J Orthop Res. 2023;41:130–40. https://doi.org/10.1002/jor.25324.
77. Jun Z, Yuping W, Yanran H, Ziming L, Yuwan L, Xizhong Z, Zhilin W, Xiaoji L. Human acellular amniotic membrane scaffolds encapsulating juvenile cartilage fragments accelerate the repair of rabbit osteochondral defects. Bone Joint Res. 2022;11:349–61. https://doi.org/10.1302/2046-3758.116.BJR-2021-0490.R1.
78. Rastegar Adib F, Bagheri F, Sharifi AM. Osteochondral regeneration in rabbit using xenograft decellularized ECM in combination with different biological products; platelet-rich fibrin, amniotic membrane extract, and mesenchymal stromal cells. J Biomed Mater Res B Appl Biomater. 2022;110:2089–99. https://doi.org/10.1002/jbm.b.35063.
79. Wang J, Li C, Zhang J, An M, Zhao G, Stark SD, Liu Y. Effect of decellularized amniotic membrane on the tendon-bone integration in rotator cuff repair: a comparative rat model study. Orthop Surg. 2025;17:575–82. https://doi.org/10.1111/os.14316.
80. Shimazaki J, Yang H-Y, Tsubota K. Amniotic membrane transplantation for ocular surface reconstruction in patients with chemical and thermal burns. Ophthalmology. 1997;104:2068–76. https://doi.org/10.1016/S0161-6420(97)30057-8.
81. Tsubota K, Satake Y, Ohyama M, Toda I, Takano Y, Ono M, Shinozaki N, Shimazaki J. Surgical reconstruction of the ocular surface in advanced ocular cicatricial pemphigoid and stevens-Johnson syndrome. Am J Ophthalmol. 1996;122:38–52. https://doi.org/10.1016/S0002-9394(14)71962-2.
82. Prabhasawat P, Barton K, Burkett G, Tseng SCG. Comparison of conjunctival autografts, amniotic membrane grafts, and primary closure for pterygium excision. Ophthalmology. 1997;104:974–85. https://doi.org/10.1016/S0161-6420(97)30197-3.
83. Tseng SCG, Prabhasawat P, Lee S-H. Amniotic membrane transplantation for conjunctival surface reconstruction. Am J Ophthalmol. 1997;124:765–74. https://doi.org/10.1016/S0002-9394(14)71693-9.
84. Lee S-H, Tseng SCG. Amniotic membrane transplantation for persistent epithelial defects with ulceration. Am J Ophthalmol. 1997;123:303–12. https://doi.org/10.1016/S0002-9394(14)70125-4.
85. Choi YS, Kim JY, Wee WR, Lee JH. Effect of the application of human amniotic membrane on rabbit corneal wound healing after excimer laser photorefractive keratectomy. Cornea. 1998;17:389–95. https://doi.org/10.1097/00003226-199807000-00009.
86. Kim JC, Tseng SC. Transplantation of preserved human amniotic membrane for surface reconstruction in severely damaged rabbit corneas. Cornea. 1995;14:473–84.
87. Fukuda K, Chikama T, Nakamura M, Nishida T. Differential distribution of subchains of the basement membrane components type IV collagen and laminin among the amniotic membrane, cornea, and conjunctiva. Cornea. 1999;18:73–9.
88. Mao Y, Protzman NM, John N, Kuehn A, Long D, Sivalenka R, Junka RA, Shah AU, Gosiewska A, Hariri RJ, Brigido SA. An in vitro comparison of human corneal epithelial cell activity and inflammatory response on differently designed ocular amniotic membranes and a clinical case study. J Biomed Mater Res. 2023;111:684–700. https://doi.org/10.1002/jbm.b.35186.

89. Bakhshandeh H, Atyabi F, Soleimani M, Taherzadeh ES, Shahhoseini S, Cohan RA. Biocompatibility improvement of artificial cornea using chitosan-dextran nanoparticles containing bioactive macromolecules obtained from human amniotic membrane. Int J Biol Macromol. 2021;169:492–9. https://doi.org/10.1016/j.ijbiomac.2020.12.125.
90. Basasoro A, Mendicute J, Rezola M, Burgos J, Fernández M, Esporrín-Ubieto D, Sonzogni A, Calderón M, Calafel I, Díaz A, De Souza J, Aiastui A, Azkargorta M, Elortza F, Vecino E, Acera A. The influence of amniotic membrane proteins on corneal regeneration when delivered directly or using hydrogel platforms. Front Med. 2025;12:1498319. https://doi.org/10.3389/fmed.2025.1498319.
91. Gulameabasse S, Gindraux F, Catros S, Fricain J-C, Fenelon M. Chorion and amnion/chorion membranes in oral and periodontal surgery: a systematic review. J Biomed Mater Res B Appl Biomater. 2021;109:1216–29. https://doi.org/10.1002/jbm.b.34783.
92. Mahheidari N, Kamalabadi-Farahani M, Nourani MR, Atashi A, Alizadeh M, Aldaghi N, Salehi M. Biological study of skin wound treated with alginate/carboxymethyl cellulose/chorion membrane, diopside nanoparticles, and botox A. NPJ Regen Med. 2024;9:1–20. https://doi.org/10.1038/s41536-024-00354-2.
93. Schneider KH, Enayati M, Grasl C, Walter I, Budinsky L, Zebic G, Kaun C, Wagner A, Kratochwill K, Redl H, Teuschl AH, Podesser BK, Bergmeister H. Acellular vascular matrix grafts from human placenta chorion: impact of ECM preservation on graft characteristics, protein composition and *in vivo* performance. Biomaterials. 2018;177:14–26. https://doi.org/10.1016/j.biomaterials.2018.05.045.
94. Falkner F, Mayer SA, Thomas B, Zimmermann SO, Walter S, Heimel P, Thiele W, Sleeman JP, Bigdeli AK, Kiss H, Podesser BK, Kneser U, Bergmeister H, Schneider KH. Acellular human placenta small-diameter vessels as a Favorable source of super-microsurgical vascular replacements: a proof of concept. Bioengineering. 2023;10:337. https://doi.org/10.3390/bioengineering10030337.
95. Oliveira TS, Smirnow I, Santee KM, Miglino MA, da Silva Nunes Barreto R. Decellularized vascular scaffolds derived from bovine placenta blood vessels. Arq Bras Cardiol. 2023;120:e20220816. https://doi.org/10.36660/abc.20220816.
96. Martins EAG, Deus IA, Gomes MC, Silva AS, Mano JF, Custódio CA. Human chorionic membrane-derived Tunable hydrogels for vascular tissue engineering strategies. Adv Healthc Mater. 2025;14:2401510. https://doi.org/10.1002/adhm.202401510.
97. Comperat L, Chagot L, Massot S, Stachowicz M-L, Dusserre N, Médina C, Desigaux T, Dupuy J-W, Fricain J-C, Oliveira H. Harnessing human placental membrane-derived bioinks: characterization and applications in bioprinting and Vasculogenesis. Adv Healthc Mater. 2024;13:2303370. https://doi.org/10.1002/adhm.202303370.
98. Go YY, Kim SE, Cho GJ, Chae S-W, Song J-J. Differential effects of amnion and chorion membrane extracts on osteoblast-like cells due to the different growth factor composition of the extracts. PLoS One. 2017;12:e0182716. https://doi.org/10.1371/journal.pone.0182716.
99. Zare-Bidaki M, Sadrinia S, Erfani S, Afkar E, Ghanbarzade N. Antimicrobial properties of amniotic and chorionic membranes: a comparative study of two human Fetal sacs. J Reprod Infertil. 2017;18:218–24.
100. Lakkireddy C, Vishwakarma SK, Raju N, Ahmed SI, Bardia A, Khan MA, Annamaneni S, Khan AA. Fabrication of decellularized amnion and chorion scaffolds to develop bioengineered cell-laden constructs. Cell Mol Bioeng. 2022;15:137–50. https://doi.org/10.1007/s12195-021-00707-7.
101. Khazaei M, Bozorgi M, Rezakhani L, Bozorgi A. Fabrication and characterization of nanohydroxyapatite/chitosan/decellularized placenta scaffold for bone tissue engineering applications. Int J Biol Macromol. 2024;281:136340. https://doi.org/10.1016/j.ijbiomac.2024.136340.
102. Kim SG. Dehydrated human amnion–chorion membrane as a bioactive scaffold for dental pulp tissue regeneration. Biomimetics (Basel). 2024;9:771. https://doi.org/10.3390/biomimetics9120771.

103. Wetzell B, Ork B, Softic D, Morse J, Hutchens W, Meng F, McLean JB, Moore MA, Qin X. Characterization of a full-thickness decellularized and lyophilized human placental membrane for clinical applications. Int Wound J. 2024;21:e14888. https://doi.org/10.1111/iwj.14888.
104. Deng X, Zhang S, Qing Q, Wang P, Ma H, Ma Q, Zhao W, Tang H, Lu M. Distinct biological characteristics of mesenchymal stem cells separated from different components of human placenta. Biochem Biophys Rep. 2024;39:101739. https://doi.org/10.1016/j.bbrep.2024.101739.
105. Miki T, Lehmann T, Cai H, Stolz DB, Strom SC. Stem cell characteristics of amniotic epithelial cells. Stem Cells. 2005;23:1549–59. https://doi.org/10.1634/stemcells.2004-0357.
106. Tamagawa T, Ishiwata I, Saito S. Establishment and characterization of a pluripotent stem cell line derived from human amniotic membranes and initiation of germ layers in vitro. Hum Cell. 2008;17:125–30. https://doi.org/10.1111/j.1749-0774.2004.tb00028.x.
107. Alviano F, Fossati V, Marchionni C, Arpinati M, Bonsi L, Franchina M, Lanzoni G, Cantoni S, Cavallini C, Bianchi F, Tazzari PL, Pasquinelli G, Foroni L, Ventura C, Grossi A, Bagnara GP. Term amniotic membrane is a high throughput source for multipotent mesenchymal stem cells with the ability to differentiate into endothelial cells in vitro. BMC Dev Biol. 2007;7:11. https://doi.org/10.1186/1471-213X-7-11.
108. Zhao P, Ise H, Hongo M, Ota M, Konishi I, Nikaido T. Human amniotic mesenchymal cells have some characteristics of cardiomyocytes. Transplantation. 2005;79:528–35. https://doi.org/10.1097/01.TP.0000149503.92433.39.
109. Parolini O, Alviano F, Bagnara GP, Bilic G, Bühring H-J, Evangelista M, Hennerbichler S, Liu B, Magatti M, Mao N, Miki T, Marongiu F, Nakajima H, Nikaido T, Portmann-Lanz CB, Sankar V, Soncini M, Stadler G, Surbek D, Takahashi TA, Redl H, Sakuragawa N, Wolbank S, Zeisberger S, Zisch A, Strom SC. Concise review: isolation and characterization of Cells from human term placenta: outcome of the first international workshop on placenta derived stem cells. Stem Cells. 2008;26:300–11. https://doi.org/10.1634/stemcells.2007-0594.
110. Savickiene J, Treigyte G, Baronaite S, Valiuliene G, Kaupinis A, Valius M, Arlauskiene A, Navakauskiene R. Human amniotic fluid mesenchymal stem Cells from second- and third-trimester amniocentesis: differentiation potential, molecular signature, and proteome analysis. Stem Cells Int. 2015;2015:1–15. https://doi.org/10.1155/2015/319238.
111. Tsai M-S. Isolation of human multipotent mesenchymal stem cells from second-trimester amniotic fluid using a novel two-stage culture protocol. Hum Reprod. 2004;19:1450–6. https://doi.org/10.1093/humrep/deh279.
112. Spitzhorn L-S, Rahman MS, Schwindt L, Ho H-T, Wruck W, Bohndorf M, Wehrmeyer S, Ncube A, Beyer I, Hagenbeck C, Balan P, Fehm T, Adjaye J. Isolation and molecular characterization of amniotic fluid-derived mesenchymal stem Cells obtained from caesarean sections. Stem Cells Int. 2017;2017:5932706. https://doi.org/10.1155/2017/5932706.
113. Wang N, Wang H, Weng D, Wang B, Wang J, He J, Mo X, Wang F, He Z. Human amniotic mesenchymal stem cells improve patency and regeneration of electrospun biodegradable vascular grafts via anti-thrombogenicity and M2 macrophage polarization. Colloids Surf B: Biointerfaces. 2025;250:114559. https://doi.org/10.1016/j.colsurfb.2025.114559.
114. Feng M, Hu S, Qin W, Tang Y, Guo R, Han L. Bioprinting of a blue light-cross-linked biodegradable hydrogel encapsulating amniotic mesenchymal stem Cells for intrauterine adhesion prevention. ACS Omega. 2021;6:23067–75. https://doi.org/10.1021/acsomega.1c02117.
115. Dai X, Yuan M, Yang Y, Dang M, Yang J, Shi J, Liu D, Li M, Yao H, Fei W. Dual cross-linked COL1/HAp bionic gradient scaffolds containing human amniotic mesenchymal stem cells promote rotator cuff tendon-bone interface healing. Biomater Adv. 2024;158:213799. https://doi.org/10.1016/j.bioadv.2024.213799.
116. Rameshbabu AP, Bankoti K, Datta S, Subramani E, Apoorva A, Ghosh P, Jana S, Manchikanti P, Roy S, Chaudhury K, Dhara S. Bioinspired 3D porous human placental derived extracellular matrix/silk fibroin sponges for accelerated bone regeneration. Mater Sci Eng C Mater Biol Appl. 2020;113:110990. https://doi.org/10.1016/j.msec.2020.110990.

117. Zhang Q, Lai D. Application of human amniotic epithelial cells in regenerative medicine: a systematic review. Stem Cell Res Ther. 2020;11:439. https://doi.org/10.1186/s13287-020-01951-w.
118. Russo V, El Khatib M, di Marcantonio L, Ancora M, Wyrwa R, Mauro A, Walter T, Weisser J, Citeroni MR, Lazzaro F, Di Federico M, Berardinelli P, Cammà C, Schnabelrauch M, Barboni B. Tendon biomimetic electrospun PLGA fleeces induce an early epithelial-mesenchymal transition and tenogenic differentiation on amniotic epithelial stem cells. Cells. 2020;9:303. https://doi.org/10.3390/cells9020303.
119. Russo V, El Khatib M, Prencipe G, Mauro A, Di Giacinto O, Haidar-Montes AA, Pulcini F, Dufrusine B, Cerveró-Varona A, Faydaver M, Di Berardino C, Dainese E, Berardinelli P, Schnabelrauch M, Barboni B. Tendon 3D scaffolds establish a tailored microenvironment instructing paracrine mediated regenerative amniotic epithelial stem cells potential. Biomedicine. 2022;10:2578. https://doi.org/10.3390/biomedicines10102578.
120. Manzari-Tavakoli A, Babajani A, Vousooghi N, Moghimi A, Tarasi R, Safaeinejad F, Norouzi S, Bahrami S, Niknejad H. Therapeutic potential of placenta-derived stem cells cultivated on noggin-loaded nanochitosan/polypyrrole-alginate conductive scaffold to restore spinal cord injury. Stem Cell Res Ther. 2024;15:497. https://doi.org/10.1186/s13287-024-04104-5.
121. Li J, Yao Y, Zhou J, Yang Z, Qiu C, Lu Y, Xie J, Liu J, Jiang T, Kou Y, Ge Z, Liang P, Qiu C, Shen L, Zhu Y, Gao C, Yu L. Epicardial transplantation of antioxidant polyurethane scaffold based human amniotic epithelial stem cell patch for myocardial infarction treatment. Nat Commun. 2024;15:9105. https://doi.org/10.1038/s41467-024-53531-8.
122. Peister A, Woodruff MA, Prince JJ, Gray DP, Hutmacher DW, Guldberg RE. Cell sourcing for bone tissue engineering: amniotic fluid stem cells have a delayed, robust differentiation compared to mesenchymal stem cells. Stem Cell Res. 2011;7:17–27. https://doi.org/10.1016/j.scr.2011.03.001.
123. Song Y, Zhang T, Shi P, Gao Y, Pang X. Exosomes derived from human amniotic mesenchymal stem cells promotes angiogenesis in hUVECs by delivering novel miRNA N-194. Mol Med. 2025;31:173. https://doi.org/10.1186/s10020-025-01192-8.
124. Fu S, Zhang H, Li X, Zhang Q, Guo C, Qiu K, Feng J, Liu X, Liu D. Exosomes derived from human amniotic mesenchymal stem Cells facilitate diabetic wound healing by angiogenesis and enrich multiple lncRNAs. Tissue Eng Regen Med. 2023;20:295–308. https://doi.org/10.1007/s13770-022-00513-w.
125. Sandonà M, Esposito F, Cargnoni A, Silini A, Romele P, Parolini O, Saccone V. Amniotic membrane-derived stromal Cells release extracellular vesicles that Favor regeneration of dystrophic skeletal muscles. Int J Mol Sci. 2023;24:12457. https://doi.org/10.3390/ijms241512457.
126. Peng Z-Q, Guan X-H, Yu Z-P, Wu J, Han X-H, Li M-H, Qu X-H, Chen Z-P, Han X-J, Wang X-Y. Human amniotic mesenchymal stem cells-derived conditioned medium and exosomes alleviate oxidative stress-induced retinal degeneration by activating PI3K/Akt/FoxO3 pathway. Exp Eye Res. 2024;244:109919. https://doi.org/10.1016/j.exer.2024.109919.
127. Hu S, Wang Z, Jin C, Chen Q, Fang Y, Jin J, Chen J, Lu L, Tian H, Xu J, Gao F, Wang J, Zhang J, Cui H-P, Xu G-T, Ou Q. Human amniotic epithelial cell-derived extracellular vesicles provide an extracellular matrix-based microenvironment for corneal injury repair. J Tissue Eng. 2022;13:20417314221122123. https://doi.org/10.1177/20417314221122123.
128. Varyani L, Ahmadpanah N, Kasiri R, Shahzamani S, Tomraee S, Jafari A, Mirjalili H, Asl NS. Human amniotic membrane hydrogel loaded with exosomes derived from human placental mesenchymal stem cells accelerate diabetic wound healing. Tissue Cell. 2024;91:102590. https://doi.org/10.1016/j.tice.2024.102590.
129. Tian L, Wang Z, Chen S, Guo K, Hao Y, Ma L, Ma K, Chen J, Liu X, Li L, Fu X, Zhang C. Ellagic acid-loaded sEVs encapsulated in GelMA hydrogel accelerate diabetic wound healing by activating EGFR on skin repair cells. Cell Prolif. 2025;58:e70064. https://doi.org/10.1111/cpr.70064.

130. Huleihel L, Hussey GS, Naranjo JD, Zhang L, Dziki JL, Turner NJ, Stolz DB, Badylak SF. Matrix-bound nanovesicles within ECM bioscaffolds. Sci Adv. 2016;2:e1600502. https://doi.org/10.1126/sciadv.1600502.
131. Kobayashi M, Negishi J, Ishida N, Hashimoto Y, Sasaki Y, Akiyoshi K, Kimura T, Kishida A. Effects of the matrix-bounded nanovesicles of high-hydrostatic pressure decellularized tissues on neural regeneration. Sci Technol Adv Mater. 2024;25:2404380. https://doi.org/10.1080/14686996.2024.2404380.
132. Ma K, Yao H, Zhang M, Guo J-J, Cheng L, Li J-H, Liu Z-J. Effect of human placental extract on proliferation of human umbilical cord blood CD34(+) cells in vitro. Zhongguo Shi Yan Xue Ye Xue Za Zhi. 2012;20:1183–6.
133. Togashi S-I, Takahashi N, Iwama M, Watanabe S, Tamagawa K, Fukui T. Antioxidative collagen-derived peptides in human-placenta extract. Placenta. 2002;23:497–502. https://doi.org/10.1053/plac.2002.0833.
134. O'Keefe EJ, Payne RE, Russell N. Keratinocyte growth-promoting activity from human placenta. J Cell Physiol. 1985;124:439–45. https://doi.org/10.1002/jcp.1041240312.
135. Hong JW, Lee WJ, Hahn SB, Kim BJ, Lew DH. The effect of human placenta extract in a wound healing model. Ann Plast Surg. 2010;65:96. https://doi.org/10.1097/SAP.0b013e3181b0bb67.
136. Nagae M, Nagata M, Teramoto M, Yamakawa M, Matsuki T, Ohnuki K, Shimizu K. Effect of porcine placenta extract supplement on skin condition in healthy adult women: a randomized, double-blind placebo-controlled study. Nutrients. 2020;12:1671. https://doi.org/10.3390/nu12061671.
137. Lee J, Kim D, Jang CH, Kim GH. Highly elastic 3D-printed gelatin/HA/placental-extract scaffolds for bone tissue engineering. Theranostics. 2022;12:4051–66. https://doi.org/10.7150/thno.73146.
138. Taweechaipaisankul A, Thumrongsiri N, Chonniyom W, Dana P, Tanyapanyachon P, Rattanatayarom M, Chinchoosak W, Saengkrit N. Alginate-based encapsulation of porcine placenta extract: preparation, enteric sustained release, biological activities, and stability. Food Hydrocoll Health. 2025;7:100194. https://doi.org/10.1016/j.fhfh.2024.100194.
139. Capella-Monsonís H, Cramer M, Turner N, Reing J, Zhang L, Kronengold RT, Bartolacci J, Badylak SF. The composition and mechanical properties of porcine placental ECM from three different breeds. Biomed Phys Eng Express. 2023;9:065012. https://doi.org/10.1088/2057-1976/acfb05.
140. Kollmetz T, Castillo-Alcala F, Veale RWF, Taghavi N, van Heeswijk VM, Persenaire M, May BCH, Dempsey SG. Comparative analysis of commercially available extracellular matrix soft tissue bioscaffolds. Tissue Eng Part A. 2024;31:442. https://doi.org/10.1089/ten.tea.2024.0076.
141. Mao Y, John N, Protzman NM, Kuehn A, Long D, Sivalenka R, Junka RA, Gosiewska A, Hariri RJ, Brigido SA. A decellularized flowable placental connective tissue matrix supports cellular functions of human tenocytes in vitro. J Exp Orthop. 2022;9:69. https://doi.org/10.1186/s40634-022-00509-4.
142. Ruiz-Muñoz M, Martinez-Barrios F-J, Lopezosa-Reca E. Placenta-derived biomaterials vs. standard care in chronic diabetic foot ulcer healing: a systematic review and meta-analysis. Diabetes Metab Syndr Clin Res Rev. 2025;19:103170. https://doi.org/10.1016/j.dsx.2024.103170.
143. Ragsdale LB, Sarhaddi D, Nathan C. Novel use of wound matrix in mastopexy complicated by pyoderma gangrenosum, aesthetic surgery journal open. Forum. 2023;5:ojad085. https://doi.org/10.1093/asjof/ojad085.
144. Fife C, LeBoutillier B, Taylor C, Marcinek BT. Real-world use and outcomes of hard-to-heal wounds managed with porcine placental extracellular matrix. Cureus. 2024;16:e76262. https://doi.org/10.7759/cureus.76262.

145. Gibbons GW. Grafix®, a cryopreserved placental membrane, for the treatment of chronic/stalled wounds. Adv Wound Care (New Rochelle). 2015;4:534–44. https://doi.org/10.1089/wound.2015.0647.
146. Du YL, Lim P, Isseroff R, Dahle S. Patterns of use of advanced wound matrices in the veterans administration clinics. Wound Repair Regen. 2024;32:118–22. https://doi.org/10.1111/wrr.13150.
147. Ganesh P, Puranik S, Abhaya M, Misra P, Guruvigneshwari M, Daniel JI. Connective tissue matrices from placental disc for wound healing: mini-review. Biotechnol Lett. 2023;45:921–9. https://doi.org/10.1007/s10529-023-03403-w.
148. Wilmas KM, Patel J, Silapunt S, Doan HQ, Migden MR. The use of a dehydrated complete human placental membrane allograft for Mohs surgical defects of the nose. Dermatologic Surg. 2023;49:343. https://doi.org/10.1097/DSS.0000000000003711.
149. McQuilling JP, Kimmerling KA, Staples MC, Mowry KC. Evaluation of two distinct placental-derived membranes and their effect on tenocyte responses in vitro. J Tissue Eng Regen Med. 2019;13:1316–30. https://doi.org/10.1002/term.2876.
150. Ditmars FS, Lind RA, Broderick TC, Fagg WS. Safety and efficacy of acellular human amniotic fluid and membrane in the treatment of non-healing wounds in a patient with chronic venous insufficiency. SAGE Open Med Case Rep. 2022;10:2050313X221100882. https://doi.org/10.1177/2050313X221100882.
151. Travé-Huarte S, Wolffsohn JS. Sutureless dehydrated amniotic membrane (Omnigen) application using a specialised bandage contact lens (OmniLenz) for the treatment of dry eye disease: a 6-month randomised control trial. Medicina (Kaunas). 2024;60:985. https://doi.org/10.3390/medicina60060985.
152. Huang Y-H, Tsai D-C, Wang L-C, Chen S-J. Comparison between cryopreserved and dehydrated human amniotic membrane graft in treating challenging cases with macular hole and macular hole retinal detachment. J Ophthalmol. 2020;2020:1–9. https://doi.org/10.1155/2020/9157518.
153. Chuck RS, Graff JM, Bryant MR, Sweet PM. Biomechanical characterization of human amniotic membrane preparations for ocular surface reconstruction. Ophthalmic Res. 2004;36:341–8. https://doi.org/10.1159/000081637.
154. Miyakoshi A, Nishida Y, Tanaka A, Hayashi A. Histological equivalence of a hyper-dry amniotic membrane and the Ambio2™ after implantation in the rabbit conjunctiva. Ophthalmic Res. 2020;63:423–6. https://doi.org/10.1159/000504579.
155. Naxer S, Horn M, Schittkowski M. Processed amniotic membrane for conjunctival reconstruction in complex strabismus surgery. Strabismus. 2018;26:191–7. https://doi.org/10.1080/09273972.2018.1502794.
156. Choi CM, Jeon HS. Clinical outcomes of in-office Sutureless amniotic membrane transplantation in persistent epithelial defect. Korean J Ophthalmol. 2022;36:87–96. https://doi.org/10.3341/kjo.2021.0095.
157. Morkin MI, Hamrah P. Efficacy of self-retained cryopreserved amniotic membrane for treatment of neuropathic corneal pain. Ocul Surf. 2018;16:132–8. https://doi.org/10.1016/j.jtos.2017.10.003.
158. Harmon KA, Kimmerling KA, Avery JT, Mowry KC. Hypothermically stored amnion is robust and provides a scaffold for supporting wound healing by retaining the characteristics of native tissue. Int J Mol Sci. 2024;25:10347. https://doi.org/10.3390/ijms251910347.
159. Snyder RJ, Shimozaki K, Tallis A, Kerzner M, Reyzelman A, Lintzeris D, Bell D, Rutan RL, Rosenblum B. A prospective, randomized, multicenter, controlled evaluation of the use of dehydrated amniotic membrane allograft compared to standard of care for the closure of chronic diabetic foot ulcer. Wounds. 2016;28:70–7.
160. Lintzeris D, Yarrow K, Johnson L, White A, Hampton A, Strickland A, Albert K, Cook A. Use of a dehydrated amniotic membrane allograft on lower extremity ulcers in patients with challenging wounds: a retrospective case series. Ostomy Wound Manage. 2015;61:30–6.

161. Barr SM. Dehydrated amniotic membrane allograft for treatment of chronic leg ulcers in patients with multiple comorbidities: a case series. J Am Coll Clin Wound Spec. 2014;6:38–45. https://doi.org/10.1016/j.jccw.2016.01.002.
162. Abdo RJ. Treatment of diabetic foot ulcers with dehydrated amniotic membrane allograft: a prospective case series. J Wound Care. 2016;25:S4–9. https://doi.org/10.12968/jowc.2016.25.Sup7.S4.
163. Rosenblum BI. A retrospective case series of a dehydrated amniotic membrane allograft for treatment of unresolved diabetic foot ulcers. J Am Podiatr Med Assoc. 2016;106:328–37. https://doi.org/10.7547/15-139.
164. Thompson P, Hanson DS, Langemo D, Anderson J. Comparing human amniotic allograft and standard wound care when using total contact casting in the treatment of patients with diabetic foot ulcers. Adv Skin Wound Care. 2019;32:272–7. https://doi.org/10.1097/01.ASW.0000557831.78645.85.
165. Boyar V, Galiczewski C. Efficacy of dehydrated human amniotic membrane allograft for the treatment of severe extravasation injuries in preterm neonates. Wounds. 2018;30:224–8.
166. Bianchi C, Cazzell S, Vayser D, Reyzelman AM, Dosluoglu H, Tovmassian G, E.V.S. Group. A multicentre randomised controlled trial evaluating the efficacy of dehydrated human amnion/chorion membrane (EpiFix®) allograft for the treatment of venous leg ulcers. Int Wound J. 2018;15:114–22. https://doi.org/10.1111/iwj.12843.
167. Glat P, Orgill DP, Galiano R, Armstrong D, Serena T, DiDomenico LA, Kaufman J, Carter MJ, Jacobs AM, Zelen CM. Placental membrane provides improved healing efficacy and lower cost versus a tissue-engineered human skin in the treatment of diabetic foot ulcerations. Plast Reconstr Surg Glob Open. 2019;7:e2371. https://doi.org/10.1097/GOX.0000000000002371.
168. Sabol TJ, Tran GS, Matuszewski J, Weston WW. Standardized reporting of amnion and amnion/chorion allograft data for wound care. Health Sci Rep. 2022;5:e794. https://doi.org/10.1002/hsr2.794.
169. Holder S. Amnioexcel® plus graft and its prospective benefits in salvaging a below- the- knee-amputation stump wound. IJCMCR. 2023;24:000593. https://doi.org/10.46998/IJCMCR.2023.24.000593.

Sex Differences

Sex Differences in Bone: Considerations for Biomaterial Design

Aleczandria Tiffany and Vasiliki Kolliopoulos

Abstract Bone provides structural support and protects vital organs in our bodies. Its structure, composition, and functionality vary across development and aging as well as across sex. In this chapter, we discuss sex-based differences in bone during different stages of development, injury, and aging and we highlight sex-based considerations one should take when designing an experiment and choosing materials and reagents. First, we provide an overview of key mediators of bone homeostasis and sex-based differences that result in changes to the composition, structure, or function of healthy, injured, and aging bone. We then summarize biomaterial design strategies to develop bone-mimetic biomaterials that recapitulate the mechanical properties and heterogeneous composition of bone. Finally, we introduce biomaterials approaches to evaluate sex-based differences in bone-mimetic microenvironments in vitro, in vivo, and ex vivo.

Keywords Bone regeneration · Biomaterials · Sex-based differences · Bone injury · Bone formation · Multicellular crosstalk · Osteoblast · Osteoclast · Homeostasis · Osteoporosis · Estrogen · Hormones

1 Introduction

Bone fractures are common and costly injuries that affect people worldwide. A 2021 study evaluated the burden of bone fractures at global levels from 1990 to 2019 for all ages in male and female individuals (intersex individuals not included). They

---

Aleczandria Tiffany and Vasiliki Kolliopoulos contributed equally to this work.

A. Tiffany
Independent Scientist, New York, NY, USA

V. Kolliopoulos (✉)
Department of Bioengineering, Rice University, Houston, TX, USA
e-mail: ak182@rice.edu

S. G. Zambuto, M. L. Oyen (eds.), *Biomaterials for Women's Health Engineering*,
https://doi.org/10.1007/978-3-032-10745-9_14

report that there were 178 million new fractures and 455 million cases of acute or long-term symptoms of a fracture that occurred globally in 2019 [1]. The total number of new fracture cases (across all ages) was higher in males (102 million) than females (76.4 million), and the age-standardized rate of fracture was higher in males (2619.8 cases per 100,000 people) than females (1943.6 cases per 100,000 people) [1].

When the data is separated by age, it reveals that older age groups are more likely to have new fractures compared to younger age groups. These fractures are due to the bone becoming more fragile with age. Furthermore, when examining fractures that occur in patients over the age of 64, the analysis reveals that females exhibit higher rates of fracture than males [1]. Several other studies have also indicated that older females are more prone to fracture than older males [2–4]. Despite experiencing fragility fractures at lower rates, males have poorer outcomes following surgical intervention from fractures in major joints (e.g., hip) [3, 4]. This would suggest that additional intervention is needed to prevent fractures in female patients and improve post-surgery care and recovery in male patients.

Clinical intervention for nonunion bone fractures, fractures unable to heal without clinical intervention [5], commonly utilize bone grafts derived from the injured patient (autograft), cadaveric human donors (allograft and demineralized bone matrix), or animals (xenograft). Autografts are effective and successful solutions to nonunion bone repair and are considered the "gold standard" for clinical use [6], but they are limited by the available bone that can be removed from the donor site without causing additional tissue injury [6, 7]. Allografts and demineralized bone matrix (allogenic tissue with the mineral component removed [8]) have concerns related to variable purification methods, differences in bone healing based on donor characteristics, and disease transmission [7]. Xenografts are plagued by poor integration with the host tissue and long-term patient complications [9, 10] and are most often refused by patients, along with allografts [11]. Engineered biomaterials are becoming more popular for nonunion bone repair and can be designed to address current limitations in bone tissue repair [12]. However, there is a significant lack of sex-aggregated data in the tissue engineering scientific literature. A 2019 review evaluated papers published in tissue engineering and found that over 95% of studies using cell lines and ~90% of studies using primary cells fail to mention the sex of the cells used during their tissue engineering experiments [13].

We mentioned that biological sex significantly impacts age-related fracture incidence and patient outcome [1–4]. This suggests that biological sex should be used as a biological variable in age-related repair studies to adequately address disparities in healing for older patients. As we will discuss in depth, biological sex also impacts bone biology during development, homeostasis, and injury. Thus, we assert that biological sex should be *ubiquitously* used as a biological variable when engineering bone biomaterials and designing all in vitro and in vivo studies.

In this chapter, we will first discuss the biology of bone and how biological sex plays a role during bone development, homeostasis, injury and subsequent healing, and aging. We will then cover existing research that evaluates biological sex in bone tissue engineering applications and discuss when and how biological sex can be incorporated into biomaterials design.

2 Developing Bone

2.1 Key Terms

- *Stem cells* are pluripotent cells originating in the bone marrow or periosteum that can differentiate into osteoblasts, chondrocytes, and adipocytes. *Differentiation* is the process by which stem cells become different cell types.
- *Osteoblasts* are bone cells that are responsible for collagen production and mineral deposition in bone tissue. Osteoblasts differentiate into osteocytes. *Osteocytes* are mature bone cells that are embedded in the surrounding collagen matrix.
- *Chondrocytes* are cartilage cells that are responsible for collagen deposition in cartilage tissue. *Adipocytes* are adipose (i.e., fat) cells that compose adipose tissue and store energy as fat.
- *Sex hormones* (also called sex steroids [14]) are chemical messengers produced by the reproductive organs (testes in males, ovaries in females), adrenal glands in males and females, and the placenta in pregnant females. The sex hormones are present in both sexes, but at varying levels. The "female sex hormones" are estrogen and progesterone, and the "male sex hormones" are testosterone and dihydrotestosterone.
- *Progesterone* is a sex hormone associated with the female reproductive system that is important during pregnancy. Progesterone is produced in the ovaries and adrenal gland in females, the placenta in pregnant females, and the testes and adrenal gland in males [15].
- *Estrogen* is a sex hormone associated with the female reproductive system. Estrogens are produced in the ovaries in females and the testes in males. There are three types of estrogens: estrone, estradiol, and estriol [16].
- *Androgens* are a group of sex hormones associated with the male reproductive system and include testosterone and dihydrotestosterone [17].
- *Testosterone* is a sex hormone associated with the male reproductive system. Testosterone is produced in the testes in males and the ovaries in females [18].
- *Dihydrotestosterone* (DHT) is a sex hormone associated with the male reproductive system and is synthesized from testosterone [18].

2.2 Section Overview

In this section, we discuss the role of sex hormones in bone development. Bone development is a complex and well-coordinated process, and there are two types of bone formation that occur during human development: *intramembranous ossification* [19–23] and *endochondral ossification* [20–24]. These two processes are also important for bone healing, which we will discuss in a later section. Sex hormones are necessary for bone development and impact bone growth, maturation, and maintenance. Furthermore, sex hormones are responsible for the physical differences in the male and female skeleton [25–27].

2.3 The Biology of Bone Formation: Intramembranous and Endochondral Ossification

Intramembranous ossification occurs in the development of flat bones, which include the bones in your skull, pelvis, and ribcage (Fig. 1). During intramembranous ossification, stem cells directly differentiate into osteoblasts, which are specialized cells responsible for building bone [19–22, 28]. The differentiation of stem cells into osteoblasts, called osteogenic differentiation, is mediated by bone morphogenic proteins (BMPs). BMPs upregulate other cytokines including the osteogenic factor runt-related transcription factor 2 (RUNX2) and the angiogenic factor vascular endothelial growth factor (VEGF). RUNX2 further interacts with Osterix, an osteoblast-specific transcription factor secreted by pre-osteoblasts, osteoblasts, and osteocytes. VEGF is critical for osteogenesis and angiogenesis, promoting osteogenic differentiation of stem cells into osteoblasts and facilitating the formation of vasculature. Mature osteoblasts secrete a non-mineralized extracellular

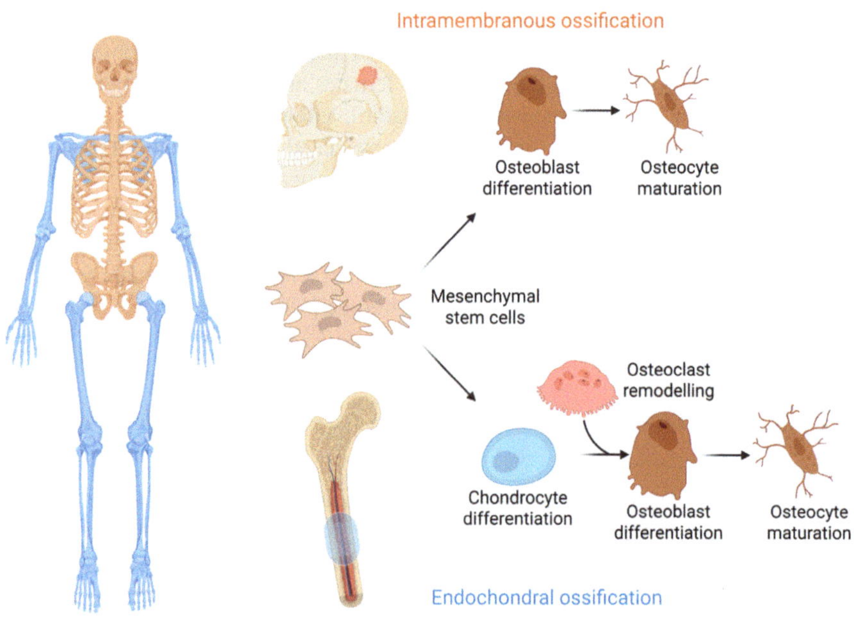

Fig. 1 Types of bone formation based on bone location. Top: Intramembranous ossification of the skull, neck, spine, and pelvis. Bottom: Endochondral ossification of the long bones

matrix composed of Type I collagen, and this matrix mineralizes once vascularization occurs. Osteoblasts encapsulated in the mineralized matrix further differentiate into osteocytes. Traditional bone tissue engineering strategies for bone regeneration induce direct bone formation, mimicking the process of intramembranous ossification [19].

Endochondral ossification occurs in the development of long bones, which include the bones in your legs and arms, and occurs at the growth plates (Fig. 1). Growth plates are temporary cartilage tissues responsible for longitudinal growth [29]. During endochondral ossification, stem cells differentiate into chondrocytes before differentiating into osteoblasts [20–24]. The differentiation of stem cells into chondrocytes, called chondrogenesis, is mediated by transforming growth factor beta (TGF-β) and BMP2. These two cytokines upregulate other cytokines including the chondrogenic factor SRY-Box Transcription Factor 9 (SOX9), further promoting endochondral ossification. Chondrocytes are stimulated by parathyroid hormone-related protein (PTHrP) to proliferate and secrete a non-mineralized extracellular matrix composed of Type II collagen. Eventually, these chondrocytes become hypertrophic and undergo apoptosis, secreting Type X collagen and releasing calcium phosphate mineral into the surrounding matrix. Stem cells in the surrounding area respond to the mineralized matrix and begin differentiating into osteoblasts. Hypertrophic chondrocytes also secrete VEGF, leading to vascularization and osteoblast invasion. Invading osteoblasts deposit Type I collagen and continue to remodel the cartilage matrix into bone matrix, eventually differentiating into osteocytes. At skeletal maturity, the growth plate is resorbed, and only bone tissue remains. Endochondral ossification is an important developmental process that may improve regenerative bone healing in biomaterials [23, 29, 30].

Key Takeaway During human skeletal development, bones form through intramembranous ossification or endochondral ossification. Intramembranous ossification is bone formation via the direct differentiation of stem cells into osteoblasts and occurs in flat bones. Endochondral ossification is bone formation via a cartilage intermediate and occurs in long bones.

2.4 Role of Sex Hormones on Bone Development

There are no apparent differences in bone and skeletal development between the sexes during fetal development [25]; however, sex hormones are necessary for bone development [17] and play a major role in bone maintenance and turnover [31–34]. Furthermore, estrogens and androgens influence bone growth and maintenance and are responsible for sexual dimorphism in the human skeleton [25–27]. Sex differences in skeletal growth become more apparent during puberty, and sex hormones play an important role in this process. Females stop growing ~2 years earlier than males and are shorter in stature, on average [25], because males continue pubertal growth for approximately 1 more year [25, 35, 36]. Further, sex differences in bone mineral content emerge in all regions of the body such that males have larger bone size and higher bone mass on average, although females have higher bone mineral content and density in the spine and pelvis [25].

Estrogen and its impact on bone development in males and females has been well studied [31]. Estrogen is critical during bone development, providing a stimulating effect on bone formation and an inhibitive effect on bone resorption [31, 32, 37]. Estrogen exerts its action by binding to estrogen receptors alpha (ERa) and beta (ERb) and G protein-coupled estrogen receptor-1 (GPER1). All three estrogen receptors are expressed in bone cells [38, 39]. Progesterone and its impact on bone development is less understood [31], but it has been shown to promote osteoblast differentiation and is implicated in bone formation [40, 41].

Androgens and their impact on bone development have been studied to a lesser extent than estrogen [31], but data suggests that androgens play an important role in the regulation of bone formation in males and females [42, 43]. Testosterone increases the lifespan of osteoblasts by inhibiting the production of interleukin-6 (IL-6) [43], which has been shown to stimulate osteoclast formation and activity [44]. It is hypothesized that testosterone affects mature osteoblasts and osteocytes, while estrogen regulates osteoblast activity at early and late stages of differentiation [32]. Furthermore, osteocalcin, a protein produced by osteoblasts during bone formation, regulates testosterone biosynthesis [43]. Dihydrotestosterone (DHT), a sex steroid that is synthesized from testosterone, has been shown to increase the proliferation and differentiation of osteoblasts in vitro [45].

Key Takeaway Sex steroids (estrogen, progesterone, androgens) are critical for bone development in males and females and are the cause for physical differences between the sexes. Androgens and estrogens have fundamental roles in regulating bone formation in males and females and positively influence growth, maturation, and maintenance of the bones [27, 42, 43].

2.5 Impact of Hormonal Treatment on Bone Health in Adolescents

Hormone therapy is used in the care of adolescents with various conditions including differences in sex development (DSD), hyper- and hypogonadism, and gender dysphoria. DSD, also called "intersex," are diverse set of conditions in which the reproductive system develops differently than what is expected [46, 47]. Examples include male chromosomes (XY) and genitalia that appears female, female chromosomes (XX) and genitalia that appears male, typical sex organs but an abnormal chromosome arrangement (XXY or XO chromosomes), and the presence of both ovarian and testicular tissue [47–50]. Hypogonadism is a condition in which there is a deficiency in the production of sex steroids, and this can occur in both adolescent males and females [48]. Gender dysphoria is when one has experienced and expressed that gender does not match their assigned-sex-at-birth [51]. Considering the impact of sex steroids on bone development and maintenance, it is important to consider the impact of hormone therapy in treatment of patients requiring estrogen or testosterone treatment.

Hyper- and hypogonadism refer to conditions in which there is an excess or deficiency in sex steroid production, respectively. Individuals with DSD individuals with DSD often require estrogen and/or testosterone therapy to ensure sexual development and puberty proceed normally and often experience hyper- and hypogonadism [48, 52]. Females with hyper- and hypogonadism require estrogen therapy to promote the progression of puberty and skeletal development [53, 54]. Estrogen can be delivered as estrogen or estradiol, and delaying estrogen replacement in females with hypogonadism will negatively impact bone health [55–58]. Males with hypergonadism are often untreated, and those with hypogonadism require testosterone treatment to ensure puberty progresses correctly [54, 59, 60]. Overall, estrogen and testosterone treatment in adolescents with hyper- and hypogonadism positively impact bone health and development, although testosterone treatment can lead to early bone closure in some cases [60].

Puberty blockers and gender affirming hormone treatment is rarely prescribed to transgender adolescents [61] and ~50% of transgender adults are receiving hormone therapy [62]. Over 70% of transgender individuals who start gender affirming hormone treatment will continue use after 4 years [63]. There can be a negative impact of long-term puberty suppression on bone mineral density, which can only partially be restored by sex steroid administration [64–66]. Transgender girls are more vulnerable than transgender boys to compromised bone health due to puberty blockers [66]. Testosterone and estrogen therapy can protect transgender men and women, respectively, against bone loss [67].

3 Healthy Bone

3.1 Key Terms

- *Stem cells* are pluripotent cells originating in the bone marrow or periosteum that can differentiate into osteoblasts, chondrocytes, and adipocytes. *Differentiation* is the process by which stem cells become different cell types.
- *Osteoblasts* are bone cells that are responsible for collagen production and mineral deposition in bone tissue. Osteoblasts differentiate into osteocytes. *Osteocytes* are mature bone cells that are embedded in the surrounding collagen matrix.
- *Osteoclasts* are bone cells that resorb bone and are critical for remodeling adult bone tissue. Osteoclasts are derived from macrophages. *Macrophages* are immune cells responsible for phagocytosis and play a critical role in healing following an injury.
- *Compact bone* is generally stronger and stiffer than *spongy bone*. Compact bone is also called cortical bone, and spongy bone is also called trabecular or cancellous bone.

3.2 Section Overview

In this section, we discuss the biology of healthy bones, including tissue mechanics, extracellular matrix and cell composition, and bone remodeling.

3.3 Compact and Spongy Bone: Tissue Structure and Mechanics

Bone is complex in both its structure and composition with two types of bone: compact and spongy. *Compact bone*, also called cortical bone, is generally stronger and stiffer than spongy bone and composes 80% of the human skeleton. Compact bone is made of closely packed haversian systems, which consist of osteonic canals surrounded by concentric rings of matrix called lamellae. Osteonic canals are microscopic tunnels for blood vessels and nerves. Osteocytes are located between these concentric rings, in spaces called lacunae. *Spongy bone*, also called trabecular or cancellous bone, is less dense than compact bone. Spongy bone consists of a highly interconnected network of pillars of bone, called trabeculae, that surround irregular cavities filled with bone marrow. Compact bone is much denser with a porosity of 5–10% and spongy bone is less dense with a porosity of 50–90% [68]. Compact bone can withstand much higher external forces than spongy bone (~150 MPa vs. ~50 MPa), while spongy bone can withstand higher structural deformation than compact bone (~50% strain vs. ~3% strain) [68].

There are no apparent sex differences in the structure of bone in healthy adults [69]; however, males have greater trabecular bone volume and higher cortical area, resulting in increased height, bone size, and strength [70]. The trabeculae in bone become thinner and lose their connectivity during aging, and this occurs more rapidly in females [25]. Bone loss in early osteoporosis occurs mainly in trabecular bone, but cortical bone becomes more porous and suffers significant bone loss as the patient ages [71].

3.4 Extracellular Matrix and Cellular Composition

The extracellular matrix in compact and spongy bone is composed of ~60% (w/w) inorganic material (i.e., calcium phosphate mineral), ~25% organic material (i.e., collagen, glycosaminoglycans), and ~5% water [72]. Hydroxyapatite is the calcium phosphate mineral phase in bone and forms as needles or thin plates. Collagen composes 90% of the organic material in bone and is deposited by osteoblasts. Type I collagen is the most abundant form of collagen found in bones. The remaining organic material is comprised of non-collagenous proteins like glycosaminoglycans, which largely consist of chondroitin and heparin sulfate. Finally, the blood supply delivers a variety of exogenously derived proteins that become sequestered within the highly porous and mineralized bone matrix. In healthy adults, there are no significant sex differences in bone composition [69]; however, bone becomes less mineralized with age and the rate of mineral loss is more significant in aging females than aging males [73].

Compact and spongy bones contain four types of bone cells: osteoblasts, osteoclasts, bone lining cells, and osteocytes. *Osteoblasts* are metabolically active bone cells that result in the formation of new bone via the deposition of Type I collagen and glycosaminoglycans and the promotion of mineralization via the secretion of matrix vesicles containing alkaline phosphatase (ALP) among other enzymes [74]. Osteoblast differentiation from mesenchymal stem cells is regulated via the core-binding factor alpha-1 transcription factor (Cbfα-1), bone morphogenetic proteins (BMPs), and Indian Hedgehog (Ihh) [72]. *Osteoclasts* are bone resorbing cells responsible for maintaining bone remodeling in response to growth or mechanical stress. Osteoclasts are derived from the monocyte–macrophage lineage in the bone marrow and are regulated by macrophage colony-stimulating factor (MCSF), osteoprotegerin (OPG), receptor activator NF-κB (RANK), and RANK-ligand (RANKL). MCSF maintains the survival and chemotactic behavior of mature osteoclasts, while the OPG/RANK/RANKL pathway is the key signal transduction pathway that regulates bone homeostasis in healthy bone. *Bone lining cells* are metabolically inactive differentiated osteoblasts that protect the surface of the bone from osteoclast-mediated resorption and can revert to osteoblasts upon extracellular matrix signaling [75]. *Osteocytes* are considered the terminal osteoblast differentiation state within the bone and are involved in the routine remodeling of the bone matrix and respond to mechanical stimuli [76].

Bone tissue is maintained through a remodeling process that is mediated by osteoclasts, osteoblasts, and osteocytes and serves to maintain the mechanical integrity of the adult skeleton. Osteoclasts resorb, or remove, bone tissue and osteoblasts deposit new matrix. The regulation of bone remodeling involves hormones, mechanical stimuli, cytokines, and growth factors [31]. Hormones critical to bone remodeling include the sex steroids (estrogen, progesterone, testosterone), parathyroid hormone (PTH), thyroid hormones, growth hormone, glucocorticoids, and 1,25-dihydroxyvitamin D [31]. Sex steroids modulate several signaling pathways important in bone remodeling including the TGF-β, OPG, RANKL, Wnt/β-catenin, Fas ligand (FasL), insulin-like growth factor (IGF), PTH, and calcitonin signaling pathways [69].

There are no apparent differences in cellular composition or cellular function in healthy adults [69]; however, sex steroids have significant impact on pathways relevant in bone remodeling, so age-related decreases in sex steroid production, as well as disorders in sex steroid secretion, will impact bone health. We will discuss the biology of aging bones in a later section.

4 Injured Bone

4.1 Key Terms

- *Macrophages* are immune cells responsible for phagocytosis and play a critical role in healing following an injury. Macrophages exist on a spectrum of inflammation in which *M1 macrophages* exhibit more pro-inflammatory phenotypes and *M2 macrophages* exhibit more anti-inflammatory/pro-healing phenotypes.
- *Inflammation* is the bodies immune response to injury, infection or irritation characterized by complex cellular signaling.
- *Osteomacs* are specialized bone-resident macrophages.
- *Mesenchymal stem cells* are pluripotent cells that can differentiate into osteoblasts, chondrocytes, and adipocytes.
- *Osteoblasts* are bone cells that are responsible for collagen production and mineral deposition in bone tissue. Osteoblasts differentiate into osteocytes. *Osteocytes* are mature bone cells that are embedded in the surrounding collagen matrix.
- *Chondrocytes* are cartilage cells that are responsible for collagen deposition in cartilage tissue. *Adipocytes* are adipose (i.e., fat) cells that compose adipose tissue and store energy as fat.
- *Osteoclasts* are bone cells that are responsible for bone resorption in bone tissue. These cells are critical in the modeling of developing bone and the remodeling of adult bone.
- *Secretome* is the combination of proteins, growth factors, cytokines, chemokines, and extracellular vesicles released by cells in the extracellular matrix.

4.2 Section Overview

In this section, we discuss the biology of injured and healing bones. Bone healing is a well-coordinated process that takes place following an injury and consists of three phases: inflammatory, regenerative, and remodeling (Fig. 2).

4.3 Phases of Bone Healing

During the *inflammatory phase* of bone healing, blood vessels rupture creating a hematoma as a provisional matrix, where immune cells such as neutrophils will beckon macrophages to the site of injury. Macrophages will polarize toward a pro-inflammatory phenotype (M1), which phagocytoses any debris or pathogens and secretes a range of inflammatory cytokines to trigger the recruitment of fibroblasts, stem cells, and osteoprogenitor cells that are involved in regeneration. Key

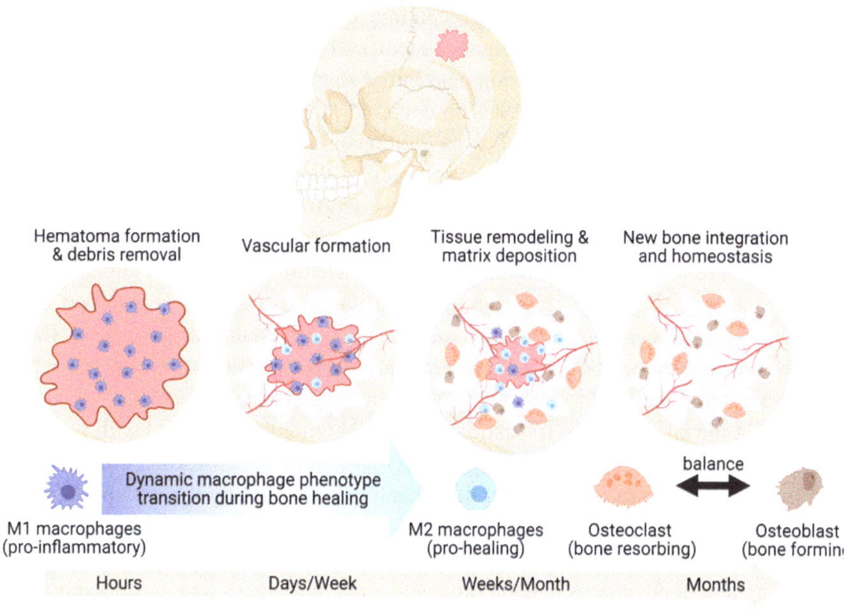

Fig. 2 Phases of bone healing: (left to right) inflammatory phase, regenerative phase, and remodeling phase. (Reproduced with permission from Kolliopoulos [118])

cytokines that are secreted in this stage include MCSF and RANKL, secreted by osteoclasts to polarize macrophages toward an M1 phenotype [77, 78]. In turn, M1 macrophages secrete cytokines including tumor necrosis factor-α (TNF-α), interleukins-1 and -6 (IL-1, IL-6), and interferon-gamma (INF-γ). TNF-α is mainly produced by monocytes (precursor immune cells to macrophages) and is believed to promote bone resorption; however, recent studies have showed that TNF-α displays peak concentrations 24 h and 4 weeks after fracture, which align with the recruitment of bone marrow stem cells and endochondral ossification, respectively [79]. IL-1 exists in different forms and plays key roles in osteoclast differentiation and formation. IL-6 has been shown to be essential for bone development and regeneration with decreased bone mineral density, fracture healing ability, and delayed mineralization observed in IL-6 knockout models [80]. Finally, IFN-γ inhibits the excessive formation of osteoclasts displaying an osteoprotective effect by inhibiting RANKL signaling [81]. An extended list of inflammatory cytokines released following injury to bone can be found elsewhere [23]. The recruited cell types induce vascular formation, relieving the hypoxic microenvironment, and inducing macrophage polarization toward an anti-inflammatory (M2) phenotype, which secrete cytokines such as IL-4, IL-10, and TGF-β, all contribute to osteoblast activation and differentiation as well as inflammatory suppression. The completion of this phase is marked by a decrease in immune cell population, and an increase in stem cells, fibroblasts, and osteoblasts. Sex differences in inflammatory markers.

In the *regenerative phase* of bone healing, the low oxygen microenvironment (i.e., hypoxia) stimulates mesenchymal stem cell (MSC) proliferation, fibroblast activation, osteogenic differentiation, and initial stages of vascularization. Recruited fibroblasts and differentiated MSCs into chondrocytes deposit matrix forming a collagen-rich fibrocartilaginous network that spans the fracture site. Chondrocytes will then undergo apoptosis, resulting in vascular invasion and migration of osteoblasts. Subsequently, a layer of woven bone is deposited by newly differentiated or infiltrating osteoblasts replacing the cartilaginous matrix [82, 83]. Following the soft callus formation, it is replaced by the hard callus via the activation of chondrocytes, osteoblasts, and osteoclasts. Here, the fibrocartilaginous network is resorbed while woven bone is further deposited. Key soluble mediators in this stage include BMPs, as they promote bone formation and stimulate the production of VEGF-A, which activates angiogenesis. In this stage, osteomacs (a subtype of macrophages) are enriched at the sites of bone formation and are commonly associated with maturing bone tissues [84, 85]. This stage can last up to 4 weeks under normal conditions.

Finally, the *remodeling phase* in bone healing is defined by the resorption of the hard callus via osteoclasts and the deposition of new compact bone centrally, as well as lamellar bone peripherally by osteoblasts [86]. This continuous state of bone resorption and deposition is called homeostasis and allows for newly formed bone to achieve the mechanical and biochemical properties of normal bone. Primary modulators of homeostasis are osteocytes, which influence remodeling via both cell–cell and paracrine interactions. Most notably, osteocytes have been shown to secrete OPG, a potent inhibitor of RANKL, directly correlating osteocyte–osteoclast regulation of bone resorption [87]. Additionally, osteocytes have been reported to secrete cytokines such as sclerostin and Dickkopf-related protein 1 (DKK1), which are both inhibitors of the Wnt/β-catenin pathway regulating osteoblast-induced bone formation [88]. These dynamic interactions of osteocytes with osteoclasts and osteoblasts have been related to mechanical stimulation/loading as well as hormonal (parathyroid hormone—PTH) stimulation [87]. Furthermore, estrogen has been shown to inhibit osteoclast-mediated bone resorption and induce osteoclast apoptosis via regulation of VEGF. On the other hand, estrogen has been shown to promote bone formation via the induction of osteoblast survival [33, 89]. This stage can last between months and years depending on the defect size and severity.

Key Takeaway Bone healing takes place in three phases: inflammatory, regenerative, and remodeling. The inflammatory phase is guided by the macrophage secretome, which directs cell recruitment and differentiation, and is eventually resolved by macrophage polarization toward a pro-healing/anti-inflammatory phenotype. The regenerative phase comprises an intricate balance of fibrocartilage remodeling and bone formation mediated by chondrocytes and osteoblasts. The remodeling phase is driven by osteoblast and osteoclast-mediated bone formation and resorption, respectively, to result in new healthy bones.

5 Aging Bone

5.1 Section Overview

In this section, we will discuss the biology of aging bones and how it differs from healthy bones (Fig. 3). Sex steroids are essential for skeletal development and the maintenance of bone health throughout adult life, and the decreasing levels of sex

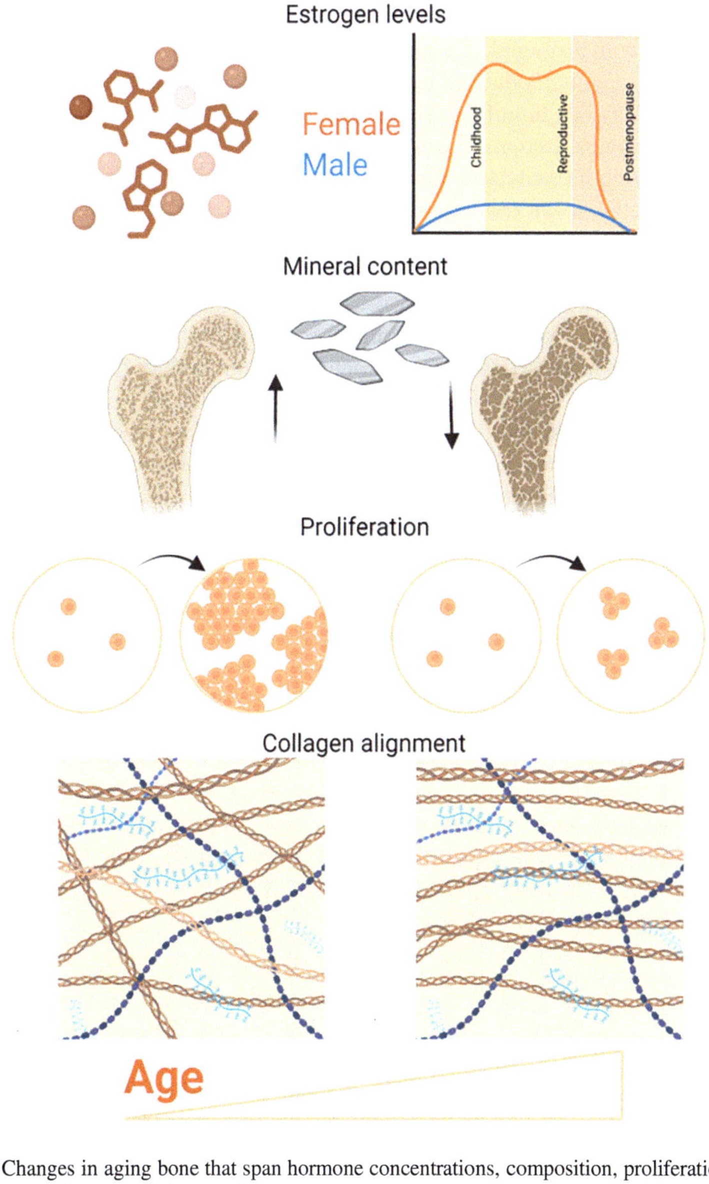

Fig. 3 Changes in aging bone that span hormone concentrations, composition, proliferation rates, and macroscopic extracellular matrix structure

steroids with age leads to a loss of bone mass and functional integrity [26, 90]. Estrogen deficiency at menopause is a major factor in the development of osteoporosis in postmenopausal females [31, 91] and is the major determinant of age-related bone loss in both sexes [31].

5.2 *Compositional Changes in Aging Bone*

As people age, cells in the bone microenvironment age, leading to a cascade of structural and compositional changes that impact bone function. All cells have a limited lifespan that is modulated by the length of their telomeres, which has been defined as the Hayflick limit [92]. This results in fewer bone marrow stem cells able to differentiate into osteoprogenitors and fewer hematopoietic stem cells able to differentiate into pre-osteoclasts. The decrease in stem cell population coupled with a decrease in cell division results in fewer cells capable of maintaining bone density.

From a compositional perspective, bone protein and mineral density change with age while structurally it has been shown that collagen alignment increases with age [93]. Bone proteins (such as collagen), which provide flexibility in bone, exhibit increased crosslinks formed by glycation or oxidation, resulting in advanced glycation end-products (AGEs) that contribute to bone fragility [94, 95]. Additionally, mineral content in bone increases with age, resulting in brittle bone and an increase in fracture risk [96]. A common metric to evaluate these changes is by quantifying bone mineral density (BMD) via micro-computed tomography (micro-CT) imaging. Studies have evaluated various species with age and show that males display faster increases in BMD in early adulthood, while females display faster decreases in BMD in late adulthood [97–99].

Key Takeaway Aging bone experiences changes in both composition and micro-architecture, resulting in changes in fragility and strength.

5.3 *The Impact of Age-Related Hormonal Changes on Bone*

Hormonal changes, such as decreases in estrogens and androgens in both men and women are known to be correlated with age. Decreases in these sex hormone levels have been linked to a decrease in the body's defense against oxidative stress, resulting in increased bone resorption [91]. Enhanced bone resorption is one of the main causes of osteoporosis, a bone disease that disproportionately affects women compared to men. While women tend to have higher rates of bone fractures than men, men show significantly greater mortality rates following a fracture compared to women (18% in men over 80 years old, 8% in women of the same age) [4]. A metanalysis showed that a potential reason for this difference in mortality rates is that men are less likely to receive treatment for osteoporosis (e.g., bisphosphonates) post bone fracture. These treatments directly impact the bone mineral density with low values of bone fragility. To better understand how to treat bone fragility and loss, a deeper understanding of how cell–ECM signaling drives an apoptotic cascade is necessary.

Estrogens are the primary hormone regulators of bone resorption in women, and there is a significant decrease in hormone levels following menopause such that the loss of bone mineral content is more significant in females than males at all skeletal sites, although the magnitude of the difference is greater in the spine and pelvis [25, 28]. Androgens and estrogens play independent and fundamental roles in regulating bone resorption in males [42]. In aging males, estrogen is the dominant sex steroid regulating bone resorption, whereas both estrogen and testosterone are important for males during bone formation [100]. Estrogen hormone therapy, including estrogen and estrogen receptor modulators, can improve bone health in both aging males and females [28].

Key Takeaway The levels of sex steroids decrease with age in both males and females, and this decrease impacts bone health. Older females are more susceptible to osteoporosis than older males.

6 Biomaterials for Bone

6.1 Key Terms

- *Osteoinductive* materials stimulate stem cell differentiation toward osteoblasts.
- *Osteoconductive* materials promote bone regeneration by allowing osteoblasts to proliferation and mineralize the surrounding tissue.
- *Hydroxyapatite* and *β-tricalcium phosphate* are calcium phosphate mineral phases commonly used in bone biomaterials. Hydroxyapatite is present in native bone tissue.
- *Secretome* is the combination of proteins, growth factors, cytokines, chemokines, and extracellular vesicles released by cells in the extracellular matrix.
- in vitro studies are conducted with cells that have been isolated from an organism. In vitro studies can be conducted in 2D (i.e., on tissue cultured plastic) or 3D (i.e., biomaterials).
- in vivo studies are conducted using whole and living organisms. Commonly used animals for in vivo biomaterial studies include mice, rabbits, and pigs.
- *Ex vivo* studies are conducted using living tissue that has been removed from the organism.

6.2 Section Overview

Age- and sex-dependent differences in bone strength have been well reported [101]. However, the driving factors behind these differences remain unknown.

Tissue engineering and regenerative medicine provide a toolbox of approaches wherein systematic and mechanistic studies can be conducted using biomaterials in vitro, ex vivo, and in vivo. To elucidate the driving factors behind these differences in bone architecture, composition, and mechanics, biomaterials can be leveraged to understand cell response to environmental stimuli. Biomaterials can be employed to evaluate cell–material interactions, cell–cell interactions, and cell–hormone interactions.

To study sex-based differences and the above interactions and develop means of modulating cell response by tuning both biomaterial properties and biomolecule signals, one must consider the necessary design parameters to achieve bone-mimetic properties. Once a bone-mimetic biomaterial has been developed, it can be employed in various schemes in vitro, ex vivo, and in vivo to evaluate the role of sex and environmental signals on cell proliferation, differentiation, and bone regeneration.

6.3 Biomaterial "Tuning Knobs" to Study Sex-Based Differences

As established earlier in this chapter, bone is a highly complex, hierarchical, multicellular tissue that is comprised of a milieu of polymeric proteins, soluble signals, and calcium phosphate mineral. Its hierarchical structure is what results in the mechanical properties of bone, simultaneously being strong and elastic. Key properties in bone-mimetic biomaterial design are biomaterial composition, structural features, and mechanics.

6.3.1 Biomaterial Composition

Here, we describe biomaterial composition as the combination of "primary" and "secondary" components. Primary components are materials that compose most of the biomaterial's composition and significantly impact its structure and function. Secondary components are supplemental materials that impart additional characteristics to the biomaterial's structure, mechanics, or biological activity. Both synthetic and naturally derived polymers can be employed in the design of bone-mimetic biomaterials as primary or secondary components. Additives such as ceramics, metals, growth factors, nanofibers, and/or therapeutics are often added as secondary components to bone-mimetic biomaterials to improve different aspects of bone regeneration (e.g., vascular formation, osteoblast function).

Synthetic polymers are commonly used because they can closely mimic the mechanical properties of bone; however, they do not inherently possess osteoinductive or osteoconductive properties. Furthermore, synthetic materials are highly tunable because they can be synthesized to possess the desired characteristics. Commonly used synthetic polymers in bone tissue engineering and biomaterial

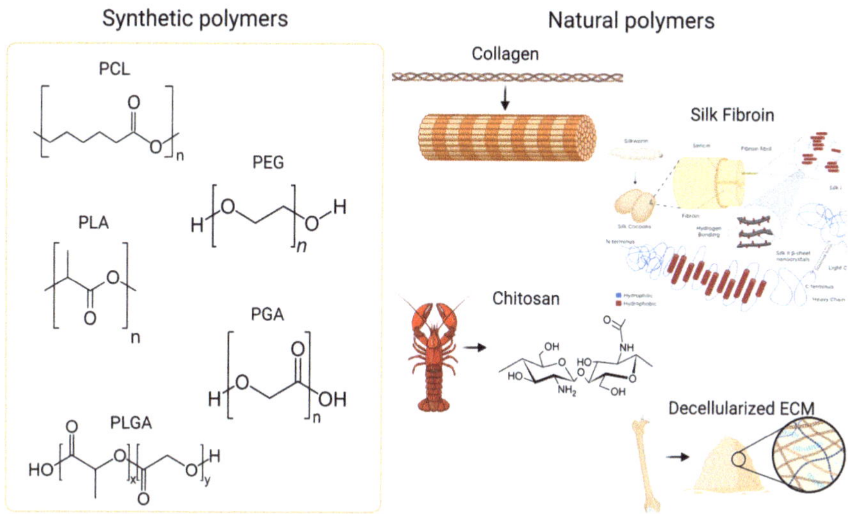

Fig. 4 Synthetic and natural polymer choices for the development and fabrication of bone-mimetic biomaterials. (Silk fibroin panel reproduced with permission from Howard et al. [119])

design include poly-(ε-caprolactone) (PCL), polyglycolic acid (PGA), polylactic acid (PLA), and poly(lactic-co-glycolic acid) (PLGA) (Fig. 4) [102–104]. As these materials are not naturally found in the body, their primary role is to restore mechanical support and function. To enhance the regenerative capacity and osteoconductivity of these biomaterials, ceramic additives such as hydroxyapatite (HA) or β-tricalcium phosphate (β-TCP) are added as a secondary component within the synthetic polymer mixture [105–107]. Although these synthetic materials are biocompatible, some release toxic or acidic by-products during their degradation, which can elicit a negative inflammatory response. Synthetic materials and composites are commonly fabricated using casting, 3D printing, and electrospinning to form solid or porous scaffolds [108]. Many examples of synthetic materials have been translated into the clinic [109], although no extensive studies have been conducted to evaluate sex-based differences in response to these materials.

Naturally derived polymers such as collagen, glycosaminoglycans, chitosan, silk fibroin, alginate, and decellularized tissue-derived extracellular matrix are attractive alternatives to synthetic polymers (Fig. 4). Natural materials lack the mechanical properties of bone but mimic the native extracellular matrix of the tissue and are biocompatible and biodegradable with harmless by-products. An important consideration when using natural materials is that these are commonly derived from mammals and by extension are also associated with a sex. Therefore, all the sex differences in bone structure and composition that were discussed earlier in this chapter would also apply to these naturally derived materials. Although a characterization of these materials as a function of sex has yet to be reported in the literature, it is critical to consider the sex of the source when evaluating cell variability as a function of sex on biomaterials. Natural biomaterials are commonly fabricated with casting, freeze-drying, particulate leaching, 3D printing, and electrospinning. There are many examples of these materials having been translated into the clinic; however, few are specifically for bone applications [109, 110].

In addition to the polymer of choice, biomolecule additives such as glycosaminoglycans, cytokines, growth factors, peptides, and RNAs can also influence cell migration, proliferation, and differentiation. These additives result in an (almost) unlimited number of combinations to impact biomaterial composition. When evaluating sex-based differences, a prominent compositional signal of interest are hormones. Hormones can be incorporated in biomaterials as soluble, matrix-bound, or encapsulated signals. The way in which hormones interact with cells can therefore be spatiotemporally tuned. These approaches can be leveraged to mimic native hormonal fluctuations as well as evaluate dosage effects.

6.3.2 Structural Features

The structural features of biomaterials can be tuned during the fabrication process, and these features may change due to cell-mediated changes. These structural features can include microstructures of the polymer or additive used (e.g., synthetic polymers with varying steric structures [111], crystal structure of hydroxyapatite mineral phase [112, 113]) as well as porosity, pore size, pore shape, and pore alignment [114]. The porous properties of biomaterials are also highly tunable and relevant for bone-mimetic biomaterial design. Depending on the fabrication technique employed for the development of the biomaterial, the size, shape, surface topography, and degree of interconnectivity of the pores can be tuned [114]. Many studies have investigated the effects of pore size and shape on osteogenesis; however, this has not been thoroughly studied as a function of sex. Surface topographical signals have been largely investigated in 2D; however, native tissues are 3D, resulting in a need for the evaluation of surface topographical effects on cell response in 3D biomaterials. In a recent study, it has been shown that osteoblast response to hormones (estrogen) is sex-dependent and surface property dependent [115, 116]. This shows the degree of complexity that biomaterial properties require to study sex-based differences as many of these appear to have interaction effects.

6.3.3 Mechanical Properties

Mechanical properties can be tuned through the choice of polymer, degree of crosslinking, spatial organization of the polymer, and introduction of additives. As mentioned above, synthetic polymers have higher mechanical properties compared to natural polymers, and these can be further tuned via their molecular weight. The higher the molecular weight of the polymer, the higher the mechanical properties. With synthetic polymers, the degree of crystallinity is directly and positively correlated with the material's mechanical properties. Both synthetic and natural polymers can have tunable mechanical properties guided by their degree of crosslinking, with higher degrees of crosslinking resulting in higher mechanical properties. The spatial organization of the polymer can also guide the mechanical properties of the biomaterial with spiral structures, resulting in higher mechanics compared to woodpile lattice structures. Finally, the addition of additives such as ceramics can also enhance the mechanical properties of biomaterials.

Metrics such as cell proliferation, cell morphometrics, cell migration, and cell response to stressors have been reported to be different as a function of sex [116, 117]. In pulmonary arterial fibroblasts, it has been shown that male cells become less activated than female cells on soft materials and more activated on stiff materials. However, female cells only followed this pattern when cultured with younger (<50 years old) serum or when older female serum (>50 years old) was supplemented with estradiol. This suggests that there is both a hormone and material property-driven effect on cell response that is not completely independent of each other [116]. In the context of bone, as females tend to suffer from osteoporosis at higher rates, the effects of mechanical stimulation and bone mechanical properties are most likely coupled with levels of sex hormones, rendering the need for greater evaluation of this dependence.

Key Takeaways Biomaterials are highly tunable in their composition, structure, and macroscopic properties. Bone-mimetic biomaterials are often designed to mimic the properties of native bone such as porosity, mechanical strength, and composition. There is not one universally accepted bone-mimetic biomaterial.

6.4 Considerations of Sex-Based Differences in Experimental Design and Cell Culture

Biomaterials are often employed as in vitro models to study cell–material and cell–cell interactions (Fig. 5). Classical approaches to evaluate cell–material interactions include direct cell seeding on the biomaterial or using material-conditioned media. Direct cell seeding involves cells being introduced to the biomaterial during its fabrication or directly pipetted onto the biomaterial after its fabrication. These types of experiments are used to evaluate the material property effects, such as topography, stiffness, pore size and shape, and composition on cell response. By conditioning media with biomaterial-released factors (e.g., growth factors, extracellular vesicles) or degradation products, and introducing this to cells, one can evaluate the effects of the released factors and degradation signals on cell response.

Cell–cell interactions are commonly interrogated on 2D surfaces; however, it is now well established that cell response is different in 2D compared to 3D constructs. Therefore, culturing cells on materials and generating cell-conditioned media or coculturing cells directly or indirectly are approaches to evaluate cell–cell interactions. As for cell-conditioned media studies, one or more cell types are exposed to media containing the secreted factors of another cell (or cells). These types of experiments are used to evaluate the effects of cell-secreted factors (the secretome)

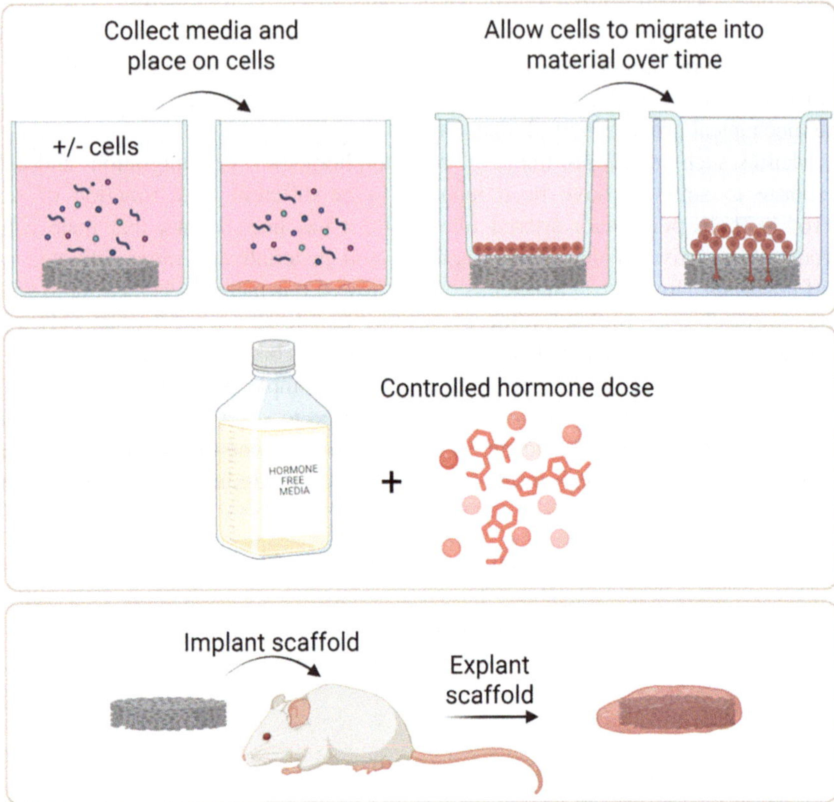

Fig. 5 Experimental designs leveraging biomaterials in vitro, in vivo, and ex vivo to understand sex-based differences in both cell–material and cell–cell interactions. Top panel illustrates experimental designs to evaluate material secretome effects on cell response via conditioned media and migration studies. The second panel illustrates the importance of evaluating hormonal levels introduced to cells within experiments. The last panel depicts standard small animal model studies to evaluate biocompatibility

on another cell (or cells) of interest. Commonly, multicellular interactions are interrogated via direct or indirect cocultures. Transwell setups are commonly used for indirect cocultures because they allow cell-secreted factors to pass between the transwell membrane while cells remain physically separated. Direct cocultures in which multiple cell types are seeded on the biomaterial simultaneously allow for the evaluation of the effect of cell–material and cell–cell interactions. These are commonly used methods, but there are many other methods that can be used to study cell–material and cell–cell interactions. Furthermore, new experimental setups are being developed and used due to the creative freedom one can take in the process of biomaterial design and experimental setup.

For multicellular studies, it is critical that cells are sex-matched unless there is a rationale for mixing sexes. If sex is mixed, a full factorial design of the experimental setup would be essential. In both cell–cell and cell–material setups, to evaluate sex-based differences, one must use both male and female cells. It is critical that if the biomaterial of choice is a natural material that the sex of the source tissue is also reported and considered as a confounding variable (e.g., the sex of the placenta matches the sex of the baby, not the sex of the mother). Data one can collect from these types of studies includes cell morphology, metabolic activity, and proliferation dynamics, as well as gene, protein, and surface marker expression as a function of material properties.

When evaluating hormonal effects as a function of sex in vitro, a necessary consideration is the composition of the media. For bone research, a common component of the media is fetal bovine serum (FBS), which provides necessary cell growth and maintenance signals in addition to hormones. Although FBS is derived from mammals (commonly cows) and is associated with the sex of the animal, it is rare that the sex of the FBS source is reported in the literature. One approach to mediate the number of hormones introduced to cells via FBS is to charcoal strip it, which removes most of the hormonal content. In this way, researchers can better probe the effects of the introduced hormones in their system. Another common constituent of the media that can have confounding effects on hormonal studies is phenol red. Phenol red is used as a pH indicator to illustrate the need for media supplementation. Phenol red, however, can behave like estrogen and induce estrogen signaling in cells. Thus, many have resulted in avoiding the use of phenol red in their media to eliminate this as a variable.

Ex vivo models are also useful in evaluating sex-based differences in bone. These can be leveraged to evaluate native cell infiltration into biomaterials in a sex-dependent manner. Furthermore, ex vivo models are useful in investigating biomaterial integration within bone defects. Implant micromotion can result in implant failure; thus, evaluating the integration of a biomaterial within a defect is essential for predicting its success. The evaluation of sex-based differences in biomaterial integration within explants remains to be studied.

Finally, in vivo models remain the gold standard in evaluating biomaterial performance and regenerative capacity. Although the sex of the animals used is reported (not always), the hormonal state of the animals is rarely evaluated. When studying sex-based differences in vivo, just reporting sex is not adequate, as the amount of patient-to-patient variability is large. Efforts should be made to profile the hormonal landscape into which the biomaterials are being implanted so that a more holistic evaluation of sex-based differences can be completed.

Key Takeaways Biomaterials can be leveraged to interrogate cell–cell and cell–material interactions, which will inform the response of cells in the native microenvironment, to treatment, and in potential implant microenvironments. Experimental designs can be formulated for in vitro, ex vivo, and in vivo setups that allow for increased biological complexity. To probe sex-based differences, both sexes must be included within the experimental design, and phenol-free and serum-free media should be used to limit the confounding effects of hormones.

6.5 Including Sex as a Biological Variable

Studying sex-based differences must move beyond the pure categorization of male and female into the realm of true complexity that sex is. Sex is guided by chromosomal, anatomical, and hormonal parameters, and so all must be considered when designing, conducting, and analyzing experimental studies. A common misconception in tissue engineering and regenerative medicine is that sex is associated with the cells and animal models used. However, sex comes into the equation in many other ways as discussed above. Sex can be associated with the material of choice and with media additives such as fetal bovine serum (FBS). It is critical that biomaterial scientists are not only aware of sex as a variable associated with these parameters but also stringent in their reporting. We are aware that this information is not always made available to the researcher, and so this serves as a call to action for labs isolating cells and companies producing these materials to fully characterize and report this information.

Furthermore, in designing biomaterials as implants for bone repair, it is pivotal that clinical data and sex-based differences are considered. There is a significant barrier in clinical data documentation as (1) sex is generally self-reported with no chromosomal confirmation, and (2) terms such as sex and gender are often used interchangeably, resulting in an unreliable association to clinical data. With the advent of hormonal therapies, there is a clinical opportunity to evaluate changes in bone health. However, this information will not result in a scientifically dependable hypothesis unless issues with the reporting mechanisms are resolved.

Acknowledgments Figures were created in BioRender. Kolliopoulos V (2025) https://BioRender.com/3cexyio.

References

1. Wu AM, Bisignano C, James SL, et al. Global, regional, and national burden of bone fractures in 204 countries and territories, 1990–2019: a systematic analysis from the Global Burden of Disease Study 2019. Lancet Healthy Longev. 2021;2. https://doi.org/10.1016/S2666-7568(21)00172-0.
2. Bergh C, Wennergren D, Möller M, Brisby H. Fracture incidence in adults in relation to age and gender: a study of 27,169 fractures in the Swedish Fracture Register in a well-defined catchment area. PLoS One. 2021;15. https://doi.org/10.1371/journal.pone.0244291.
3. Kannegaard PN, van der Mark S, Eiken P, Abrahamsen B. Excess mortality in men compared with women following a hip fracture. National analysis of comedications, comorbidity and survival. Age Ageing. 2010;39. https://doi.org/10.1093/ageing/afp221.
4. Cawthon PM. Gender differences in osteoporosis and fractures. Clin Orthop Relat Res. 2011;469. https://doi.org/10.1007/s11999-011-1780-7.
5. Marsh D. Concepts of fracture union, delayed union, and nonunion. Clin Orthop Relat Res. 1998;355. https://doi.org/10.1097/00003086-199810001-00004.
6. Schmidt AH. Autologous bone graft: Is it still the gold standard? Injury. 2021;52. https://doi.org/10.1016/j.injury.2021.01.043.

7. Betz RR. Limitations of autograft and allograft: new synthetic solutions. Orthopedics. 2002;25. https://doi.org/10.3928/0147-7447-20020502-04.
8. Gruskin E, Doll BA, Futrell FW, Schmitz JP, Hollinger JO. Demineralized bone matrix in bone repair: history and use. Adv Drug Deliv Rev. 2012;64. https://doi.org/10.1016/j.addr.2012.06.008.
9. Bracey DN, Cignetti NE, Jinnah AH, et al. Bone xenotransplantation: a review of the history, orthopedic clinical literature, and a single-center case series. Xenotransplantation. 2020;27. https://doi.org/10.1111/xen.12600.
10. Rodriguez AE, Nowzari H. The long-term risks and complications of bovine-derived xenografts: a case series. J Indian Soc Periodontol. 2019;23. https://doi.org/10.4103/jisp.jisp_656_18.
11. Fernández RF, Bucchi C, Navarro P, Beltrán V, Borie E. Bone grafts utilized in dentistry: an analysis of patients' preferences. BMC Med Ethics. 2015;16. https://doi.org/10.1186/s12910-015-0044-6.
12. Battafarano G, Rossi M, De Martino V, et al. Strategies for bone regeneration: from graft to tissue engineering. Int J Mol Sci. 2021;22. https://doi.org/10.3390/ijms22031128.
13. James BD, Guerin P, Allen JB. Let's talk about sex—biological sex is underreported in biomaterial studies. Adv Healthc Mater. 2021;10. https://doi.org/10.1002/adhm.202001034.
14. Pillerová M, Borbélyová V, Hodosy J, et al. On the role of sex steroids in biological functions by classical and non-classical pathways. An update. Front Neuroendocrinol. 2021;62. https://doi.org/10.1016/j.yfrne.2021.100926.
15. Cable JK, Grider MH. Physiology, Progesterone. Treasure Island: StatPearls [Internet]; 2020.
16. Delgado BJ, Lopez-Ojeda W. Estrogen continuing education activity. StatPearls: Published online; 2022.
17. Handa RJ, Pak TR. Androgen action. Amsterdam: Encyclopedia of Stress, Elsevier; 2007. https://doi.org/10.1016/B978-012373947-6.00032-5.
18. Nassar GN, Leslie SW. Physiology, testosterone. Treasure Island: StatPearls [Internet]; 2018.
19. Ko FC, Sumner DR. How faithfully does intramembranous bone regeneration recapitulate embryonic skeletal development? Dev Dyn. 2021;250. https://doi.org/10.1002/dvdy.240.
20. Breeland G, Sinkler MA, Menezes RG. Embryology, bone ossification. Treasure Island: StatPearls [Internet]; 2023.
21. Galea GL, Zein MR, Allen S, Francis-West P. Making and shaping endochondral and intramembranous bones. Dev Dyn. 2021;250. https://doi.org/10.1002/dvdy.278.
22. Gilbert SF. Osteogenesis: the development of bones. In: Developmental biology. 6th ed. Sunderland: Sinauer Associates; 2000. (Hall 1988).
23. Zhu G, Zhang T, Chen M, et al. Bone physiological microenvironment and healing mechanism: basis for future bone-tissue engineering scaffolds. Bioact Mater. 2021;6. https://doi.org/10.1016/j.bioactmat.2021.03.043.
24. Fu R, Liu C, Yan Y, Li Q, Huang RL. Bone defect reconstruction via endochondral ossification: a developmental engineering strategy. J Tissue Eng. 2021;12. https://doi.org/10.1177/20417314211004211.
25. Plotkin LI, Bruzzaniti A, Pianeta R. Sexual dimorphism in the musculoskeletal system: sex hormones and beyond. J Endocr Soc. 2024;8. https://doi.org/10.1210/jendso/bvae153.
26. Carson JA, Manolagas SC. Effects of sex steroids on bones and muscles: similarities, parallels, and putative interactions in health and disease. Bone. 2015;80. https://doi.org/10.1016/j.bone.2015.04.015.
27. Fitzpatrick LA. Sex differences in skeletal development. Adv Mol Cell Biol. 2004;34. https://doi.org/10.1016/S1569-2558(03)34016-0.
28. Zhang YY, Xie N, Sun XD, et al. Insights and implications of sexual dimorphism in osteoporosis. Bone Res. 2024;12:8. https://doi.org/10.1038/s41413-023-00306-4.
29. Tiffany AS, Harley BAC. Growing pains: the need for engineered platforms to study growth plate biology. Adv Healthc Mater. 2022;11. https://doi.org/10.1002/adhm.202200471.

30. Dennis SC, Berkland CJ, Bonewald LF, Detamore MS. Endochondral ossification for enhancing bone regeneration: converging native extracellular matrix biomaterials and developmental engineering in vivo. Tissue Eng Part B Rev. 2015;21. https://doi.org/10.1089/ten.teb.2014.0419.
31. Compston JE. Sex steroids and bone. Physiol Rev. 2001;81:419–47. https://doi.org/10.1152/physrev.2001.81.1.419.
32. Syed F, Khosla S. Mechanisms of sex steroid effects on bone. Biochem Biophys Res Commun. 2005;328. https://doi.org/10.1016/j.bbrc.2004.11.097.
33. Manolagas SC, Kousteni S, Jilka RL. Sex steroids and bone. Recent Prog Horm Res. 2002;57. https://doi.org/10.1210/rp.57.1.385.
34. Riggs BL, Khosla S, Melton LJ. Sex steroids and the construction and conservation of the adult skeleton. Endocr Rev. 2002;23. https://doi.org/10.1210/edrv.23.3.0465.
35. Ortona E, Pagano MT, Capossela L, Malorni W. The role of sex differences in bone health and healing. Biology (Basel). 2023;12. https://doi.org/10.3390/biology12070993.
36. Wells JCK. Sexual dimorphism of body composition. Best Pract Res Clin Endocrinol Metab. 2007;21. https://doi.org/10.1016/j.beem.2007.04.007.
37. Khosla S, Oursler MJ, Monroe DG. Estrogen and the skeleton. Trends Endocrinol Metab. 2012;23. https://doi.org/10.1016/j.tem.2012.03.008.
38. Lara-Castillo N. Estrogen signaling in bone. Appl Sci. 2021;11. https://doi.org/10.3390/app11104439.
39. Karlafti E, Lampropoulou-Adamidou K, Tournis S, Trovas G, Triantafyllopoulos IK. Effect of estrogen on bone cells: what is new? J Res Pract Musculoskelet Syst. 2019;3. https://doi.org/10.22540/jrpms-03-113.
40. Seifert-Klauss V, Prior JC. Progesterone and bone: actions promoting bone health in women. J Osteoporos. 2010;2010. https://doi.org/10.4061/2010/845180.
41. Prior JC. Progesterone as a bone-trophic hormone. Endocr Rev. 1990;11. https://doi.org/10.1210/edrv-11-2-386.
42. Leder BZ, LeBlanc KM, Schoenfeld DA, Eastell R, Finkelstein JS. Differential effects of androgens and estrogens on bone turnover in normal men. J Clin Endocrinol Metab. 2003;88. https://doi.org/10.1210/jc.2002-021036.
43. Karsenty G. The mutual dependence between bone and gonads. J Endocrinol 2012;213. https://doi.org/10.1530/JOE-11-0452.
44. Sims NA. Influences of the IL-6 cytokine family on bone structure and function. Cytokine. 2021;146. https://doi.org/10.1016/j.cyto.2021.155655.
45. Thu HE, Mohamed IN, Hussain Z, Shuid AN. Dihydrotestosterone, a robust promoter of osteoblastic proliferation and differentiation: understanding of time-mannered and dose-dependent control of bone forming cells. Iran J Basic Med Sci. 2017;20. https://doi.org/10.22038/ijbms.2017.9111.
46. Beale JM, Creighton SM. Long-term health issues related to disorders or differences in sex development/intersex. Maturitas. 2016;94. https://doi.org/10.1016/j.maturitas.2016.10.003.
47. Ahmed SF, Achermann JC, Arlt W, et al. Society for Endocrinology UK guidance on the initial evaluation of an infant or an adolescent with a suspected disorder of sex development (Revised 2015). Clin Endocrinol (Oxf). 2016;84. https://doi.org/10.1111/cen.12857.
48. Nordenström A, Ahmed SF, van den Akker E, et al. Pubertal induction and transition to adult sex hormone replacement in patients with congenital pituitary or gonadal reproductive hormone deficiency: an Endo-ERN clinical practice guideline. Eur J Endocrinol. 2022;186. https://doi.org/10.1530/EJE-22-0073.
49. Differences in sex development – NHS. https://www.nhs.uk/conditions/differences-in-sex-development/. Accessed 23 July 2025.
50. Disorders of Sexual Development (DSDs). https://my.clevelandclinic.org/health/diseases/disorders-of-sexual-development. Accessed 23 July 2025.

51. Marconi E, Monti L, Marfoli A, et al. A systematic review on gender dysphoria in adolescents and young adults: focus on suicidal and self-harming ideation and behaviours. Child Adolesc Psychiatry Ment Health. 2023;17. https://doi.org/10.1186/s13034-023-00654-3.
52. Nordenström A. Puberty in individuals with a disorder of sex development. Curr Opin Endocr Metab Res. 2020;14:42–51. https://doi.org/10.1016/J.COEMR.2020.05.004.
53. Klein KO, Phillips SA. Review of hormone replacement therapy in girls and adolescents with hypogonadism. J Pediatr Adolesc Gynecol. 2019;32:460–8. https://doi.org/10.1016/J.JPAG.2019.04.010.
54. Viswanathan V, Eugster EA. Etiology and treatment of hypogonadism in adolescents. Pediatr Clin N Am. 2011;58:1181. https://doi.org/10.1016/J.PCL.2011.07.009.
55. Dural Ö, Poyrazoğlu Ş. Hormone replacement therapy in a patient with hypogonadism and coexisting medical conditions. JCRPE J Clin Res Pediatr Endocrinol. 2020;12. https://doi.org/10.4274/jcrpe.galenos.2020.2019.S0021.
56. Benetti-Pinto CL, Bedone A, Magna LA, Marques-Neto JF. Factors associated with the reduction of bone density in patients with gonadal dysgenesis. Fertil Steril. 2002;77. https://doi.org/10.1016/S0015-0282(01)03215-0.
57. Gussinyé M, Terrades P, Yeste D, Vicens-Calvet E, Carrascosa A. Low areal bone mineral density values in adolescents and young adult Turner syndrome patients increase after long-term transdermal estradiol therapy. Horm Res. 2000;54:131–5. https://doi.org/10.1159/000053246.
58. Nabhan ZM, DiMeglio LA, Qi R, Perkins SM, Eugster EA. Conjugated oral versus transdermal estrogen replacement in girls with Turner syndrome: a pilot comparative study. J Clin Endocrinol Metab. 2009;94. https://doi.org/10.1210/jc.2008-2123.
59. Rey RA. Recent advancement in the treatment of boys and adolescents with hypogonadism. Ther Adv Endocrinol Metab. 2022;13. https://doi.org/10.1177/20420188211065660.
60. Varnum AA, van Leeuwen L, Velasquez DA, et al. Testosterone replacement therapy in adolescents and young men. J Mens Health. 2024;20:24–31. https://doi.org/10.22514/JOMH.2024.164/HTM.
61. Hughes LD, Charlton BM, Berzansky I, Corman JD. Gender-affirming medications among transgender adolescents in the US, 2018–2022. JAMA Pediatr. 2025;179:342–4. https://doi.org/10.1001/JAMAPEDIATRICS.2024.6081.
62. Stroumsa D, Crissman HP, Dalton VK, Kolenic G, Richardson CR. Insurance coverage and use of hormones among transgender respondents to a national survey. Ann Fam Med. 2020;18:528–34. https://doi.org/10.1370/AFM.2586.
63. Roberts CM, Klein DA, Adirim TA, Schvey NA, Hisle-Gorman E. Continuation of gender-affirming hormones among transgender adolescents and adults. J Clin Endocrinol Metab. 2022;107. https://doi.org/10.1210/clinem/dgac251.
64. Hembree WC, Cohen-Kettenis PT, Gooren L, et al. Endocrine treatment of gender-dysphoric/gender-incongruent persons: an endocrine society clinical practice guideline. J Clin Endocrinol Metab. 2017;102. https://doi.org/10.1210/jc.2017-01658.
65. Schagen SEE, Wouters FM, Cohen-Kettenis PT, Gooren LJ, Hannema SE. Bone development in transgender adolescents treated with gnrh analogues and subsequent gender-affirming hormones. J Clin Endocrinol Metab. 2020;105. https://doi.org/10.1210/clinem/dgaa604.
66. Ciancia S, Dubois V, Cools M. Impact of gender-affirming treatment on bone health in transgender and gender diverse youth Endocr Connect. 2022;11. https://doi.org/10.1530/EC-22-0280.
67. Davidge-Pitts C, Clarke BL. Transgender bone health. Maturitas. 2019;127:35–42. https://doi.org/10.1016/j.maturitas.2019.05.002.
68. Lin CY, Kang JH. Mechanical properties of compact bone defined by the stress-strain curve measured using uniaxial tensile test: a concise review and practical guide. Materials (Basel). 2021;14. https://doi.org/10.3390/ma14154224.

69. Chen S, Patel J, Katzmeyer T, Pei M. Sex-dependent variation in bone adaptation: from degeneration to regeneration. J Orthop Transl. 2025;52:325–43. https://doi.org/10.1016/J.JOT.2025.04.011.
70. Riggs BL, Melton LJ, Robb RA, et al. Population-based study of age and sex differences in bone volumetric density, size, geometry, and structure at different skeletal sites. J Bone Miner Res. 2004;19. https://doi.org/10.1359/JBMR.040916.
71. Osterhoff G, Morgan EF, Shefelbine SJ, Karim L, McNamara LM, Augat P. Bone mechanical properties and changes with osteoporosis. Injury. 2016;47:S11. https://doi.org/10.1016/S0020-1383(16)47003-8.
72. Mohamed AMFS. An overview of bone cells and their regulating factors of differentiation. Malays J Med Sci. 2008;15:4–12.
73. Alswat KA. Gender disparities in osteoporosis. J Clin Med Res. 2017;9:382. https://doi.org/10.14740/JOCMR2970W.
74. Anderson HC. Vesicles associated with calcification in the matrix of epiphyseal cartilage. J Cell Biol. 1969;41. https://doi.org/10.1083/jcb.41.1.59.
75. Miller SC, De Saint-Georges L, Bowman BM, Jee WSS. Bone lining cells: structure and function. Scanning Microsc. 1989;3:953–60.
76. Tresguerres FGF, Torres J, López-Quiles J, Hernández G, Vega JA, Tresguerres IF. The osteocyte: a multifunctional cell within the bone. Ann Anat. 2020;227:151422. https://doi.org/10.1016/j.aanat.2019.151422.
77. Huang R, Wang X, Zhou Y, Xiao Y. RANKL-induced M1 macrophages are involved in bone formation. Bone Res. 2017;5. https://doi.org/10.1038/boneres.2017.19.
78. Sierra-Filardi E, Nieto C, Domínguez-Soto Á, et al. CCL2 shapes macrophage polarization by GM-CSF and M-CSF: identification of CCL2/CCR2-dependent gene expression profile. J Immunol. 2014;192. https://doi.org/10.4049/jimmunol.1302821.
79. Maruyama M, Rhee C, Utsunomiya T, et al. Modulation of the inflammatory response and bone healing. Front Endocrinol (Lausanne). 2020;11:1–14. https://doi.org/10.3389/fendo.2020.00386.
80. Yang X, Ricciardi BF, Hernandez-Soria A, Shi Y, Pleshko Camacho N, Bostrom MPG. Callus mineralization and maturation are delayed during fracture healing in interleukin-6 knockout mice. Bone. 2007;41. https://doi.org/10.1016/j.bone.2007.07.022.
81. Takayanagi H, Sato K, Takaoka A, Taniguchi T. Interplay between interferon and other cytokine systems in bone metabolism. Immunol Rev. 2005;208. https://doi.org/10.1111/j.0105-2896.2005.00337.x.
82. Elhawary H, Baradaran A, Abi-Rafeh J, Vorstenbosch J, Xu L, Efanov JI. Bone healing and inflammation: principles of fracture and repair. Semin Plast Surg. 2021;35. https://doi.org/10.1055/s-0041-1732334.
83. Kenkre JS, Bassett JHD. The bone remodelling cycle. Ann Clin Biochem. 2018;55. https://doi.org/10.1177/0004563218759371.
84. Miron RJ, Bosshardt DD. OsteoMacs: key players around bone biomaterials. Biomaterials. 2016;82. https://doi.org/10.1016/j.biomaterials.2015.12.017.
85. Batoon L, Millard SM, Raggatt LJ, Pettit AR. Osteomacs and bone regeneration. Curr Osteoporos Rep. 2017;15. https://doi.org/10.1007/s11914-017-0384-x.
86. Al-Aql ZS, Alagl AS, Graves DT, Gerstenfeld LC, Einhorn TA. Molecular mechanisms controlling bone formation during fracture healing and distraction osteogenesis. J Dent Res. 2008;87. https://doi.org/10.1177/154405910808700215.
87. Kramer I, Halleux C, Keller H, et al. Osteocyte Wnt/β-catenin signaling is required for normal bone homeostasis. Mol Cell Biol. 2010;30:3071. https://doi.org/10.1128/mcb.01428-09.
88. Baron R, Kneissel M. WNT signaling in bone homeostasis and disease: from human mutations to treatments. Nat Med. 2013;19. https://doi.org/10.1038/nm.3074.
89. Kousteni S, Bellido T, Plotkin LI, et al. Nongenotropic, sex-nonspecific signaling through the estrogen or androgen receptors: dissociation from transcriptional activity. Cell. 2001;104. https://doi.org/10.1016/s0092-8674(01)00268-9.

90. Emmanuelle NE, Marie-Cécile V, Florence T, et al. Critical role of estrogens on bone homeostasis in both male and female: from physiology to medical implications. Int J Mol Sci. 2021;22. https://doi.org/10.3390/ijms22041568.
91. Manolagas SC. From estrogen-centric to aging and oxidative stress: a revised perspective of the pathogenesis of osteoporosis. Endocr Rev. 2010;31. https://doi.org/10.1210/er.2009-0024.
92. Martin GM, Sprague CA, Epstein CJ. Replicative life-span of cultivated human cells. Effects of donor's age, tissue, and genotype. Lab Investig. 1970;23:86–92.
93. Campagnola PJ, Loew LM. Second-harmonic imaging microscopy for visualizing biomolecular arrays in cells, tissues and organisms. Nat Biotechnol. 2003;21:1356. https://doi.org/10.1038/nbt894.
94. Nyman JS, Roy A, Acuna RL, et al. Age-related effect on the concentration of collagen crosslinks in human osteonal and interstitial bone tissue. Bone. 2006;39:1210. https://doi.org/10.1016/j.bone.2006.06.026.
95. Nyman JS, Roy A, Tyler JH, Acuna RL, Gayle HJ, Wang X. Age-related factors affecting the postyield energy dissipation of human cortical bone. J Orthop Res. 2007;25:646. https://doi.org/10.1002/jor.20337.
96. Currey JD. The relationship between the stiffness and the mineral content of bone. J Biomech. 1969;2:477. https://doi.org/10.1016/0021-9290(69)90023-2.
97. Schneider S, Breit SM, Grampp S, et al. Comparative assessment of bone mineral measurements obtained by use of dual-energy x-ray absorptiometry, peripheral quantitative computed tomography, and chemical-physical analyses in femurs of juvenile and adult dogs. Am J Vet Res. 2004;65:891. https://doi.org/10.2460/ajvr.2004.65.891.
98. Duque G, Rivas D, Li W, et al. Age-related bone loss in the LOU/c rat model of healthy ageing. Exp Gerontol. 2009;44:183. https://doi.org/10.1016/j.exger.2008.10.004.
99. Somerville JM, Aspden RM, Armour KE, Armour KJ, Reid DM. Growth of C57Bl/6 mice and the material and mechanical properties of cortical bone from the tibia. Calcif Tissue Int. 2004;74:469. https://doi.org/10.1007/s00223-003-0101-x.
100. Falahati-Nini A, Riggs BL, Atkinson EJ, O'Fallon WM, Eastell R, Khosla S. Relative contributions of testosterone and estrogen in regulating bone resorption and formation in normal elderly men. J Clin Invest. 2000;106:1553. https://doi.org/10.1172/JCI10942.
101. Carriero A, Javaheri B, Bassir Kazeruni N, Pitsillides AA, Shefelbine SJ. Age and sex differences in load-induced tibial cortical bone surface strain maps. JBMR Plus. 2021;5: e10467. https://doi.org/10.1002/jbm4.10467.
102. Kumar A, Mir SM, Aldulijan I, et al. Load-bearing biodegradable PCL-PGA-beta TCP scaffolds for bone tissue regeneration. J Biomed Mater Res Part B Appl Biomater. 2021;109:193. https://doi.org/10.1002/jbm.b.34691.
103. Benatti ACB, Pattaro AF, Rodrigues AA, et al. Bioreabsorbable polymers for tissue engineering: PLA, PGA, and their copolymers. In: Materials for biomedical engineering: hydrogels and polymer-based scaffolds. Amsterdam: Elsevier; 2019. https://doi.org/10.1016/B978-0-12-816901-8.00004-3.
104. Lü JM, Wang X, Marin-Muller C, et al. Current advances in research and clinical applications of PLGA-based nanotechnology. Expert Rev Mol Diagn. 2009;9:325. https://doi.org/10.1586/erm.09.15.
105. Owen GR, Dard M, Larjava H. Hydoxyapatite/beta-tricalcium phosphate biphasic ceramics as regenerative material for the repair of complex bone defects. J Biomed Mater Res Part B Appl Biomater. 2018;106:2493. https://doi.org/10.1002/jbm.b.34049.
106. Smith BT, Bittner SM, Watson E, et al. Multimaterial dual gradient three-dimensional printing for osteogenic differentiation and spatial segregation. Tissue Eng Part A. 2020;26:0204. https://doi.org/10.1089/ten.tea.2019.0204.
107. Knabe C, Mele A, Kann PH, et al. Effect of sex-hormone levels, sex, body mass index and other host factors on human craniofacial bone regeneration with bioactive tricalcium phosphate grafts. Biomaterials. 2017;123:48. https://doi.org/10.1016/j.biomaterials.2017.01.035.

108. Shi C, Yuan Z, Han F, Zhu C, Li B. Polymeric biomaterials for bone regeneration. Ann Jt. 2016;1:27. https://doi.org/10.21037/AOJ.2016.11.02.
109. Girón J, Kerstner E, Medeiros T, et al. Biomaterials for bone regeneration: an orthopedic and dentistry overview. Braz J Med Biol Res. 2021;54:e11055. https://doi.org/10.1590/1414-431X2021E11055.
110. Gillman CE, Jayasuriya AC. FDA-approved bone grafts and bone graft substitute devices in bone regeneration. Mater Sci Eng C. 2021;130:112466. https://doi.org/10.1016/j.msec.2021.112466.
111. Yu B, Cao Y, Sun H, Han J. The structure and properties of biodegradable PLLA/PDLA for melt-blown nonwovens. J Polym Environ. 2017;25:510. https://doi.org/10.1007/s10924-016-0827-y.
112. Ran J, Jiang P, Sun G, et al. Comparisons among Mg, Zn, Sr, and Si doped nano-hydroxy-apatite/chitosan composites for load-bearing bone tissue engineering applications. Mater Chem Front. 2017;1:900. https://doi.org/10.1039/c6qm00192k.
113. Szterner P, Antosik A, Pagacz J, Tymowicz-Grzyb P. Morphology control of hydroxyapatite as a potential reinforcement for orthopedic biomaterials: the hydrothermal process. Crystals. 2023;13:793. https://doi.org/10.3390/cryst13050793.
114. Peng W, Liu Y, Wang C. Definition, measurement, and function of pore structure dimensions of bioengineered porous bone tissue materials based on additive manufacturing: a review. Front Bioeng Biotechnol. 2023;10:1081548. https://doi.org/10.3389/fbioe.2022.1081548.
115. Olivares-Navarrete R, Hyzy SL, Chaudhri RA, Zhao G, Boyan BD, Schwartz Z. Sex dependent regulation of osteoblast response to implant surface properties by systemic hormones. Biol Sex Differ. 2010;1:4. https://doi.org/10.1186/2042-6410-1-4.
116. Berger MB, Cohen DJ, Olivares-Navarrete R, et al. Human osteoblasts exhibit sexual dimorphism in their response to estrogen on microstructured titanium surfaces. Biol Sex Differ. 2018;9:30. https://doi.org/10.1186/s13293-018-0190-x.
117. Kolliopoulos V, Tiffany A, Polanek M, Harley BAC. Donor sex and passage conditions influence msc osteogenic response in mineralized collagen scaffolds. Adv Healthc Mater. 2024;13:e2400039. https://doi.org/10.1002/adhm.202400039.
118. Kolliopoulos V. Employing mineralized collagen scaffolds in a patient-centric approach for improved craniomaxillofacial bone repair. Doctoral dissertation, University of Illinois at Urbana-Champaign; 2023.
119. Howard FH, et al. Silk fibroin nanoparticles: a biocompatible multi-functional polymer for drug delivery. In: Biotechnology-biosensors, biomaterials and tissue engineering annual, vol. 2023. IntechOpen; 2023.

Hormonal and Pregnancy-Related Changes on Bone Mechanical Properties: Considerations for Biomaterial Design

Laura C. Bowman, Heather C. M. Allaway, Patricia K. Thomas, and Anthony G. Lau

Abstract During a female's reproductive lifecycle, hormones such as estrogen, progesterone, and follicle-stimulating hormone (FSH) play crucial roles in bone health. Their levels fluctuate significantly from puberty through menopause, influencing the bone remodeling process and the risk of osteoporosis and fracture. Pregnancy and breastfeeding require a significant amount of calcium, which is temporarily withdrawn from the mother's bones to support the fetus/infant, but is typically fully recovered during weaning. In the long run, the changes to bone during pregnancy set the trajectory of bone health leading up to the menopause transition. Menopause and the 1–2 years leading up to a woman's last period are characterized by a sharp decline in estrogen and progesterone, triggering rapid bone loss. While the major consequences to skeletal health due to the loss of estrogen in postmenopausal women is well understood, the impact of hormonal fluctuations to bone strength and structure during other lifecycle stages is less well studied. In addition, the alterations in bone morphology, material properties, and hormonal status warrant further investigation as they are important factors to consider when designing and optimizing the biomaterials used in implants for women.

Keywords Bone · Estrogen · Progesterone · Prolactin · Menstrual cycle · Pregnancy · Lactation · Menopause

---

L. C. Bowman · A. G. Lau (✉)
Department of Biomedical Engineering, The College of New Jersey, Ewing, NJ, USA
e-mail: BowmanL@tcnj.edu; Anthony.Lau@tcnj.edu

H. C. M. Allaway
School of Kinesiology, Louisiana State University, Baton Rouge, LA, USA
e-mail: hallaway@lsu.edu

P. K. Thomas
Department of Biomedical Engineering, Wake Forest University School of Medicine, Winston-Salem, NC, USA
e-mail: Patricia.Thomas@wfusm.edu

S. G. Zambuto, M. L. Oyen (eds.), *Biomaterials for Women's Health Engineering*,
https://doi.org/10.1007/978-3-032-10745-9_15

1 Introduction

The mechanical and material properties of bone are fundamental to the ability of the skeleton to withstand and transfer loading during everyday activities. Bone is extremely metabolically active, undergoing continuous cycles of old bone removal and new tissue formation to maintain bone strength, adapt to changes in loading conditions, and repair injuries. The remodeling process is regulated by a complex interplay of reproductive hormones, cytokines, and growth hormones. The changing hormone levels that occur throughout each reproductive life stage impact the health and function of all tissues of the body, whether it is increasing joint laxity or affecting bone strength [1–4].

While the fundamental aspects of bone are similar between males and females, sex and hormonal status play a large role on bone mass and strength. However, sexual dimorphism in bone structure and regenerative capacity are often overlooked and, until recently, sex differences have been largely ignored. Differences in bone properties are detectable starting in childhood with differential growth patterns between males and females linked to the accrual of bone mineral [5] and are largely due to the introduction of sex hormones during puberty [6].

Skeletal sexual dimorphism is also present in animal models. 3D reconstruction of microcomputed tomography (microCT) data reveals significant differences in the trabecular bone microarchitecture of the proximal tibia of 9-month-old male and female Long-Evans rats (Fig. 1). While the total bone volume in this proximal tibia region (cortical + trabecular) was similar between males and females, the distribution

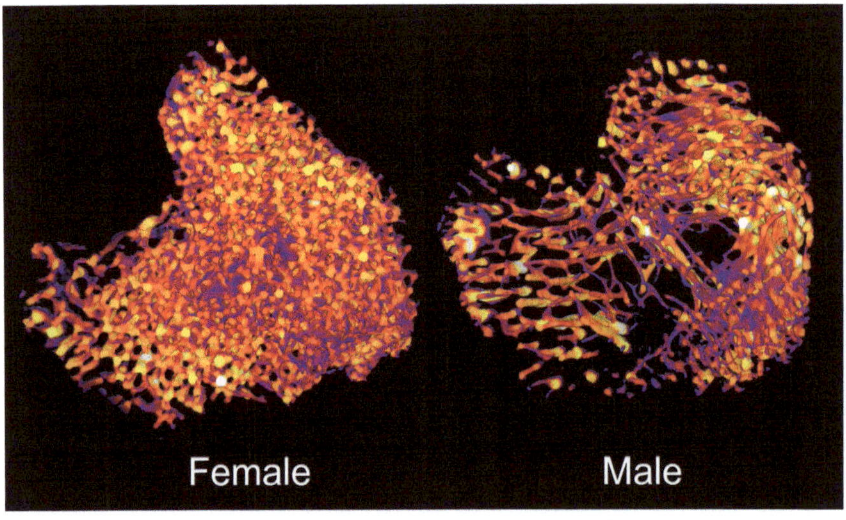

Fig. 1 Trabecular thickness maps of the proximal tibia region of a female (left) and male (right) Long-Evans rat. Female rats have significantly greater density of trabecular bone compared with males. (Images were generated in Fiji/BoneJ using microCT data (manuscript in preparation))

between cortical vs. trabecular diverged. Males had higher cortical bone volume compared to females, while females had higher trabecular compartmental bone volume fraction (BV/TV) [7].

2 Hormonal Changes Related to Reproductive Status

Hormones fluctuate throughout a female's reproductive life cycle, from puberty to menopause. Following birth but prior to puberty, reproductive hormone levels (follicle-stimulating hormone [FSH], luteinizing hormone [LH], estradiol [E2], and progesterone [P4]) are consistently low [8, 9]. At the onset of puberty, secretion of FSH and LH slowly rise and hormone levels begin to oscillate at regular monthly intervals [8]. At menarche, the first incidence of menses, the reproductive years in a female's life begins. The menstrual cycle takes time to stabilize into a consistent monthly occurrence, and in some females, it never stabilizes to a consistent monthly occurrence.

The menstrual cycle is an external signal of the hormonal communications between the brain and the ovaries, where the objective is to grow a healthy ovarian follicle. This includes the egg and leads to the development of an appropriate uterine environment for growth of a fetus, should fertilization occur. During the menstrual cycle, FSH secretion begins with the withdrawal of E2 and P4 at the previous menstrual cycle. FSH recruits a cohort of ovarian follicles that were quiescent to begin growth. As follicles grow, they begin to secrete E2, which suppresses the pituitary secretion of FSH. The suppression of the FSH secretion results in the atresia of all but the follicle that is dominant and will eventually ovulate. The dominant follicle continues to secrete E2 at increasing concentrations, which results in the mid-cycle LH and FSH surge, causing ovulation and the release of the egg. Ovulation separates the menstrual cycle into the follicular (first half) and luteal (second half) phases (Fig. 2). The cells of the follicle that remain in the ovary following ovulation become the corpus luteum, a hormone-secreting group of cells that are maintained if pregnancy occurs [10]. The release of FSH mid-cycle recruits a cohort of follicles that grow and secrete E2, while the corpus luteum secretes P4 and a small amount of E2. If fertilization of the egg does not occur, the E2 and P4 levels begin to decline, which removes the inhibition of these hormones on the pituitary secretion of FSH and LH [11].

2.1 Pregnancy and Lactation

If fertilization occurs, there is a pattern of hormonal secretion changes across the 37–42 week duration of a typical pregnancy. The hormones secreted are essential to support and maintain a healthy pregnancy, facilitate the growth and development of the fetus, and enable lactation following delivery. During the first trimester of

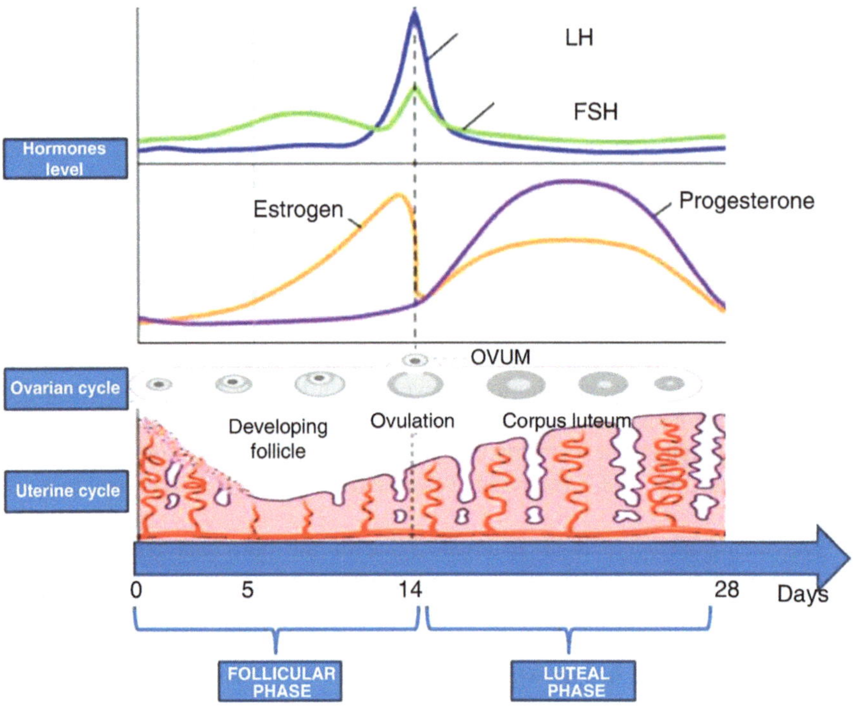

Fig. 2 LH, FSH, E2, and P4 levels over the course of the menstrual cycle with ovulation denoted as a dashed line. (Reproduced with permission from Ref. [12])

pregnancy, the corpus luteum continues to secrete P4 to maintain the uterine lining for implantation. For a successful implantation of the fertilized egg at the blastocyst stage, human chorionic gonadotropin (hCG) levels need to increase within 4 days of ovulation to maintain the corpus luteum [13]. During pregnancy, P4 plays a role in implantation and pregnancy maintenance. The corpus luteum produces most of the P4 until 10 weeks gestation, when the placenta starts to produce P4. Throughout the pregnancy, P4 and E2 levels increase, as seen in Fig. 3 [14]. Estrogens contribute to uterine vessel dilation and placental angiogenesis, but likely contribute to the risk of preeclampsia [14, 15]. Since both hormones are produced by the placenta during pregnancy, after the delivery of the placenta, both hormone levels drop [16].

Many other hormones are also involved throughout pregnancy, including relaxin and prolactin. Relaxin is responsible for collagen remodeling, allowing for pelvic ligament relaxation [17]. The levels of relaxin increase in the first trimester and are maintained until postpartum, when the levels drop, as it is primarily produced by the corpus luteum and placenta during pregnancy. During non-pregnancy, relaxin levels are cyclic, with peak levels observed in the serum near the end of the cycle at days 21–24 [17]. Prolactin promotes lactation and breast development, and since prolactin production is stimulated by estrogen levels, prolactin levels also increase throughout the pregnancy duration [18]. The anterior pituitary gland is a primary source of

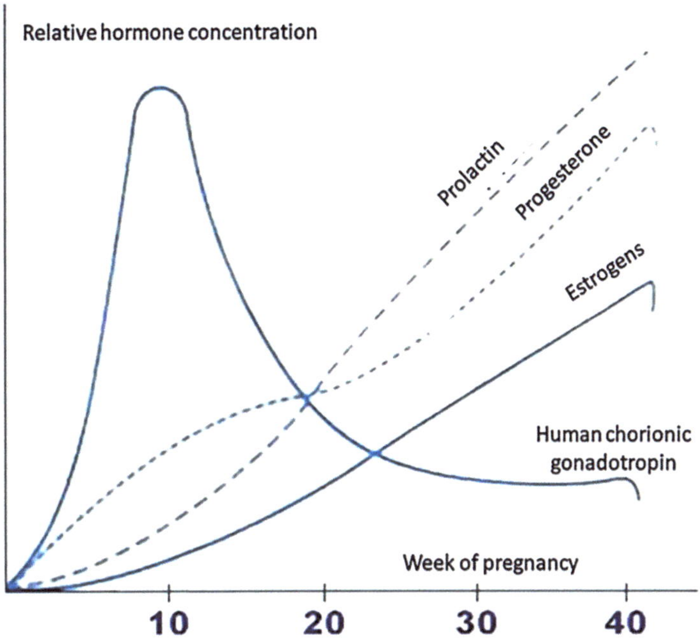

Fig. 3 Hormone levels throughout the duration of pregnancy. (Reproduced with permission from Ref. [12])

prolactin; however, other organs such as the uterus and mammary glands also produce prolactin. Prolactin production can also be stimulated by breastfeeding, leading to varying levels postpartum based on if and how long the parent chooses to breastfeed the infant [19]. In contrast, during nonpregnant periods of a female's reproductive life cycle, prolactin levels are undetectable in blood serum.

2.2 *Menopause*

At the end of a woman's reproductive lifespan, hormone secretion during the menstrual cycle becomes erratic, with FSH levels rising and E2 levels declining. The menopause transition is a broad time period that varies among females, but is divided into early and late menopause transition stages, characterized by distinct hormonal changes. According to the 2012 Stages of Reproductive Aging Workshop, the early menopause transition typically occurs between the late 30's to about 45 and is defined as a "persistent difference of 7 or more days in length for consecutive menstrual cycles" and no more than 59 days between menses [20]. The late menopause transition typically occurs after the age of 46 years and is defined as "no menses for 60 days and up to 12 months of no menses." Entry into the postmenopausal time period occurs after the final menstrual period (FMP), which is established retrospectively after 12 months of no menses. The natural occurrence of the FMP is observed at an average age of 51.4 years [21, 22], but can vary widely from 40 to 58 years [23]. In addition to the reproductive hormone changes, there is an increase in chronic systemic inflammation as humans age [24], with some of the inflammatory changes occurring as a result of the loss of E2 in females postmenopause [25–28]. When E2 levels are chronically low, as observed during postmenopause, there is an elevation in pro-inflammatory signals (i.e., Tumor Necrosis Factor-alpha (TNF-a), Interleukin-1-beta (IL-1b), Interleukin-17 (IL-17)) and reactive oxygen species production [29–37], with a lack of stimulation of anti-inflammatory signals [38].

3 Hormonal Contributions to Bone Properties

The importance of estrogen exposure in bone accrual and maintenance is well known. Under adequate estrogen exposure, bone resorption and formation signals are balanced. Estrogen signaling decreases Receptor Activator of Nuclear Factor B Ligand (RANKL) and increases Osteoprotegerin (OPG) production, thus decreasing osteoclastogenesis [39, 40] and serum markers of resorption, such as carboxyterminal telopeptide (CTx) [41]. Estrogen has been shown to decrease sclerostin [39, 40, 42], a potent inhibitor of Wnt signaling and of osteoblastogenesis [42–44], resulting in reductions in bone resorption. One well-researched area of hypoestrogenism is functional hypothalamic amenorrhea (FHA) [45, 46]. The hypoestrogenism that is hallmark of FHA contributes to low bone mass [47, 48] by dysregulating bone remodeling signals [49–53] and reducing expression of estrogen receptor alpha (ERα) [54], leading to increased osteoclastogenesis and osteoblast and osteocyte apoptosis [55, 56], thus increasing fracture risk [57–62]. ERα is an important factor in translating the mechanotransduction signals in bone. Ulnar periosteal and endosteal bone formation rates following bouts of mechanical loading are reduced threefold in ERα knock-out mice [63]. It is speculated that estradiol suppression below adequate concentrations required for ERα expression may lead to a decrease in the number of functional ERα and the inability to process the cell strain response [64]. Functional ERα are needed to activate osteoblasts in response to strain and cause proliferation of osteoblasts in response to dynamic strain [64, 65]. Specifically, exercising women with FHA have increased sclerostin and reduced bone formation markers compared with normally cycling exercising women and non-exercising women [51, 66].

For example, the cyclic rise in E2 during the follicular phase of the menstrual cycle is associated with increased joint laxity in sports medicine [1]. However, these sex-specific changes in reproductive hormones secretion are not the only hormones affecting these tissues. Other hormone levels, such as calcitonin and parathyroid hormone (PTH), which both regulate osteoclast activity in bone, have been shown to change over the course of pregnancy [3, 67]. Most female bone health research has

Table 1 Summary of changes in human maternal hormone levels during pregnancy, lactation, and menopause and the general impact on bone health

	Pregnancy	Lactation	Menopause	Effect to bone
Estradiol (E2)	↑	↓	↓	↑ Formation Limits OC activity Enhances intestinal calcium absorption
Progesterone (P4)	↑	↓	↓	↑ Formation Stimulates OB differentiation and formation
Follicle-stimulating hormone (FSH)	↓	↔	↑	Stimulates OC formation
Parathyroid hormone (PTH)	↓	↓	↔ *to* ↑	↑ Resorption Stimulates conversion of vitamin D to calcitriol
Parathyroid hormone-related protein (PTHrP)	↑	↑	↔	↑ Resorption Replaces PTH during pregnancy
Serum calcium	↓	↔	↔	Low levels stimulate PTH release High levels stimulate calcitonin release
Calcitriol, 1,25(OH)D	↑	↔	↓	↓ Resorption Antagonist to PTH and PTHrP Increases calcium absorption
Calcitonin	↑	↑	↓	↓ Resorption Inhibits OC activity
Relaxin	↑	↔	↓	Increases ligament flexibility and joint laxity
Prolactin	↑	↑	↓	↑ Resorption Indirectly stimulates OCs

OB osteoblast, *OC* osteoclast
↔ Normal levels, ↑ Increased, ↓ Decreased

been focused on the postmenopausal period of life [68], with limited studies on the bone changes that occur during pregnancy. The bone changes around pregnancy are important to understand, as they can set the trajectory of bone health, leading up to the menopause transition. Table 1 summarizes the physiological changes in hormone levels during the human reproductive lifecycle and the impact on skeletal health.

3.1 Pregnancy

During pregnancy, there are many physiological and hormonal changes that can impact bone health. Significant changes to both bone metabolism and maternal calcium are required to fulfill the calcium requirements of the fetal skeleton, which peaks in the third trimester. This increased calcium need is primarily met through increased calcium absorption in the intestines via either an active, rapid, transcellular pathway or a passive, slower, paracellular pathway [69]. Ionized calcium levels and phosphate levels in the blood are constant throughout the pregnancy in humans, while total serum calcium, which includes ionized, complexed, and albumin bound fractions of calcium, decreases [4, 67, 70–73]. In both animals and humans, the bulk of calcium absorption is through the passive route, with the active route becoming more important in cases of limited calcium in the maternal diet [74, 75]. Both pathways are stimulated by calcitriol, the hormonal form and most active metabolite of vitamin D, which can reach triple prepregnancy levels by the third trimester in humans [4, 67, 71, 72, 76, 77].

Other hormones not directly involved in calcium absorption that impact bone are also altered during pregnancy. Parathyroid hormone (PTH) is replaced by parathyroid hormone-related protein (PTHrP), which both prevents secondary and tertiary hyperthyroidism and promotes bone resorption. PTHrP levels rise over the course of the pregnancy before dropping drastically following labor [78]. Levels of E2, the most potent and abundant form of estrogen, also rise up to 100-fold in humans during gestation [79, 80].

Most of the data from humans indicate an overall neutral effect of pregnancy to maternal bone [69]. However, one study in humans found that urinary cross-linked Type I collagen N-telopeptide (NTx), a biomarker for bone resorption, peaked in the third trimester and postpartum [70]. The study also noted that estrogens also increased throughout pregnancy with further increases after birth. Along with estrogen increase, there was a decrease in total calcium levels in the serum. In humans, areal bone mineral density (aBMD) in the lumbar spine and trochanter of the femur was also found to decrease significantly between preconception and postpartum [70]. The hip and femoral neck BMD did not change significantly, likely due to Wolff's law compensating for the increased weight on these bones.

Studies in rodent models are more mixed. Several rodent studies have assessed the effect of pregnancy on bone mass through dual-energy X-ray absorptiometry (DXA) measurements. The majority only compare prepregnancy and end-of-pregnancy bone mineral content (BMC) or aBMD, and there is wide variation in the results depending on skeletal site examined and the mouse strain used. On average, C57BL/6 mice lose around 3% and 18% of whole body and lumbar spine BMC, respectively, while gaining 6–7% in the hindlimbs [81]. In contrast, CD-1 mice had no change in mineral content at any skeletal site [82, 83] and Black Swiss mice increased whole body BMC by 10–12% during gestation [77, 84].

In pregnant rats, no significant differences in torsional mechanical properties of femora were found until day 20 of a 22-day gestation [4]. However, the pregnant rats had smaller fracture angles, greater stiffness, and lower shear moduli compared to controls. Histologically, there were larger bone crystals at day 20 compared to controls. This leads to fewer crystals in the same volume, allowing for fractures to propagate more easily, even though the mineral content was not significantly different. There was also an increase in vasculature in the cortical bone of pregnant samples, which would also affect the material properties that were not directly tested [4].

While mice and rats are frequently used to model maternal adaptations throughout the female reproductive cycle, there are some significant differences between animal and human models that should be considered. Rodents have a much shorter gestational cycle than humans and the calcium demands on a pregnant rat or mouse will be proportionally greater than a pregnant woman due to the increased average number of fetuses per pregnancy [69]. Rats can bear 6–12 fetuses per litter compared to the typical single fetus carried per pregnancy for most human females. This means that, over the course of the pregnancy, while a human fetus will receive ~5–10% of the mother's circulating calcium, the rat litter requires ~80% of circulating maternal calcium [85].

3.2 *Lactation and Postpartum*

Maternal bone is preferentially resorbed to meet high calcium demands during lactation. After birth, E2 levels drop sharply while nursing maintains high levels of PTHrP. This appears to play a key role in increased resorption during lactation and subsequent bone loss. In rodents, treatment with estradiol and ablation of PTHrP receptors in mammary tissue were shown to reduce bone loss during lactation [83, 86]. Conversely, while treatment with PTHrP infusion combined with ovariectomy-induced estrogen deficiency (OVX) reduced BMD by a similar amount to lactation in the femur (17%), it did not completely reproduce the effects of lactation on BME at the spine (lactation: 23%, OVX+PTHrP:11%) [87]. In humans, the role of E2 is less clear with high levels of PTHrP, contributing more toward loss of bone mass.

Human females will typically lose 3–10% of bone mass while nursing with the majority of the bone loss happening from trabecular bone and endocortical surfaces [88, 89]. In humans, most of the bone loss occurs in the first 4–6 months after birth during the period before the introduction of solid food (exclusive breastfeeding). In this timeframe, human females typically lose 5% of bone mass from the lumbar spine [90]. Several longitudinal studies have shown that aBMD returns to prepregnancy or early postpartum levels within 12 months of weaning. In contrast, mice and rats typically lose 25–35% of bone mineral between birth and weaning [91–94]. In one study using a rat model, after 21 days of lactation, maximum load on lumbar vertebrae and vertebral flexural rigidity decreased 64% and 56%, respectively. This was followed by almost complete recovery by 8 weeks after weaning [3].

Historically, it has been assumed that osteoclastic resorption was the main driver of bone loss during lactation. Recent studies have demonstrated that lactation also induces osteolytic osteolysis where osteocytes behave as osteoclasts and resorb small amounts of bone matrix from the surrounding lacunae [95, 96]. One study showed elastic modulus of the mid-shaft femur, as determined by microindentation, was decreased by 10% and 13% in the posterior and anterior locations, respectively, in mice after 2 weeks of lactation [97]. Lacunar volume and canalicular space were increased and there was no indication of intracortical resorption. In the same study, complete recovery of elastic modulus was achieved by 1-week postweaning.

3.3 *Menopause*

The menopause transition is a time of significant bone loss in human females, with the greatest loss occurring over a 3-year period that begins during the late menopause transition (Fig. 4). This 3-year period begins with the 1 year that precede the FMP and the 2 years following the FMP, and is termed transmenopause [98–100]. During this time period, females lose more bone at the hip and spine than at any other time in their lives [98–100]. There are very distinct differences in bone health in females across the early versus late menopause transition, as first demonstrated through the Study of Women's Health Across the Nation (SWAN) [101]. The major aBMD loss occurring during the transmenopause period increases the risk for postmenopausal osteoporosis development. There was no appreciable decline in aBMD at the lumbar spine or femoral neck in females prior to the start of the late menopause transition [99].

Starting with the late menopause transition, human females lose an estimated 10% of aBMD [102], and postmenopausal human females will continue to lose approximately 1.2% aBMD per year [103]. Human females over 60 years are four times as likely to develop osteoporosis and have almost double the lifetime risk of fragility fracture compared with men [104, 105].

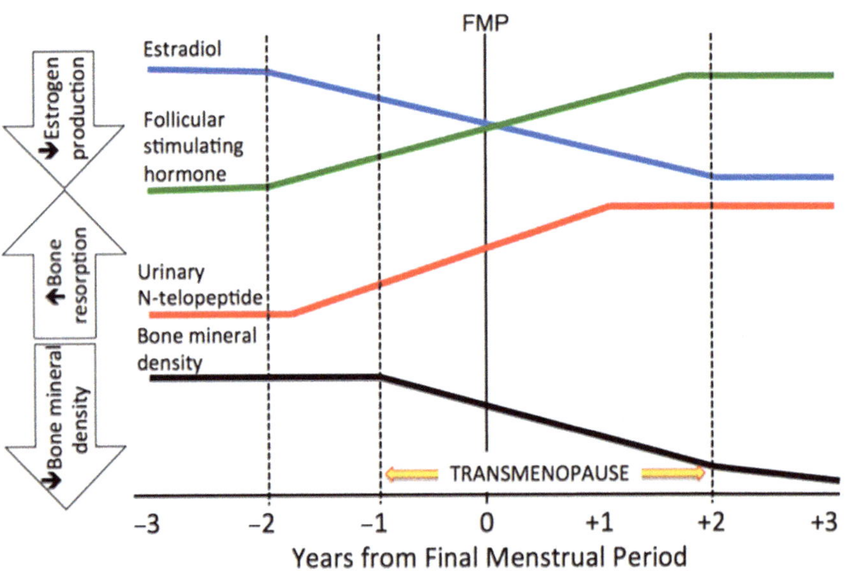

Fig. 4 Changes in sex steroid hormones (E2, FSH), bone resorption marker (U-NTX), and BMD over the menopause transition period. Blue: estradiol (E2); Green: follicular-stimulating hormone (FSH), Red: urinary N-telopeptide (U-NTX); Black: bone mineral density (BMD). (Reproduced with permission from Ref. [106])

4 Implications for Biomaterial Design and Concluding Remarks

The design of biomaterials for bone tissue engineering and implant development must consider sex differences in bone, particularly in the hormonal responses of the trabecular and cortical bone throughout the female reproductive cycle, and impact on bone health and strength as well as risk of fracture. It is essential to consider these differences when designing implants and biomaterials to mimic the natural bone's microstructural and material properties. These changes are not necessarily captured by the existing standard clinical and research assays, which limit our knowledge for designing novel biomaterials optimized for bone tissue. In addition, the interpretation of traditional bone health assays for male and female subjects must be carefully considered, as hormonal changes during pregnancy and lactation are known to have effects on the bone at the material, microarchitectural, and structural length scales.

Traditional methods of bone health assessment, such as clinical bone mineral density with Dual-Energy X-Ray Absorptiometry (DXA) or high resolution microCT quantitative imaging in a research setting, may not accurately reflect these changes at the material level. Direct evaluation of material level properties, using micro/nano indentation techniques [97, 107–111] is crucial to understand these material level changes. Furthermore, the design of implant interfaces must consider the differences in cortical and trabecular bone distribution. The interface must be tailored to accommodate these differences to ensure proper integration of the implant with the surrounding bone tissue.

In conclusion, the design of biomaterials and implants for bone tissue engineering must consider the sex-specific differences in bone structure and function to ensure optimal implant performance and bone health. By considering these differences, biomaterials can be designed to mimic the natural bone structure, and implants can be tailored to accommodate the specific needs of male and female patients.

References

1. Shultz SJ, Sander TC, Kirk SE, Perrin DH. Sex differences in knee joint laxity change across the female menstrual cycle. J Sports Med Phys Fitness. 2005;45:594–603.
2. Marnach ML, Ramin KD, Ramsey PS, et al. Characterization of the relationship between joint laxity and maternal hormones in pregnancy. Obstet Gynecol. 2003;101:331–5.
3. Vajda EG, Bowman BM, Miller SC. Cancellous and cortical bone mechanical properties and tissue dynamics during pregnancy, lactation, and postlactation in the rat. Biol Reprod. 2001;65:689–95.
4. Leopold SS, Boskey AL, Doty SB, et al. Diminished material properties and altered bone structure in rat femora during pregnancy. J Orthop Res. 1995;13:41–9.
5. Wells JCK. Sexual dimorphism of body composition. Best Pract Res Clin Endocrinol Metab. 2007;21:415–30.
6. Chen S, Patel J, Katzmeyer T, Pei M. Sex-dependent variation in bone adaptation: from degeneration to regeneration. J Orthop Translat. 2025;52:325–43.

7. Vander Wiele SS, Cavallero NJ, Felipe JT, et al. Bone microstructural changes in rat tibias exposed to space radiation. 2023.
8. Howard SR. Interpretation of reproductive hormones before, during and after the pubertal transition-identifying health and disordered puberty. Clin Endocrinol. 2021;95:702–15.
9. Zec I, Kučak I, Begčević I, et al. Reference intervals for reproductive hormones in prepubertal children on the automated Roche cobas e 411 analyzer. Clin Biochem. 2012;45:1206–12.
10. Reynolds LP, Redmer DA. Growth and development of the corpus luteum. J Reprod Fertil Suppl. 1999;54:181–91.
11. Baerwald AR, Adams GP, Pierson RA. Ovarian antral folliculogenesis during the human menstrual cycle: a review. Hum Reprod Update. 2012;18:73–91.
12. Gianfaldoni S, Tchernev G, Tirant M, et al. Skin and skin disease throughout life. In: Atlas of dermatology, dermatopathology and venereology. Cham: Springer; 2022. p. 405–28.
13. Kumar P, Magon N. Hormones in pregnancy. Niger Med J. 2012;53:179–83.
14. Berkane N, Liere P, Oudinet J-P, et al. From pregnancy to preeclampsia: a key role for estrogens. Endocr Rev. 2017;38:123–44.
15. Zinaman MJ, Johnson S, Warren G. HCG and FSH levels during early pregnancy and reproductive aging [24A]. Obstet Gynecol. 2020;135:14S.
16. Hendrick V, Altshuler LL, Suri R. Hormonal changes in the postpartum and implications for postpartum depression. Psychosomatics. 1998;39:93–101.
17. Marshall SA, Senadheera SN, Parry LJ, Girling JE. The role of relaxin in normal and abnormal uterine function during the menstrual cycle and early pregnancy. Reprod Sci. 2017;24:342–54.
18. Al-Chalabi M, Bass AN, Alsalman I. Physiology, prolactin. Treasure Island: StatPearls; 2025.
19. Noel GL, Suh HK, Frantz AG. Prolactin release during nursing and breast stimulation in postpartum and nonpostpartum subjects. J Clin Endocrinol Metab. 1974;38:413–23.
20. Harlow SD, Gass M, Hall JE, et al. Executive summary of the stages of reproductive aging workshop + 10: addressing the unfinished agenda of staging reproductive aging. Menopause. 2012;19:387–95.
21. Shifren J, Gass M. The North American Menopause Society recommendations for clinical care of midlife women. Menopause. 2014;21:1038–62.
22. Gold EB, Bromberger J, Crawford S, et al. Factors associated with age at natural menopause in a multiethnic sample of midlife women. Am J Epidemiol. 2001;153:865–74.
23. Faubion SS, Enders F, Hedges MS, et al. Impact of menopause symptoms on women in the workplace. Mayo Clin Proc. 2023;98:833–45.
24. Franceschi C, Garagnani P, Parini P, et al. Inflammaging: a new immune–metabolic viewpoint for age-related diseases. Nat Rev Endocrinol. 2018;14:576–90.
25. Sharma N, Sharma RK, Tewari S, et al. Association of periodontal inflammation, systemic inflammation, and duration of menopausal years in postmenopausal women. Quintessence Int. 2018;49:123–31.
26. Kim OY, Chae JS, Paik JK, et al. Effects of aging and menopause on serum interleukin-6 levels and peripheral blood mononuclear cell cytokine production in healthy nonobese women. Age (Dordr). 2012;34:415–25.
27. Singh T, Newman AB. Inflammatory markers in population studies of aging. Ageing Res Rev. 2011;10:319–29.
28. Yasui T, Maegawa M, Tomita J, et al. Changes in serum cytokine concentrations during the menopausal transition. Maturitas. 2007;56:396–403.
29. Pacifici R. Estrogen, cytokines, and pathogenesis of postmenopausal osteoporosis. J Bone Miner Res. 1996;11:1043–51.
30. Sapir-Koren R, Livshits G. Postmenopausal osteoporosis in rheumatoid arthritis: the estrogen deficiency-immune mechanisms link. Bone. 2017;103:102–15.
31. Roggia C, Gao Y, Cenci S, et al. Up-regulation of TNF-producing T cells in the bone marrow: a key mechanism by which estrogen deficiency induces bone loss in vivo. Proc Natl Acad Sci USA. 2001;98:13960–5.

32. Pietschmann P, Grisar J, Thien R, et al. Immune phenotype and intracellular cytokine production of peripheral blood mononuclear cells from postmenopausal patients with osteoporotic fractures. Exp Gerontol. 2001;36:1749–59.
33. Manolagas SC. From estrogen-centric to aging and oxidative stress: a revised perspective of the pathogenesis of osteoporosis. Endocr Rev. 2010;31:266–300.
34. Scheidt-Nave C, Bismar H, Leidig-Bruckner G, et al. Serum interleukin 6 is a major predictor of bone loss in women specific to the first decade past menopause. J Clin Endocrinol Metab. 2001;86:2032–42.
35. Molnár I, Bohaty I, Somogyiné-Vári É. High prevalence of increased interleukin-17A serum levels in postmenopausal estrogen deficiency. Menopause. 2014;21:749–52.
36. Ginaldi L, Di Benedetto MC, De Martinis M. Osteoporosis, inflammation and ageing. Immun Ageing. 2005;2:14.
37. Cenci S, Toraldo G, Weitzmann MN, et al. Estrogen deficiency induces bone loss by increasing T cell proliferation and lifespan through IFN-gamma-induced class II transactivator. Proc Natl Acad Sci USA. 2003;100:10405–10.
38. Harnish DC, Scicchitano MS, Adelman SJ, et al. The role of CBP in estrogen receptor cross-talk with nuclear factor-kappaB in HepG2 cells. Endocrinology. 2000;141:3403–11.
39. Khosla S, Oursler MJ, Monroe DG. Estrogen and the skeleton. Trends Endocrinol Metab. 2012;23:576–81.
40. Compston JE. Sex steroids and bone. Physiol Rev. 2001;81:419–47.
41. Mozzanega B, Gizzo S, Bernardi D, et al. Cyclic variations of bone resorption mediators and markers in the different phases of the menstrual cycle. J Bone Miner Metab. 2013;31:461–7.
42. Mödder UI, Hoey KA, Amin S, et al. Relation of age, gender, and bone mass to circulating sclerostin levels in women and men. J Bone Miner Res. 2011;26:373–9.
43. Wijenayaka AR, Kogawa M, Lim HP, et al. Sclerostin stimulates osteocyte support of osteoclast activity by a RANKL-dependent pathway. PLoS One. 2011;6:e25900.
44. Mirza FS, Padhi ID, Raisz LG, Lorenzo JA. Serum sclerostin levels negatively correlate with parathyroid hormone levels and free estrogen index in postmenopausal women. J Clin Endocrinol Metab. 2010;95:1991–7.
45. Berga SL, Mortola JF, Girton L, et al. Neuroendocrine aberrations in women with functional hypothalamic amenorrhea. J Clin Endocrinol Metab. 1989;68:301–8.
46. Yen SS, Rebar R, VandenBerg G, Judd H. Hypothalamic amenorrhea and hypogonadotropinism: responses to synthetic LRF. J Clin Endocrinol Metab. 1973;36:811–6.
47. Grinspoon S, Miller K, Coyle C, et al. Severity of osteopenia in estrogen-deficient women with anorexia nervosa and hypothalamic amenorrhea. J Clin Endocrinol Metab. 1999;84:2049–55.
48. Warren MP, Stiehl AL. Exercise and female adolescents: effects on the reproductive and skeletal systems. J Am Med Womens Assoc. 1999;54:115–20, 138
49. Maïmoun L, Guillaume S, Lefebvre P, et al. Role of sclerostin and dickkopf-1 in the dramatic alteration in bone mass acquisition in adolescents and young women with recent anorexia nervosa. J Clin Endocrinol Metab. 2014;99:E582–90.
50. Faje AT, Fazeli PK, Katzman D, et al. Inhibition of Pref-1 (preadipocyte factor 1) by oestradiol in adolescent girls with anorexia nervosa is associated with improvement in lumbar bone mineral density. Clin Endocrinol. 2013;79:326–32.
51. Fazeli PK, Ackerman KE, Pierce L, et al. Sclerostin and Pref-1 have differential effects on bone mineral density and strength parameters in adolescent athletes compared with non-athletes. Osteoporos Int. 2013;24:2433–40.
52. Fazeli PK, Bredella MA, Misra M, et al. Preadipocyte factor-1 is associated with marrow adiposity and bone mineral density in women with anorexia nervosa. J Clin Endocrinol Metab. 2010;95:407–13.
53. Ohwada R, Hotta M, Sato K, et al. The relationship between serum levels of estradiol and osteoprotegerin in patients with anorexia nervosa. Endocr J. 2007;54:953–9.
54. Hoyland JA, Baris C, Wood L, et al. Effect of ovarian steroid deficiency on oestrogen receptor alpha expression in bone. J Pathol. 1999;188:294–303.

55. Weitzmann MN, Pacifici R. Estrogen deficiency and bone loss: an inflammatory tale. J Clin Invest. 2006;116:1186–94.
56. Syed F, Khosla S. Mechanisms of sex steroid effects on bone. Biochem Biophys Res Commun. 2005;328:688–96.
57. Johansson H, Kanis JA, Odén A, et al. A meta-analysis of the association of fracture risk and body mass index in women: a meta-analysis of the association of fracture risk and BMI in women. J Bone Miner Res. 2014;29:223–33.
58. Mallinson RJ, Williams NI, Hill BR, De Souza MJ. Body composition and reproductive function exert unique influences on indices of bone health in exercising women. Bone. 2013;56:91–100.
59. Ackerman KE, Nazem T, Chapko D, et al. Bone microarchitecture is impaired in adolescent amenorrheic athletes compared with eumenorrheic athletes and nonathletic controls. J Clin Endocrinol Metab. 2011;96:3123–33.
60. Vestergaard P, Emborg C, Støving RK, et al. Fractures in patients with anorexia nervosa, bulimia nervosa, and other eating disorders–a nationwide register study: eating disorders and fracture. Int J Eat Disord. 2002;32:301–8.
61. Lucas AR, Melton LJ 3rd, Crowson CS, O'Fallon WM. Long-term fracture risk among women with anorexia nervosa: a population-based cohort study. Mayo Clin Proc. 1999;74:972–7.
62. Miller KK, Klibanski A. Clinical review 106: amenorrheic bone loss. J Clin Endocrinol Metab. 1999;84:1775–83.
63. Lee K, Jessop H, Suswillo R, et al. Endocrinology: bone adaptation requires oestrogen receptor-alpha: endocrinology. Nature. 2003;424:389.
64. Armstrong VJ, Muzylak M, Sunters A, et al. Wnt/beta-catenin signaling is a component of osteoblastic bone cell early responses to load-bearing and requires estrogen receptor alpha. J Biol Chem. 2007;282:20715–27.
65. Jessop HL, Suswillo RFL, Rawlinson SCF, et al. Osteoblast-like cells from estrogen receptor alpha knockout mice have deficient responses to mechanical strain. J Bone Miner Res. 2004;19:938–46.
66. Zanker CL, Swaine IL. Bone turnover in amenorrhoeic and eumenorrhoeic women distance runners. Scand J Med Sci Sports. 1998;8:20–6.
67. Kovacs CS. Calcium and bone metabolism during pregnancy and lactation. J Mammary Gland Biol Neoplasia. 2005;10:105–18.
68. Osterhoff G, Morgan EF, Shefelbine SJ, et al. Bone mechanical properties and changes with osteoporosis. Injury. 2016;47 Suppl 2:S11–20.
69. Kovacs CS. Maternal mineral and bone metabolism during pregnancy, lactation, and post-weaning recovery. Physiol Rev. 2016;96:449–547.
70. Ulrich U, Miller PB, Eyre DR, et al. Bone remodeling and bone mineral density during pregnancy. Arch Gynecol Obstet. 2003;268:309–16.
71. Bordeau A, Manganella G, Thil-Trubert CL, Cournot G. Bioactive parathyroid hormone in pregnant rats and fetuses. Am J Physiol. 1990;258:E549–54.
72. Quan-Sheng D, Miller SC. Calciotrophic hormone levels and calcium absorption during pregnancy in rats. Am J Phys. 1989;257:E118–23.
73. Marie PJ, Cancela L, Le Boulch N, Miravet L. Bone changes due to pregnancy and lactation: influence of vitamin D status. Am J Phys. 1986;251:E400–6.
74. Diaz de Barboza G, Guizzardi S, Tolosa de Talamoni N. Molecular aspects of intestinal calcium absorption. World J Gastroenterol. 2015;21:7142–54.
75. Christakos S. Mechanism of action of 1,25-dihydroxyvitamin D3 on intestinal calcium absorption. Rev Endocr Metab Disord. 2012;13:39–44.
76. Olmos-Ortiz A, Avila E, Durand-Carbajal M, Díaz L. Regulation of calcitriol biosynthesis and activity: focus on gestational vitamin D deficiency and adverse pregnancy outcomes. Nutrients. 2015;7:443–80.

77. Kirby BJ, Ma Y, Martin HM, et al. Upregulation of calcitriol during pregnancy and skeletal recovery after lactation do not require parathyroid hormone: PTH during pregnancy and lactation. J Bone Miner Res. 2013;28:1987–2000.
78. Ardawi MS, Nasrat HA, BA'Aqueel HS. Calcium-regulating hormones and parathyroid hormone-related peptide in normal human pregnancy and postpartum: a longitudinal study. Eur J Endocrinol. 1997;137:402–9.
79. Møller UK, Streym S, Mosekilde L, et al. Changes in calcitropic hormones, bone markers and insulin-like growth factor I (IGF-I) during pregnancy and postpartum: a controlled cohort study. Osteoporos Int. 2013;24:1307–20.
80. O'Leary P, Boyne P, Flett P, et al. Longitudinal assessment of changes in reproductive hormones during normal pregnancy. Clin Chem. 1991;37:667–72.
81. Kirby BJ, Ardeshirpour L, Woodrow JP, et al. Skeletal recovery after weaning does not require PTHrP. J Bone Miner Res. 2011;26:1242–51.
82. Ardeshirpour L, Dann P, Adams DJ, et al. Weaning triggers a decrease in receptor activator of nuclear factor-kappaB ligand expression, widespread osteoclast apoptosis, and rapid recovery of bone mass after lactation in mice. Endocrinology. 2007;148:3875–86.
83. VanHouten JN, Wysolmerski JJ. Low estrogen and high parathyroid hormone-related peptide levels contribute to accelerated bone resorption and bone loss in lactating mice. Endocrinology. 2003;144:5521–9.
84. Fudge NJ, Kovacs CS. Pregnancy up-regulates intestinal calcium absorption and skeletal mineralization independently of the vitamin D receptor. Endocrinology. 2010;151:886–95.
85. Comar CL. Radiocalcium studies in pregnancy. Ann N Y Acad Sci. 1956;64:281–98.
86. VanHouten JN, Dann P, Stewart AF, et al. Mammary-specific deletion of parathyroid hormone-related protein preserves bone mass during lactation. J Clin Invest. 2003;112: 1429–36.
87. Ardeshirpour L, Brian S, Dann P, et al. Increased PTHrP and decreased estrogens alter bone turnover but do not reproduce the full effects of lactation on the skeleton. Endocrinology. 2010;151:5591–601.
88. Sowers M. Pregnancy and lactation as risk factors for subsequent bone loss and osteoporosis. J Bone Miner Res. 1996;11:1052–60.
89. Kovacs CS, Kronenberg HM. Maternal-fetal calcium and bone metabolism during pregnancy, puerperium, and lactation. Endocr Rev. 1997;18:832–72.
90. Møller UK, Við Streym S, Mosekilde L, Rejnmark L. Changes in bone mineral density and body composition during pregnancy and postpartum. A controlled cohort study. Osteoporos Int. 2012;23:1213–23.
91. Gillies BR, Ryan BA, Tonkin BA, et al. Absence of calcitriol causes increased lactational bone loss and lower milk calcium but does not impair post-lactation bone recovery in Cyp27b1 null mice. J Bone Miner Res. 2018;33:16–26.
92. Gonen E, Sahin I, Ozbek M, et al. Effects of pregnancy and lactation on bone mineral density, and their relation to the serum calcium, phosphorus, calcitonin and parathyroid hormone levels in rats. J Endocrinol Investig. 2005;28:322–6.
93. Zeni SN, Di Gregorio S, Mautalen C. Bone mass changes during pregnancy and lactation in the rat. Bone. 1999;25:681–5.
94. Nishiwaki M, Yasumizu T, Hoshi K, Ushijima H. Effect of pregnancy, lactation and weaning on bone mineral density in rats as determined by dual-energy X-ray absorptiometry. Endocr J. 1999;46:711–6.
95. Wysolmerski JJ. Osteocytes remove and replace perilacunar mineral during reproductive cycles. Bone. 2013;54:230–6.
96. Qing H, Ardeshirpour L, Pajevic PD, et al. Demonstration of osteocytic perilacunar/canalicular remodeling in mice during lactation. J Bone Miner Res. 2012;27:1018–29.
97. Kaya S, Basta-Pljakic J, Seref-Ferlengez Z, et al. Lactation-induced changes in the volume of osteocytc lacunar-canalicular space alter mechanical properties in cortical bone tissue. J Bone Miner Res. 2017;32:688–97.

98. Finkelstein JS, Lee H, Karlamangla A, et al. Antimullerian hormone and impending menopause in late reproductive age: the study of women's health across the nation. J Clin Endocrinol Metab. 2020;105:e1862–71.
99. Greendale GA, Sowers M, Han W, et al. Bone mineral density loss in relation to the final menstrual period in a multiethnic cohort: results from the study of women's health across the nation (SWAN). J Bone Miner Res. 2012;27:111–8.
100. Finkelstein JS, Brockwell SE, Mehta V, et al. Bone mineral density changes during the menopause transition in a multiethnic cohort of women. J Clin Endocrinol Metab. 2008;93:861–8.
101. Harlow SD, Burnett-Bowie S-AM, Greendale GA, et al. Disparities in reproductive aging and midlife health between black and white women: the study of women's health across the nation (SWAN). Womens Midlife Health. 2022;8:3.
102. Ji M-X, Yu Q. Primary osteoporosis in postmenopausal women. Chronic Dis Transl Med. 2015;1:9–13.
103. Lang TF, Sigurdsson S, Karlsdottir G, et al. Age-related loss of proximal femoral strength in elderly men and women: the age gene/environment susceptibility study–Reykjavik. Bone. 2012;50:743–8.
104. Alswat KA. Gender disparities in osteoporosis. J Clin Med Res. 2017;9:382–7.
105. Nguyen ND, Ahlborg HG, Center JR, et al. Residual lifetime risk of fractures in women and men. J Bone Miner Res. 2007;22:781–8.
106. Karlamangla AS, Burnett-Bowie S-AM, Crandall CJ. Bone health during the menopause transition and beyond. Obstet Gynecol Clin N Am. 2018;45:695–708.
107. Thomas PK, Sullivan LK, Dickinson GH, et al. The effect of helium ion radiation on the material properties of bone. Calcif Tissue Int. 2021;108:808–18.
108. Heveran CM, Schurman CA, Acevedo C, et al. Chronic kidney disease and aging differentially diminish bone material and microarchitecture in C57Bl/6 mice. Bone. 2019;127:91–103.
109. Lau A, Oyen ML, Kent RW, et al. Indentation stiffness of aging human costal cartilage. Acta Biomater. 2008;4:97–103.
110. Mattice JM, Lau AG, Oyen ML, Kent RW. Spherical indentation load-relaxation of soft biological tissues. J Mater Res. 2006;21:2003–10.
111. Oyen ML. Nanoindentation hardness of mineralized tissues. J Biomech. 2006;39:2699–702.

Biomaterial Design to Interrogate Sex-Biased Effects and Deliver Sex Hormones for Therapeutic Treatments in Orthopedic Tissues

Jennifer L. Robinson

Abstract While the musculoskeletal system is not typically the first considered in the context of sex-biased biology, emerging evidence shows that it exhibits profound sex-based differences in both structure and function. This chapter explores these differences in orthopedic tissues, with a focus on how biomaterial systems can be used to interrogate cellular mechanisms and deliver sex hormones in a spatially and temporally controlled manner to promote regeneration and homeostasis. Further, these biomaterials can be used to determine how structural and mechanical cues from the tissue microenvironment drive cell behavior and can be capitalized on for applications in cell migration and regeneration, considering sex as a biological variable for more personalized regenerative engineering strategies. While advancements have been made in biomaterial design for hormone release and sex-specific regeneration, there are several limitations that still exist to ensure scientific conclusions are sound and biomaterial devices are rigorous and reproducible. The main caveats are complexities with sex hormones in cell culture media confounding the impact of hormone dosing in controlled studies, the wide variance in hormone levels from person to person and daily/month/yearly within a single person, and adequately powered study designs to confidently contribute differences to biological sex and not donor variability. The goal is to highlight opportunities in biomaterial design that support discovery and therapeutic innovation for sex-informed approaches after injury and to promote lifetime musculoskeletal health.

Keywords Sex differences · Orthopedic tissues · Sex steroid hormones · Estrogen (17β-estradiol, E2) · Testosterone · Progesterone · Tissue remodeling · Biomaterials · Controlled hormone release · Selective estrogen receptor modulators (SERMs) · Tissue-specific hormone production · Sex hormone bioavailability · Sex-informed biomaterial design

J. L. Robinson (✉)
Department of Orthopaedic Surgery and Sports Medicine, Department of Mechanical Engineering, University of Washington, Seattle, WA, USA
e-mail: jrobins1@uw.edu

S. G. Zambuto, M. L. Oyen (eds.), *Biomaterials for Women's Health Engineering*,
https://doi.org/10.1007/978-3-032-10745-9_16

1 Anatomical and Physiological Sex Differences in Orthopedic Tissues

Biological sex innately impacts anatomical size, shape, and features of orthopedic tissues (Fig. 1). Herein, bone, adipose, muscle, and fibrous connective tissues (tendon, ligament, cartilage, and fibrocartilage) will be featured. Male and female bone differ in anatomical shape and size [1] (Fig. 1a). Cortical and cancellous bone tissues across skeletal regions—particularly in long bones such as the femur—exhibit different remodeling responses influenced by hormonal signaling, mechanical loading, and site-specific properties (e.g., diaphysis vs. epiphysis). Specifically, estrogen plays a crucial role in load-induced remodeling and maintenance of bone mass, a process essential in both males and females. Further, female sex is a major risk factor for compromised bone repair during fracture healing [6, 7] and decreased osseointegration of implants [8]. Lastly, postmenopausal women experience osteoporosis significantly more than age-matched men, suggesting the influence of estrogen in bone remodeling and subsequent strength [9, 10].

While bone has arguably been the most widely studied of the orthopedic tissues, sex-based differences have been shown in nearly all tissues assessed. Adipose or fat tissue displays sex-biased characteristics, particularly in the type and location. Females store more subcutaneous fat, particularly around the hips and thighs, termed gluteofemoral fat (Fig. 1b)—regions associated with metabolic reserves required during energetically demanding periods such as pregnancy and lactation that provide necessary nutrients such as specific fatty acids for fetal brain and eye development

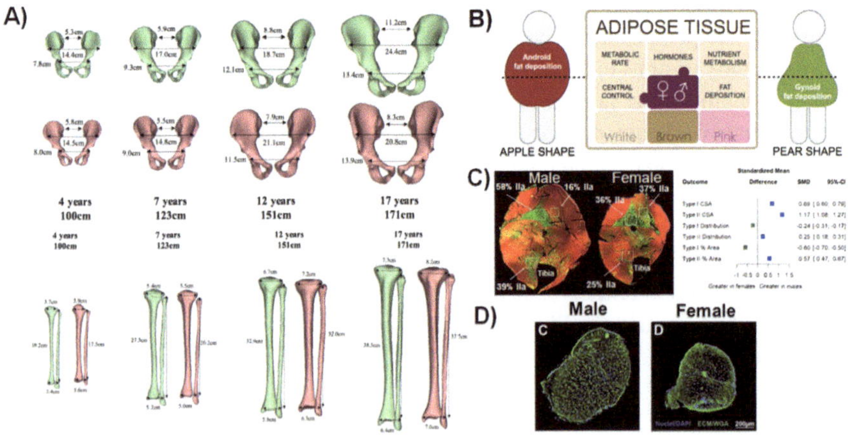

Fig. 1 Anatomical sex differences in male and female orthopedic tissue. (**a**) Bone size significantly differs comparing male and female structures. (Reprint from Carman et al. [1]). (**b**) Male and female fat type and distribution differs. (Reprint from Valencak et al. [2]). (**c**) The distribution of muscle type I and II differs. (Reprint from Haizlip et al. [3]; James et al. [4]). (**d**) Cross-sectional area differs in male and female tendons. (Reprint from Sarver et al. [5])

[11]. This sexually dimorphic fat distribution supports different metabolic strategies and may also influence biomechanical loading and tissue regeneration in orthopedic contexts. Additionally, sex differences have been observed in comparing the lipid-storing, endocrine-signaling, metabolically active anti-inflammatory white fat (WAT) vs. heat-generating brown fat (BAT) [12]. Females have more WAT compared to males, resulting in poorer metabolic and anti-inflammatory signaling in males. These sex-based discrepancies are reduced during and after menopause, suggesting a role of sex hormones [13].

Sex differences in muscle exist specifically in the composition of muscle fiber types and function and regeneration potential. In general, males have greater muscle mass and strength and greater aerobic capacity, whereas females exhibit less muscle fatigability and faster recovery during endurance exercise [14]. Women typically have a higher proportion of slow-twitch (Type I) fibers relative to fast-twitch (Type II) fibers [14], with larger Type I fibers in females and larger Type II fibers in males [15, 16], resulting in enhanced endurance performance (Fig. 1c). This biological advantage aligns with evolutionary demands and is supported by sex hormone signaling pathways that regulate muscle metabolism and fatigue resistance. Further, evaluation of rotator cuff muscles with age and across sexes revealed increased fatty infiltration in females [17]. At the cell level, female muscle-derived stem cells (MDSCs) exhibited higher regeneration efficiency of skeletal muscle in a diseased dystrophic mdx mouse model, suggesting this is partly due to sex-biased effects with MDSC response to oxidative stress [18].

Fibrous connective tissues, including ligaments, tendons, articular cartilage, and fibrocartilage, are likewise impacted by sex. While there are not many studies investigating anatomical or physiological differences in male and female connective tissue, it has been shown that male murine plantar-flexor tendons have a larger diameter than females [2] (Fig. 1d), sex differences occur in Achilles tendon mechanical properties with age [19], and male bovine articular cartilage exhibit more crosslinked tissue and consequential higher compressive modulus compared to female tissue [20]. Research has shown that hormonal fluctuations influence the mechanical properties and extracellular matrix (ECM) organization of these tissues. For instance, anterior cruciate ligament (ACL) injuries are more prevalent in females [21, 22], with worst outcomes after reconstructive surgery. Evidence suggests that hormonal modulation of ligament cell biology [23], anatomy, and neuromuscular and muscle composition differences [24] all contribute to this disparity. At the stem cell level, young (3-week-old) male and female murine MDSCs were assessed for chondrogenic differentiation potential and articular cartilage regeneration in rat femoral full thickness defect [25]. Male MDSCs produced larger pellets with ECM indicative of cartilage (e.g., rich in glycosaminoglycans) and contributed to more complete articular cartilage regeneration compared to female MDSCs. Similar findings were shown in human MDSCs with male cells resulting in more chondrogenic and osteogenic potential with both young and old skeletal muscle tissue donors [26]. Recent studies, including work on fibrocartilage, have begun to uncover sex-based variations in cell behavior and tissue remodeling potential, further supporting the need for sex-informed strategies in biomaterials research.

2 Sex Hormone Influences on Orthopedic Tissue Properties and Remodeling Capacity

Sex steroid hormone impact on the soft tissues of the musculoskeletal system is critical during development and homeostasis in both biological males and females [27]. Most of what we understand comes from gonadectomized mouse models—with removal of ovaries in the female and testes in the male mice. In general, removal of these major hormone-producing tissues results in catabolic effects with orthopedic tissue degradation and reduced growth. Sex hormones impact orthopedic cell processes including proliferation, metabolism, differentiation capacity, senescence, and matrix remodeling and repair [28]. In general, concentrations of E2 comparable to right before ovulation in the female body menstrual cycle results in increased proliferation, reduced senescence, and increased differentiation capacity for adult stem cells including ASCs, MSCs, and tissue-specific progenitors [28]. There are many excellent review articles that articulate these influences in more detail [28–30].

The sex hormones of interest in this chapter, including progesterone (P4), testosterone, and 17β-estradiol (E2), are all derived from cholesterol. Cholesterol is a master precursor to three main classes of molecules: mineralocorticoids (i.e., aldosterone, corticosterone), glucocorticoids (i.e., cortisol), and sex steroid hormones. Of particular importance are the connections of P4, testosterone, and E2. P4, through multiple biochemical reactions, is converted to testosterone, which can then be cleaved via aromatase to generate E2, which is a precursor to other isoforms of estrogen detailed below. In young, healthy adults, these reactions occur primarily in the ovaries in biological females and testes in biological males. However, there is also local tissue production of these sex hormones including from the adrenal glands, adipose tissue, and placenta (during pregnancy), and this tissue-specific production becomes more predominant with aging and menopause. Additional details of the biochemical reactions that result in hormones of interest are discussed below.

2.1 *Estrogen*

There are four main isoforms of estrogen in the human body: estrone (E1), 17-β-estradiol (E2), estriol (E3), and estetrol (E4) (Fig. 2a). Both males and females produce E1–3 but males produce them at much lower concentrations (Fig. 2b) [43]. E1 is synthesized from androstenedione by aromatase (CYP19A1) in both females and males and is the predominant estrogen produced in postmenopausal women. E2 is the most widely studied isoform as it is the most abundant in premenopausal women; therefore, it will be the main isoform discussed in this chapter. E2 is synthesized from E1 by the enzyme HSD17B1, which occurs primarily in the ovaries of premenopausal women and testes in men [44]. It can also be synthesized from testosterone by aromatase (CYP19). Similar to E1 production,

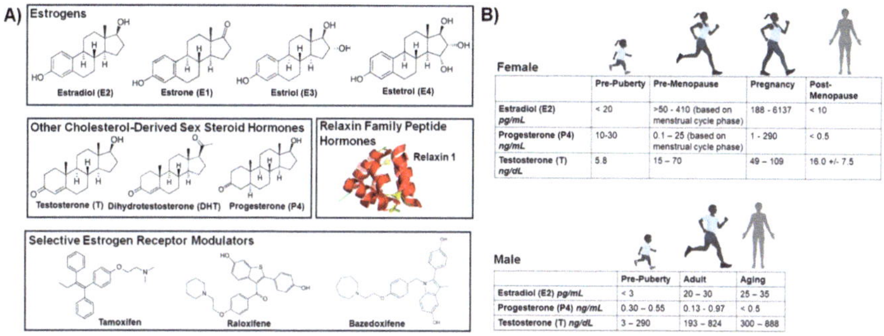

Fig. 2 Sex steroid hormones, peptide hormones, and receptor modulators in the male and female system throughout life stages. (**a**) Chemical structure of estrogens and other sex steroid hormones, peptide hormones, and selective estrogen receptor modulators. (**b**) Total serum levels, not bioavailable levels, of E2, P4, and T at life stages in male and female bodies. (References for E2 [31–36], P4 [37–39], and T [35, 40–42] values)

these reactions occur primarily in ovaries and testes, but also in adipose, muscle, brain, liver, breast, skin, endothelium, bone, and gastric parietal cells [27, 45, 46]. To reach nonreproductive tissues via the bloodstream, E2 must avoid becoming metabolized at the site of production. As such, most of the E2-based effects on nonreproductive tissues are based on local production typically via enzymatic activity [34].

Estriol (E3) is derived mainly as a metabolite from the hydroxylation of E2 and E1. Large amounts are produced by the placenta during pregnancy. Although it has been historically considered as the least potent form of estrogen, the impacts of E3 on epigenetic regulation [47] and immunomodulation [48, 49] are starting to emerge. Estetrol (E4) is produced exclusively by the human fetal liver during pregnancy [50, 51] and circulates through both the maternal and fetal bloodstream. Because of tissue-specific activity and reduced off-target effects, E4 is of interest for estrogen therapies.

2.2 *Testosterone*

Testosterone (T) (Fig. 2a) is primarily produced in the gonads with smaller amounts synthesized in the adrenal cortex and skin [44, 52–54]. Overall, testosterone is roughly 5–20 times higher in concentration in males compared to females [55, 56] (Fig. 2b). Like estrogens, testosterone can be locally produced through enzymatic activity and this is known to occur in brain and adipose tissues [57–60]. Testosterone levels are highest during early adulthood and decline with age in both males and females. Testosterone can be metabolized to dihydrotestosterone (DHT) by the enzyme 5-alpha-reductase mostly in the liver, but also in the skin. Progesterone is another source of both DHT and T. DHT can be even more potent than testosterone and is the only androgen that cannot be converted to E2.

2.3 Progesterone

Progesterone (P4) (Fig. 2) is primarily produced in the ovaries after ovulation, by the placenta during pregnancy, and from the adrenal glands in men and women in lower concentrations. Progesterone metabolites, including 5α-dihydroprogesterone and 20α-dihydroprogesterone, do have important functions including regulation of the menstrual cycle. Each of these cholesterol-derived hormones have different routes of metabolism depending on concentration of precursor hormones and enzymes that determine the molecular mechanism of action. P4 is synthesized from pregnenolone (P5) by CYP11A1 in the cytoplasm and endoplasmic reticulum. Through a series of biochemical reactions, P4 can then be further converted into testosterone. Alternatively, P5 can be used by a different enzyme, CYP17A1, to produce 17-α-hydroxypregnenolone and dehydroepiandrosterone (DHEA), and then to androstenedione.

In general, sex hormones including estrogen, testosterone, and progesterone impact cell cycle processes including proliferation and metabolism, cell phenotype, and differentiation [28, 61]. Also, these hormones impact tissue remodeling [28], tissue mechanical properties and resistance to strain, and homeostasis. Because most of the research has been on estrogen signaling and its impacts, that is the focus in this chapter. Estrogen signals through two predominant pathways including the canonical, genomic pathway, and rapid signaling through receptors at the plasma membrane [29]. Selective estrogen receptor modulators (SERMs) are small molecules that specifically interact with estrogen receptors as agonists or antagonists and promote specific activity of the receptors. The chemical structure of common selective estrogen receptor modulators (SERMs) is shown in Fig. 2.

2.4 Bioavailability

Many factors contribute to the bioavailability of sex steroid hormones. In general, serum half-lives of freely available hormones range from single minutes to multiple hours and can be significantly altered with enzymatic activity, illustrating the dynamic nature of hormone concentration. E2 has a half-life of 2–4 h in the circulation [62, 63], but most of it is metabolized in the liver or converted to estrone rapidly, decreasing availability in the rest of the body. Estriol and estrone have half-lives of 10–30 min [64, 65] and 30–70 min [66, 67], respectively. Of relevance to in vitro, mechanistic studies, E2, P4, and T are lipophilic compounds that can adsorb to lab-relevant glass, plastics, and tissue culture vessels. The use of low-adsorption materials and serum have been shown effective in reducing this adsorption and ensuring adequate availability for cell culture experiments [68].

Testosterone, dihydrotestosterone, and E2 circulate in the bloodstream bound to albumin and sex hormone-binding globulin (SHBG) [69, 70], with only a small fraction unbound and biologically active [71, 72]. SHBG levels vary according to many factors including physical activity, obesity, and hormone levels [73, 74] and bioavailability can be inferred from SHBG levels [69, 73, 74]. SHBG levels are about twice as high in women as in men, a mechanism to reduce and limit exposure to androgens and estrogens.

The levels of steroid hormones in the synovial fluid where many connective musculoskeletal tissues reside are thought to be correlated to the blood concentration, but there is limited human data determining the hormone concentration at any given time within a musculoskeletal tissue. Interestingly, LC-MS results from male and female synovial fluid have illustrated sex differences in metabolites such as cervonyl carnitine, highlighting the possibility of obtaining sex steroid hormone levels from similar samples [75]. Given the production of hormones from adipose tissue, it is also possible that hormone levels vary in synovial joints with nearby fat pads and bursa. Further, macromolecule transport through the synovium and into the intra-articular space of joints is less studied relative to transport to and through other tissue and organ compartments [76–79], suggesting significant differences in steroid hormone levels dependent on the transport kinetics.

Regardless of the exposure, there are also likely tissue-specific differences in steroid processing and/or metabolism that impact concentrations within the tissue proper. For example, E2 has been found to be loosely bound in the uterus and vagina for several hours after administration, whereas the metabolism to water-soluble derivatives happens quickly in the liver [80]. In addition, the presence of hormone precursors in different tissues has been reported, suggesting a potential for tissue-specific hormone production. Aromatase, the enzyme that converts androgens into estrogens has been found in many tissues including fat, brain, and bone [32] and shown to be produced by immune cells including macrophages [81] and B and T lymphocytes [82, 83] in response to microenvironmental changes. The knowledge of transport and resulting bioavailability is critical for biomaterial design to recapitulate the relative native concentrations in vitro to understand the impact of concentration, chemistry, and timing on cell and tissue response.

2.5 Goals for Biomaterial Design

To engineer biomaterials for controlled release of hormones, a target concentration as a function of time is required. While this is still unknown for many tissues in the human system, recent work has focused on distilling this information for multiple tissues in the mouse during phases of the estrous cycle [84]. Mice were assessed for stage of estrous cycle using vaginal cytology and then they were sacrificed in each distinct phase of the cycle (proestrus, estrus, diestrus—analogous to the follicular phase, ovulation, and luteal phase of the human menstrual cycle, respectively) and after ovariectomy (OVX) as a control. At this point, 16 different tissues were prepared for high-performance liquid chromatography-mass spectroscopy (HPLC-MS), and relative concentrations of 17β-estradiol (E2), testosterone, androstenedione, and progesterone were assessed. Overall, hormone distribution in tissues differed during each phase of the estrous cycle with most tissues having maximum concentrations of E2, testosterone, and androstenedione during the proestrus cycle and most tissues having the highest progesterone in estrus and diestrus. Also, hormone concentrations differed significantly when comparing tissues. Further, cell and tissue sensitivity to varying E2 levels differs based on cell and tissue type and the signaling mechanisms and displays a hermetic response [85]. These results highlight the significant differences in hormone concentrations across tissues and the dynamic, cyclic nature of the levels—all of which must be considered in biomaterial design.

3 Biomaterial Applications: Hormone Delivery

Polymeric-based biomaterials with tunable chemical and physical properties are advantageous for controlled and localized hormone delivery. Table 1 highlights biomaterial approaches for controlled hormone release for orthopedic tissue applications. Early and translational work on sustained release of sex steroid hormones focused on using biomaterials as drug depots with controlled delivery capabilities for long-term contraceptive release. In general, these implantable devices release hormones over the course of 3–5 years, providing critical design information for controlled, localized release to specific cells and tissues [94]. Further, drug delivery devices have been formulated for hormone replacement therapy with the same goal of long-term release [95].

Studies in the early 2000s were the first to look at encapsulation and release of E2 for applications outside of contraception using nano- and microparticles to increase biological transport and tune the release rate and/or porous scaffolds to support cell and tissue ingrowth and health. Birnbaum et al. investigated the impact of E2 solubility in dichloromethane (DCM), 9:1 DCM:methanol, and ethyl acetate and encapsulated in PLGA microparticles. From this study, it was determined that solvated E2 released slower and at a more controlled rate compared to solid E2, with total release over 40–50 days [96]. The impact of E2 solubility on release rate and profile was further investigated using Carbopol/surfactant dispersions and the chemistry of the surfactant in the dispersion and whether surfactant was in the release reservoir media was shown to significantly delay E2 release [97]. Cyclodextrin hydrogels with high affinity for E2 were fabricated and controlled release for up to 1 week based on cyclodextrin chemistry [98].

Regarding the release of sex steroid hormones for tissue remodeling and regeneration in the musculoskeletal systems, majority of studies have focused on E2 for osteogenesis and bone regeneration—primarily to reduce osteoporosis. Hong et al. fabricated E2-encapsulated PLGA microparticles with cationic poly(amidoamine) dendrimers (PAMAP) for increased cellular uptake and investigated the impact of intracellular E2 release from human bone marrow-derived mesenchymal stromal cells (hMSCs) [87]. E2 release occurred over 7 days with ~55% in the first 24 h, and E2 increased osteogenesis based on increased mRNA transcript levels of alkaline

Table 1 Biomaterial applications: hormone delivery for orthopedic applications

Biomaterial system	Cell type, biological sex	Tissue	Species	Hormone, concentration	Study
Mesoporous silica nanoparticles embedded in gelatin/chitosan multilayers, coated on titanium films	Osteoblasts (calvaria), sex not disclosed	NA	Rat	E2, 50 μM	Hu et al. [86]
PLGA microparticles with surface modification of cationic polyamidoamine dendrimers for cell uptake	Bone marrow mesenchymal stromal cells (MSCs), sex not disclosed	NA	Human	E2, 10 mg/ 200 mg PLGA	Hong et al. [87]
PLGA nanoparticles (NPs) in chitosan–hydroxyapatite foams	Adipose-derived stem cells (ASCs), male	NA	Rat	E2, 0.1 mg/ 2 mg NPs	Irmak et al. [88]
PLGA nanoparticles in chitosan–hydroxyapatite foam	ASCs, sex not disclosed	Calvarial critical size bone defect	Rat, sex not disclosed	E2, 10%, w/w to PLGA	Calis et al. [89]
Nanodiamonds in chitosan hydrogel	NA	Palatal expansion, bone remodeling for cleft palette	Rat, female	E2, 2 mg	Hong et al. [90]
PLGA (BMP-2) and PLA (E2) microspheres in Pluronic F127/ Tetrone 1307 and alpha-cyclodextrin supramolecular gel	NA	OVX-induced "osteoporosis," calvarial critical size bone defect	Rat, female	E2, 4 mg/ 200 mg PLA	Segredo-Morales et al. [91]
PCL/silk fibroin electrospun fibers	MC3T3-E1 preosteoblasts, male RAW 264.7 primed to osteoclasts, male	NA	Mouse	E2, 0.1%, 1%, 5%	Steffi et al. [92]
Mesoporous bioactive glass NPs modified with β-cyclodextrin in silk fibroin electrospun fibers	MC3T3-E1 preosteoblasts, male RAW 264.7 primed to osteoclasts, male	NA	Mouse	E2, 50 μg/ mL (25% EtOH) in 40 mg NPs	Wang et al. [93]

phosphatase (ALP) and core binding factor alpha (Cbfa-1) compared to osteogenic differentiation media. Hu et al. fabricated polyelectrolyte layers of chitosan and gelatin with E2-loaded mesoporous nanoparticles embedded within that was then functionalized on the surface of titanium implants to facilitate osseointegration [86]. Wang et al. encapsulated E2 in β-cyclodextrin-modified mesoporous bioactive glass nanoparticles and then included in silk electrospun fibers and showed delayed release compared to E2 directly encapsulated in silk fibers [93]. E2 released from the nanoparticles in silk fibers reduced osteoclast activity of RAW 264.7 cells and resulted in comparable MC3T3-E1 preosteoblast activity compared to the nanoparticle fiber control group without E2 released. Similarly, Steffi et al. fabricated PCL/silk fibroin electrospun fibers encapsulating E2 at different concentrations and observed delayed release over 3 weeks based on the E2 concentration [92]. While MC3T3-E1 preosteoblast activity outcomes including ALP and collagen levels did not differ in E2-loaded fibers compared to control fibers, TRAP activity of RAW 264.7 cells decreased in a concentration-dependent manner with E2-loaded fibers. E2-loaded PLGA microspheres (65:35) were loaded onto chitosan–hydroxyapatite foams either during or after the foaming process with delayed release occurring if incorporated during foaming [88]. While there was an increase in osteocalcin, a marker of osteoblast maturity, at Day 7 in the E2-loaded groups, all other assessments did not show an impact of E2 on osteogenesis compared to blank scaffolds. Unfortunately, in all these studies, the biological sex of the cells was not disclosed and there were no comparisons between sex of the cells, limiting our understanding of the impact of tunable release kinetics of sex hormones, namely E2, on cell behavior in males and females, respectively.

Similar biomaterial-based models have been investigated for osteogenic impact in preclinical models. Calis et al. fabricated E2-loaded chitosan–hydroxyapatite scaffolds that were implanted in a critical-size calvarial defect model in Sprague-Dawley rats (sex not reported) with the inclusion of adipose-derived stromal cells (ASCs) [89]. Increased mineralized matrix formation was observed after 12 weeks in the scaffold with E2 and ASCs compared to the scaffold with only E2 or ASCs. The impact of E2 on osteoporotic bone remodeling was assessed with a cranial defect model in ovariectomized Sprague-Dawley female rates. In situ forming Pluronic F127–Tetrone 1307 and α-cyclodextrin supramolecular hydrogels were synthesized with BMP-2 and E2 encapsulated in PLGA or PLA microspheres, respectively [91]. The burst release of BMP-2 and E2 was reduced by encapsulation in the microspheres. Bone formation in the osteoporotic models, as assessed by histomorphometry and collagen staining, was increased in the groups with BMP-2 and E2 compared to BMP-2 alone. Nanodiamond-E2 nanoparticles embedded in methacrylated glycol chitosan hydrogels were employed to promote bone remodeling during maxillary expansion techniques for patients with cleft lip and/or palate [90]. Female Sprague-Dawley rats underwent an expansion procedure and gels with E2/ND were injected and compared to ND without E2. Overall, a reduction in relapse was observed in the E2/ND groups with an increase in osteoblast number, bone mineral density, and bone volume. While localized, controlled release of E2 using biomaterial systems has not been investigated in soft orthopedic tissues including muscle and connective tissues, there is convincing evidence that E2 concentration and timing significantly impacts these tissues [23, 99, 100].

Other systems have been tested for applications in gynecological tissues, breast, epidermis, pelvic floor, and the central nervous system. Of immense interest, pro-drugs can be fabricated using polymer engineering and released at precise time points for years [101]. Specifically, a novel poly(pro-E2) chemistry, a polymerized pro-drug, was electrospun into nanofibers and exhibited nanomolar E2 release over the course of 1–10 years in vitro. These materials promoted and guided neurite extension ex vivo and reduced oxidative stress in vitro. This approach highlights the ability for engineered biomaterials to promote reduced inflammation and enhanced regeneration for years, an exciting possibility moving forward in orthopedic tissues. Maghraby et al. synthesized deformable liposomes encapsulating E2 for skin delivery by investigating the impact of formulations of cholesterol, soybean PC, and/or DPPC lipids with surfactants in some of the formulations on delivery efficacy [102]. Lastly, multiple examples from the MacNeil research group have illustrated the importance of controlled E2 release from electrospun fibers and hydrogels on pelvic floor and urogenital reconstruction [103–105]. In general, E2 release increased extracellular matrix production of human ASCs and angiogenesis and new blood vessel formation when released from polyester-based nanofibers. Further, using GelMA/MeHA hydrogels that released E2 over the course of 21 days for applications in soft tissue interposition for urogenital reconstruction, E2 hydrogels resulted in more collagen production from human dermal fibroblasts (HDFs) and enhanced blood vessel ingrowth in a chicken embryo chorioallantoic membrane (CAM) assay [103]. Applying these technologies to orthopedic applications holds great promise for cell-specific targeting of hormone release at desired concentrations without negative side effects.

Further, biomaterials can be used to locally deliver selective estrogen receptor modulators (SERMs), with predominant focus on targeting and killing ER+ breast cancer cells. Much like the small molecule sex hormones, SERMs exhibit poor water solubility and bioavailability [106]. As such, biomaterial systems must be designed to encapsulate these hydrophobic compounds and maintain their structure for localized release to be advantageous as carriers and drug delivery vehicles. To encapsulate the hydrophobic, small molecule SERMs and maintain their bioavailability for the site of delivery, polymer and solvent interactions are heavily considered for nanoparticle synthesis. A series of novel, biodegradable poly(ethylene succinate-*co*-propylene adipate) (P(ESu-*co*-Pad)) polyesters were synthesized and clear candidates were used to encapsulate raloxifene into nanoparticles using a polycondensation method [107]. Raloxifene was shown to have minimal interaction with the polymer/solvent phases, maintain a crystalline morphology, and release with an initial burst followed by linear release that was tuned by the copolymer ratio. Further, mesoporous silica nanoparticles with pH-responsive chitosan tethers were synthesized for the release of raloxifene [108]. The cumulative release of raloxifene from the nanoparticles was reduced from ~80% after 60 h in pH 5.6 to ~50% after 60 h in pH of 7.4 and this tunability was shown to be important for viability of MCF-7 breast cancer cells [108]. Tamoxifen, one of the most widely used SERMs, is most commonly used for breast cancer prevention [109, 110]. Interestingly, this small molecule acts as a nonspecific estrogen receptor antagonist is breast tissue but as an agonist in other tissues including bone [111]. Further, tamoxifen's activity is dependent on ovarian status; tamoxifen reduces estrogen-deficient bone loss in ovariectomized rats but contributes to bone loss in ovary intact rats [111]. Pinzón-García et al. developed electrospun PCL nanofibers for the release of tamoxifen citrate, showing total release after 14 h and cytotoxic effects to MCF-7 breast tumor cells [112]. Fan et al. fabricated tamoxifen-containing polysaccharide-based nanoparticle prodrug conjugates with a reactive oxygen species (ROS)-sensitive linker for release after uptake in cancer cells that on average have ~10X ROS compared to other cell types [113]. These nanoparticles (NPs) resulted in targeted cytotoxicity in MCF-7 breast cancer cells but did not induce hepatotoxicity in liver organoid models, at low E2 concentrations.

The release of SERMs for orthopedic tissues has also been done. Kavas et al. investigated the impact of tunable concentrations of raloxifene conjugated to PEG and encapsulated in PCL or PCL/PLGA blend microspheres for the potential to promote osteogenesis with ASCs in culture [114]. Overall, tuning the microsphere system to increase the hydrolytic degradation rate of the microspheres and increase the water solubility of the raloxifene allowed for tuning of the cumulative release profile and osteogenic differentiation. Cellulose/cyclodextrin lyophilized foams with raloxifene encapsulated were pursued for bone regeneration [115]. Distinct formulations resulted in controlled release and evidence of proliferation and enhanced ALP activity and calcium ion production, albeit using Saos-2 cells from an 11-year-old female osteosarcoma. A similar approach was taken with raloxifene encapsulated in PLGA microspheres and then embedded in a lyophilized collagen/chitosan/β-tricalcium phosphate scaffold [116]. Raloxifene microspheres embedded in the scaffold exhibited slower release profiles and promoted enhanced calcium deposition and ALP activity from MC3T3-E1 preosteoblast cells. Controlled release of SERMs to rheumatic rat joints was employed to reduce inflammation and reduce negative off-target effects. PCL microspheres with either triamcinolone, raloxifene, or both were employed in a rat adjuvant-induced arthritis model [117]. Due to poor solubility in the PCL, raloxifene was released slowly if encapsulated on its own but more quickly in the dual-loaded groups. The microsphere-loaded triamcinolone and raloxifene resulted in superior lesion scores in the knee joint compared to injections of the compounds alone with the best results in the dual-loaded microsphere group.

4 Biomaterial Applications: Tissue Mimetic Constructs for Mechanistic Studies and Tissue Engineering

Table 2 highlights biomaterial approaches as in vitro systems to determine sex-biased influences on tissue regeneration and for use in tissue engineering strategies. While there has been effort in localized and controllable sex hormone release, investigation of biomaterials as tissue mimetics that model chemical, physical, and mechanical cues to determine sex-biased effects have been minimal.

Modeling native ECM is the major goal of biomaterial systems for in vitro mechanistic studies. Wu et al. sought to determine the optimal denatured ECM scaffold, in comparing male and female porcine articular, tracheal, and auricular cartilage, for cartilage tissue engineering [125]. While this study concluded that there were not significant sex differences in male and female cartilage denaturation properties or response of female human ASCs to either ECM, increased donors are needed to increase power to determine differences across sexes and also investigate the impact of cartilage sources on male ASCs as a direct comparison. This is in light of what has already been discussed in differences in articular cartilage mechanical properties between sexes [20]. Additionally, collagen isolated from male and female porcine and bovine skin and tendon was fabricated into sponges and resulting mechanical properties and impact on human adult dermal fibroblast and THP-1 cell viability and metabolism was assessed [123]. Overall, there were no significant differences in most outcomes except for compressive properties, which were higher in female tissues than male tissues when comparing in the same species and tissue. As can be seen, there are many factors that drive sex differences in ECM properties and incorporating all these factors is difficult to capture in experimental study design.

Majority of the studies using biomaterial platforms to investigate the impact of hormones or innate sex differences on tissue regeneration have been focused on bone—similar to the controlled release of E2. In vitro human osteoblasts from three male and three female donors were cultured on titanium discs with varying surface profiles including smooth, etched, and increased hydrophilicity [121]. Female cells on all titanium surfaces and tissue culture polystyrene (TCPS) controls exhibited increased ALP activity and protein levels of osteocalcin (OCN) and both latent and active TGFβ1, whereas male cells showed increased protein levels of osteoprotegerin (OPG). After cells became confluent on each respective disc formulation, media with 1 nM E2 was added for 24 h. On nearly every condition, E2 treatment increased ALP and protein levels of OCN, OPG, and TGFβ1 with female cells exhibiting higher levels than males across the board, highlighting the importance of biomaterial surface properties on sex-biased response to hormone levels. In a similar study, increases in human osteoblast ALP activity, OCN, TGFβ1, and prostaglandin E2 (PDGE2) were shown to be E2 dose-dependent with increased signal at 100 nM compared to 10 nM and titanium surface roughness having a significant influence [130]. Of note, this was in a single female donor. Male and female rat osteoblasts on the same treated titanium discs exhibited some similarities and some differences compared to the human osteoblast response [118], noting potential differences across species. Ueno et al. were interested in determining whether there were sex-biased effects in biomaterial-mediated femoral bone healing [124]. Gelatin microribbon scaffolds, unmodified or with IL-4 overexpressing MSCs encapsulated, were implanted into male and female Balb/c murine critical size femoral defects and healing assessed via μCT and immunohistochemistry. The only statistically significant difference comparing outcomes in male and female

Table 2 Biomaterial applications: tissue mimetic constructs for mechanistic studies and tissue engineering

Biomaterial system	Cell type, biological sex	Tissue	Species	Hormone, concentration	Study
Titanium discs with surface roughness	Osteoblasts, male and female	NA	Sprague-Dawley rats, male and female	17β-estradiol (1 nM) or 1α,25 (OH)2D3 (10 nM) for 24 h	Olivares-Navarrete et al. [118]
Poly(L-lactide)/poly(-ε-caprolactone) electrospun mesh	Myogenically differentiated adipose-derived stem cells (MD-ASCs); smooth muscle cells from urinary bladder	NA	Sprague-Dawley rats	E2, 10 pM–100 nM	Feng et al. [119]
Nano-hydroxyapatite/collagen/poly(L-lactic acid) scaffold (nHAC/PLA)	Periodontal ligament stem cells (PDLSCs), female	Subcutaneous implantation	Sprague-Dawley rats, female Osteoporotic tissue after 3 months post OVX (cells); SCID mice	E2, 100 nM	Ling-Ling et al. (2016)
Bioactive tricalcium phosphate bone graft	NA	Bone biopsy from grafted maxillary alveolar process and residual native crest	Human, male and female ($n = 60$ each)	NA	Knabe et al. [120]
Titanium discus with surface modulation (surface roughness, hydrophilicity)	Osteoblasts, female ($n = 3$) and male ($n = 3$)	NA	Human	17β-estradiol (1 nM) or 1α,25 (OH)2D3 (10 nM)	Berger et al. [121]
PEG, collagen type 1, and Matrigel hydrogels	MCF-7 breast cancer cell line, female	NA	Human, female	E2, 1 nM for 48 h	Livingston et al. [122]
Collagen sponges	Adult dermal fibroblasts; leukemic monocyte cells (THP-1)	Skin and tendon	Human (cells); bovine and porcine (tissue), male and female	NA	Sorushanova et al. [123]

Gelatin-based microribbon hydrogels	Bone marrow-derived mesenchymal stromal cells, female and male (Balb/c mice)	Femoral critical sized defect	Balb/c mice (cells and bone tissue)	NA	Ueno et al. [124]
Collagen II lyophilized foams	Adipose-derived stem cells (ASCs), female	Articular cartilage, tracheal cartilage, auricular cartilage, male and female	Human (cells); pig (cartilage)	NA	Wu et al. [125]
Collagen type 1 scaffold (bovine)	Meniscal fibrochondrocytes	NA	Human, male and female (four donors each)	NA	Ma et al. [126]
Poly(ethylene) microparticles and titanium rod (mimic wear particles)	Bone marrow-derived mesenchymal stromal cells (MSCs)	Femur (bone)	Balb/c mice, male and female	NA	Shen et al. [127]
Poly(acrylamide) hydrogels	Tenocytes	Flexor tendon	Mice, male and female	NA	El Sherif et al. [128]
Collagen hydroxyapatite with magnesium ions (MaioRegen) and filtered bone marrow aspirate	NA, female ($n = 40$) and male ($n = 50$)	Knee joint surface lesions	Human (clinical trial)	NA	Kolar et al. [129]

mice was enhanced ALP positive area in male mice with MSCs overexpressing IL-4—albeit there was a trend of male mice performing better in most outcomes with the IL-4 overexpression in MSC group. In humans, the impact of biological sex and hormones on craniofacial bone regeneration using tricalcium phosphate (TCP) bone grafting material (CEROS TCP®) after sinus floor augmentation procedures was assessed in 60 males and 60 females [120]. Interestingly, in males, higher E2 levels and higher BMI-enhanced TCP-mediated bone repair effects not observed in females.

Beyond bone, the impact of the biomaterial microenvironment and E2 release impacts other musculoskeletal cells. Periodontal ligament cells from ovariectomized and sham-treated female Sprague-Dawley rats were cultured on nano-hydroxyapatite/collagen/poly(L-lactide) (nHAC/PLA) scaffolds and assessed in vitro and implanted subcutaneously on the back of immunodeficient SCID mice [131]. E2 treatment to OVX cells reduced proliferation and increased mRNA expression of ALP, OCN, Erα, and ERβ in vitro and enhanced bone growth in vivo. Human male and female meniscal cells, isolated from partial meniscectomies, were cultured in collagen type 1 hydrogels with chondrogenic media and subjected to simulated microgravity (SMG) or cyclic hydrostatic pressure (CHP) with static controls to assess the impact of unloading on osteoarthritis (OA) [126]. SMG was shown to induce an OA-like phenotype and CHP-promoted chondrogenesis, with transcriptional differences based on the sex of the cells. Further, sex differences in male and female meniscal cell response to compressive stiffness has been observed, with male cells becoming more spread, fibroblast-like morphology on hyaluronic acid-based hydrogels that mimic the stiffest region of the meniscus and female cells maintaining a chondrocyte-like morphology [132, 133]. Myogenically differentiated adipose stem cells (MD-ASCs) from rat inguinal subcutaneous fat were seeded on E2-encapsulated PLA/PCL electrospun fibers and were investigated for muscle tissue engineering after stress urinary incontinence complications in postmenopausal women [119]. Fibers releasing E2 increased MD-ASC proliferation and myogenic differentiation.

There are recognizable caveats to study design in investigating sex-biased effects in engineered biomaterials. The strikingly obvious one is the lack of knowledge of sex hormone levels in different locations or compartments in the body, as mentioned earlier in the chapter. Unfortunately, most of the data is based on blood serum levels, which does not reflect levels in all tissues, especially those that are relatively avascular.

5 Caveats for Sex-Biased and Hormone-Based Studies

When designing model systems for in vitro and ex vivo studies, limitations will inevitably exist. In the context of understanding sex hormone signaling, the traditional cell culture media, which has been optimized for each cell type to promote cell proliferation and metabolic health, contains hormones or hormone-mimetic compounds that can influence cell behavior [61]. With more studies focused on the impact of biological sex on a particular outcome, specific consideration on rigor and reproducibility must be considered to ensure conclusions are sound. A particular error that occurs in sex differences research, coined the "difference in sex-specific significance" or DISS, whereby differences between biological sexes is determined when statistical significance in a particular outcome is found in one sex but not the other [134]. Best practices and methods for study design and statistical analysis must be followed to ensure true understanding of sex-biased effects [134–136]. Further, the studies discussed in this chapter focused on estrogen and SERMs. However, the impact of dual hormones including progesterone and testosterone is significant and must be further studied.

6 Current Outlook

The past decade has brought increased interest in sex differences and sex hormone influences in nonreproductive tissues and the impact this has on injury, regeneration, and overall health. With that, the use of biomaterial systems to understand these mechanisms with adequate controls has been critical. However, there is much work to do. Bridging disciplines to bring together biomaterial scientists and engineers with polymer chemists, biochemists, cell biologists, endocrinologist, orthopedic surgeons, kinesiologists, physical therapists, and so on is crucial to ensure the biomaterial systems being developed and applications for testing are scientifically and clinically sound. Further, a major point for the future efficacy of this work is the need for all studies to have biological sex reported and to use cells, tissues, and in vivo systems from both XX and XY. As noted in this chapter, a large portion of the previous studies did not disclose sex, only used a single sex, or pooled sexes, all limiting our understanding of sex-biased effects of biomaterial systems and hormone release. Per the NIH SABV policy, pilot studies to investigate whether an outcome exhibits a sex-biased effect are required. If it is determined that sex does not impact the outcome of interest, then samples of both biological sexes can be because the outcome is not dependent on biological sex. If the outcome does depend on biological sex, then further studies are required with adequately powered sample sizes to determine the impact of sex on the outcome. By understanding the physiological functions of sex hormones and the sex-biased impacts of the cell microenvironment, the next decades will bring advances in biomaterial design for tissue engineering, regenerative medicine, and hormone replacement applications.

Acknowledgments The author wishes to thank Aidan Alemifar, Nandita Annamaneni, John Bradford, and Kyley Burkey for reviewing and summarizing the literature used in this chapter.

References

1. Carman L, Besier T, Stott NS, Choisne J. Sex differences in linear bone measurements occur following puberty but do not influence femoral or tibial torsion. Sci Rep. 2023;13:11733.
2. Valencak TG, Osterrieder A, Schulz TJ. Sex matters: The effects of biological sex on adipose tissue biology and energy metabolism. Redox Biol. 2017;12:806–813. https://doi.org/10.1016/j.redox.2017.04.012. Epub 2017 Apr 13. PMID: 28441629; PMCID: PMC5406544
3. Haizlip KM, Harrison BC, Leinwand LA. Sex-based differences in skeletal muscle kinetics and fiber-type composition. Physiology (Bethesda). 2015;30(1):30–9. https://doi.org/10.1152/physiol.00024.2014. PMID: 25559153; PMCID: PMC4285578.
4. James JJ, Mellow ML, Bueckers EP, Gutsch SB, Wrucke DJ, Pearson AG, Smith AE, Hunter SK. Sex differences in human skeletal muscle fiber types and the influence of age, physical activity, and muscle group: A systematic review and meta-analysis. Physiol Rep. 2025;13:e70616.
5. Sarver DC, et al. Sex differences in tendon structure and function. J Orthop Res. 2017;35:2117–26.
6. Parker MJ, Raghavan R, Gurusamy K. Incidence of fracture-healing complications after femoral neck fractures. Clin Orthop Relat Res. 2007;458:175–9.
7. Strube P, et al. Sex-specific compromised bone healing in female rats might be associated with a decrease in mesenchymal stem cell quantity. Bone. 2009;45:1065–72.
8. Pien DM, Olmedo DG, Guglielmotti MB. Influence of age and gender on peri-implant osteogenesis. Age and gender on peri-implant osteogenesis. Acta Odontol Latinoam. 2001;14:9.
9. Ejiri S, et al. Estrogen deficiency and its effect on the jaw bones. J Bone Miner Metab. 2008;26:409–15.
10. Cawthon PM. Gender differences in osteoporosis and fractures. Clin Orthop Relat Res. 2011;469:1900–5.
11. Brenna JT, Lapillonne A. Background paper on fat and fatty acid requirements during pregnancy and lactation. Ann Nutr Metab. 2009;55:97–122.
12. Kaikaew K, Grefhorst A, Visser JA. Sex differences in Brown adipose tissue function: sex hormones, glucocorticoids, and their crosstalk. Front Endocrinol (Lausanne). 2021;12:652444.
13. Bloor ID, Symonds ME. Sexual dimorphism in white and brown adipose tissue with obesity and inflammation. Horm Behav. 2014;66:95–103.
14. Bassett AJ, et al. The biology of sex and sport. JBJS Rev. 2020;8:e0140.
15. Staron RS, et al. Fiber type composition of the vastus lateralis muscle of young men and women. J Histochem Cytochem. 2000;48:623–9.
16. Trevino MA, et al. Sex-related differences in muscle size explained by amplitudes of higher-threshold motor unit action potentials and muscle fibre typing. Acta Physiol. 2019;225:e13151-n/a.
17. Riem L, et al. Objective analysis of partial three-dimensional rotator cuff muscle volume and fat infiltration across ages and sex from clinical MRI scans. Sci Rep. 2023;13:14345.
18. Deasy BM, et al. A role for cell sex in stem cell–mediated skeletal muscle regeneration: female cells have higher muscle regeneration efficiency. J Cell Biol. 2007;177:73–86.
19. Sprague AL, Awokuse D, Pohlig RT, Cortes DH, Grävare Silbernagel K. Relationship between mechanical properties (shear modulus and viscosity), age, and sex in uninjured Achilles tendons. Transl Sports Med. 2020;3:321–7.
20. Hernandez PA, et al. Sexual dimorphism in the extracellular and pericellular matrix of articular cartilage. Cartilage. 2022;13:19476035221121792.
21. The female ACL. Why is it more prone to injury? J Orthop. 2016;13:A1–4.
22. Chidi-Ogbolu N, Baar K. Effect of Estrogen on musculoskeletal performance and injury risk. Front Physiol. 2018;9:1834.

23. Lee CA, et al. Estrogen inhibits lysyl oxidase and decreases mechanical function in engineered ligaments. J Appl Physiol. 2015;118:1250–7.
24. Bruder AM, et al. Let's talk about sex (and gender) after ACL injury: a systematic review and meta-analysis of self-reported activity and knee-related outcomes. Br J Sports Med. 2023;57: 602–10.
25. Matsumoto T, et al. The influence of sex on the chondrogenic potential of muscle-derived stem cells: implications for cartilage regeneration and repair. Arthritis Rheum. 2008;58:3809–19.
26. Scibetta AC, et al. Characterization of the chondrogenic and osteogenic potential of male and female human muscle-derived stem cells: implication for stem cell therapy. J Orthop Res. 2019;37:1339–49.
27. Cooke PS, Nanjappa MK, Ko C, Prins GS, Hess RA. Estrogens in male physiology. Physiol Rev. 2017;97:995–1043.
28. Knewtson KE, Ohl NR, Robinson JL. Estrogen signaling dictates musculoskeletal stem cell behavior: sex differences in tissue repair. Tissue Eng Part B Rev. 2022;28:789–812.
29. Arnal J-F, et al. Membrane and nuclear Estrogen receptor alpha actions: from tissue specificity to medical implications. Physiol Rev. 2017;97:1045–87.
30. Manolagas SC, O'Brien CA, Almeida M. The role of estrogen and androgen receptors in bone health and disease. Nat Rev Endocrinol. 2013;9:699–712.
31. Hall J. Guyton and Hall: textbook of medical physiology. Elsevier; 2011.
32. Simpson ER. Aromatase: biologic relevance of tissue-specific expression. Semin Reprod Med. 2004;22:11–23.
33. Labrie F. Intracrinology. Mol Cell Endocrinol. 1991;78:C113–8.
34. Vrtačnik P, Ostanek B, Mencej-Bedrač S, Marc J. The many faces of estrogen signaling. Biochem Med (Zagreb). 2014;24:329–42.
35. Albin A-K, Norjavaara E. Pubertal growth and serum testosterone and Estradiol levels in boys. Horm Res Paediatr. 2013;80:100–10.
36. Jasuja GK, et al. Age trends in estradiol and estrone levels measured using liquid chromatography tandem mass spectrometry in community-dwelling men of the Framingham heart study. J Gerontol A Biol Sci Med Sci. 2013;68:733–40.
37. Burtis CA, et al. Tietz textbook of clinical chemistry. 3rd ed. Philadelphia: W.B. Saunders; 1999. NLM Catalog – NCBI. https://www.ncbi.nlm.nih.gov/nlmcatalog?cmd=PureSearch&term=9713073%5Bnlmid%5D.
38. Oettel M, Mukhopadhyay A. Progesterone: the forgotten hormone in men? Aging Male. 2004;7:236–57.
39. Lee PA, Migeon CJ. Puberty in boys: correlation of plasma levels of gonadotropins (LH, FSH), androgens (testosterone, androstenedione, dehydroepiandrosterone and its Sulfate), Estrogens (estrone and Estradiol) and progestins (progesterone and 17-hydroxyprogesterone). J Clin Endocrinol Metab. 1975;41:556–62.
40. Mouritsen A, et al. Longitudinal changes in circulating testosterone levels determined by LC-MS/MS and by a commercially available radioimmunoassay in healthy girls and boys during the pubertal transition. Horm Res Paediatr. 2014;82:12–7.
41. Feldman HA, et al. Age trends in the level of serum testosterone and other hormones in middle-aged men: longitudinal results from the Massachusetts male aging study. J Clin Endocrinol Metab. 2002;87:589–98.
42. Laughlin GA, Barrett-Connor E, Kritz-Silverstein D, von Mühlen D. Hysterectomy, oophorectomy, and endogenous sex hormone levels in older women: the rancho Bernardo Study1. J Clin Endocrinol Metab. 2000;85:645–51.
43. Hess RA. Estrogen in the adult male reproductive tract: a review. Reprod Biol Endocrinol. 2003;1:52.
44. Payne AH, Hales DB. Overview of steroidogenic enzymes in the pathway from cholesterol to active steroid hormones. Endocr Rev. 2004;25:947–70.
45. Fuentes N, Silveyra P. Estrogen receptor signaling mechanisms. Adv Protein Chem Struct Biol. 2019;116:135–70.

46. Rochira V, Carani C. Estrogens, male reproduction and beyond. In: Feingold KR, et al., editors. Endotext. South Dartmouth: MDText.com, Inc.; 2000.
47. Zhou Y, et al. The steroid hormone estriol (E3) regulates epigenetic programming of fetal mouse brain and reproductive tract. BMC Biol. 2022;20:93.
48. Lang TJ. Estrogen as an immunomodulator. Clin Immunol. 2004;113:224–30.
49. Ali ES, Mangold C, Peiris AN. Estriol: emerging clinical benefits. Menopause. 2017;24:1081.
50. Holinka CF, Diczfalusy E, Coelingh Bennink HJT. Estetrol: a unique steroid in human pregnancy. J Steroid Biochem Mol Biol. 2008;110:138–43.
51. Stanczyk FZ, Archer DF. Biosynthesis of estetrol in human pregnancy: potential pathways. J Steroid Biochem Mol Biol. 2023;232:106359.
52. Chen W, Thiboutot D, Zouboulis CC. Cutaneous androgen metabolism: basic research and clinical perspectives. J Invest Dermatol. 2002;119:992–1007.
53. Udhane SS, Flück CE. Regulation of human (adrenal) androgen biosynthesis-new insights from novel throughput technology studies. Biochem Pharmacol. 2016;102:20–33.
54. Thiboutot D, Gilliland K, Light J, Lookingbill D. Androgen metabolism in sebaceous glands from subjects with and without acne. Arch Dermatol. 1999;135:1041–5.
55. Vesper HW, Wang Y, Vidal M, Botelho JC, Caudill SP. Serum Total testosterone concentrations in the US household population from the NHANES 2011-2012 study population. Clin Chem. 2015;61:1495–504.
56. Handelsman DJ, Hirschberg AL, Bermon S. Circulating testosterone as the hormonal basis of sex differences in athletic performance. Endocr Rev. 2018;39:803–29.
57. Quinkler M, et al. Androgen generation in adipose tissue in women with simple obesity–a site-specific role for 17beta-hydroxysteroid dehydrogenase type 5. J Endocrinol. 2004;183:331–42.
58. Steckelbroeck S, et al. Characterization of 17beta-hydroxysteroid dehydrogenase activity in brain tissue: testosterone formation in the human temporal lobe. J Neuroendocrinol. 1999;11: 457–64.
59. Jaffe RB. Testosterone metabolism in target tissues. Hypothalamic and pituitary tissues of the adult rat and human fetus, and the immature rat epiphysis. Steroids. 1969;14:483–98.
60. Bélanger C, Luu-The V, Dupont P, Tchernof A. Adipose tissue intracrinology: potential importance of local androgen/estrogen metabolism in the regulation of adiposity. Horm Metab Res. 2002;34:737–45.
61. Bradford JC, Robinson JL. Endogenous estrogen-mimetic compounds in cell culture media influence human mesenchymal stromal cell (hMSC) processes and differentiation in a sex-biased manner. 2025. Preprint at https://doi.org/10.1101/2025.05.27.656455.
62. Ginsburg ES, Gao X, Shea BF, Barbieri RL. Half-life of estradiol in postmenopausal women. Gynecol Obstet Investig. 1998;45:45–8.
63. O'Connell MB. Pharmacokinetic and pharmacologic variation between different estrogen products. J Clin Pharmacol. 1995;35:18S–24S.
64. Voss HF. Saliva as a fluid for measurement of estriol levels. Am J Obstet Gynecol. 1999;180: S226–31.
65. Klopper A, Buchan P, Wilson G. The plasma half-life of placental hormones. Br J Obstet Gynaecol. 1978;85:738–47.
66. Hembree WC, Bardin CW, Lipsett MB. A study of estrogen metabolic clearance rates and transfer factors. J Clin Invest. 1969;48:1809–19.
67. Longcope C, Layne DS, Tait JF. Metabolic clearance rates and interconversions of estrone and 17beta-estradiol in normal males and females. J Clin Invest. 1968;47:93–106.
68. McManus JM, Sharifi N. Structure-dependent retention of steroid hormones by common laboratory materials. J Steroid Biochem Mol Biol. 2020;198:105572.
69. Rosner W, Hryb DJ, Kahn SM, Nakhla AM, Romas NA. Interactions of sex hormone-binding globulin with target cells. Mol Cell Endocrinol. 2010;316:79–85.
70. Pearlman WH, Fong IF, Tou JH. A further study of a testosterone-binding component of human pregnancy serum. J Biol Chem. 1969;244:1373–80.

71. Jin M, Wener MH, Bankson DD. Evaluation of automated sex hormone binding globulin immunoassays. Clin Biochem. 2006;39:91–4.
72. Goldman AL, et al. A reappraisal of testosterone's binding in circulation: physiological and clinical implications. Endocr Rev. 2017;38:302–24.
73. Vermeulen A. Physiology of the testosterone-binding globulin in man. Ann N Y Acad Sci. 1988;538:103–11.
74. Pugeat M, Crave JC, Tourniaire J, Forest MG. Clinical utility of sex hormone-binding globulin measurement. Horm Res. 1996;45:148–55.
75. Welhaven HD, et al. Metabolic phenotypes reflect patient sex and injury status: a cross-sectional analysis of human synovial fluid. Osteoarthr Cartil. 2024;32:1074–83.
76. Guang Y, et al. Combined experimental approach and finite element Modeling of small molecule transport through joint synovium to measure effective diffusivity. J Biomech Eng. 2020;142:0410101–8.
77. Wigginton SM, Chu BC, Weisman MH, Howell SB. Methotrexate pharmacokinetics after intraarticular injection in patients with rheumatoid arthritis. Arthritis Rheum. 1980;23:119–22.
78. Soma LR, et al. Pharmacokinetics of methylprednisolone acetate after intra-articular administration and its effect on endogenous hydrocortisone and cortisone secretion in horses. Am J Vet Res. 2006;67:654–62.
79. Owen SG, Francis HW, Roberts MS. Disappearance kinetics of solutes from synovial fluid after intra-articular injection. Br J Clin Pharmacol. 1994;38:349–55.
80. Jensen E, Jacobson H. Basic guides to the mechanism of estrogen action. Recent Prog Horm Res. 1962;18:387–414.
81. Mor G, et al. Macrophages, estrogen and the microenvironment of breast cancer. J Steroid Biochem Mol Biol. 1998;67:403–11.
82. Samy TS, et al. Divergent immune responses in male and female mice after trauma-hemorrhage: dimorphic alterations in T lymphocyte steroidogenic enzyme activities. Endocrinology. 2001;142:3519–29.
83. Straub RH. The complex role of estrogens in inflammation. Endocr Rev. 2007;28:521–74.
84. Unger CA, et al. A novel tissue-specific insight into sex steroid fluctuations throughout the murine Estrous cycle. Endocrinology. 2023;165:bqad175.
85. Fontaine C, et al. The tissue-specific effects of different 17β-estradiol doses reveal the key sensitizing role of AF1 domain in ERα activity. Mol Cell Endocrinol. 2020;505:110741.
86. Hu Y, Cai K, Luo Z, Jandt KD. Layer-by-layer assembly of β-estradiol loaded mesoporous silica nanoparticles on titanium substrates and its implication for bone homeostasis. Adv Mater. 2010;22:4146–50.
87. Hong L, et al. Intracellular release of 17-β estradiol from cationic polyamidoamine dendrimer surface-modified poly (lactic-co-glycolic acid) microparticles improves osteogenic differentiation of human mesenchymal stromal cells. Tissue Eng Part C Methods. 2011;17:319–25.
88. Irmak G, Demirtaş TT, Çetin Altındal D, Çalış M, Gümüşderelioğlu M. Sustained release of 17β-estradiol stimulates osteogenic differentiation of adipose tissue-derived mesenchymal stem cells on chitosan-hydroxyapatite scaffolds. Cells Tissues Organs. 2014;199:37–50.
89. Calis M, et al. Estrogen as a novel agent for induction of adipose-derived mesenchymal stem cells for osteogenic differentiation: in vivo bone tissue-engineering study. Plast Reconstr Surg. 2014;133:499e–510e.
90. Hong C, et al. Reducing posttreatment relapse in cleft lip palatal expansion using an injectable estrogen-nanodiamond hydrogel. Proc Natl Acad Sci USA. 2017;114:E7218–25.
91. Segredo-Morales E, Reyes R, Arnau MR, Delgado A, Évora C. In situ gel-forming system for dual BMP-2 and 17β-estradiol controlled release for bone regeneration in osteoporotic rats. Drug Deliv Transl Res. 2018;8:1103–13.
92. Steffi C, et al. Estradiol-loaded poly(ε-caprolactone)/silk fibroin electrospun microfibers decrease osteoclast activity and retain osteoblast function. ACS Appl Mater Interfaces. 2018;10:9988–98.

93. Wang D, et al. Beta-cyclodextrin modified mesoporous bioactive glass nanoparticles/silk fibroin hybrid nanofibers as an implantable estradiol delivery system for the potential treatment of osteoporosis. Nanoscale. 2018;10:18341–53.
94. Palomba S, Falbo A, Di Cello A, Materazzo C, Zullo F. Nexplanon: the new implant for long-term contraception. A comprehensive descriptive review. Gynecol Endocrinol. 2012;28:710–21.
95. Yoo J-W, Lee CH. Drug delivery systems for hormone therapy. J Control Release. 2006;112:1–14.
96. Birnbaum DT, Kosmala JD, Henthorn DB, Brannon-Peppas L. Controlled release of beta-estradiol from PLAGA microparticles: the effect of organic phase solvent on encapsulation and release. J Control Release. 2000;65:375–87.
97. Barreiro-Iglesias R, Alvarez-Lorenzo C, Concheiro A. Controlled release of estradiol solubilized in Carbopol/surfactant aggregates. J Control Release. 2003;93:319–30.
98. Rodriguez-Tenreiro C, Alvarez-Lorenzo C, Rodriguez-Perez A, Concheiro A, Torres-Labandeira JJ. Estradiol sustained release from high affinity cyclodextrin hydrogels. Eur J Pharm Biopharm. 2007;66:55–62.
99. Collins BC, Laakkonen EK, Lowe DA. Aging of the musculoskeletal system: how the loss of estrogen impacts muscle strength. Bone. 2019;123:137–44.
100. Collins BC, et al. Estrogen regulates the satellite cell compartment in females. Cell Rep. 2019;28:368–381.e6.
101. D'Amato AR, et al. Vastly extended drug release from poly(pro-17β-estradiol) materials facilitates in vitro neurotrophism and neuroprotection. Nat Commun. 2019;10:4830.
102. El Maghraby GM, Williams AC, Barry BW. Skin hydration and possible shunt route penetration in controlled estradiol delivery from ultradeformable and standard liposomes. J Pharm Pharmacol. 2001;53:1311–22.
103. Mangır N, et al. An estradiol releasing, proangiogenic hydrogel as a candidate material for use in soft tissue interposition. Neurourol Urodyn. 2019;38:1195–202.
104. Mangır N, Hillary CJ, Chapple CR, MacNeil S. Oestradiol-releasing biodegradable mesh stimulates collagen production and angiogenesis: an approach to improving biomaterial integration in pelvic floor repair. Eur Urol Focus. 2019;5:280–9.
105. Shafaat S, Mangir N, Regureos SR, Chapple CR, MacNeil S. Demonstration of improved tissue integration and angiogenesis with an elastic, estradiol releasing polyurethane material designed for use in pelvic floor repair. Neurourol Urodyn. 2018;37:716–25.
106. Kim N, Lukong KE. Treating ER-positive breast cancer: a review of the current FDA-approved SERMs and SERDs and their mechanisms of action. Oncol Rev. 2025;19:1564642.
107. Bikiaris D, Karavelidis V, Karavas E. Novel biodegradable polyesters. Synthesis and application as drug carriers for the preparation of raloxifene HCl loaded nanoparticles. Molecules. 2009;14:2410–30.
108. Shah PV, Rajput SJ. Facile synthesis of chitosan capped mesoporous silica nanoparticles: a pH responsive smart delivery platform for raloxifene hydrochloride. AAPS PharmSciTech. 2018;19:1344–57.
109. Howell A, Howell SJ. Tamoxifen evolution. Br J Cancer. 2023;128:421–5.
110. Cuzick J, et al. Tamoxifen for prevention of breast cancer: extended long-term follow-up of the IBIS-I breast cancer prevention trial. Lancet Oncol. 2015;16:67–75.
111. Sibonga JD, Evans GL, Hauck ER, Bell NH, Turner RT. Ovarian status influences the skeletal effects of tamoxifen in adult rats. Breast Cancer Res Treat. 1996;41:71–9.
112. Pinzón-García AD, Sinisterra R, Cortes M, Mesa F, Ramírez-Clavijo S. Polycaprolactone nanofibers as an adjuvant strategy for tamoxifen release and their cytotoxicity on breast cancer cells. PeerJ. 2021;9:e12124.
113. Fan M, Zheng J, Huang Y, Lu H, Lu M. Efficacy and hepatotoxicity of tamoxifen-loaded fructose-based nanodrug for breast cancer treatment. J Mater Chem B. 2025;13:8229–38.

114. Kavas A, Keskin D, Altunbaş K, Tezcaner A. Raloxifene−/raloxifene-poly(ethylene glycol) conjugate-loaded microspheres: a novel strategy for drug delivery to bone forming cells. Int J Pharm. 2016;510:168–83.
115. Kamel R, El-Wakil NA, Abdelkhalek AA, Elkasabgy NA. Nanofibrillated cellulose/cyclodextrin based 3D scaffolds loaded with raloxifene hydrochloride for bone regeneration. Int J Biol Macromol. 2020;156:704–16.
116. Zhang M-L, Cheng J, Xiao Y-C, Yin R-F, Feng X. Raloxifene microsphere-embedded collagen/chitosan/β-tricalcium phosphate scaffold for effective bone tissue engineering. Int J Pharm. 2017;518:80–5.
117. Ocal Y, et al. Characterization and evaluation of triamcinolone, raloxifene, and their dual-loaded microspheres as prospective local treatment system in rheumatic rat joints. J Pharm Sci. 2014;103:2396–405.
118. Olivares-Navarrete R, et al. Sex dependent regulation of osteoblast response to implant surface properties by systemic hormones. Biol Sex Differ. 2010;1:4.
119. Feng C, et al. Association of 17-β Estradiol with adipose-derived stem cells: new strategy to produce functional myogenic differentiated cells with a Nano-scaffold for tissue engineering. PLoS One. 2016;11:e0164918.
120. Knabe C, et al. Effect of sex-hormone levels, sex, body mass index and other host factors on human craniofacial bone regeneration with bioactive tricalcium phosphate grafts. Biomaterials. 2017;123:48–62.
121. Berger MB, et al. Human osteoblasts exhibit sexual dimorphism in their response to estrogen on microstructured titanium surfaces. Biol Sex Differ. 2018;9:30.
122. Livingston MK, et al. Evaluation of PEG-based hydrogel influence on estrogen receptor driven responses in MCF7 breast cancer cells. ACS Biomater Sci Eng. 2019;5:6089–98.
123. Sorushanova A, Skoufos I, Tzora A, Mullen AM, Zeugolis DI. The influence of animal species, gender and tissue on the structural, biophysical, biochemical and biological properties of collagen sponges. J Mater Sci Mater Med. 2021;32:12.
124. Ueno M, et al. Sex differences in mesenchymal stem cell therapy with Gelatin-based microribbon hydrogels in a murine long bone critical-size defect model. Front Bioeng Biotechnol. 2021;9:755964.
125. Wu Z, et al. In the quest of the optimal tissue source (porcine male and female articular, tracheal and auricular cartilage) for the development of collagen sponges for articular cartilage. Biomed Eng Adv. 2021;1:100002.
126. Ma Z, et al. Engineered human meniscus in Modeling sex differences of knee osteoarthritis in vitro. Front Bioeng Biotechnol. 2022;10:823679.
127. Shen H, et al. Sex differences in the therapeutic effect of unaltered versus NFκB sensing IL-4 over-expressing mesenchymal stromal cells in a murine model of chronic inflammatory bone loss. Front Bioeng Biotechnol. 2022;10:962114.
128. El Sherif N, et al. Investigating sex-dependent differences in tensional homeostasis. 2024. https://doi.org/10.11159/icbb24.121.
129. Kolar M, Veber M, Girandon L, Drobnič M. A biomimetic osteochondral scaffold augmented with filtered bone marrow aspirate for the treatment of joint surface lesions in the knee. Am J Sports Med. 2024;52:1826–33.
130. Lohmann CH, et al. Response of normal female human osteoblasts (NHOst) to 17β-estradiol is modulated by implant surface morphology. J Biomed Mater Res. 2002;62:204–13.
131. Ling-Ling E, et al. Estrogen enhances the bone regeneration potential of periodontal ligament stem cells derived from osteoporotic rats and seeded on nano-hydroxyapatite/collagen/poly (L-lactide). Int J Mol Med. 2016;37:1475–86.
132. Burkey K, et al. Modulating pentenoate-functionalized hyaluronic acid hydrogel network properties for meniscal fibrochondrocyte mechanotransduction. J Biomed Mater Res A. 2023;111:1525–37. https://doi.org/10.1002/jbm.a.37551.
133. Burkey K, Meinhold KL, Knewtson KE, Stackhouse B, Robinson JL. Biomaterial tools to interrogate sex differences in knee connective tissue regeneration. Daegu; 2024.

134. Maney DL, Rich-Edwards JW. Sex-inclusive biomedicine: are new policies increasing rigor and reproducibility? Womens Health Issues. 2023;33:461–4.
135. Pape M, et al. Sex contextualism in laboratory research: enhancing rigor and precision in the study of sex-related variables. Cell. 2024;187:1316–26.
136. Rich-Edwards JW, Maney DL. Best practices to promote rigor and reproducibility in the era of sex-inclusive research. elife. 2023;12:e90623.

Sex-Based Insights into Aortic Valve Disease and Scaffold Design

Joshita Suresh, Nafeesah Ibrahim, and Kristyn S. Masters

Abstract Calcific aortic valve disease (CAVD) affects over 25% of individuals over the age of 65, making it the most prevalent valvular disease. Advanced age is the primary risk factor for CAVD, but biological sex follows close behind, wherein males are twice as likely as females to develop CAVD (Alushi et al. Front Pharmacol 11:685, 2020). This sex difference in disease prevalence has long been recognized, but ongoing research continues to reveal myriad cellular-scale sex differences that underlie the pathogenesis of this disease. Some of these cellular-scale sex differences are present at birth, while others are acquired, often in response to sex hormone signaling. Ultimately, sex differences in valvular function manifest in CAVD, taking a different form in men vs. women: in men, valvular stiffening is associated with calcification, while in women it is primarily due to fibrosis (Simard et al. Circ Res 120:681–91, 2017). This chapter discusses the complex interplay between different types of valvular cells, the extracellular matrix, aging processes, and sex differences in the development of CAVD. These characteristics are also discussed in the context of constructing valvular biomaterials, as engineered tissue models provide a promising avenue for furthering our understanding of disease pathogenesis, sexual dimorphisms, and potential therapeutic targets to mitigate CAVD severity.

Joshita Suresh and Nafeesah Ibrahim contributed equally to this work.

J. Suresh · N. Ibrahim
Department of Chemical and Biological Engineering, University of Colorado-Boulder, Boulder, CO, USA
e-mail: joshita.suresh@cuanschutz.edu; nafeesah.ibrahim@colorado.edu

K. S. Masters (✉)
Department of Biomedical Engineering, University of Colorado-Denver, Anschutz, Aurora, CO, USA
e-mail: kristyn.masters@cuanschutz.edu

S. G. Zambuto, M. L. Oyen (eds.), *Biomaterials for Women's Health Engineering*,
https://doi.org/10.1007/978-3-032-10745-9_17

Keywords Calcific aortic valve disease (CAVD) · Endothelial dysfunction · Extracellular matrix (ECM) · Fibrosis · Inflammation · Mechanical signaling · Myofibroblast activation · Osteogenic differentiation · Sex differences · Biomaterials · Biofabrication · Organ-on-a-chip

1 The Aortic Valve: Extracellular Matrix (ECM) Structure and Cellular Composition

1.1 Anatomy and ECM of the Healthy Aortic Valve

The aortic valve is comprised of three avascular leaflets, separating the left ventricle and the aorta [1, 2]. The leaflets respond to pressure differences between systole and diastole, opening during systole to allow blood flow through the aorta and circulate around the body. During diastole, the leaflets close, preventing backflow of fluid while the left ventricle is resupplied with oxygenated blood. Healthy, mature aortic valves are typically 300 μm in thickness and have been identified to contain three sublayers within its structure that each provide a unique purpose to the overall function of the valve [1, 3]. The proximal layer is referred to as the fibrosa layer and is composed of collagen fibers, specifically 75% type I and 25% type III. These collagen fibers are oriented circumferentially, providing the tensile strength and mechanical support necessary to withstand immense hemodynamic stresses [3, 4]. On the ventricle side, another layer aptly named the ventricularis is comprised of both collagen fibers and elastin, which is positioned perpendicular to the fibers present in the fibrosa. Elastin plays a critical role in the leaflets' ability to recoil once the hemodynamic pressure is alleviated between heartbeats. In between the fibrosa and the ventricularis lies a section of the valve referred to as the spongiosa, home to glycosaminoglycans (GAGs) and proteoglycans (PGs), which provide cushioning and lubrication to the valve [3]. Each of these layers and the molecules that are comprised within them provide crucial mechanical and biological functions that maintain healthy valvular cell phenotypes and a soundly functioning aortic valve. An overview of valve anatomy is presented in Fig. 1.

1.2 Cell Types in the Aortic Valve

Among the most critical cell types within the valve are valvular interstitial cells (VICs) and valvular endothelial cells (VECs). These cell populations work in concert to regulate homeostasis, respond to mechanical stresses, and prevent pathological changes. Their dysfunction is a central feature in the development of calcific aortic valve disease (CAVD), particularly in the context of aging and hormonal changes such as those occurring during menopause.

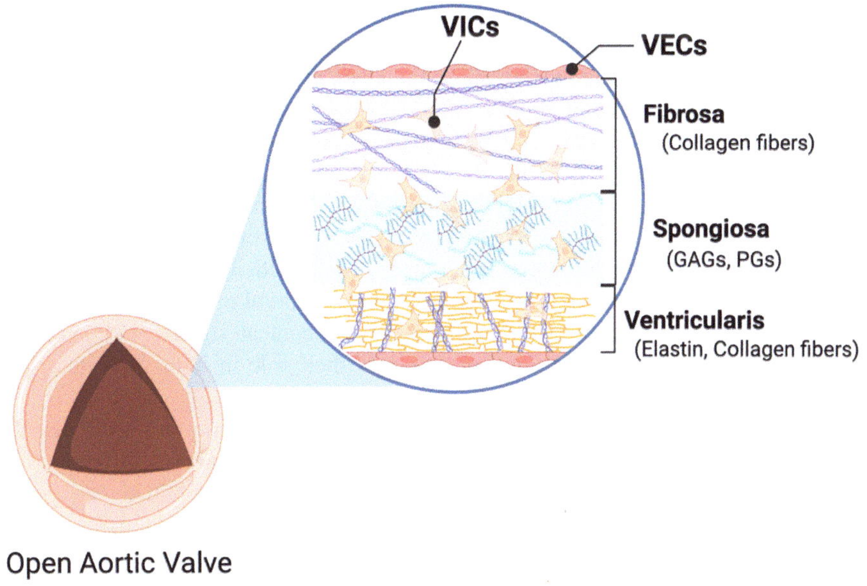

Fig. 1 Overview of aortic heart valve anatomy. The aortic heart valve is comprised of three distinct layers of extracellular matrix (fibrosa, spongiosa, and ventricularis), as well as two distinct cell types (valvular interstitial cells and valvular endothelial cells). (Created in https://BioRender.com)

1.2.1 Valvular Interstitial Cells (VICs): Phenotype, Sexual Dimorphism, and Role in CAVD

VICs are the principal cellular constituents of heart valve leaflets, distributed throughout the fibrosa, spongiosa, and ventricularis layers. Their primary physiological function is the regulation of extracellular matrix (ECM) turnover, which is essential for maintaining leaflet structure and biomechanical function over the lifespan of the valve. VICs synthesize key matrix components such as collagen, elastin, and proteoglycans and are responsible for the enzymatic degradation and remodeling of these components when necessary.

VICs exhibit significant phenotypic plasticity, allowing them to transition between quiescent, activated, myofibroblastic, and osteoblastic-like states depending on environmental cues [5]. In healthy adult valves, VICs are typically quiescent and display a fibroblast-like phenotype. However, in response to injury, inflammation, or mechanical strain, they can transition into a more active myofibroblast phenotype. This transformation is marked by increased proliferative and synthetic activity, elevated expression of α-SMA, and enhanced production of matrix metalloproteinases (MMPs), which facilitate tissue remodeling. This myofibroblastic activation plays a role in wound healing and adaptive tissue repair but becomes pathogenic when prolonged, contributing to fibrosis and valve stiffening. In pathological contexts such as CAVD, VICs may undergo further phenotypic modulation toward an osteoblast-like lineage.

The dynamic nature of VIC phenotype is reflected in their diverse marker profile. Quiescent VICs predominantly express vimentin and fibroblast-specific protein-1 (FSP-1), indicating their mesenchymal origin. Upon myofibroblastic activation, they upregulate α-SMA, smooth muscle 22α, and calponin, indicating a contractile phenotype. In contrast, osteogenic VICs express markers typically associated with bone cells, such as osteopontin and RUNX2, and show mineral deposition capabilities when cultured under pro-calcific conditions [6]. Notably, even within healthy valves, VICs display a range of phenotypic states, suggesting a population of cells poised to respond to microenvironmental cues. This plasticity, while necessary for adaptive tissue maintenance, also positions VICs as central mediators of pathological remodeling in CAVD. Their response to mechanical signals, inflammatory mediators, and biochemical stimuli underscores their role in both valve integrity and degeneration.

Although CAVD has long been associated with a sex disparity in overall disease prevalence, it was only in 2012 that the existence of cellular-scale sex differences in VIC gene expression was first described [7]. Investigators identified 183 genes whose expression levels were significantly distinct between male and female porcine VICs. Genes correlated to ECM remodeling, angiogenesis, calcification, lipid metabolism, cell proliferation, and cell migration were found to demonstrate sexual dimorphism, with upregulation in male VICs compared to females [7]. These sex differences persist in cell culture, as male VICs have been found to express increased levels of α-SMA, transforming growth factor-β1 (TGF-β1), and MMPs, which are correlated with myofibroblast differentiation of VICs [8]. Many of these findings are consistent with observations from human VICs isolated from stenotic valves. A recent study found that male human VICs from diseased valves exhibited higher inflammatory activity and collagen I production compared to female VICs [9]. While information on the influence of sex hormones on VIC function is still emerging, there is evidence that some of these sex differences may be linked to sex chromosomes [10]. Transcriptomic analysis from cells cultured in vitro resulted in at least 28 X-chromosome-linked genes that were differentially regulated between myofibroblast and fibroblast populations of VICs, further providing insight into sex-based gene regulation. The Rho-associated protein kinase (RhoA/ROCK) signaling pathway, which regulates myofibroblast activation along with α-SMA activation, was shown to be responsive to inhibitory proteins in a sex-based manner as well as in response to environmental cues, and Rho inhibition reduced α-SMA only in activated male VICs [10].

1.2.2 Valvular Endothelial Cells (VECs): Phenotype, Sexual Dimorphism, and Role in CAVD

VECs line the surface of heart valves and play a central role in maintaining valve homeostasis, mechanosensing, and immune modulation [11]. Unlike vascular endothelial cells (ECs), which primarily facilitate nutrient exchange and barrier function in blood vessels, VECs are adapted to the unique biomechanical environment of the cardiac valves, characterized by constant deformation, oscillatory flow, and pressure fluctuations. VECs are crucial for valve integrity, mediating interactions between blood flow and the underlying VICs. They regulate VIC behavior by secreting signaling molecules, including nitric oxide (NO), TGF-β, and bone morphogenetic proteins (BMPs), thus influencing ECM remodeling and calcification processes [12]. VECs also contribute to anti-thrombotic and anti-inflammatory environments via production of prostacyclin (PGI2) and other bioactive agents. Their response to shear stress is essential in maintaining valve function: laminar flow tends to preserve quiescence, while disturbed or oscillatory flow can promote pathological activation. Hence, VECs from different sides of the valve exhibit distinct phenotypes, with those on the aortic side being more prone to dysfunction due to exposure to disturbed flow patterns [13]. Normal VEC function is associated with the expression of endothelial markers such as VE-cadherin, CD31, and endothelial nitric oxide synthase (eNOS), which contribute to maintaining an anti-inflammatory and anti-calcific microenvironment. However, under conditions of oxidative stress or pro-inflammatory signaling, VECs can undergo endothelial-to-mesenchymal transition (EndMT), leading to increased VIC activation and fibrotic or calcific remodeling of the valve [14].

Few studies have examined sex differences in VECs. Under healthy in vitro culture conditions, porcine VECs exhibited few sex differences, with similar metabolic activity and tubulogenesis outcomes, although male VEC proliferation was significantly higher than females [15]. Similar to VICs, male VECs isolated from human diseased valves demonstrate increased inflammatory activity compared to female VECs [9]. There are likely many more sex differences in VEC functions, but this remains a nascent line of investigation. However, many sex differences have been documented in vascular ECs [16, 17], which are likely to be highly relevant to VECs. Vascular ECs exhibit sex differences at birth, as well as acquired sex differences. At birth, female ECs exhibit enrichment of activation pathways such as endothelial-to-mesenchymal transition (EMT), hypoxia, and NFkB signaling [18]. Human female ECs also exhibit higher levels of ROS production and mitochondrial damage, as well as expression of genes associated with inflammation and apoptosis [19]. The acquired sex differences in ECs also have significant overlap with pathways regulated by sex hormones. Estrogen has many effects on ECs, including elevation of NO [17] and PGl2 [20, 21], and enhancement of EC barrier functions via strengthening of tight junctions [22, 23]. Androgens such as testosterone and dihydrotestosterone have also been observed to induce activation of NO secretion in ECs. Broadly, both estrogen and testosterone increase the proliferation and migration of ECs as well as promote angiogenesis [24, 25].

Homeostasis within the aortic valve is tightly regulated by the interplay between VICs and VECs, ensuring that minor mechanical and biochemical perturbations do not result in permanent structural damage. Under normal conditions, VECs release NO and other signaling molecules that inhibit VIC activation and fibrosis [26]. Likewise, VICs maintain a balanced ECM composition by regulating protease and inhibitor activity. However, chronic inflammation, oxidative stress, and altered hemodynamic forces can disrupt this homeostasis, triggering pathological cascades that drive valve thickening and calcification [27].

2 Aortic Valve Aging and Disease

2.1 A Brief History of Calcific Aortic Valve Disease (CAVD)

Physician Lazare Riviere is credited with providing one of the first descriptions of aortic stenosis, in 1663 [28]. Riviere, Bonet, and many other physicians in the mid-1600s describe accounts of autopsies performed on men that died suddenly in which "white ossific nodules" were observed on the aortic valve. Proceeding hypotheses and theories marked the beginnings of understanding CAVD. Early scientists were quick to infer that heart failure in patients with calcified aortic valves was most likely due to the inability of blood to be pumped through the boney, rigid valve, thus leading to abnormal palpitations of the heart, difficulty breathing, and eventual death [28].

However, despite CAVD first being described over 350 years ago, uncovering the pathogenesis of this disease has been hampered by the long-standing assumption that it was a passive, degenerative disease—i.e., a natural consequence of "healthy" aging [3]. It was only in the late 1990s that it became widely accepted that CAVD arose from an active disease process, causing a shift in mindset about the pathophysiology and curability of the disease. Age-related pathways, however, may still contribute to the initial onset of disease in the aortic valve. Decreased activity of telomerases and endothelial cell senescence leading to production of reactive oxygen species (ROS) are two age-related pathways that may lead to valvular vulnerability and prime the tissue for disease progression [29].

2.2 Aortic Valve Aging and Sex Hormones

Healthy tissue aging is associated with myriad changes and remains incompletely characterized for many tissues. As noted above, age-related changes in aortic valves were historically conflated with CAVD development, as the latter was long thought to just be a consequence of normal aging. However, many years of aging research have revealed cellular-level aging processes that generally apply to most cells in the body. Briefly, cellular aging is associated with shortening of telomeres, disruption in the gene transcription, issues with transportation of information through the nuclear envelope via the eukaryotic nuclear pore complex, maladaptive protein translation, haphazard maintenance and denaturation of proteins, decreased clearance/recycling of damaged proteins and organelles through autophagy, and damage to mitochondrial functions [30]. Among these many disruptions, increased ROS production accelerates the progression toward dysfunction that may potentiate the path toward chronic disease in older populations [30–32]. Although cellular aging is a complex factor to decipher, inferences on tissue health can also be made by observing changes in the ECM.

Tissue thickening and stiffening are common consequences of aging, both in heart valve tissues [33, 34] and beyond [35]. Expression and regulation of collagen is positively correlated with age, along with dysregulation in collagen glycosylation, which leads to misalignment of collagen fibers [30, 36, 37]. Collagen deposition has been named as a driving factor for VIC differentiation and disease progression [37]; as noted above, collagen production is also different across the sexes [8, 9]. Analysis of healthy patient valves demonstrated a significant increase in valve thickness in both biological males and females after age 50, further illustrating ECM changes with age [1, 38]. In addition to collagen, other valve ECM constituents such as elastin have also been observed to deteriorate with age, causing weakening of tissues and loss of elasticity [39, 40]. In human valves, overall GAGs decrease in aging from adolescence to adulthood, although these studies did not extend to ages associated with CAVD [34]. Analyses of porcine valves at different life stages indicated that not just GAG amount but also GAG composition changes with age [41]. Ultimately, the functional consequence of these combined ECM changes tends to be tissue stiffening, which itself can initiate multiple pathological pathways. Tissue stiffness alters blood flow hemodynamics, which, in turn, stimulates EC dysfunction [35]. VICs in stiff environments are also prone to myofibroblastic differentiation [42, 43]. It is through these changes that normal aging appears to set the stage for the onset of valvular pathology.

In the context of aortic heart valves, it is yet to be determined whether a healthy, aged male valve has different ECM and mechanical properties compared to a healthy, aged female valve. Additionally, it is challenging to decouple the effects of aging vs. the effects of changes in sex hormones (i.e., menopause). In the last decade, the field of cardiovascular disease has come to the broad conclusion that estrogen provides cardioprotective and immunoprotective properties [1, 44–47]. In other fibrotic tissue models, estrogen decreases TGF-β gene expression through suppression of the Smad signaling pathways; as noted earlier, TGF-β is a significant driving factor in CAVD [48, 49]. Circulating lipoproteins, which are also promoters of VIC differentiation [49, 50], dramatically increase in females after menopause and are thought to correlate with the sudden rise in cardiovascular disease diagnoses in postmenopausal women [51]. Consistent with these observations, meta-analyses of heart disease vulnerabilities show that CAVD affects postmenopausal women at significantly higher rates than premenopausal women [47]. However, the rates of severe CAVD development are still significantly lower in postmenopausal women compared to their age-matched male counterparts, which may suggest the involvement of nonhormonal pathways in regulating disease susceptibility [47, 52]. A key question in CAVD research is defining the point at which the disease process diverges between the sexes—i.e., whether aged male and female valves significantly differ in their composition prior to disease onset, or if the sex differences in CAVD appearance manifest during the disease process. Further research on age-associated changes in aortic heart valves, and whether these are associated with sex differences, are needed to address these questions.

2.3 *CAVD Pathophysiology: Early-Stage Disease*

2.3.1 Cellular Changes in CAVD

The earliest indications of CAVD include endothelial dysfunction, mild inflammatory infiltration, and ECM remodeling (Fig. 2). VECs that line the aortic valve leaflets experience increased oxidative stress and pro-inflammatory signaling [53], leading to an initial loss of their protective functions. Shear stress alterations, especially in regions of low or disturbed flow, contribute to endothelial permeability changes, allowing inflammatory cells such as macrophages to infiltrate the valve tissue [54]. These immune cells release cytokines, including TNF-α and interleukin-6 (IL-6), which promote VIC activation and transition into osteogenic and myofibroblastic phenotypes [55].

At this stage, VICs begin transitioning from a quiescent fibroblast-like state to an activated myofibroblast phenotype. This shift is characterized by increased expression of α-SMA and heightened ECM synthesis [55], often driven by TGF-β1 [29]. TGF-β1 is produced by both inflammatory cells and VICs themselves and acts to promote inflammation, leading to eventual fibrosis/calcific deposition in valvular ECM [3, 50]. As noted above, these responses exhibit sexual dimorphism, with males tending to have a lower threshold for disease induction [8, 49, 56, 57]. While this response is initially reparative, chronic activation can lead to excessive ECM remodeling and fibrosis, laying the groundwork for calcific lesions.

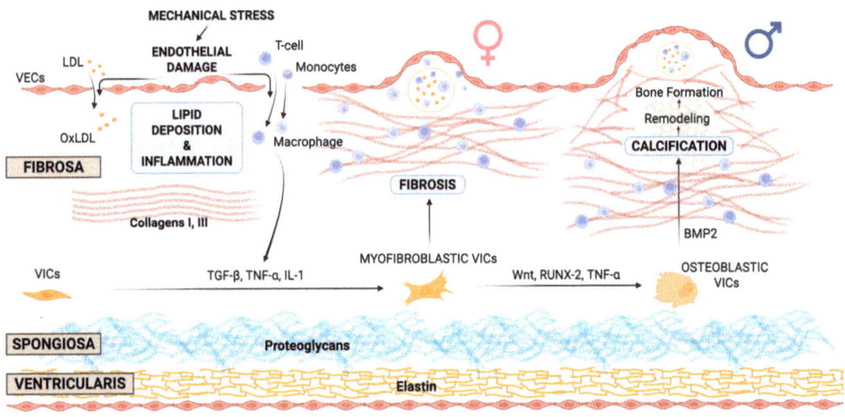

Fig. 2 Schematic representation of sex-specific mechanisms in calcific aortic valve disease (CAVD). Endothelial injury and mechanical stress initiate lipid deposition, oxidation of LDL, and inflammatory cell recruitment, activating valvular interstitial cells (VICs) via cytokines such as TGF-β, TNF-α, and IL-1. Activated VICs adopt myofibroblastic phenotypes, leading to extracellular matrix remodeling and fibrosis, which predominates in females. In males, signaling through Wnt, RUNX-2, and BMP2 drives osteogenic VIC differentiation and calcific nodule formation. While males typically exhibit greater calcification and females more fibrosis, both processes share overlapping inflammatory and mechanical triggers and often coexist within diseased valve tissue. (Created in https://BioRender.com)

Activated VICs also exhibit increased production of proteolytic enzymes, such as MMPs, which degrade ECM components and contribute to disorganized tissue structure [58]. Additionally, activated VICs produce pro-inflammatory cytokines that further exacerbate immune cell recruitment and tissue damage, creating a self-perpetuating cycle of inflammation and remodeling [59].

Understanding the complex interactions between VICs and VECs provides insight into potential therapeutic approaches for CAVD. Strategies that aim to restore endothelial function, such as NO donors or anti-inflammatory agents, could help maintain VEC integrity and prevent VIC activation [60]. Additionally, targeting pathways involved in EndMT and osteogenic differentiation, such as TGF-β inhibitors or Wnt signaling modulators, may offer promising avenues for slowing disease progression.

2.3.2 ECM Changes in CAVD

In early CAVD, ECM composition is altered due to dysregulated VIC activity and chronic inflammation [58]. Early signs of CAVD include increased presence of PGs and GAGs, which lead to valvular thickening [61, 62]. Decorin, hyaluronic acid, and versican are among the earliest GAGs and PGs to increase in concentration past homeostatic amounts, leading to not only thickening of the valve but also sequestering oxidized phospholipids that further promote disease progression [62, 63]. Other ECM molecules such as collagens, lumican, biglycan, aggrecan, laminin, fibronection, periostin, and prolargin are also enriched in diseased valves [61].

Fibrillar collagen deposition has been associated with early onset of fibrosis, specifically in the spongiosa [58, 64]. The overproduction of collagen types I and III ultimately leads to increased stiffness, and, when combined with elastic fiber degradation, reduces the valve's elastic recoil properties [58]. Another hallmark feature of early CAVD is the misalignment of collagen fibers, which disrupts the normal architecture of the valve and contributes to leaflet stiffness [65]. Collagen fibers, primarily composed of type I and III collagen, become disorganized and lose their parallel alignment, reducing the valve's ability to withstand hemodynamic stress [66]. Disrupted collagen alignment in the fibrosa and ventricularis are also evident and become more pronounced as CAVD progresses [16]. Alterations to collagen fibers have been observed in both in vitro and in vivo histology sections and may be attributed to the increase of MMPs such as MMP-1, 9, 10, 12, and 28, which are all known to be upregulated in end-stage, stenotic valves [67–70]. Fibrotic tissue deposition in the valve is more prevalent in females than in males, however [71], and in vitro cell culture experiments corroborate this observation. Sex-separated studies conducted with porcine VICs found upregulation of collagen-associated genes in females compared to males as well as increased collagen content in the conditioned media. Further investigation into proteins associated with ECM remodeling revealed that male samples contained higher levels of collagenase and gelatinase, which are enzymes associated with ECM degradation [8]. Activated male

VICs also present myofibroblast-like phenotypes compared to females as well as higher levels of osteogenic markers that promote calcium deposition in the surrounding ECM [8, 72]. Other sex-based variations in VIC ECM regulation have been found to contribute to pro-fibrotic deposition in female samples versus pro-calcific/osteogenic behavior in males [72]. Specifically, MMP variations in female and male groups contributed to decreased collagen fibers observed in males who also showed significantly higher positive staining for osteogenic markers such as BMP-9 and Sox-9, among others [72].

In addition to collagen disorganization, elastic fiber fragmentation is another key structural change observed in early CAVD. Elastin, which provides elasticity and resilience to the valve, undergoes degradation due to the upregulation of MMPs, specifically MMP-2 and MMP-9 [73]. Fragmentation of elastin not only compromises the valve's elasticity but also creates bioactive elastin peptides that can promote inflammation and calcification [74, 75]. This combination of collagen misalignment and elastin fragmentation contributes to the pathological remodeling of the aortic valve, setting the stage for calcific nodule formation and valve stiffening.

As the disease progresses, the ability of VICs to regulate ECM turnover diminishes, and calcified nodules form within the valve leaflets, ultimately impairing valve function. This calcification is further exacerbated in postmenopausal women, where the absence of estrogen-mediated protective mechanisms accelerates VIC osteogenic differentiation and increases susceptibility to CAVD [76]. Additionally, disturbed flow patterns resulting from calcification can create a positive feedback loop, further promoting endothelial dysfunction and VIC activation.

2.3.3 Other Contributors to Disease Progression

Inflammation and Lipid Deposition

The innate immune system's initial role in CAVD is thought to be analogous to that seen in atherosclerosis, which is characterized by chronic inflammation [77, 78]. Standard innate immune responses are initiated by an insult or injury that releases damage-associated molecular patterns, followed by neutrophil infiltration, monocyte and macrophage recruitment, and chronic inflammation of the wound site [79]. In CAVD and atherosclerosis, damage to ECs is hypothesized to allow immune cell infiltration and increased lipoprotein presence in the area [50, 80, 81]. As a result of oxidized lipid deposition, additional immune cell recruitment occurs, creating an inflammatory environment that promotes angiogenesis and continued progression into fully calcified leaflets [50].

VEC disruption on the aortic side of the valve may be an initiating factor in CAVD onset [50]. The disturbance to the VEC lining leads to accumulation of lipoproteins, red blood cells, and immune cells at the site of injury [50]. Lipoproteins can also directly influence valve cell function, and clinical studies have shown a significant correlation between lipoprotein (a) (Lp(a)) serum levels and CAVD severity [80, 81]. Lp(a) promotes VIC differentiation and its function as a carrier of oxidized phospholipids (ox-PLs) [80, 81], which contribute to macrophage polarization [82]. Research has also shown that Lp(a) stimulation of VICs in vitro increases known pro-osteogenic factors such as IL-6, BMP2, and RUNX2 [82]. The production of Lp(a) is species-specific and found only in humans and primates, leading to limitations of typical in vivo murine, rodent, and rabbit models. 3D in vitro models thus provide a convenient, cost-effective, and tunable platform for further investigating Lp(a) function in CAVD progression.

Low-density lipoproteins (LDLs) are structurally similar to Lp(a) and also infiltrate the valve following endothelial layer injury [50]. Oxidized LDLs (ox-LDLs) have been observed in early stages of disease development, contributing to increased production of sulfated GAGs such as chondroitin sulfate via stimulation of VICs [50, 63, 70]. These lipoproteins also indirectly increase production of biglycans, molecules correlated to stenotic severity and have the capacity to stimulate VICs down the path of osteogenic differentiation [70, 83].

The inflammatory environment now present in the valve leads to the recruitment of multiple different immune cells such as macrophages, mast cells, and T-cells [50]. Macrophages, stimulated into an M1 pro-inflammatory phenotypes, are another key player and potential therapeutic target to be understood in the context of CAVD. These cells produce cytokines such as TNF-α and IL-6, further contributing to chronic inflammation, and secrete enzymes such as MMPs, specifically MMP-1, -2, -3, -9, and -10, along with cathepsins that allow for continued remodeling of the surrounding environment [50]. Extracellular vesicles discharged by these cells contribute to nucleation sites for calcium deposition [50]. Although immune cells typically function to phagocytose damaged tissue and undergo apoptosis once their mission is accomplished, in CAVD, immune cell apoptosis results in the formation of nucleation sites that further exacerbate calcification [70].

Hypoxia and Angiogenesis

Native, healthy valve tissue is typically avascular with nutrients being supplied to cells through diffusion. However, as ECM deposition increases with disease progression, oxygen diffusion into the valve is compromised. This decrease in oxygen availability causes cellular stress and upregulates hypoxia-inducible factor-α (HIF-α) [84, 85], which is found to be enriched in diseased human valves [86]. Non-hypoxia signals can also upregulate HIF-1α production, as treatment with inflammatory stimuli interferon-gamma and lipopolysaccharide also stimulated HIF-1α production by VICs [87]. HIF-α proteins translocate into the nucleus and function to upregulate genes that produce insulin-like growth factor-2 (IGF-2) and transforming growth factor-α (TGF-α) that act to promote glucose transportation and cell survival [86]. Other genes are also upregulated to increase VEGF levels that manifest in increased angiogenesis [70, 88]. The HIF-α subtypes present in hypoxic environments are determined by the activation of the macrophages in the surrounding area, resulting in higher levels of hypoxic proteins in inflammatory environments [70, 86, 88].

Inflammatory cells are believed to be a dominant source of stimuli that promote angiogenesis in the diseased valve. Their production of cytokines such as TNF-α and

IL-1β can directly activate HIF-1α [89]. Macrophage-mediated ECM remodeling has also been hypothesized as an indirect avenue for VIC activation, resulting in the production of angiogenic growth factors such as VEGF, driving subsequent neovascularization in the diseased, thickening tissue [50]. Angiotensin II synthesis also results from the inflammatory response, further driving neovascularization, and bringing more RBCs, lipoproteins, and immune cells to the area [50]. Increased HIF-1α via flow-driven cascades was not observed in vitro when porcine VICs were treated with a hypoxic protein inhibitor, suggesting that hypoxia observed in aortic leaflets may result not only from increased ECM density but also from disruptions in blood circulation parameters [84, 86]. The role of HIF-2α is predominantly as a transcription factor released from immune cells recruited to the injury site and increases production of Runx2 and Sox9, both of which are observed in CAVD progression [86].

There is emerging evidence that valvular angiogenesis is a sexually dimorphic event. In vitro studies of porcine cells suggest sexual dimorphism in angiogenic factors secreted from VICs and consequent effects on VECs. Angiogenic factors produced by both male and female porcine VICs in both activated and quiescent phenotypes were quantified; key findings from this study included increased production of several pro-angiogenic growth factors by male VICs, as well as differential sequestration of these molecules in the ECM by males vs. females [15]. There was also significant, sex-specific variance in thrombospondin-2 secretion, a glycoprotein known to regulate fibrosis [15]. Sex hormones are also likely to play a role in regulating angiogenesis in the valve. As mentioned in previous sections, estrogen is a significant influencer of vascular tone and promotes vasodilation through NO production [17, 85]. In human-derived cell culture models of non-inflammatory activation of HIF-1α, male samples produced significantly higher expression levels of pro-angiogenic genes and proteins than females, although estrogen has been known to promote angiogenesis via stimulation of VEGF and eNOS production [49, 90].

2.4 *CAVD Pathophysiology: Late-Stage Disease, Sex Differences, Diagnostics, and Treatments*

In the absence of treatment, CAVD progresses to severe aortic stenosis with significant clinical consequences. The narrowing of the aortic valve increases afterload on the left ventricle, initiating a compensatory hypertrophic response. While left ventricular hypertrophy may preserve systolic function initially, it is associated with reduced diastolic compliance, increased myocardial oxygen demand, and eventual decompensation [91]. Once patients develop symptoms such as exertional dyspnea, syncope, or angina, the prognosis declines substantially. Longitudinal studies have demonstrated that symptomatic severe aortic stenosis is associated with a mortality rate of approximately 50% at 2 years without valve replacement [92].

Both cellular and ECM changes discussed in previous sections ultimately lead to unchecked mineral deposition, either of calcium or fibrillar collagen, ultimately leading to aortic valve stenosis. At this end-stage, patients tend to be in critical condition with poor prognoses. The resulting rigid, osteogenic-like structure of diseased valve tissue is unable to appropriately function under physiological hemodynamic stresses nor appropriately recoil during diastole. The decrease in valve opening area has been reported to be under 1 cm^2 while normal functioning valves are able to reach orifice areas between 2.5 and 4.5 cm^2 [59]. Emerging evidence also highlights sex-specific differences in the pathophysiology and clinical presentation of CAVD (Table 1). Men with aortic stenosis are more likely to exhibit extensive leaflet calcification, which correlates with higher aortic valve calcium scores on

Table 1 Sex-based differences in CAVD progression

Stage/feature	Male response	Female response
Early CAVD	Greater myofibroblast activation of VICs (↑α-SMA, TGF-β1, MMPs) Increased osteogenic signaling (RUNX2, BMPs) Pro-calcific ECM remodeling Elevated inflammatory cytokine production	More ECM accumulation (↑collagen types I/III) Less osteogenic but more matrix stiffening Pro-fibrotic responses (↑collagen gene expression) Lower MMP activity than males
ECM changes	Disorganized collagen and elastin High collagenase/gelatinase activity Earlier onset of calcium deposition	Increased proteoglycans and glycosaminoglycans (e.g., decorin, HA, versican) Higher overall collagen content and tissue stiffness
Angiogenesis	VICs secrete more pro-angiogenic factors (VEGF, thrombospondin-2) Greater hypoxia-induced gene expression	ECM composition leads to sequestration of angiogenic factors Slightly reduced angiogenic signaling
Late CAVD	Heavy valve calcification High aortic valve calcium scores on CT Presence of bone-like nodules	Dense fibrotic valve tissue Lower calcium scores despite severe hemodynamic impairment
Clinical imaging	CT imaging effectively detects disease severity via calcium quantification	CT underestimates disease severity due to lower calcium burden
Functional impact	Severe calcification reduces leaflet mobility and contributes to obstruction	Fibrotic thickening leads to valve stiffening and impaired motion despite low calcification
Valve replacement outcomes	Higher leaflet calcification may necessitate more invasive procedures	Despite increased procedural risk, females often have comparable or better outcomes post-TAVR

Summary of the sex-specific differences in valvular interstitial cell (VIC) responses and tissue remodeling during early and late stages of calcific aortic valve disease (CAVD). Differences in extracellular matrix (ECM) composition, angiogenesis, disease manifestation, and treatment outcomes are highlighted between male and female phenotypes computed tomography (CT) imaging [93]. In contrast, women tend to present with a predominantly fibrotic phenotype, characterized by collagen-rich, thickened valve leaflets with relatively lower calcium burden [93]. Despite these differences in tissue composition, women often have similar or even more severe hemodynamic obstruction compared to men. These findings suggest that imaging techniques relying heavily on calcium quantification may underestimate disease severity in women, potentially leading to delays in diagnosis and treatment.

Total valve replacement remains the only solution to aortic valve stenosis. The introduction of surgical aortic valve replacement (SAVR) and transcatheter aortic valve replacement (TAVR) has significantly altered the natural history of CAVD. In appropriately selected patients, valve replacement improves symptoms, functional capacity, and survival. One-year survival following TAVR typically exceeds 80–90%, depending on patient age, comorbidities, and procedural risk [94]. Nevertheless, a substantial proportion of patients with aortic stenosis remain undiagnosed or are diagnosed late in the disease course. This is partly due to the asymptomatic nature of early disease and limitations in clinical assessment, particularly in elderly individuals with overlapping comorbid conditions. Additionally, some diagnosed patients may not undergo intervention due to perceived surgical risk or underestimation of disease severity. Furthermore, sex differences may influence clinical outcomes following valve replacement. Some studies have reported that women, despite having a higher procedural risk profile, experience similar or better long-term survival after TAVR compared to men [95]. The underlying mechanisms remain under investigation but may involve differences in myocardial remodeling, comorbid conditions, and vascular biology.

In addition to limited treatments, diagnostic tools for determining severity have also been reported to lack standardization [59, 96, 97]. As is evident in earlier sections of this chapter, it continues to be a challenge not only to determine early-stage onset of CAVD but also to diagnose patients prior to signs of irreversible ECM remodeling with inevitable disease progression. Only within the past decade has aortic valve research begun to consider sexual dimorphisms in disease progression, another area that necessitates further investigation.

3 Biomaterials and Tissue Engineering Approaches in CAVD

3.1 Motivation for 3D Valve Models

Because the only treatment for CAVD is surgical replacement, the field has a long history of creating tissue-engineered heart valves (TEHVs) for use as tissue-based valve replacements [98, 99]. Dating back several decades, these studies have provided a foundation for heart valve biomaterials and tissue engineering, with materials ranging from synthetic elastomers to natural hydrogels to decellularized lab-grown tissues being examined as potential scaffolds. Although many large animal studies with these engineered tissues have yielded promising results, TEHVs have not yet reached approval for use in humans, as they tend to suffer from premature calcification and contraction.

However, the propensity of TEHVs to exhibit disease characteristics renders them highly useful in the context of in vitro disease modeling. Over the past 20 years, the heart valve tissue engineering field has experienced a significant shift, with the majority of engineered valve work now being focused on mechanistic disease studies, rather than direct valve replacement. This disease-mimicking focus may also yield nearer-term clinical impact compared to TEHVs for valve replacement, as disease-inspired tissue engineering has the potential to identify new treatment targets and act as a testing platform for various therapeutics.

Moreover, the use of tissue-engineered platforms to study CAVD is also rooted in logistical practicalities. CAVD is believed to have a "point of no return," after which disease progression may be too far gone to be halted. Thus, there is a need to study early stages of disease, but acquiring human valve samples with early disease is challenging, as valves are only replaced in late-stage disease. And, while animals serve as good models for many other diseases, their drawbacks in mimicking CAVD can be significant. Limitations for rodent models include lack of the three-layered valve leaflet structure; the strikingly different ECM structure and consequent biomechanics can make it difficult to extrapolate rodent-based findings to human systems [100]. Rabbit models are more favorable as they overcome the major limitation in murine valve structure, but they do not metabolize lipids in the same fashion as humans [100]. Porcine models are popular for cardiac-based research due to similarities in heart structure and lipid metabolism to humans, but high costs, low throughput, and prolonged duration for adequate research significantly limit the use of such animal models [101, 102]. Even when predisposed to CAVD development via genetic mutation, pigs tend to be 1–2 years old by the time they display early signs of CAVD [103], at which point their cost is several thousand dollars per animal.

In vitro systems include 2D and 3D models, which are much more cost-effective and provide more controlled platforms for cellular-level studies. Monolayer cell culture systems provide a cost-effective alternative to investigate behavioral changes in both VICs and VECs when cultured with disease stimuli. The resulting outputs can be measured through a variety of standardized bioassays such as ELISAs, PCR, and Western Blots. However, 2D models do not allow for cross-talk between cells growing in different planes within a tissue section and often are cultured on much stiffer platforms than is physiologically relevant, resulting in mechanical cues that may alter the behavior of the cells, providing data that may not correlate with natural disease progression. Due to these limitations, 3D models have gained popularity in tissue engineering research, especially in the context of CAVD in which the ECM plays a vital role in both cell homeostasis and disease progression. Table 2 summarizes some of the main approaches for bioengineering aortic heart valve tissues.

Table 2 Bioengineering approaches for modeling sex-based aortic valve disease

Approach	Relevance to aortic valve disease/scaffold design	Representative references
ECM-inspired hydrogels	Mimics native ECM composition; allows tuning of stiffness and enzymatic degradability; replicates GAG remodeling seen in CAVD; supports VIC/VEC interactions	Porras et al. [64], Buppathong et al. [117], Dahal et al. [110]
3D bioprinting	Enables leaflet-scale geometry and patient-specific structures; multi-material bioinks (e.g., Me-HA/Me-Gel) allow spatial control of VIC/VEC co-localization	Duan et al. [118], Bhandari et al. [119], Mathur et al. [120]
Photolithography/ micropatterning	Enables microscale anisotropy and stiffness gradients mimicking native leaflet fiber architecture; guides cellular alignment and mechanosensing	Zhang et al. [121, 122]
Electrospinning (and melt-electrowriting)	Produces fiber-aligned scaffolds with native-like anisotropic mechanics; hybrid systems (e.g., PCL + GelMA/CSMA) combine mechanical and bioactive features	Xu et al. [123], Stadelmann et al. [124]
Hydrogel coculture (VICs + VECs)	Captures endothelial–interstitial cross-talk; models shear-dependent regulation of VIC activation and sex-based differences in fibrotic signaling	Tandon et al. [125], Dahal et al. [110]
Microfluidics/ organ-on-a-chip	Allows fine control of shear stress, cyclic strain, and transmural gradients; enables real-time visualization of VIC/VEC response to mechanical cues	Wang et al. [126], Monteduro et al. [127]
Sex-based design anchors	Sex differences guide scaffold design: e.g., women show fibrosis-dominant phenotype; men show calcification-dominant phenotype; scaffold stiffness and mineralization cues can be tuned accordingly	DesJardin et al. [128], Matilla et al. [73], Mascherbauer et al. [129]

Summary of key bioengineering strategies developed to replicate the extracellular matrix composition, mechanical environment, and cellular interactions underlying CAVD progression. Approaches such as ECM-based hydrogels, advanced microfabrication, coculture, and organ-on-chip systems provide complementary insights into disease remodeling and sex-specific pathophysiology. ECM-inspired hydrogels mimic the fibrosis prominent in female-dominant disease, while 3D printing, photolithography, and electrospinning enable precise spatial and mechanical control to model valve microarchitecture. Coculture and microfluidic systems integrate dynamic shear, inflammatory signaling, and endothelial–interstitial crosstalk to capture both fibrotic and calcific processes observed across sexes

3.2 Design Considerations for 3D Valve Biomaterial Platforms

Stiffness tunability plays a pivotal role in regulating cell behavior, particularly that of VICs. Understanding how variations in substrate stiffness influence VIC function is essential for improving tissue-engineered models and developing interventions for CAVD. Under physiological conditions, VICs maintain a quiescent fibroblast-like state, ensuring ECM homeostasis. However, deviations in matrix stiffness can induce VIC activation, leading to pathological processes such as fibrosis and calcification. Studies have demonstrated that VICs cultured on stiff substrates (>5 kPa) exhibit increased myofibroblast activation, characterized by the upregulation of α-SMA and heightened ECM production [104]. This process is mediated by mechanotransduction signaling pathways, including focal adhesion kinase (FAK), Yes-associated protein (YAP), and TGF-β signaling [105]. Elevated stiffness also promotes VIC differentiation into osteoblast-like cells, contributing to the formation of calcific nodules within the valve.

Conversely, softer substrates (~3 kPa) maintain VICs in a native fibroblast-like phenotype, similar to that observed in healthy valve tissue, reducing pathological ECM remodeling and minimizing the risk of fibrosis [104]. By fine-tuning substrate stiffness, tissue-engineered models can be optimized to study early-stage disease processes or to develop interventions that prevent VIC activation. The ability to modulate stiffness in 3D tissue-engineered models has significant implications for both basic research and translational applications. Disease models with tunable mechanical properties enable researchers to simulate pathological conditions such as CAVD and test potential treatments targeting VIC mechanotransduction pathways. Additionally, bioengineered valve replacements with optimized stiffness properties hold promise for improving long-term functionality and integration with native tissues.

Another design consideration for engineered valve tissues is ECM composition and structure. For such a thin tissue, the ECM of the aortic valve is remarkably complex. Moreover, the valve ECM appears to be highly influential in modulating VIC phenotype and expression of disease hallmarks. For example, when tissue-engineered platforms were made to mimic the GAG enrichment that occurs in early CAVD, it was found that increased GAGs affected the secretion of angiogenic factors by the VICs and allowed for the deposition of oxLDL, which promoted a pro-inflammatory VIC phenotype [63]. Thus, engineered valve structures should also consider ECM composition and structure in their design.

3.3 *Scaffold Systems for Valve Tissue Engineering*

Hydrogel-based models have become the most common platform for mimicking the microenvironment of VICs. Hydrogels provide many benefits for in vitro modeling due to the diverse array of materials that can be utilized for fabrication, their ability to incorporate native ECM molecules, and their tunable stiffness. Decellularized scaffolds, in which aortic valves from other animals are decellularized and seeded with a controlled set of cells, have also been employed for 3D culturing of VICs. However, challenges in reintroducing VICs to the system has remained the limiting step in utilizing decellularized scaffolds for CAVD research [101].

Hydrogels made from unmodified natural materials, such as collagen or fibrin, support good cell viability and function, but typically lack adequate mechanical stiffness for mimicking a diseased valve environment [101]. Thus, hybrid hydrogels that incorporate both natural and synthetic elements have become commonly used for heart valve tissue engineering (TE). With respect to our scaffold design considerations, hybrid hydrogels can be tailored to include multiple native ECM components, as well as tuned to possess a range of stiffnesses. By adjusting crosslinking density, polymer composition, and percent ECM incorporation, scaffolds that resemble the ECM and mechanics of the native valve environment can be created.

Methacrylated gelatin (GelMA)-based gels are the most prevalent scaffold for in vitro 3D modeling due to their biocompatibility and tunable mechanical properties, allowing for more accurate recapitulation of the native valve [101, 106]. Relevant GAGs and PGs can also be incorporated into these engineered scaffolds to provide more appropriate chemical characteristics to the microenvironment. Isolated VICs and VECs can then be encapsulated in or seeded onto the crosslinked hydrogels, creating cocultures to assess cell and ECM behavior under diseased or healthy conditions [101, 102, 107]. Stiffness of GelMA-based hydrogels can be controlled through the amount of methacrylic anhydride added during the synthesis of the material, with higher concentrations typically leading to higher stiffnesses of the final, formed hydrogel [106]. In addition, photoinitiator concentration and exposure time to adequate light influence hydrogel stiffness. GelMA also has the advantage of being biodegradable, allowing cells to remodel their microenvironment through secretion of MMPs as they are naturally inclined to do in response to external stimuli [101, 106].

Recent advances in biofabrication techniques, including 3D bioprinting and electrospinning, have further enhanced the ability to generate spatially heterogeneous scaffolds that replicate the layered architecture of the aortic valve (Fig. 3) [108]. These models provide an invaluable platform for investigating VIC behavior under physiologically relevant conditions and testing therapeutic strategies aimed at modulating cellular responses to mechanical stimuli. Biofabrication techniques currently in practice include standard pipetting into disc-shaped molds, bioprinting, lithography, and microfluidics [106]. 3D-bioprinting may be particularly attractive for recapitulating the complex ECM layering of the valve, as it allows for deliberate placement of hydrogels and encapsulated cells, although maintaining viability remains a hurdle. Immohr et al. revealed a bioprinting technique in 2023 that made progress on this limitation, achieving >60% cell viability over a period of 21 days in culture [107]. The researchers also tested a sandwich-and-tube design in which VECs were seeded on top of, or on either side of, encapsulated VICs, providing further physiological relevance for better understanding VIC–VEC interactions during CAVD [107]. Lithography allows for specified patterning of materials and the capacity to build 3D structures in a bottom-up approach, resulting in homogenous cell-laden structures [106]. Stereolithography allows for automated scale-up, an advantage when compared to other hydrogel fabrication methods; however, it is limited to one resin type, thus decreasing the ability to incorporate key GAGs and PGs into the model's design [106].

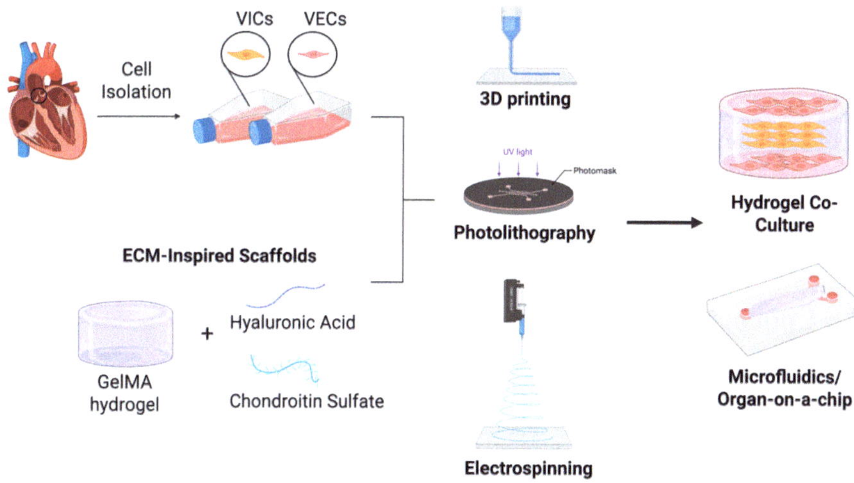

Fig. 3 Schematic overview of advanced bioengineering approaches to model calcific aortic valve disease (CAVD). Valvular interstitial cells (VICs) and valvular endothelial cells (VECs) are isolated from native heart valves and incorporated into biomimetic platforms. Example materials include hydrogels composed of GelMA, hyaluronic acid, and chondroitin sulfate, which can be fabricated into 3D constructs using techniques such as 3D printing, photolithography, and electrospinning. The resulting systems support coculture of valve cell types within structured microenvironments, enabling development of hydrogel-based models and integration into microfluidic or organ-on-a-chip platforms for disease modeling and mechanistic studies. (Created in https://BioRender.com)

Current research efforts utilizing 3D bioengineered CAVD tissues strive to further understanding of how mechanical stresses and chemical stimuli affect VIC behavior, subsequently leading to these cells remodeling the surrounding ECM. Given the importance of ECM components, many researchers have incorporated GAGs such as hyaluronic acid (HA) and chondroitin sulfate (CS) to investigate the role of these molecules in maladaptive behaviors in valve cells. For example, a coculture model containing GAGs was compared to stiffness-varied collagen gels, with the latter reported to have a more significant impact on ALP activity [109]. The presence of CS in the model significantly increased calcified nodule formation without needing external pro-osteogenic minerals [109, 110]. HA seems to play a more homeostatic role in the presence of VECs in hydrogel models while inclusion of HA on polyacrylamide hydrogels results in increased calcification [110, 111].

3D hydrogels have also been used to develop platforms for therapeutic testing. For example, a high-throughput screening model with the capacity to study VIC behavior in response to stimuli and mechanical stress was recently described [112]. This novel platform uses a 48-well plate within which VICs encapsulated in collagen type I hydrogels are formed around two PDMS posts. When exposed to osteogenic growth media, visible contraction of the neo-tissue was observed and allowed for calculation of stress measurements. Immunofluorescent staining of the neo-tissues also indicated patterned αSMA presence, further indicating the importance of mechanobiology in the behavior of VICs [112]. Valve-on-chip models are a more recent development, incorporating another layer of physiological relevance through shear stress and tensile strain applied to cells encapsulated within hydrogels [113, 114]. Bioengineered tissues continue to evolve at a rapid rate and, with each novel technique reported in literature, significant insights into CAVD disease progression and potential therapeutic targets are unveiled for further discovery.

4 Conclusion and Future Directions

Over the past 20 years, substantial progress has been made to understand the cellular and molecular level processes that contribute to the progression of CAVD to aortic valve stenosis. It is evident that not only age but also sex differences manifest in varied cellular pathways, leading to more calcium deposition in male valves versus fibrotic tissue development in female valves. Driving factors leading to valve thickening include damage to valve endothelial lining, activation of typically quiescent VICs, increased ECM deposition of molecules such as collagen and chondroitin sulfate, and the development of an inflammatory environment through recruitment of immune cells. Adding to these complexities are both intrinsic (chromosomal) cellular-scale sex differences as well as sex hormone-driven cell behaviors.

Tissue engineering approaches are uniquely able to allow for separation of the many variables that influence CAVD pathogenesis, enabling researchers to gain targeted mechanistic insight that is not possible using in vivo specimens. Utilizing biomimetic 3D platforms to study CAVD pathogenesis continues to shed light on critical pathways that may lead to not only therapeutic targets but also markers for earlier diagnostics. Future directions for these biomaterials may include closer attention to mimicking not just ECM composition but also ECM architecture, as the arrangement of collagen fibers can influence cell behaviors [115]. The next generations of scaffold environments could also include stiffness gradients to better replicate the heterogeneous nature of the valve ECM. Incorporating dynamic mechanical cues, such as cyclic stretch and fluid shear stress, may further enhance the physiological relevance of these models and provide deeper insights into VIC mechanobiology. Additionally, as we uncover more about sex differences in valvular ECM composition, creating biomimetic environments may entail construction of sex-specific scaffolds in order to accurately represent native tissue differences [116]. Finally, utilizing sex-specific cultures along with hormone treatment regimens could be critical for further distinguishing pathophysiology in males versus females and lead to more individualized diagnosis and treatment downstream.

Acknowledgments The authors were supported by funding from the National Institutes of Health (R01 HL172046 to K.S.M.). Figures were created using BioRender software.

References

1. Sahasakul Y, et al. Age-related changes in aortic and mitral valve thickness: implications for two-dimensional echocardiography based on an autopsy study of 200 normal human hearts. Am J Cardiol. 1988;62:424–30.
2. Kraler S, et al. Calcific aortic valve disease: from molecular and cellular mechanisms to medical therapy. Eur Heart J. 2022;43:683–97.
3. Scott AJ, et al. Engineering the aortic valve extracellular matrix through stages of development, aging, and disease. J Mol Cell Cardiol. 2021;161:1–8.
4. Chen JH, Simmons CA. Cell-matrix interactions in the pathobiology of calcific aortic valve disease: critical roles for matricellular, matricrine, and matrix mechanics cues. Circ Res. 2011;108:1510–24.
5. Fayet C, Bendeck MP, Gotlieb AI. Cardiac valve interstitial cells secrete fibronectin and form fibrillar adhesions in response to injury. Cardiovasc Pathol. 2007;16:203–11.
6. Zhang XW, et al. Twist-related protein 1 negatively regulated osteoblastic transdifferentiation of human aortic valve interstitial cells by directly inhibiting runt-related transcription factor 2. J Thorac Cardiovasc Surg. 2014;148:1700–1708 e1.
7. McCoy CM, Nicholas DQ, Masters KS. Sex-related differences in gene expression by porcine aortic valvular interstitial cells. PLoS One. 2012;7:e39980.
8. Simon LR, et al. Cellular-scale sex differences in extracellular matrix remodeling by valvular interstitial cells. Heart Vessel. 2023;38:122–30.
9. Tiraplegui C, et al. Sex differences in aortic valve inflammation and remodeling in chronic severe aortic regurgitation. Am J Physiol Heart Circ Physiol. 2025;328:H693–710.
10. Aguado BA, et al. Genes that escape X chromosome inactivation modulate sex differences in valve myofibroblasts. Circulation. 2022;145:513–30.
11. Wang H, Leinwand LA, Anseth KS. Cardiac valve cells and their microenvironment–insights from in vitro studies. Nat Rev Cardiol. 2014;11:715–27.
12. Fan L, et al. Beyond VICs: shedding light on the overlooked VECs in calcific aortic valve disease. Biomed Pharmacother. 2024;178:117143.
13. Deb N, Lacerda CMR. Valvular endothelial cell response to the mechanical environment-a review. Cell Biochem Biophys. 2021;79:695–709.
14. Ma X, et al. Endothelial-to-mesenchymal transition in calcific aortic valve disease. Acta Cardiol Sin. 2020;36:183–94.
15. Nelson V, et al. Angiogenic secretion profile of valvular interstitial cells varies with cellular sex and phenotype. Front Cardiovasc Med. 2021;8:736303.
16. Mudrovcic N, et al. Endothelial maintenance in health and disease: importance of sex differences. Pharmacol Res. 2017;119:48–60.
17. Robert J. Sex differences in vascular endothelial cells. Atherosclerosis. 2023;384:117278.
18. Hartman RJG, et al. Intrinsic transcriptomic sex differences in human endothelial cells at birth and in adults are associated with coronary artery disease targets. Sci Rep. 2020;10:12367.
19. Shin J, et al. Unraveling the role of sex in endothelial cell dysfunction: evidence from lineage tracing mice and cultured cells. Arterioscler Thromb Vasc Biol. 2024;44:238–53.
20. Ospina JA, Krause DN, Duckles SP. 17beta-estradiol increases rat cerebrovascular prostacyclin synthesis by elevating cyclooxygenase-1 and prostacyclin synthase. Stroke. 2002;33:600–5.
21. Marcantoni E, et al. Effects of estrogen on endothelial prostanoid production and cyclooxygenase-2 and heme oxygenase-1 expression. Prostaglandins Other Lipid Mediat. 2012;98:122–8.
22. Burek M, et al. Claudin-5 as a novel estrogen target in vascular endothelium. Arterioscler Thromb Vasc Biol. 2010;30:298–304.
23. Shin JA, et al. Activation of classical estrogen receptor subtypes reduces tight junction disruption of brain endothelial cells under ischemia/reperfusion injury. Free Radic Biol Med. 2016;92:78–89.

24. Liu P, et al. Testosterone promotes tube formation of endothelial cells isolated from veins via activation of Smad1 protein. Mol Cell Endocrinol. 2017;446:21–31.
25. Morales DE, et al. Estrogen promotes angiogenic activity in human umbilical vein endothelial cells in vitro and in a murine model. Circulation. 1995;91:755–63.
26. Shapero K, et al. Reciprocal interactions between mitral valve endothelial and interstitial cells reduce endothelial-to-mesenchymal transition and myofibroblastic activation. J Mol Cell Cardiol. 2015;80:175–85.
27. Rutkovskiy A, et al. Valve interstitial cells: the key to understanding the pathophysiology of heart valve calcification. J Am Heart Assoc. 2017;6:e006339.
28. Vaslef SN, Roberts WC. Early descriptions of aortic valve stenosis. Am Heart J. 1993;125: 1465–74.
29. Côté N, Pibarot P, Clavel MA. Aortic stenosis: what is the role of aging processes? Aging (Albany NY). 2019;11:1085–6.
30. DiLoreto R, Murphy CT. The cell biology of aging. Mol Biol Cell. 2015;26:4524–31.
31. Muchir A, et al. Identification of mutations in the gene encoding lamins A/C in autosomal dominant limb girdle muscular dystrophy with atrioventricular conduction disturbances (LGMD1B). Hum Mol Genet. 2000;9:1453–9.
32. Nikolova-Krstevski V, et al. Nesprin-1 and actin contribute to nuclear and cytoskeletal defects in lamin A/C-deficient cardiomyopathy. J Mol Cell Cardiol. 2011;50:479–86.
33. Oomen PJ, et al. Age-dependent changes of stress and strain in the human heart valve and their relation with collagen remodeling. Acta Biomater. 2016;29:161–9.
34. van Geemen D, et al. Age-dependent changes in geometry, tissue composition and mechanical properties of fetal to adult cryopreserved human heart valves. PLoS One. 2016;11:e0149020.
35. Kohn JC, Lampi MC, Reinhart-King CA. Age-related vascular stiffening: causes and consequences. Front Genet. 2015;6:112.
36. Ringstrom N, et al. Framing heartaches: the cardiac ecm and the effects of age. Int J Mol Sci. 2023;24:4713.
37. Tvaroska I. Glycosylation modulates the structure and functions of collagen: a review. Molecules. 2024;29:1417.
38. Seki A, Fishbein MC. Chapter 2 – Age-related cardiovascular changes and diseases. In: Buja LM, Butany J, editors. Cardiovascular pathology. 4th ed. San Diego: Academic Press; 2016. p. 57–83.
39. Kular JK, Basu S, Sharma RI. The extracellular matrix: structure, composition, age-related differences, tools for analysis and applications for tissue engineering. J Tissue Eng. 2014;5: 2041731414557112.
40. Damodarasamy M, et al. Collagen extracts derived from young and aged mice demonstrate different structural properties and cellular effects in three-dimensional gels. J Gerontol A Biol Sci Med Sci. 2010;65:209–18.
41. Stephens EH, Chu CK, Grande-Allen KJ. Valve proteoglycan content and glycosaminoglycan fine structure are unique to microstructure, mechanical load and age: relevance to an age-specific tissue-engineered heart valve. Acta Biomater. 2008;4:1148–60.
42. Duan B, et al. Active tissue stiffness modulation controls valve interstitial cell phenotype and osteogenic potential in 3D culture. Acta Biomater. 2016;36:42–54.
43. Yip CY, et al. Calcification by valve interstitial cells is regulated by the stiffness of the extracellular matrix. Arterioscler Thromb Vasc Biol. 2009;29:936–42.
44. St Pierre SR, Peirlinck M, Kuhl E. Sex matters: a comprehensive comparison of female and male hearts. Front Physiol. 2022;13:831179.
45. Parks RJ, Howlett SE. Sex differences in mechanisms of cardiac excitation-contraction coupling. Pflugers Arch. 2013;465:747–63.
46. Wittnich C, et al. Sex differences in myocardial metabolism and cardiac function: an emerging concept. Pflugers Arch. 2013;465:719–29.
47. Iorga A, et al. The protective role of estrogen and estrogen receptors in cardiovascular disease and the controversial use of estrogen therapy. Biol Sex Differ. 2017;8:33.

48. Avouac J, et al. Estrogens counteract the profibrotic effects of TGF-β and their inhibition exacerbates experimental dermal fibrosis. J Invest Dermatol. 2020;140:593–601.e7.
49. Willemars MMA, et al. Evaluation of the interaction of sex hormones and cardiovascular function and health. Curr Heart Fail Rep. 2022;19:200–12.
50. Broeders W, et al. Innate immune cells in the pathophysiology of calcific aortic valve disease: lessons to be learned from atherosclerotic cardiovascular disease? Basic Res Cardiol. 2022;117:28.
51. Stevenson JC. Mechanisms whereby oestrogens influence arterial health. Eur J Obstet Gynecol Reprod Biol. 1996;65:39–42.
52. Cramariuc D, et al. Sex differences in cardiovascular outcome during progression of aortic valve stenosis. Heart. 2015;101:209–14.
53. Hulin A, et al. Advances in pathophysiology of calcific aortic valve disease propose novel molecular therapeutic targets. Front Cardiovasc Med. 2018;5:21.
54. Baratchi S, et al. Transcatheter aortic valve implantation represents an anti-inflammatory therapy via reduction of shear stress-induced, piezo-1-mediated monocyte activation. Circulation. 2020;142:1092–105.
55. Grim JC, et al. Secreted factors from proinflammatory macrophages promote an osteoblast-like phenotype in valvular interstitial cells. Arterioscler Thromb Vasc Biol. 2020;40:e296–308.
56. Jiang S, et al. Testosterone attenuates hypoxia-induced hypertension by affecting NRF1-mediated transcriptional regulation of ET-1 and ACE. Hypertens Res. 2021;44:1395–405.
57. Wakasugi M, et al. The effects of sex hormones on the synthesis of prostacyclin (PGI2) by vascular tissues. Prostaglandins. 1989;37:401–10.
58. Di Vito A, et al. Extracellular matrix in calcific aortic valve disease: architecture, dynamic and perspectives. Int J Mol Sci. 2021;22:913.
59. Alushi B, et al. Calcific aortic valve disease-natural history and future therapeutic strategies. Front Pharmacol. 2020;11:685.
60. Liu Z, et al. Endothelial cell-derived tetrahydrobiopterin prevents aortic valve calcification. Eur Heart J. 2022;43:1652–64.
61. Anousakis-Vlachochristou N, et al. Focusing on the native matrix proteins in calcific aortic valve stenosis. JACC Basic Transl Sci. 2023;8:1028–39.
62. Otto CM, et al. Characterization of the early lesion of 'degenerative' valvular aortic stenosis. Histological and immunohistochemical studies. Circulation. 1994;90:844–53.
63. Porras AM, et al. Creation of disease-inspired biomaterial environments to mimic pathological events in early calcific aortic valve disease. Proc Natl Acad Sci USA. 2018;115:E363–71.
64. Hutson HN, et al. Calcific aortic valve disease is associated with layer-specific alterations in collagen architecture. PLoS One. 2016;11:e0163858.
65. Baugh L, et al. Influence of collagen fiber architecture on calcific aortic valve disease progression. In: 2014 40th annual northeast bioengineering conference (NEBEC). IEEE; 2014.
66. Korossis S. Structure-function relationship of heart valves in health and disease. In: Kırali K, editor. Structural insufficiency anomalies in cardiac valves. IntechOpen: Rijeka; 2018.
67. Edep ME, et al. Matrix metalloproteinase expression in nonrheumatic aortic stenosis. Cardiovasc Pathol. 2000;9:281–6.
68. Fondard O, et al. Extracellular matrix remodelling in human aortic valve disease: the role of matrix metalloproteinases and their tissue inhibitors. Eur Heart J. 2005;26:1333–41.
69. Kaden JJ, et al. Expression and activity of matrix metalloproteinase-2 in calcific aortic stenosis. Z Kardiol. 2004;93:124–30.
70. Scott Patterson AJ, et al. Extracellular matrix dynamics in aortic valve health and disease: insights into fibrocalcific remodeling and creation of biomimetic platforms. J Heart Valve Soc. 2024;1:10.1177/30494826241296675.
71. Voisine M, et al. Age, sex, and valve phenotype differences in fibro-calcific remodeling of calcified aortic valve. J Am Heart Assoc. 2020;9:e015610.
72. Matilla L, et al. Sex-differences in aortic stenosis: mechanistic insights and clinical implications. Front Cardiovasc Med. 2022;9:818371.

73. Vijayakumar A, Wang M, Kailasam S. The senescent heart-“Age doth wither its infinite variety”. Int J Mol Sci. 2024;25:3581.
74. Perrotta I, et al. New evidence for a critical role of elastin in calcification of native heart valves: immunohistochemical and ultrastructural study with literature review. Histopathology. 2011;59:504–13.
75. Halsey G, et al. Role of elastic fiber degradation in disease pathogenesis. Biochim Biophys Acta Mol Basis Dis. 2023;1869:166706.
76. Zhang B, Miller VM, Miller JD. Influences of sex and estrogen in arterial and valvular calcification. Front Endocrinol (Lausanne). 2019;10:622.
77. Dweck MR, Boon NA, Newby DE. Calcific aortic stenosis: a disease of the valve and the myocardium. J Am Coll Cardiol. 2012;60:1854–63.
78. New SE, Aikawa E. Molecular imaging insights into early inflammatory stages of arterial and aortic valve calcification. Circ Res. 2011;108:1381–91.
79. Marshall JS, et al. An introduction to immunology and immunopathology. Allergy Asthma Clin Immunol. 2018;14:49.
80. Tintut Y, Hsu JJ, Demer LL. Lipoproteins in cardiovascular calcification: potential targets and challenges. Front Cardiovasc Med. 2018;5:172.
81. Hu J, et al. Lipoprotein(a), a lethal player in calcific aortic valve disease. Front Cell Dev Biol. 2022;10:812368.
82. Koschinsky ML, Boffa MB. Oxidized phospholipid modification of lipoprotein(a): epidemiology, biochemistry and pathophysiology. Atherosclerosis. 2022;349:92–100.
83. Zhu X, et al. Oxidized phospholipids facilitate calcific aortic valve disease by elevating ATF4 through the PERK/eIF2alpha axis. Aging (Albany NY). 2023;15:6834–47.
84. Salim MT, et al. miR-214 is stretch-sensitive in aortic valve and inhibits aortic valve calcification. Ann Biomed Eng. 2019;47:1106–15.
85. Raberin A, et al. Women at altitude: sex-related physiological responses to exercise in hypoxia. Sports Med. 2024;54:271–87.
86. Georgy M, et al. Role of hypoxia inducible factor HIF-1alpha in heart valves. Glob Cardiol Sci Pract. 2023;2023:e202309.
87. Parra Izquierdo I, et al. A novel non-hypoxic and sex-biased mechanism of HIF-1alpha in human aortic valve interstitial cells: crosstalk between JAK-STAT and TLR pathways. Eur Heart J. 2017;39:P5363.
88. Abe H, Semba H, Takeda N. The roles of hypoxia signaling in the pathogenesis of cardiovascular diseases. J Atheroscler Thromb. 2017;24:884–94.
89. Imtiyaz HZ, Simon MC. Hypoxia-inducible factors as essential regulators of inflammation. Curr Top Microbiol Immunol. 2010;345:105–20.
90. Parra-Izquierdo I, et al. Lipopolysaccharide and interferon-gamma team up to activate HIF-1alpha via STAT1 in normoxia and exhibit sex differences in human aortic valve interstitial cells. Biochim Biophys Acta Mol Basis Dis. 2019;1865:2168–79.
91. Lorell BH, Carabello BA. Left ventricular hypertrophy: pathogenesis, detection, and prognosis. Circulation. 2000;102:470–9.
92. Coeytaux RR, et al. Percutaneous heart valve replacement for aortic stenosis: state of the evidence. Ann Intern Med. 2010;153:314–24.
93. Simard L, et al. Sex-related discordance between aortic valve calcification and hemodynamic severity of aortic stenosis: is valvular fibrosis the explanation? Circ Res. 2017;120:681–91.
94. Strange JE, et al. Mortality at one year after transcatheter aortic valve replacement – relation of age and comorbidities. Int J Cardiol Heart Vasc. 2022;43:101157.
95. Caponcello MG, et al. Gender differences in aortic valve replacement: is surgical aortic valve replacement riskier and transcatheter aortic valve replacement safer in women than in men? J Thorac Dis. 2020;12:3737–46.
96. Genereux P, et al. The mortality burden of untreated aortic stenosis. J Am Coll Cardiol. 2023;82:2101–9.

97. Shvartz V, et al. Predictors of mortality following aortic valve replacement in aortic stenosis patients. Pathophysiology. 2022;29:106–17.
98. Albert BJ, Butcher JT. Future prospects in the tissue engineering of heart valves: a focus on the role of stem cells. Expert Opin Biol Ther. 2023;23:553–64.
99. Mendelson K, Schoen FJ. Heart valve tissue engineering: concepts, approaches, progress, and challenges. Ann Biomed Eng. 2006;34:1799–819.
100. Sider KL, Blaser MC, Simmons CA. Animal models of calcific aortic valve disease. Int J Inflamm. 2011;2011:364310.
101. Zhu Z, et al. Models for calcific aortic valve disease in vivo and in vitro. Cell Regen. 2024;13: 6.
102. Bogdanova M, et al. Models and techniques to study aortic valve calcification in vitro, ex vivo and in vivo. An overview. Front Pharmacol. 2022;13:835825.
103. Porras AM, et al. Development of aortic valve disease in familial hypercholesterolemic swine: implications for elucidating disease etiology. J Am Heart Assoc. 2015;4:e002254.
104. Ma H, et al. Myofibroblastic activation of valvular interstitial cells is modulated by spatial variations in matrix elasticity and its organization. Biomaterials. 2017;131:131–44.
105. Hjortnaes J, et al. Valvular interstitial cells suppress calcification of valvular endothelial cells. Atherosclerosis. 2015;242:251–60.
106. Klotz BJ, et al. Gelatin-methacryloyl hydrogels: towards biofabrication-based tissue repair. Trends Biotechnol. 2016;34:394–407.
107. Immohr MB, et al. Three-dimensional bioprinting of ovine aortic valve endothelial and interstitial cells for the development of multicellular tissue engineered tissue constructs. Bioengineering (Basel). 2023;10:787.
108. Freystetter B, et al. Combining 3D-printing and electrospinning to manufacture biomimetic heart valve leaflets. J Vis Exp. 2022;181:63604.
109. Bramsen JA, et al. Glycosaminoglycans affect endothelial to mesenchymal transformation, proliferation, and calcification in a 3D model of aortic valve disease. Front Cardiovasc Med. 2022;9:975732.
110. Dahal S, et al. Chondroitin sulfate promotes interstitial cell activation and calcification in an in vitro model of the aortic valve. Cardiovasc Eng Technol. 2022;13:481–94.
111. Baugh L, et al. Knockdown of CD44 expression decreases valve interstitial cell calcification in vitro. Am J Physiol Heart Circ Physiol. 2019;317:H26–36.
112. Shih JY, et al. Biomechanical remodeling of aortic valve interstitial cells during calcified lesion formation in vitro. Ann Biomed Eng. 2024;52:1270–9.
113. Mendoza M, et al. Shear and endothelial induced late-stage calcific aortic valve disease-on-a-chip develops calcium phosphate mineralizations. Lab Chip. 2022;22:1374–85.
114. Tandon I, et al. A three-dimensional valve-on-chip microphysiological system implicates cell cycle progression, cholesterol metabolism and protein homeostasis in early calcific aortic valve disease progression. Acta Biomater. 2024;186:167–84.
115. Abbaspour A, et al. Collagen fiber density observed in metastatic ovarian cancer promotes tumor cell adhesion. Acta Biomater. 2025;200:299–312.
116. Borelli A, Masters K. Developing sex-accurate cell culture environments. Nat Rev Bioeng. 2024;3:2–3.
117. Bupphathong S, et al. Gelatin methacrylate hydrogel for tissue engineering applications-a review on material modifications. Pharmaceuticals (Basel). 2022;15:171.
118. Duan B, et al. Three-dimensional printed trileaflet valve conduits using biological hydrogels and human valve interstitial cells. Acta Biomater. 2014;10:1836–46.
119. Bhandari S, et al. Trends and challenges in the development of 3D-printed heart valves and other cardiac implants: a review of current advances. Cureus. 2023;15:e43204.
120. Mathur V, et al. Innovative bioinks for 3D bioprinting: exploring technological potential and regulatory challenges. J Tissue Eng. 2025;16:20417314241308022.
121. Zhang X, et al. Application of hydrogels in heart valve tissue engineering. J Long-Term Eff Med Implants. 2015;25:105–34.

122. Zhang X, et al. Integrating valve-inspired design features into poly(ethylene glycol) hydrogel scaffolds for heart valve tissue engineering. Acta Biomater. 2015;14:11–21.
123. Xu C, et al. Melt-electrowriting-enabled anisotropic scaffolds loaded with valve interstitial cells for heart valve tissue engineering. J Nanobiotechnol. 2024;22:378.
124. Stadelmann K, et al. Development of a bi-layered cryogenic electrospun polylactic acid scaffold to study calcific aortic valve disease in a 3D co-culture model. Acta Biomater. 2022;140:364–78.
125. Tandon I, et al. Aortic valve cell microenvironment: considerations for developing a valve-on-chip. Biophys Rev (Melville). 2021;2:041303.
126. Wang X, et al. Phenotype transformation of aortic valve interstitial cells due to applied shear stresses within a microfluidic chip. Ann Biomed Eng. 2017;45:2269–80.
127. Monteduro AG, et al. Organs-on-chips technologies – a guide from disease models to opportunities for drug development. Biosens Bioelectron. 2023;231:115271.
128. DesJardin JT, et al. Sex differences and similarities in valvular heart disease. Circ Res. 2022;130:455–73.
129. Mascherbauer J, et al. Sex-related differences in severe native valvular heart disease: the ESC-EORP valvular heart disease II survey. Eur Heart J. 2024;45:3818–33.

Drug Delivery

Engineering Biomaterial-Based Drug Delivery Technologies to Interface with the Placenta During Pregnancy

Kelsey L. Swingle

Abstract Many biomaterial-based delivery technologies–such as inorganic, polymeric, and lipid-based nanoparticles, as well as chemically-modified drugs–have successfully navigated the pathway from invention to the clinic for therapeutic applications including cancer, genetic disorders, autoimmune diseases, and imaging. Although, the field has yet to witness the translational potential of these technologies in the context of obstetric disorders during pregnancy. In this chapter, we discuss recent preclinical research advances at the interface of biomaterials science and placental biology. First, in an effort to highlight the opportunity to repurpose clinically-approved technologies toward obstetric applications, we provide an overview of various biomaterial-based delivery technologies and their current regulatory status. We then discuss efforts to engineer delivery technologies to interface with the placenta in several ways: (i) to enable delivery of a therapeutic payload to the placenta itself, (ii) to harness the placenta as a biological barrier and enable drug retention in maternal circulation, or (iii) to facilitate transplacental drug transport to enable therapeutic payload delivery to the fetus in utero. Finally, we examine the existing literature to date that explores the therapeutic efficacy of these engineered biomaterial-based delivery technologies to treat obstetric conditions such as pre-eclampsia, fetal growth restriction, and gestational trophoblast disease.

Keywords Drug delivery · Placenta · Nanoparticles · Biomaterials science · Pregnancy · Reproductive biology · Nucleic acids · Biological barriers · Biodistribution · Physicochemical properties

---

K. L. Swingle (✉)
Department of Bioengineering, Rice University, Houston, TX, USA
e-mail: ks282@rice.edu

S. G. Zambuto, M. L. Oyen (eds.), *Biomaterials for Women's Health Engineering*,
https://doi.org/10.1007/978-3-032-10745-9_18

1 Introduction to Biomaterial-Based Delivery Technologies and Their Pathway from Invention to the Clinic

There are a wide variety of biomaterial-based technologies that have a rich history in the preclinical and clinical settings for in vivo drug delivery, including nanoparticles (NPs), modified drugs, hydrogels, films, patches, implants, and injectables [1], though many of these technologies have administration route- or application-specific use cases that are not relevant here in the context of pregnancy and the placenta. In this chapter, we will mainly discuss biomaterial-based modifications to drugs such as small molecules and nucleic acids (Sect. 1.1), as well as different NP technologies and their subclasses—that is, inorganic, polymeric, and lipid-based NPs (Sect. 1.2).

We highlight the pathway of these drug delivery technologies from invention to the clinic (Fig. 1). While biomaterial-modified drugs and NPs have been limitedly explored in the context of pregnancy for delivery to the placenta, many of these platforms have demonstrated safety and efficacy in human patients, enabling their regulatory approval for other therapeutic applications. Redesigning and repurposing these technologies for applications in pregnant patients presents a unique opportunity to accelerate the translation of biomaterial-based drugs to treat a range of obstetric disorders.

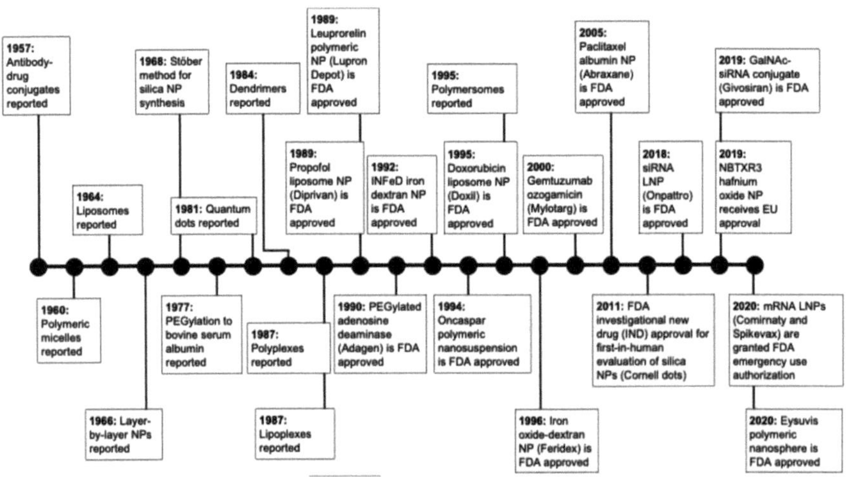

Fig. 1 From invention to approval: a timeline of biomaterial-based drug delivery technologies. The path from discovery to translation in humans had spanned more than 60 years, with many therapeutic technologies garnering U.S. Food and Drug Administration (FDA) approval over the last several decades

1.1 Biomaterial-Modified Drugs

While some therapeutic payloads, including small molecule drugs, can be effective when administered as simple intravenous (*i.v.*) injections or oral tablet formulations, biomaterial modifications have been extensively explored and implemented in the clinical setting. In particular, biomaterial-modified drugs offer several advantages in terms of increased trafficking to a target tissue of interest, prolonged circulation time, and improved stability compared to their free-drug counterparts. In this section, we will discuss the evolution of antibody–drug conjugates, PEGylation, and siRNA conjugates.

1.1.1 Antibody–Drug Conjugates

Over 100 years ago, Paul Ehrlich proposed the concept of a "magic bullet," which has sparked a century-long quest for the fields of science and medicine to develop personalized drugs that specifically target cancer cells [2]. At the time, Ehrlich proposed "magic bullet" technologies that we now know as monoclonal antibodies and antibody–drug conjugates: "antibodies are in a way magic bullets that identify and target themselves without harming the organism" [2]. This vision paved the way for others to develop personalized cancer immunotherapies, including Georges Mathé, who showed the utility of antibody–drug conjugates in 1957 against L1210 leukemia cancer cells [3]. In this work, Mathé coupled the chemotherapeutic small molecule drug methotrexate to an anti-leukemia 1210 immunoglobulin and demonstrated anti-cancer effects [3].

For antibody–drug conjugates, the pathway to the clinic was accelerated in 1975 with the successful production of monoclonal antibodies [3]. The first Food and Drug Administration (FDA) approved antibody–drug conjugate (gemtuzumab ozogamicin, also known as Mylotarg) was brought to market in 2000 to treat patients with $CD33^{+}$ acute myeloid leukemia. Now, there are more than a dozen antibody–drug conjugates on the market for various cancer conditions, demonstrating the untapped potential for this technology beyond cancer immunotherapy toward the treatment of disorders during pregnancy.

1.1.2 PEGylation

A tremendous breakthrough for the field of drug delivery was the discovery and implementation of PEGylation. This technology is based on the covalent attachment of the hydrophilic polymer poly(ethylene glycol) to drugs or NP platforms in an effort to improve biocompatibility, reduce protein adsorption, and increase circulation times [4]. Given its hydrophilic nature, water tends to colocalize with PEG molecules, creating a water sheath around the PEGylated drug or NP; as it is thermodynamically unfavorable to displace these colocalized water molecules, PEGylation consequently reduces protein adsorption on the drug or NP [4].

PEGylation was initially reported in 1977, where Abraham Abuchowski and Frank Davis demonstrated its covalent attachment to bovine serum albumin [5]. The authors compared the pharmacokinetic profiles of free albumin and PEGylated albumin following *i.v.* administration in rabbits and observed reduced immunogenicity—as measured via the presence of anti-albumin antibodies in serum—for the modified albumin treatment [5]. The first drug product containing PEG was introduced to the clinic less than two decades later; Adagen or PEGylated adenosine deaminase was brought to market in 1990 [4]. More recently, the field has begun to explore other synthetic, hydrophilic polymers to serve as PEG alternatives due to concerns over anti-PEG antibodies, which are particularly relevant in the context of redosing [6, 7]. Discussions regarding anti-PEG antibodies were highly relevant following the global COVID-19 vaccination campaign, as over 1 billion doses of SARS-CoV-2 mRNA vaccines containing PEGylated lipids were administered around the world [7].

1.1.3 siRNA Conjugates

RNA interference (i.e., gene silencing and RNAi) via small interfering RNA (siRNA) delivery was reported in 1998 by Andrew Fire and Craig Mello [8]. In this work, the authors demonstrated more effective gene interference using double-stranded RNA than either single-stranded RNA molecule in the nematode *Caenorhabditis elegans* model. A few years later, RNAi using 21-nucleotide siRNA duplexes was reported by the laboratory of Thomas Tuschl in human embryonic kidney (HEK-293) and human cervical cancer (HeLa) immortalized mammalian cells [9]. Shortly after publishing their seminal article, Fire and Mello were awarded the Nobel Prize in Physiology or Medicine in 2006.

These discoveries and early preclinical successes launched tremendous interest and funding for RNAi over the last two decades. Alnylam—a leading biotechnology company in RNAi—was founded in 2002 by Thomas Tuschl and others, aiming to translate siRNA therapeutics to the clinic. Although, the field rapidly realized that upon systemic administration, unmodified or slightly modified siRNA constructs induced undesirable toxicities and limited gene knockdown in the target cells of interest [10]. This spurred significant efforts to modify the therapeutic siRNA molecules to improve stability, which was partially accelerated by the nucleic acid chemistries that had been previously developed for antisense oligonucleotide therapeutics [10].

Simultaneously, the field explored the design of siRNA conjugates to promote intracellular nucleic acid delivery to target tissues of interest, namely, the liver. As liver hepatocytes abundantly express the asialoglycoprotein receptor (ASGPR), researchers conjugated siRNA to *N*-acetylgalactosamine (GalNAc)—the ligand for ASGPR—and demonstrated in vivo siRNA-mediated gene silencing in 2014 [11]. A few years later, in 2019, a GalNAc–siRNA conjugate was approved by the U.S. FDA (Alnylam's Givosiran) for the treatment of acute hepatic porphyria. Over the last several years, several other siRNA conjugate therapeutics by Alnylam, Novo Nordisk, and Sanofi have received regulatory approval as well, with multiple other technologies currently being evaluated in clinical trials.

1.2 Nanoparticles

Historically, NPs have been divided into three main classes based on their material composition—inorganic, polymeric, and lipid-based NP systems [12]. These can be further divided into multiple subclasses, each of which has advantages and disadvantages for the delivery of therapeutic cargo.

1.2.1 Inorganic NPs

Inorganic NPs were the first class of NPs to be identified more than 150 years ago, although they were not recognized as NPs until much more recently. This class includes a broad range of carrier systems, such as metallic (e.g., gold and silver), iron oxide, and mesoporous silica NPs, as well as quantum dots. In preclinical research, these platforms are applied for the delivery of small molecules, proteins, and nucleic acids [13], whereas in the clinic, inorganic NPs are primarily used for imaging and diagnostic applications and for the treatment of iron deficiency [12, 14]. For example, INFeD is an iron dextran NP that was approved by the U.S. FDA in 1992 for iron replacement therapy. In the years since, numerous similar iron-based inorganic NPs have been approved for iron deficiency [14]. The utility of inorganic NPs in these applications is facilitated by the ability to formulate these carriers in a highly precise and reproducible manner to possess a range of physicochemical properties [15].

Solid gold NPs, one of the most widely studied inorganic platforms, are a highly tunable carrier platform that can be formulated to possess different geometries, including nanospheres, nanoshells, nanorods, and nanocages [15]. For example, reduction of chloroauric acid ($H[AuCl_4]$) can be used to formulate nearly monodisperse spherical gold NPs with diameters ranging from 2 to 100 nm [15]. Seed-mediated synthesis is an alternative method to formulate gold NPs with unique geometries that relies on growth from small seed particles of gold in the presence of surfactant [15]. Precise gold NP formulation enables facile and reproducible surface modification with various chemistries to promote stability in various solvents [15], drug conjugation [16–18], or functionalization with a targeting moiety [16].

Besides tunability, inorganic NPs can have other advantageous magnetic, electronic, or optical properties by virtue of their material composition. For example, Feridex is a dextran-coated iron oxide NP that was approved by the U.S. FDA in 1996 as a magnetic resonance imaging (MRI) contrast agent [19]. The Feridex formulation enables MRI of the liver due to its superparamagnetic properties and NP sizes ranging from 120 to 180 nm; following *i.v.* administration, the iron-oxide NPs preferentially accumulate in the liver [19]. For similar imaging applications, in 2011, the FDA granted investigational new drug (IND) approval for the first-in-human evaluation of silica NPs, coined Cornell dots [20, 21]. These core–shell 6–7 nm silica NPs are functionalized with an arginine-glycine-aspartate (RGD) peptide derivative to enable accumulation in integrin-expressing tumors, and are labeled with ^{124}I for detection via positron emission tomography imaging [21]. In clinical trials, Cornell dots have been investigated for molecular imaging of metastatic melanoma [21], as well as image-guided detection of sentinel lymph nodes in patients with head and neck melanoma [22]. A redesigned version of this Cornell dots platform functionalized with peptides targeting malignant melanoma cells has been shown to induce programmed cell death in cancer-bearing mice [23]; a similar drug conjugate technology based on a folic acid peptide-targeted Cornell dot platform recently began its Phase I/II clinical trial in 2021 [24], indicating the potential of silica NPs for therapeutic applications too. Despite these advances, no approvals for a Cornell dots-based imaging agent or therapeutic have been granted to date, with Elucida Oncology, the biotechnology firm leading the translation of these drugs, ceasing operations in late 2024 due to insufficient funding.

NBTXR3 is another NP therapeutic that exploits an inorganic material, specifically hafnium oxide, to promote cancer cell death during radiotherapy via increased energy deposition. NBTXR3 is a radioenhancer approximately 50 nm in diameter that can be administered directly into a tumor before ionizing radiotherapy. In 2019, NBTXR3 received European Union approval for squamous cell carcinoma [14] and was granted fast-track designation by the U.S. FDA in 2020 for head and neck cancer [25]. Similarly, AuroShell—PEG-coated silica-gold nanoshells—enables thermal ablation of solid tumors. Recent promising results from a pilot study for the treatment of prostate cancer have been reported [26], but this inorganic NP system has not yet been granted FDA approval.

1.2.2 Polymeric NPs

Polymeric NPs include micelles, polymersomes, nanospheres, layer-by-layer (LbL) NPs, dendrimers, and polyplexes. The first polymeric NPs were reported in 1960 in a study that quantified the critical micelle concentration of the polymer cetomacrogol [27]. At and above the critical micelle concentration, amphiphilic polymers self-assemble into nanoscale micelle structures with a hydrophobic core and a hydrophilic shell [4]. Micelles were one of the first polymeric NP drug delivery systems due to the ease with which lipophilic drugs could be loaded in the hydrophobic core [28]. A handful of polymeric micelle technologies have been evaluated in clinical trials for the delivery of small molecule chemotherapeutics [29]; however, challenges surrounding in vivo stability have limited their broad utilization. Micelles helped pave the way for the invention of polystyrene polymersomes—an aqueous dispersion of self-assembled amphiphilic block copolymers with a bilayer structure [30]—by two separate groups in 1995 [31, 32]. By virtue of their bilayer structure, polymersomes can encapsulate both hydrophilic drugs—in the size-adjustable aqueous core—and hydrophobic drugs—in the polymer layer—making them advantageous delivery systems for payloads of various hydrophobicity and size [33]. Despite these advantages, no polymersome NP formulations have been commercialized to date due to limitations in manufacturability and biocompatibility of non-degradable polymers [33].

Other polymeric NPs are often distinguished by their structure. One of the most common is nanospheres, which are solid particles formed of crosslinked or aggregated polymer with entrapped drug inside or adsorbed on the surface [34]. Poly (lactic-co-glycolic) acid NPs are a pioneering example, with the first therapy based on them—Lupron Depot—receiving FDA approval in 1989. This hormone therapy is widely used for the treatment of conditions including prostate cancer, uterine fibroids, and endometriosis [35]. More recently, in 2020, the FDA approved Eysuvis, a 300-nm poloxamer 407 NP, for the ocular delivery of a corticosteroid to treat dry eye. This approval was supported by decades of research demonstrating that decorating polymeric NPs with a dense coating of low-molecular-weight PEG establishes a mucoinert NP surface and effective mucus penetrating particles [36, 37].

LbL and dendrimer NPs are other polymeric platforms that rely on stepwise synthesis processes. LbL NPs were reported in 1966 and are formulated by incubating a core–shell in polyelectrolyte solutions of alternating charges [38]. Payloads can be incorporated in the different layers of LbL NPs depending on the size, charge, and hydrophobicity of the cargo. LbL NPs have shown promise in preclinical research, particularly in the context of tuning polymer surface chemistry to promote ovarian cancer cell homing and delivery [39]. Dendrimers are three-dimensional, hyperbranched particles with a central core, branches, and terminal functional groups [40] that can be synthesized via cascade synthesis methods [41]. Dendrimer NPs are often drug-loaded via chemical conjugation to terminal functional groups or via electrostatic complexation. Dendrimers, along with other polymeric NPs, are advantageous in that they enable simple surface modification with peptides or antibodies to promote targeting to a cell type of interest. Finally, polyplexes are a NP platform first reported in 1987 that rely on electrostatic complexation with charged payloads such as nucleic acids [42]. Cationic NPs formulated with polyethylenimine (PEI) are one of the most widely investigated polyplex technologies that have been employed in numerous clinical trials for in vivo nucleic acid delivery [43]; however, enthusiasm surrounding this delivery system has dampened due to safety and tolerability concerns surrounding the high and persistent cationic charge density of PEI NPs [43].

To date, most FDA-approved polymeric NPs are nanosuspensions formulated from protein or drug molecules that have been covalently linked to PEG to extend the drug's circulation half-life [44]. The first such technology—PEGylated asparaginase—was approved in 1994 for the treatment of acute lymphoblastic leukemia [12]. In the years since, similar PEGylated polymeric NPs have been approved, including Plegridy [45] (2014) for multiple sclerosis, as well as Adynovate [46] (2015) and Rebinyn [47] (2017) for the treatment of hemophilia.

1.2.3 Lipid-Based NPs

To date, lipid-based NPs are the most common class of FDA-approved nanomedicines [12, 14]. Liposomes were the first in the class of lipid-based NPs to be reported, in 1964 [48]. Formulated from various lipid components, including phospholipid, cholesterol, and lipid-PEG, liposomes imitate cellular membranes and therefore are often associated with superior biocompatibility compared to inorganic NPs [49]. Liposomes can be distinguished from other lipid-based NP systems due to their bilayer structure; in this vesicle-based system, a lipophilic bilayer is sandwiched between two hydrophilic or aqueous layers [50]. As a result, liposomes are a versatile drug delivery platform, in that lipophilic drugs can be loaded in the membrane bilayer and hydrophilic drugs can be encapsulated in the aqueous compartment [49]. The first liposome-based therapy, the anesthetic propofol (Diprivan), received FDA approval in 1989 [51]. This was followed in 1997 by a liposomal formulation of the chemotherapeutic doxorubicin, which is approved for treating ovarian cancer, Kaposi's sarcoma, and multiple myeloma [51].

While the majority of lipid-based carriers in the clinic are liposomal formulations for the delivery of small-molecule drugs, this NP class suffers from low drug loading compared to inorganic and polymeric NPs. As a result, when efforts began to apply liposomal NPs for the encapsulation and delivery of larger payloads, namely, nucleic acids [52–54], it became clear that alterations to this lipid-based delivery technology would be required to improve transfection efficiency. Lipoplexes—positively charged NPs formed from a lipid dispersion containing cationic and helper lipids [55]—were reported in 1987 in a study on the delivery of DNA using NPs incorporating the novel cationic lipid DOTMA (*N*-[1-(2,3-dioleyloxy)propyl]-*N*,*N*,*N*-trimethylammonium chloride) [56]. This cationic lipid not only enabled complexation with the negatively charged nucleic acid molecules but also facilitated intracellular uptake via cellular membrane fusion and endosomal escape [55, 56].

However, the field quickly realized the potential for significant lipoplex-induced cellular toxicity due to the permanently charged cationic lipid and subsequently developed an ionizable lipid DODAP (1,2-dioleoyl-3-dimethylammonium propane) in 1994 [57]. This ionizable lipid, along with a massive assortment of other ionizable lipid structures that have since been designed and evaluated [58], aims to reduce the cellular toxicity associated with permanently-charged cationic lipids. To this end, ionizable lipids possess a neutral charge at physiological pH; rather, in the acidic endosomal compartment following cellular uptake, these lipids adopt a positive charge, facilitating fusion with and rupture of the endosomal membrane for delivery of the nucleic acid cargo to the cytosol [55]. Beyond the ionizable lipid component, this NP platform—known as ionizable LNPs—contains other lipid excipients including phospholipid, cholesterol, and a lipid-anchored PEG [59]. LNPs have been applied in the siRNA therapy patisiran (Onpattro) for transthyretin-mediated amyloidosis, which was approved in 2018, and the two mRNA vaccines for COVID-19, tozinameran (Comirnaty) and elasomeran (Spikevax), which were both emergency use authorized by the FDA in 2020 and granted full approval in 2021 and 2022, respectively.

The global COVID-19 mRNA vaccination campaign helped illuminate many advantages of LNPs, including safety and tolerability, effective encapsulation of large nucleic acid payloads, capacity for redosing, and modular design [55]. Expanding on this recent clinical success, there are numerous ongoing clinical trials using LNPs for cancer vaccines [60] (mRNA-4157), for cystic fibrosis [61] (VX-522), and for the delivery of gene editing machinery to treat heterozygous familial hypercholesterolemia and atherosclerotic cardiovascular disease [62] (VERVE-101 and VERVE-102), to name a few. Despite these advances, the clinical application of LNPs beyond vaccines has been limited to liver-based disorders to date, due to their preferential uptake by hepatocytes in the liver upon systemic administration [63].

Finally, extracellular vesicles (EVs) have recently emerged as a promising lipid-based carrier for the delivery of macromolecules such as nucleic acids, lipids, and proteins [64]. While it was initially thought that EVs only enabled the disposal of cellular waste, these nanosized vesicles are released by nearly all cells and can facilitate the transfer of biological information between neighboring cells [64]. EVs have been explored in preclinical models for a range of applications, including cancer, neurological disorders, and inflammatory conditions [65–69], but challenges with isolation, purification, cargo loading, and targeting have limited their translation to the clinic to date.

2 Understanding NP Biodistribution and Drug Transport During Pregnancy

The placenta is a tissue unique to pregnancy that facilitates the exchange of nutrients, oxygen, and waste between maternal and fetal circulation. To this end, the placenta serves as a biological barrier, separating the two blood supplies through a series of cell layers, including the syncytiotrophoblast, cytotrophoblast cells, and endothelial cells [70, 71] (Fig. 2). By exploiting this biological barrier, it therefore might be possible to engineer biomaterial-based drug delivery technologies to interface with the placenta in several ways, including (i) delivery to the placenta itself, (ii) limiting transplacental drug transport from maternal blood, and (iii) promoting transplacental drug transport to fetal circulation (Fig. 3). Although, before intentional biomaterial design, it is essential to first understand and evaluate drug and NP biodistribution and safety in pregnancy (Sect. 2.1). In this section, we will describe the unique biomaterial design considerations to achieve delivery to the placenta (Sect. 2.2), retention in maternal circulation (Sect. 2.3), or transport to fetal blood (Sect. 2.4).

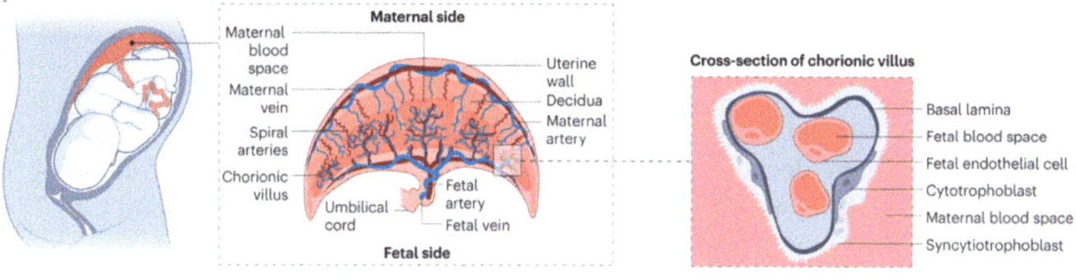

Fig. 2 The placenta as a biological barrier. By separating maternal and fetal circulation with a series of cell layers–the syncytiotrophoblast, cytotrophoblast cells, and endothelial cells–the placenta serves as an effective biological barrier to biomaterial-based drug delivery during pregnancy. (Adapted with permission from Ref. [71])

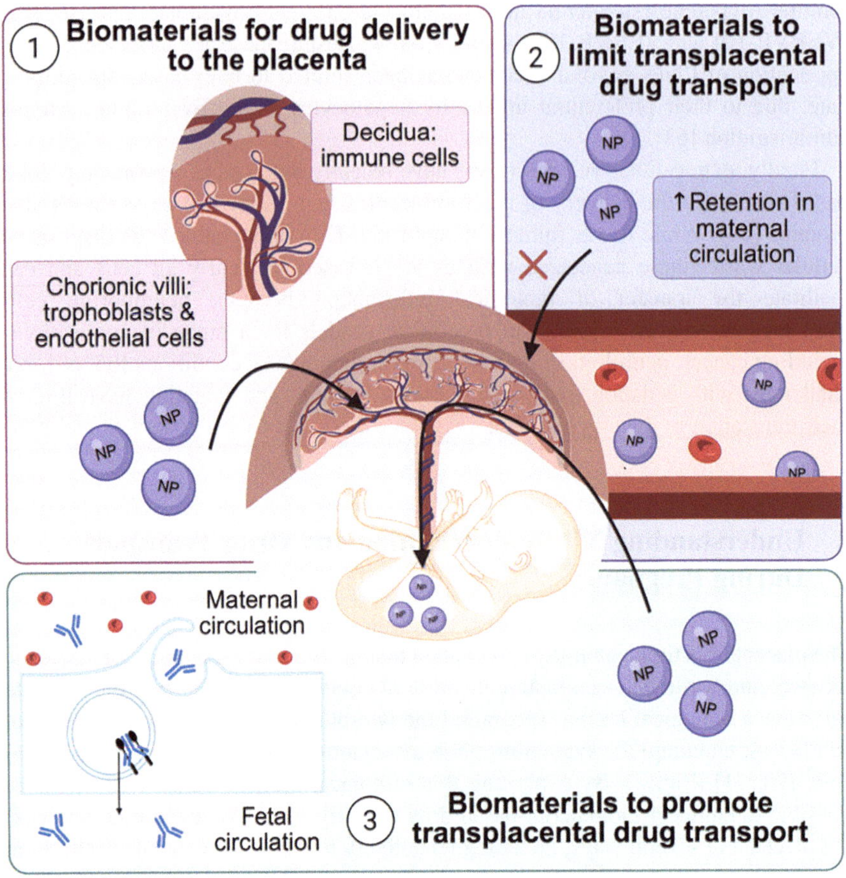

Fig. 3 Exploiting the placenta as a biological barrier for biomaterial-based drug delivery during pregnancy. Preclinical studies such as those highlighted in this chapter have engineered biomaterial-based delivery technologies to interface with the placenta in several ways: (1) for delivery to the placenta itself, (2) for limiting transplacental drug transport from maternal blood, and (3) for promoting transplacental drug transport to fetal circulation

2.1 Understanding Drug and NP Biodistribution in Pregnancy

NP biodistribution and toxicity assessments have been performed in the context of pregnancy for many decades. A large body of literature exists on the evaluation of inorganic-based NPs—including gold [72, 73], silver [74, 75], iron oxide [76, 77], and titanium dioxide [78–80] NPs—as well as polymeric [81–85] platforms during pregnancy.

Some of these works exist in the context of assessing environmental exposure to particulate matter during pregnancy; these inorganic or polymeric (i.e., plastic)

particulates can measure less than 1000 nm in diameter and are therefore often characterized as "NPs" [85]. Pregnant patients can be exposed to these NP particulates via inhalation from the air due to global increases in aerosolized particulate matter [78] or via consumption or utilization of consumer products [75, 84] (e.g., food storage containers, toothpaste, and cosmetics). For example, micro- and nanoplastic particulates of polystyrene [84] and polyamide [85] were administered to pregnant Sprague–Dawley rats and have been shown to cross the placental barrier following ingestion and inhalation, respectively. In both of these studies, the polymeric micro- and nanoplastic particles were identified in fetal tissues using histological techniques and hyperspectral dark-field microscopy [84, 85]. Similarly, studies have noted titanium dioxide deposition in the rat placenta following whole-body inhalation exposure to titanium dioxide particulates throughout gestation [78]. The authors note potential concerns around pregnant patients being exposed to poor air quality and the potential for impacts on adverse pregnancy outcomes [78], although the real-world impact of these studies may not be fully understood or appreciated until similar large, long-term studies are performed in humans.

Besides evaluating particulate exposure during pregnancy, the biodistribution of biomaterial-based drug delivery systems has also been explored in preclinical pregnancy models. In these studies, groups have sought to establish structure–function relationships to correlate biomaterial physicochemical properties such as size [72, 83, 86], charge [76], and material chemistry [73, 86, 87] with accumulation in maternal and fetal tissues as a function of gestational age [72, 73]. For instance, recent work has compared the biodistribution of PEG-coated 15-nm gold NPs and 150-nm silica core/gold nanoshells as a function of gestational age in pregnant mice [72]. Using a combination of mass spectrometry and histology, the study found that both 15-nm gold NPs and 150-nm gold nanoshells demonstrated greater placental and fetal accumulation when administered on gestational day E9.5 than E14.5 [72]. These results are consistent with a previous report describing the biodistribution and placental transport of 13-nm gold NPs with various surface modifications; in this work, gold NP accumulation in fetal tissues declined substantially when administered after gestational day E11.5 [73].

Given changes in placental development and barrier integrity as a function of gestational age, establishing these structure–function relationships in the context of NP size has perhaps been the most successful. Elucidating the role of material chemistry, surface modification, and charge has been more challenging. Some works report greater NP accumulation in placental and fetal tissues with near-neutrally charged gold NPs compared to anionic platforms [73], though with an iron oxide technology, positively charged NPs showed greater delivery to the fetal liver [76]. While it is possible that the impact of these physicochemical properties on delivery to placental and fetal tissues will always depend on the precise delivery technology in question, there is currently not yet enough literature in the context of drug and NP biodistribution in pregnancy to establish robust structure–function relationships.

2.2 Biomaterials for Drug Delivery to the Placenta

When considering the body of literature on engineered biomaterials for interfacing with the placenta, the design and evaluation of technologies for drug delivery to the placenta itself has been perhaps most robustly explored. A majority of these technologies are polymeric [88–90] or lipid-based NPs, including liposomes [91–94] and LNPs [95–100], with some literature exploring the potential for peptide-drug conjugates [101] for delivery to the placenta as well. This section will highlight the decades-long research by some groups in the field of placenta drug delivery and the more recent advancements in LNP technologies for nucleic acid delivery to the placenta.

Dr. Lynda K. Harris and her research group have pioneered several key works in this field, including a seminal piece published in 2016 that demonstrates the utility of tumor-homing peptides for targeted drug delivery to the placenta [85]. Using a bioinspired approach, this work capitalizes on the numerous similarities between solid tumors and the developing placenta, including the capacity for rapid proliferation and the invasive nature of extravillous trophoblasts in the placenta. Tumor-targeting peptide sequences, including the cyclic peptide iRGD (Cys-Arg-Gly-Asp-Lys-Gly-Pro-Asp-Cys), demonstrated selective binding to mouse and human placentas, which were then used to decorate the surface of liposomes to deliver insulin-like growth factor 2 (IGF-2) protein to the mouse placenta [94]. The Harris group has since utilized this tumor-targeting peptide platform to engineer placenta-tropic microRNA inhibitor drug conjugates and for liposome-mediated delivery of a small molecule vasodilatory payload [92]. Tropism to the placenta and the therapeutic efficacy of these technologies has been evaluated in animal models of fetal growth restriction (FGR), which will be reviewed thoroughly in Sect. 3.1.

In a similar vein, the research of Dr. Helen Jones' laboratory is also seminal in the field of placenta drug delivery, particularly in the context of NP-mediated gene therapy in the placenta. In an initial work published in 2015, the group engineers a diblock copolymer NP technology for the delivery of plasmid DNA (pDNA) to the placenta [90]. To further promote selective delivery to the placenta, this insulin-like growth factor 1 (IGF-1) pDNA construct was designed with trophoblast-specific promoters. The group has had tremendous success with this technology, demonstrating promising results in larger animal models, including guinea pigs [102–104] and non-human primates [105, 106]. Following ultrasound-guided intra-placental injection of these polymeric pDNA NPs in pregnant macaques, the team has shown uptake and *IGF-1* gene expression in the placenta syncytiotrophoblast using in situ hybridization and fluorescence microscopy [105]. As with the peptide-targeted technology described above, this IGF-1 pDNA NP platform has been extensively evaluated in animal models of FGR (Sect. 3.1).

Following the widespread commercialization of LNPs for nucleic acid delivery, several works, including my own, have sought to explore the potential for LNP delivery to the placenta. Over the last several years, several studies have emerged in this area that evaluate LNP libraries with varied lipid chemistries and excipient compositions to promote mRNA delivery to the placenta [95–98, 107]. These works have employed screening methodologies including design-of-experiments optimization [96, 97] and high-throughput in vivo screening [100] to identify placenta-tropic LNPs, which can then be further functionalized with active targeting motifs [e.g., antibodies targeting epithelial growth factor receptor (EGFR)] to further enhance delivery to the placenta [99]. Most recently, my work has proposed potential mechanism by which these LNPs enable delivery to the placenta, which suggests that the serum protein β_2-glycoprotein I adsorbs on the LNP surface following *i.v.* administration and could facilitate tropism to the placenta [100]. To date, these LNP platforms have been used for the delivery of vascular endothelial growth factor (VEGF) [95, 100] mRNA and placental growth factor [97] mRNA, as well as cytokine-encoding [interleukin (IL)-4 and IL-13] [107] mRNAs with potential applications in treating pre-eclampsia (Sect. 3.1) and facilitating local immunomodulation, respectively.

2.3 *Biomaterials to Limit Transplacental Drug Transport*

While placenta-tropic biomaterials can have therapeutic applications in treating obstetric disorders with well-characterized pathologies in the placenta, there is a substantial need for engineered technologies that can limit transplacental transport of drugs from maternal to fetal circulation. Despite the fact that 60% of pregnant patients take one or more medications, over 90% of clinically approved drugs lack appropriate labeling information for pregnant and lactating women [108], predominantly due to fetal teratogenicity concerns. Most drugs are small molecules and are known to readily transport across the placenta to fetal circulation [109]. The safety of prescription and over-the-counter medication usage during pregnancy could be substantially improved with rationally engineered technologies that limit transplacental drug transport.

Over the last several years, several studies have demonstrated the potential for polymeric conjugate technologies to reduce transplacental drug transport [83, 109, 110]. Given its regulatory approval status and high degree of biocompatibility, drug conjugation to PEG has emerged as a promising biomaterial-based solution [109, 110]. In one study, conjugating PEG to either the fluorescent molecule Cy5.5 or the small molecule drug haloperidol reduced uptake by about 40-fold in term placental explants [110]. In another study, fluorescently-labeled PEG conjugates with larger molecular weights (PEG_{40000} vs. PEG_{5000}) more effectively reduced transplacental transport to the fetus in pregnant mice as measured using an in vivo imaging system (IVIS) [109]. It is important to note here the impact of the models being used to evaluate transplacental transport of these biomaterial-based drug conjugates. For example, while the ex vivo human placental perfusion model is perhaps the gold standard for studying placental transport [109, 111], in vivo models offer the advantage of more closely recapitulating the complex physiological environment in the body. However, differences in placental structure across species can also limit the extrapolation of results from rodents to humans. While human placentas have a hemomonochorial structure—a single layer of syncytiotrophoblast separating maternal and fetal circulation—rodents such as mice and rats have a hemotrichorial structure with two layers of cytotrophoblast cells surrounding the syncytiotrophoblast layer [71]. These differences have the potential for significant impacts in assessments of placental transport, which researchers should carefully consider when interpreting and discussing their results.

Besides PEG-based drug conjugates, studies have utilized other biomaterial technologies to study transplacental drug transport, including elastin-like polypeptide platforms [83]. When administered to pregnant Sprague–Dawley rats, fluorescently-labeled elastin-like polypeptides demonstrated increased accumulation in the placenta with increased polypeptide molecular weight (25–86 kDa); elastin-like polypeptides were not detected in fetuses regardless of molecular weight [83]. Liver accumulation also increased with increased polypeptide molecular weight, while kidney clearance decreased. The results suggest that larger-molecular-weight elastin-like polypeptides can decrease drug clearance rate from plasma, offering the potential to promote drug retention in maternal circulation and limit transplacental drug transport.

2.4 Biomaterials to Promote Transplacental Drug Transport

Converse to limiting transplacental transport and promoting drug retention in maternal circulation, engineering biomaterial-based technologies to enable transport across the placenta might be desirable for prenatal therapies [112]. For instance, there are a number of congenital disorders that can result in fetal morbidity and mortality before birth; early in utero intervention for these disorders offers the potential to partially address the congenital disorder to improve fetal development [113, 114]. To this end, there is a growing body of literature that explores the potential for biomaterial-based technologies to promote the transport of therapeutic payloads across the placenta from maternal to fetal circulation [113, 115–117].

Given the genetic nature of these disorders, in utero gene therapies to partially restore or correct abnormal gene expression could be a particularly favorable therapeutic modality. This can include transplacental delivery of pDNA [117], DNA constructs for CRISPR-Cas9-mediated gene editing [115], or siRNA [113]. For example, liposomal NPs have been shown to facilitate transplacental pDNA delivery to neonatal brains when administered *i.v.* in near-term pregnant mice [117]. While this study focused on evaluating reporter (i.e., luciferase and beta-galactosidase) transgene expression, the authors demonstrated the potential for therapeutic transplacental gene therapy.

Several studies have explored modifying the surface of NPs with immunoglobulin G (IgG) antibodies [113, 116, 118] to leverage the innate mechanism by which the placenta facilitates the exchange of IgG from maternal to fetal circulation to

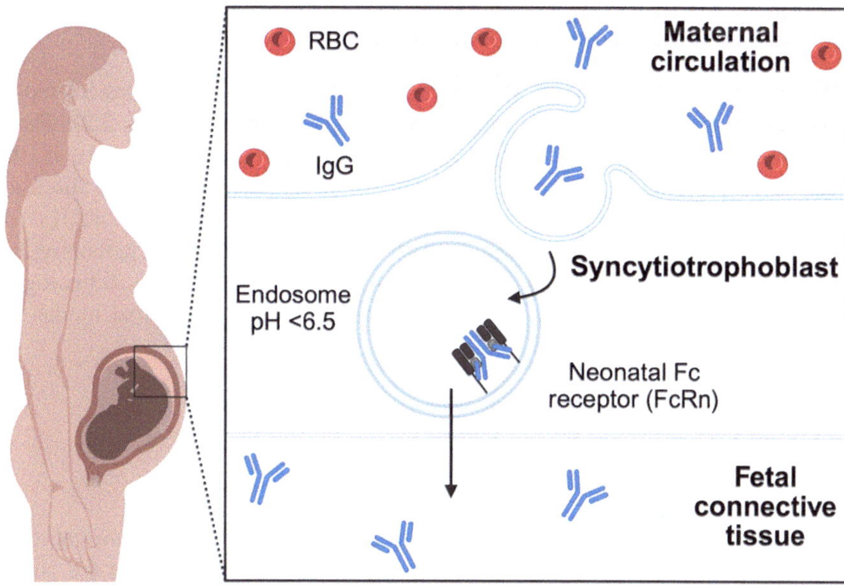

Fig. 4 Mechanism of IgG transport from maternal circulation to the fetus via the FcRn. IgG antibodies are internalized in the placental syncytiotrophoblast via pinocytosis; IgG binding to the FcRn in the acidified endosome results in antibody transport to the fetal side of the syncytiotrophoblast

provide the fetus with passive immunity. Specifically, IgG antibodies from maternal circulation are internalized by the syncytiotrophoblast in the placenta via pinocytosis, following which endosomal acidification induces IgG binding to neonatal Fc receptor (FcRn) [116, 119]. This internalization and FcRn binding process results in IgG release on the fetal side of the syncytiotrophoblast [116] (Fig. 4).

When leveraging this biological process, researchers have demonstrated that IgG-modified chitosan NPs demonstrate more than 2.5-fold greater transport across the syncytiotrophoblast in an in vitro transwell model compared to unmodified NPs [116]. A similar study using an in vitro transwell model functionalized LNPs with IgG antibodies and showed that LNP transport varied as a function of IgG orientation on the LNP surface [113]. To study this effect, the authors utilized different modified lipid-PEG molecules (i.e., lipid-PEG-NH_2, lipid-PEG-COOH, and lipid-PEG-maleimide) in the LNP formulation to chemically bind IgG antibodies to the LNP surface in different orientations. IgG LNPs formulated with lipid-PEG-COOH and lipid-PEG-maleimide achieved significantly greater in vitro transport; the authors hypothesize that these conjugation chemistries reduce steric hindrance near the Fc portion of IgG antibodies, therefore increasing interactions with the FcRn in the immortalized syncytiotrophoblast cells.

3 Clinical Applications for Drug Delivery to the Placenta

In this section, we will discuss several obstetric disorders, including pre-eclampsia and FGR (Sect. 3.1), as well as gestational trophoblast disease (Sect. 3.2). These conditions are all associated with a well-characterized pathophysiology in the placenta or placenta-like tissue (in the case of gestational trophoblast disease), which suggests the therapeutic potential of biomaterial-based technologies for drug delivery to the placenta. Given the well-characterized placental pathophysiology associated with pre-eclampsia, the majority of biomaterial-based technologies for delivery to the placenta have been evaluated in preclinical animal models of pre-eclampsia.

3.1 *Pre-eclampsia and FGR*

Pre-eclampsia affects up to 5% of all pregnancies and is a significant cause of maternal and fetal morbidity and mortality during pregnancy [120]. In the clinic, pre-eclampsia is diagnosed by the onset of gestational hypertension after 20 weeks of pregnancy, accompanied by one or more of the following conditions: proteinuria, acute kidney or liver injury, neurological and hematological complications, and uteroplacental dysfunction [120].

The pathology of pre-eclampsia is frequently described as a two-stage paradigm of placental-dysfunction (Fig. 5). The first stage is associated with aberrant remodeling of the uterine vasculature, whereby extravillous trophoblasts do not successfully migrate from the placenta to invade the myometrium of the uterus [120, 121]. Instead of a high-capacitance, low resistance environment at the maternal-fetal interface that promotes sufficient blood exchange, pre-eclampsia is characterized by a high velocity, turbulent blood flow environment, which results in the second stage of pre-eclampsia: placental ischemia and oxidative stress [120]. Turbulent blood flow damages the chorionic villi in the placenta, leading to abnormal expression of pro- and anti-angiogenic proteins. For example, soluble fms-like tyrosine kinase-1 (sFlt-1) is an anti-angiogenic protein typically elevated in the serum of pre-eclamptic patients; sFlt-1 binds VEGF, preventing the transmission of vasorelaxation signals to endothelial cells, both locally in the placenta and systemically as well [120]. This abnormal placental development also helps to explain why FGR is often observed concurrently with pre-eclampsia [120].

When pregnant patients are diagnosed with pre-eclampsia, the disorder is often progressive with a deterioration in tissue function both locally in the placenta and in systemic organs as well [120]. As no drug or therapeutic has reached the clinic that can slow or stop disease progression, practitioners work with the patient to manage delivery of the placenta and fetus—the only known "cure" for pre-eclampsia. Depending on the gestational age of the pregnancy at which pre-eclampsia is diagnosed, the provider may initiate birth or manage the symptoms with medications

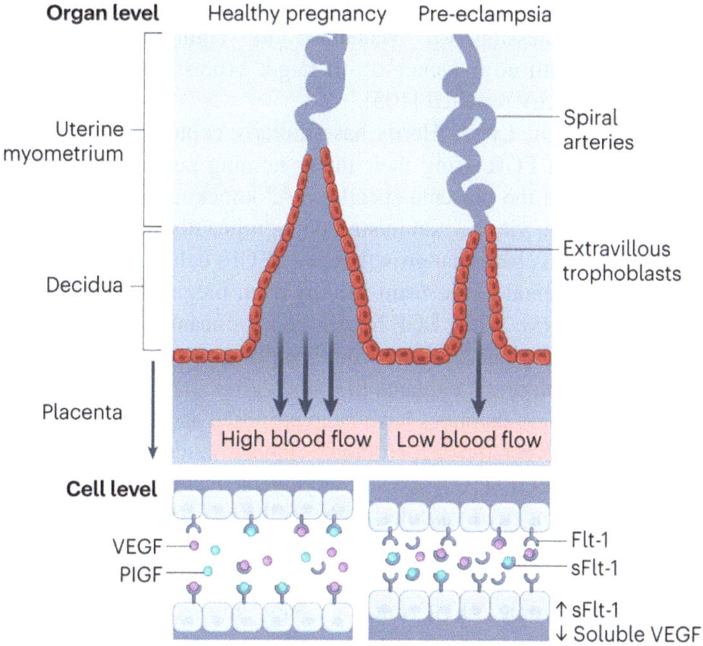

Fig. 5 The two-stage paradigm of placental dysfunction in pre-eclampsia. In Stage 1, impaired uterine remodeling at the tissue level reduces blood flow to the placenta, increases maternal blood pressure, and results in a high-velocity, turbulent blood flow environment. This subsequently causes stage two of pre-eclampsia at the cellular level, where anti-angiogenic factors such as sFlt-1 are upregulated and consequently sequester pro-angiogenic factors like VEGF from facilitating vasorelaxation. (Adapted with permission from Ref. [71])

until the fetus has reached a more advanced gestational age [120]. For instance, the provider may prescribe medications to manage blood pressure (e.g., labetalol and nifedipine), prevent seizures (e.g., magnesium sulfate), and promote fetal lung maturity (e.g., corticosteroids) [120].

Many biomaterial-based platforms have been engineered to enable local gene therapy and modulation in the placenta as a potential therapeutic modality for pre-eclampsia. For example, the laboratory of Dr. Helen Jones has pioneered the application of IGF-1 gene therapy in preclinical animal models of FGR [102–105]. IGF signaling is essential for various aspects of placental development, including cell proliferation, vasculature structure, nutrient transport, and hormone production, and IGF-1 is downregulated in human fetal growth restriciton [103]. Using a guinea pig maternal nutrient restriction model of FGR, studies have demonstrated the therapeutic potential of IGF-1 pDNA polymeric NPs delivered via ultrasound-guided intra-placental injection [102–104]. The biomaterial-based delivery technology has been shown to correct fetal weight compared to diseased controls, with the potential for fetal-sex-dependent effects [103, 104]. The platform has advanced toward larger animal models, including pregnant macaques, to assess gene delivery to trophoblasts in the placenta following intra-placental injections [105]. Transgene expression was visualized and confirmed in the placental syncytiotrophoblast with no evidence of off-target expression in maternal or fetal tissues or adverse toxicity reported [105].

The laboratory of Dr. Lynda Harris has similarly explored therapeutic growth factor delivery to treat FGR using their tumor-homing peptide-targeted liposome technology [93, 94]. In the placenta-specific *Igf-2* knockout mouse, IGF-2 protein delivery to the placenta via *i.v.* administration significantly improved fetal weight [94]. Similarly, ex vivo epidermal growth factor (EGF) delivery to the placenta has been explored in placental tissue from healthy term pregnancies and pregnancies complicated by FGR [93]. While EGF liposomes significantly increased amino acid transporter activity in explants isolated from healthy term placentas, this effect was not observed in FGR placental explants [93].

Other gene modulation therapies have been proposed and evaluated preclinically in animal models of pre-eclampsia, particularly toward modulating the imbalance of pro-angiogenic (i.e., VEGF) [100] and anti-angiogenic factors (i.e., sFlt-1) [89, 122–124]. To address the impaired vascularization in the pre-eclamptic placenta, I have demonstrated the therapeutic potential of VEGF mRNA LNPs in both inflammation- and hypoxia-induced mouse models of pre-eclampsia [100]. Following a single *i.v.* injection of placenta-tropic VEGF mRNA LNPs, this technology was shown to resolve maternal hypertension through the end of gestation and improve fetal weight and placental vasodilation at the model endpoint (gestational day 17) [100]. Notably, these promising results were only observed with the placenta-tropic LNP technology and not a liver-tropic, clinically approved platform, which was only able to temporarily ameliorate hypertension in pre-eclamptic mice, after which the pregnant mice again became hypertensive until the end of pregnancy [100]. These results suggest the importance of engineering biomaterial-based delivery technologies that traffic and home to the placenta to maximize the potential therapeutic effect.

Conversely, polymer- and polymer-lipid-based NPs have been explored for therapeutic RNA interference to treat pre-eclampsia via sFlt-1 and/or nuclear factor-erythroid 2-like 2 (Nrf2) siRNA delivery to the placenta [89, 122]. In a pregnancy-associated hypertension genetically-modified mouse model of pre-eclampsia, polymer-LNPs co-delivering sFlt-1 siRNA and Nrf2 siRNA demonstrated the greatest improvements in pre-eclampsia symptoms compared to either payload alone [122]. Besides NP delivery technology, chemical stabilization in the form of sFlt-1 siRNA conjugates has also been explored for the treatment of pre-eclampsia [123, 124]. Hydrophobic cholesterol-conjugated sFlt-1 siRNA enabled accumulation in the murine placenta, though the authors note that cholesterol conjugation did not provide placenta selectivity [123]. In the baboon uterine artery ischemia model of pre-eclampsia, this cholesterol-conjugated sFlt-1 siRNA reduced plasma levels of this anti-angiogenic factor as well as systolic blood pressure compared to pre-eclamptic control animals [123]. Given the demonstrated promise of this technology in both rodent and non-human primate models of pre-eclampsia, Comanche Biopharma is currently in the process of pursuing the clinical viability of this biomaterial-based drug product.

3.2 Gestational Trophoblast Disease

Gestational trophoblast disease is a class of obstetric disorders that encompasses complete and partial hydatidiform mole, invasive mole, choriocarcinoma, and placental-site trophoblastic tumor [125]. While in a healthy pregnancy trophoblasts from the placenta must invade the uterine vasculature, these pregnancy-related disorders are characterized by the formation of highly invasive and vascular tumors due to a failure in regulatory mechanisms [125]. Given that the majority of the literature that exists at the interface of biomaterial-based delivery technologies and gestational trophoblast disease explores applications in treating choriocarcinoma, we will focus on this specific pregnancy-related disorder in this section.

Choriocarcinoma most commonly affects pregnant patients who have a molar pregnancy, whereby the sperm and egg incorrectly join and form a hydatidiform mole; however, choriocarcinoma can also happen after an ectopic pregnancy, miscarriage, or even after a full-term pregnancy resulting in a birth. While the placenta is the tissue source for all gestational trophoblast disease, choriocarcinoma in particular is derived from villous trophoblast [125]. These malignant, epithelial tumors abundantly produce human chorionic gonadotropin (hCG), and therefore, monitoring levels of this hormone in plasma and urine is essential for managing choriocarcinoma [125].

Assuming that patients are first diagnosed with a hydatidiform mole and want to preserve their fertility, the initial standard of care for treating choriocarcinoma is uterine evacuation since the fetus is non-viable [121]. Hysterectomy is another, less recommended, treatment option for women who do not wish to preserve their fertility to stop the risk of local invasion, though this route does not eliminate the potential need for subsequent chemotherapy interventions [125]. Monochemotherapy is the standard of care for low-risk patients with choriocarcinoma; if first-line therapy fails due to resistance, second-line or even sometimes third-line chemotherapy is often successful, resulting in overall cure rates exceeding 98% [125]. Although choriocarcinoma can rapidly spread and metastasize to tissues in the rest of the body, including the lung (most common), liver, kidneys, brain, and lymph nodes, radiography, computed tomography, and MRI can be used if metastases are suspected or observed to appropriately adjust the treatment plan.

Given that choriocarcinoma is derived from placental tissue, groups have utilized similar delivery technologies to those described in Sect. 2.2 to evaluate therapeutic efficacy in preclinical models of choriocarcinoma [126–130]. For example, the laboratory of Xiujun Fan has employed a bioinspired approach to target such placenta-derived tissue based on the mechanism of *Plasmodium falciparum* (i.e., malaria parasite) infection during pregnancy [126, 128]; *P. falciparum*-infected red blood cells (RBCs) sequester in the placenta via VAR2CSA, which is expressed on the RBC surface [128]. VAR2CSA adheres to chondroitin sulfate A (CSA), which is exclusively expressed in placental trophoblasts. In multiple studies, the authors design a CSA-binding peptide derived from VAR2CSA and use it to decorate the surface of polymeric NPs to engineer a placenta-targeted delivery technology [126, 128].

Many of these studies employ mouse xenograft models where immortalized JEG-3 choriocarcinoma cells are implanted subcutaneously, and tumor reduction is assessed following treatment with engineered delivery technologies [126, 128–130]. In this model, systemically administered (i.e., *i.v.* via tail vein injection) NPs decorated with the CSA-binding peptides more effectively reduced tumor burden than the untargeted NP technology with a significant reduction in tumor weight [128]. Similar studies have designed EGFR-targeted nanospheres and evaluated their capacity for doxorubicin delivery to JEG-3 choriocarcinoma xenograft tumors [130]. Again, mice treated *i.v.* with EGFR-targeted nanospheres loaded with doxorubicin showed reduced tumor volumes compared to the untargeted nanosphere platform and free doxorubicin alone [130].

While these xenograft models can be readily implemented, they fail to closely recapitulate the local microenvironment and invasion into the uterine tissue. To address this limitation, other studies have employed a surgically-induced, orthotopic choriocarcinoma mouse model whereby JEG-3 cells are injected directly into the uterine myometrium in mice [127]. In this chapter, hyaluronic acid, cisplatin, and the near-infrared fluorescent dye indocyanine green were used to formulate NPs via self-assembly, which were subsequently encapsulated in choriocarcinoma cell membranes to improve homing [127]. Converse to the traditional systemic *i.v.* chemotherapies, the authors explore the potential for therapeutic administration via intrauterine perfusion to further promote targeted delivery to and retention in the reproductive tract [127]. When combined with ultrasound irradiation, this therapy demonstrated significant promise in treating orthotopic choriocarcinoma tumors [127].

4 Outlook on the Application of Drug Delivery Technologies During Pregnancy

Biomaterial-based delivery technologies—including chemically modified drugs and NP platforms—have demonstrated success in the preclinical setting for interfacing with the placenta, yet significant work remains to translate these technologies to the clinic. One of the major hurdles for translation was highlighted by a recent article in the *American Journal of Obstetrics and Gynecology* published in 2025; in a meta-analysis, the authors reported that fewer than 1% of clinical drug trials performed in the U.S. enroll pregnant patients [131]. This statistic can be partially explained by the complex social, ethical, and historical constructs that surround the process of enrolling a pregnant patient in a clinical trial for an IND.

While the barrier to clinical entry for biomaterial-based drugs to treat pre-eclampsia, FGR, or gestational trophoblast disease might be substantially higher than for many other therapeutic applications, the value and impact of this effort would be invaluable for pregnant patients. For example, for many obstetric conditions like pre-eclampsia, there are no therapeutics available in the clinic that slow or stop disease progression. Herein lies a unique opportunity to repurpose and redesign the biomaterial-based delivery technologies that have already garnered regulatory approval (Sect. 1) for novel therapeutic applications to treat obstetric disorders. Successfully translating therapeutic technologies to the clinic will require significant interdisciplinary efforts among engineers, clinicians, scientists, advocates, and policy experts over the next several decades.

References

1. Vargason AM, Anselmo AC, Mitragotri S. The evolution of commercial drug delivery technologies. Nat Biomed Eng. 2021;5:951–67.
2. Strebhardt K, Ullrich A. Paul Ehrlich's magic bullet concept: 100 years of progress. Nat Rev Cancer. 2008;8:473–80.
3. Zaro JL, Wang J. Antibody-drug conjugates: the 21st century magic bullets for cancer. Springer Nature; 2025.
4. Stiepel RT, Duggan E, Batty CJ, Ainslie KM. Micro and nanotechnologies: the little formulations that could. Bioeng Transl Med. 2023;8:e10421.
5. Abuchowski A, van Es T, Palczuk NC, Davis FF. Alteration of immunological properties of bovine serum albumin by covalent attachment of polyethylene glycol. J Biol Chem. 1977;252: 3578–81.
6. Sanchez AJDS, et al. Substituting poly(ethylene glycol) lipids with poly(2-ethyl-2-oxazoline) lipids improves lipid nanoparticle repeat dosing. Adv Healthc Mater. 2024;13:2304033.
7. Ju Y, et al. Anti-PEG antibodies boosted in humans by SARS-CoV-2 lipid nanoparticle mRNA vaccine. ACS Nano. 2022;16:11769–80.
8. Fire A, et al. Potent and specific genetic interference by double-stranded RNA in *Caenorhabditis elegans*. Nature. 1998;391:806–11.
9. Elbashir SM, et al. Duplexes of 21-nucleotide RNAs mediate RNA interference in cultured mammalian cells. Nature. 2001;411:494–8.
10. Khvorova A, Watts JK. The chemical evolution of oligonucleotide therapies of clinical utility. Nat Biotechnol. 2017;35:238–48.
11. Nair JK, et al. Multivalent N-acetylgalactosamine-conjugated siRNA localizes in hepatocytes and elicits robust RNAi-mediated gene silencing. J Am Chem Soc. 2014;136:16958–61.
12. Mitchell MJ, et al. Engineering precision nanoparticles for drug delivery. Nat Rev Drug Discov. 2020;20:101–24. https://doi.org/10.1038/s41573-020-0090-8.
13. Luther DC, et al. Delivery of drugs, proteins, and nucleic acids using inorganic nanoparticles. Adv Drug Deliv Rev. 2020;156:188–213.
14. Anselmo AC, Mitragotri S. Nanoparticles in the clinic: an update post COVID-19 vaccines. Bioeng Transl Med. 2021;6:e10246.
15. Heo DN, et al. Chapter 24: Scale-up production of theranostic nanoparticles. In: Chen X, Wong S, editors. Cancer theranostics. Oxford: Academic Press; 2014. p. 457–70. https://doi.org/10.1016/B978-0-12-407722-5.00024-4.
16. Wang L, et al. Intranasal delivery of Temozolomide-conjugated gold nanoparticles functionalized with anti-EphA3 for glioblastoma targeting. Mol Pharm. 2021;18:915–27.
17. Miao D, Yu Y, Chen Y, Liu Y, Su G. Facile construction of i-motif DNA-conjugated gold Nanostars as near-infrared and pH dual-responsive targeted drug delivery systems for combined cancer therapy. Mol Pharm. 2020;17:1127–38.
18. Jiang X, Du B, Huang Y, Yu M, Zheng J. Cancer photothermal therapy with ICG-conjugated gold nanoclusters. Bioconjug Chem. 2020;31:1522–8.

19. Wang Y-XJ. Superparamagnetic iron oxide based MRI contrast agents: current status of clinical application. Quant Imaging Med Surg. 2011;1:35.
20. Janjua TI, Cao Y, Yu C, Popat A. Clinical translation of silica nanoparticles. Nat Rev Mater. 2021;6:1072–4.
21. Phillips E, et al. Clinical translation of an ultrasmall inorganic optical-PET imaging nanoparticle probe. Sci Transl Med. 2014;6:260ra149.
22. Zanoni DK, et al. Use of ultrasmall core-shell fluorescent silica nanoparticles for image-guided sentinel lymph node biopsy in head and neck melanoma: a nonrandomized clinical trial. JAMA Netw Open. 2021;4:e211936.
23. Kim SE, et al. Ultrasmall nanoparticles induce ferroptosis in nutrient-deprived cancer cells and suppress tumour growth. Nat Nanotechnol. 2016;11:977–85.
24. Ma WW, et al. Abstract CT255: ELU-FRα-1: a study to evaluate ELU001 in patients with solid tumors that overexpress folate receptor alpha (FRα). Cancer Res. 2023;83:CT255.
25. Shen C, et al. Efficacy from the ongoing phase I trial study 1100 with NBTXR3 activated by radiotherapy in combination with nivolumab or pembrolizumab in patients with locoregionally recurrent or metastatic HNSCC. J Clin Oncol. 2023;41:6038.
26. Rastinehad AR, et al. Gold nanoshell-localized photothermal ablation of prostate tumors in a clinical pilot device study. Proc Natl Acad Sci. 2019;116:18590–6.
27. Elworthy PH. The critical micelle concentration of Cetomacrogol 1000. J Pharm Pharmacol. 1960;12:293–9.
28. Ghezzi M, et al. Polymeric micelles in drug delivery: an insight of the techniques for their characterization and assessment in biorelevant conditions. J Control Release. 2021;332:312–36.
29. Oerlemans C, et al. Polymeric micelles in anticancer therapy: targeting, imaging and triggered release. Pharm Res. 2010;27:2569.
30. Hasannia M, et al. Synthesis of block copolymers used in polymersome fabrication: application in drug delivery. J Control Release. 2022;341:95–117.
31. van Hest JCM, Delnoye DAP, Baars MWPL, van Genderen MHP, Meijer EW. Polystyrene-dendrimer amphiphilic block copolymers with a generation-dependent aggregation. Science. 1995;268:1592–5.
32. Zhang L, Eisenberg A. Multiple morphologies of 'crew-cut' aggregates of polystyrene-b-poly (acrylic acid) block copolymers. Science. 1995;268:1728–31.
33. Gouveia MG, et al. Polymersome-based protein drug delivery—quo vadis? Chem Soc Rev. 2023;52:728–78.
34. Madej M, Kurowska N, Strzalka-Mrozik B. Polymeric nanoparticles—tools in a drug delivery system in selected cancer therapies. Appl Sci. 2022;12:9479.
35. Kim G-Y, et al. In vitro and in vivo evaluations of a 3-month sustained-release microsphere depot formulation of leuprolide acetate. J Pharm Investig. 2022;52:129–38.
36. Wang Y-Y, et al. Addressing the PEG Mucoadhesivity paradox to engineer nanoparticles that "slip" through the human mucus barrier. Angew Chem Int Ed. 2008;47:9726–9.
37. Ensign LM, et al. Mucus-penetrating nanoparticles for vaginal drug delivery protect against herpes simplex virus. Sci Transl Med. 2012;4:138ra79.
38. Iler RK. Multilayers of colloidal particles. J Colloid Interface Sci. 1966;21:569–94.
39. Correa S, et al. Tuning nanoparticle interactions with ovarian cancer through layer-by-layer modification of surface chemistry. ACS Nano. 2020;14:2224–37.
40. An H, Deng X, Wang F, Xu P, Wang N. Dendrimers as Nanocarriers for the delivery of drugs obtained from natural products. Polymers. 2023;15:2292.
41. Abbasi E, et al. Dendrimers: synthesis, applications, and properties. Nanoscale Res Lett. 2014;9:247.
42. Wu GY, Wu CH. Receptor-mediated in vitro gene transformation by a soluble DNA carrier system. J Biol Chem. 1987;262:4429–32.
43. Casper J, et al. Polyethylenimine (PEI) in gene therapy: current status and clinical applications. J Control Release. 2023;362:667–91.

44. Konkle BA, et al. Pegylated, full-length, recombinant factor VIII for prophylactic and on-demand treatment of severe hemophilia a. Blood. 2015;126:1078–85.
45. Calabresi PA, et al. Pegylated interferon beta-1a for relapsing-remitting multiple sclerosis (ADVANCE): a randomised, phase 3, double-blind study. Lancet Neurol. 2014;13:657–65.
46. Mullins ES, et al. Extended half-life pegylated, full-length recombinant factor VIII for prophylaxis in children with severe haemophilia a. Haemophilia. 2017;23:238–46.
47. Young G, et al. Nonacog beta pegol (N9-GP) in haemophilia B: a multinational phase III safety and efficacy extension trial (paradigm™4). Thromb Res. 2016;141:69–76.
48. Bangham AD, Horne RW. Negative staining of phospholipids and their structural modification by surface-active agents as observed in the electron microscope. J Mol Biol. 1964;8:660–8.
49. Antimisiaris SG, et al. Overcoming barriers by local drug delivery with liposomes. Adv Drug Deliv Rev. 2021;174:53–86.
50. Shah S, Dhawan V, Holm R, Nagarsenker MS, Perrie Y. Liposomes: advancements and innovation in the manufacturing process. Adv Drug Deliv Rev. 2020;154–155:102–22.
51. Anselmo AC, Mitragotri S. Nanoparticles in the clinic. Bioeng Transl Med. 2016;1:10–29.
52. Ostro MJ, Giacomoni D, Dray S. Incorporation of high molecular weight RNA into large artificial lipid vesicles. Biochem Biophys Res Commun. 1977;76:836–42.
53. Dimitriadis GJ. Translation of rabbit globin mRNA introduced by liposomes into mouse lymphocytes. Nature. 1978;274:923–4.
54. Ostro MJ, Giacomoni D, Lavelle D, Paxton W, Dray S. Evidence for translation of rabbit globin mRNA after liposomemediated insertion into a human cell line. Nature. 1978;274:921–3.
55. Cullis PR, Felgner PL. The 60-year evolution of lipid nanoparticles for nucleic acid delivery. Nat Rev Drug Discov. 2024;23:709–22. https://doi.org/10.1038/s41573-024-00977-6.
56. Felgner PL, et al. Lipofection: a highly efficient, lipid-mediated DNA-transfection procedure. Proc Natl Acad Sci. 1987;84:7413–7.
57. Bailey AL, Cullis PR. Modulation of membrane fusion by asymmetric transbilayer distributions of amino lipids. Biochemistry. 1994;33:12573–80.
58. Han X, et al. An ionizable lipid toolbox for RNA delivery. Nat Commun. 2021;12:7233.
59. Swingle KL, Hamilton AG, Mitchell MJ. Lipid nanoparticle-mediated delivery of mRNA therapeutics and vaccines. Trends Mol Med. 2021;27:616–7.
60. Khattak A, et al. Abstract CT001: a personalized cancer vaccine, mRNA-4157, combined with pembrolizumab versus pembrolizumab in patients with resected high-risk melanoma: efficacy and safety results from the randomized, open-label phase 2 mRNA-4157-P201/Keynote-942 trial. Cancer Res. 2023;83:CT001.
61. Castaños C. The past 10 years of cystic fibrosis treatment: the road to cure. Lancet Respir Med. 2023;11:864–5.
62. Lee RG, et al. Efficacy and safety of an investigational single-course CRISPR base-editing therapy targeting PCSK9 in nonhuman primate and mouse models. Circulation. 2023;147: 242–53.
63. Witzigmann D, et al. Lipid nanoparticle technology for therapeutic gene regulation in the liver. Adv Drug Deliv Rev. 2020;159:344–63.
64. Vader P, Mol EA, Pasterkamp G, Schiffelers RM. Extracellular vesicles for drug delivery. Adv Drug Deliv Rev. 2016;106:148–56.
65. Herrmann IK, Wood MJA, Fuhrmann G. Extracellular vesicles as a next-generation drug delivery platform. Nat Nanotechnol. 2021;16:748–59.
66. Ricklefs FL, et al. Immune evasion mediated by PD-L1 on glioblastoma-derived extracellular vesicles. Sci Adv. 2018;4:eaar2766.
67. Alvarez-Erviti L, et al. Delivery of siRNA to the mouse brain by systemic injection of targeted exosomes. Nat Biotechnol. 2011;29:341–5.
68. Choi H, et al. Exosome-based delivery of super-repressor IκBα relieves sepsis-associated organ damage and mortality. Sci Adv. 2020;6:eaaz6980.

69. Haney MJ, et al. Exosomes as drug delivery vehicles for Parkinson's disease therapy. J Control Release. 2015;207:18–30.
70. Aengenheister L, et al. An advanced human in vitro co-culture model for translocation studies across the placental barrier. Sci Rep. 2018;8:5388.
71. Swingle KL, Ricciardi AS, Peranteau WH, Mitchell MJ. Delivery technologies for women's health applications. Nat Rev Bioeng. 2023;3:408–25. https://doi.org/10.1038/s44222-023-00040-w.
72. Irvin-Choy NS, Nelson KM, Dang MN, Gleghorn JP, Day ES. Gold nanoparticle biodistribution in pregnant mice following intravenous administration varies with gestational age. Nanomedicine. 2021;36:102412.
73. Yang H, et al. Effects of gestational age and surface modification on materno-fetal transfer of nanoparticles in murine pregnancy. Sci Rep. 2012;2:847.
74. Austin CA, et al. Distribution of silver nanoparticles in pregnant mice and developing embryos. Nanotoxicology. 2012;6:912–22.
75. Austin CA, et al. Distribution and accumulation of 10 nm silver nanoparticles in maternal tissues and visceral yolk sac of pregnant mice, and a potential effect on embryo growth. Nanotoxicology. 2016;10:654–61.
76. Di Bona KR, et al. Surface charge and dosage dependent potential developmental toxicity and biodistribution of iron oxide nanoparticles in pregnant CD-1 mice. Reprod Toxicol. 2014;50:36–42.
77. Bolandparvaz A, et al. Biodistribution and toxicity of epitope-functionalized dextran iron oxide nanoparticles in a pregnant murine model. J Biomed Mater Res A. 2020;108:1186–202.
78. D'Errico JN, Doherty C, Reyes George JJ, Buckley B, Stapleton PA. Maternal, placental, and fetal distribution of titanium after repeated titanium dioxide nanoparticle inhalation through pregnancy. Placenta. 2022;121:99–108.
79. Stapleton PA, et al. Maternal engineered nanomaterial inhalation during gestation alters the fetal transcriptome. Part Fibre Toxicol. 2018;15:3.
80. Hathaway QA, et al. Maternal-engineered nanomaterial exposure disrupts progeny cardiac function and bioenergetics. Am J Phys Heart Circ Phys. 2017;312:H446–58.
81. Cary CM, et al. Single pulmonary nanopolystyrene exposure in late-stage pregnancy dysregulates maternal and fetal cardiovascular function. Toxicol Sci. 2024;199:149–59.
82. Ho D, et al. Maternal-placental-fetal biodistribution of multimodal polymeric nanoparticles in a pregnant rat model in mid and late gestation. Sci Rep. 2017;7:2866.
83. Kuna M, Waller JP, Logue OC, Bidwell GL. Polymer size affects biodistribution and placental accumulation of the drug delivery biopolymer elastin-like polypeptide in a rodent pregnancy model. Placenta. 2018;72–73:20–7.
84. Cary CM, et al. Ingested polystyrene Nanospheres translocate to placenta and Fetal tissues in pregnant rats: potential health implications. Nano. 2023;13:720.
85. Moreno GM, et al. Identification of micro- and nanoplastic particles in postnatal Sprague-dawley rat offspring after maternal inhalation exposure throughout gestation. Sci Total Environ. 2024;951:175350.
86. Muoth C, et al. Impact of particle size and surface modification on gold nanoparticle penetration into human placental microtissues. Nanomedicine. 2017;12:1119–33.
87. Aengenheister L, et al. Gold nanoparticle distribution in advanced in vitro and ex vivo human placental barrier models. J Nanobiotechnol. 2018;16:79.
88. Li L, et al. Trophoblast-targeted Nanomedicine modulates placental sFLT1 for preeclampsia treatment. Front Bioeng Biotechnol. 2020;8:64.
89. Yu J, Jia J, Guo X, Chen R, Feng L. Modulating circulating sFlt1 in an animal model of preeclampsia using PAMAM nanoparticles for siRNA delivery. Placenta. 2017;58:1–8.
90. Ellah NA, et al. Development of non-viral, trophoblast-specific gene delivery for placental therapy. PLoS One. 2015;10:e0140879.
91. Alfaifi AA, et al. Megalin-targeting liposomes for placental drug delivery. J Control Release. 2020;324:366–78.

92. Cureton N, et al. Selective targeting of a novel vasodilator to the uterine vasculature to treat impaired Uteroplacental perfusion in pregnancy. Theranostics. 2017;7:3715–31.
93. Renshall LJ, et al. Targeted delivery of epidermal growth factor to the human placenta to treat fetal growth restriction. Pharmaceutics. 2021;13:1778.
94. King A, et al. Tumor-homing peptides as tools for targeted delivery of payloads to the placenta. Sci Adv. 2016;2:e1600349.
95. Swingle KL, et al. Ionizable lipid nanoparticles for in vivo mRNA delivery to the placenta during pregnancy. J Am Chem Soc. 2023;145:4691–706.
96. Safford HC, et al. Orthogonal design of experiments for engineering of lipid nanoparticles for mRNA delivery to the placenta. Small. 2023;20:e2303568.
97. Young RE, et al. Systematic development of ionizable lipid nanoparticles for placental mRNA delivery using a design of experiments approach. Bioact Mater. 2024;34:125–37.
98. Chaudhary N, et al. Lipid nanoparticle structure and delivery route during pregnancy dictate mRNA potency, immunogenicity, and maternal and fetal outcomes. Proc Natl Acad Sci. 2024;121:e2307810121.
99. Geisler HC, et al. EGFR-targeted ionizable lipid nanoparticles enhance *in vivo* mRNA delivery to the placenta. J Control Release. 2024;371:455–69.
100. Swingle KL, et al. Placenta-tropic VEGF mRNA lipid nanoparticles ameliorate murine pre-eclampsia. Nature. 2025;637:412–21. https://doi.org/10.1038/s41586-024-08291-2.
101. Beards F, Jones LE, Charnock J, Forbes K, Harris LK. Placental homing peptide-microRNA inhibitor conjugates for targeted enhancement of intrinsic placental growth Signaling. Theranostics. 2017;7:2940–55.
102. Wilson RL, Lampe K, Gupta MK, Duvall CL, Jones HN. Nanoparticle-mediated transgene expression of insulin-like growth factor 1 in the growth restricted Guinea pig placenta increases placenta nutrient transporter expression and fetal glucose concentrations. Mol Reprod Dev. 2022;89:540–53.
103. Davenport BN, Wilson RL, Williams AA, Jones HN. Placental nanoparticle-mediated IGF1 gene therapy corrects fetal growth restriction in a Guinea pig model. Gene Ther. 2025;32:255–65. https://doi.org/10.1038/s41434-024-00508-3.
104. Davenport BN, Williams A, Regnault TRH, Jones HN, Wilson RL. Placenta hIGF1 nanoparticle treatment in Guinea pigs mitigates FGR-associated fetal sex-dependent effects on liver metabolism-related signaling pathways. Am J Physiol Endocrinol Metab. 2025;328: E395–409.
105. Wilson RL, et al. Placental gene therapy in nonhuman primates: a pilot study of maternal, placental, and fetal response to non-viral, polymeric nanoparticle delivery of IGF1. Mol Hum Reprod. 2024;30:gaae038.
106. Schmidt JK, et al. Nanoparticle-mediated delivery of placental gene therapy via uterine artery catheterization in a pregnant rhesus macaque. Placenta. 2025;166:103–8. https://doi.org/10.1016/j.placenta.2024.09.013.
107. Hofbauer SI, et al. Cytokine mRNA delivery and local immunomodulation in the placenta using lipid nanoparticles. bioRxiv. 2025. https://doi.org/10.1101/2025.02.07.637086.
108. Ren Z, Bremer AA, Pawlyk AC. Drug development research in pregnant and lactating women. Am J Obstet Gynecol. 2021;225:33–42.
109. Fein KC, Arral ML, Kim JS, Newby AN, Whitehead KA. Placental drug transport and fetal exposure during pregnancy is determined by drug molecular size, chemistry, and conformation. J Control Release. 2023;361:29–39.
110. Dodd A, et al. Conjugation to PEG as a strategy to limit the uptake of drugs by the placenta: potential applications for drug Administration in Pregnancy. Mol Pharm. 2022;19:345–53.
111. Figueroa-Espada CG, Hofbauer S, Mitchell MJ, Riley RS. Exploiting the placenta for nanoparticle-mediated drug delivery during pregnancy. Adv Drug Deliv Rev. 2020;160: 244–61.
112. Labouta HI. Defining the landscape of prenatal nanomedicine and a roadmap for future research. Nanomedicine. 2025;20:1647–51.

113. Abostait A, et al. Optimizing lipid nanoparticles for fetal gene delivery in vitro, ex vivo, and aided with machine learning. J Control Release. 2024;376:678–700.
114. Palanki R, Peranteau WH, Mitchell MJ. Delivery technologies for in utero gene therapy. Adv Drug Deliv Rev. 2021;169:51–62.
115. Nakamura S, et al. Transplacental delivery of genome editing components causes mutations in embryonic cardiomyocytes of mid-gestational murine fetuses. IUBMB Life. 2019;71:835–44.
116. Hei Tse W, et al. The maternal-fetal transfer of passive immunity as a mechanism of transplacental nanoparticle drug delivery for prenatal therapies. *Biomaterials*. Science. 2022;10:5243–53.
117. Cornford EM, et al. Non-invasive gene targeting to the fetal brain after intravenous administration and transplacental transfer of plasmid DNA using PEGylated immunoliposomes. J Drug Target. 2016;24:58–67.
118. Gruber MM, et al. Plasma proteins facilitates placental transfer of polystyrene particles. J Nanobiotechnol. 2020;18:128.
119. Pyzik M, Kozicky LK, Gandhi AK, Blumberg RS. The therapeutic age of the neonatal fc receptor. Nat Rev Immunol. 2023;23:415–32.
120. Chappell LC, Cluver CA, Kingdom J, Tong S. Pre-eclampsia. Lancet. 2021;398:341–54.
121. Geisler HC, Safford HC, Mitchell MJ. Rational design of nanomedicine for placental disorders: birthing a new era in women's reproductive health. Small. 2024;20:e2300852. https://doi.org/10.1002/smll.202300852.
122. Li L, et al. Nanoparticle-mediated simultaneous downregulation of placental Nrf2 and sFlt1 improves maternal and Fetal outcomes in a preeclampsia mouse model. ACS Biomater Sci Eng. 2020;6:5866–73.
123. Turanov AA, et al. RNAi modulation of placental sFLT1 for the treatment of preeclampsia. Nat Biotechnol. 2018;36:1164–73.
124. Davis SM, et al. Chemical optimization of siRNA for safe and efficient silencing of placental sFLT1. Mol Ther Nucleic Acids. 2022;29:135–49.
125. Seckl MJ, Sebire NJ, Berkowitz RS. Gestational trophoblastic disease. Lancet. 2010;376:717–29.
126. Zhang B, et al. Targeted delivery of doxorubicin by CSA-binding nanoparticles for choriocarcinoma treatment. Drug Deliv. 2018;25:461–71.
127. Zhao H, et al. Intrauterine perfusion of versatile Nanotherapeutics for revolutionizing Sonochemotherapeutic treatment of Orthotopic Choriocarcinoma. Adv Funct Mater. 2025;35: 2422357.
128. Zhao K, et al. Targeted delivery prodigiosin to choriocarcinoma by peptide-guided dendrigraft poly-l-lysines nanoparticles. Int J Mol Sci. 2019;20:5458.
129. Yu H, et al. A biomimetic nanoreactor for combinational chemo/chemodynamic therapy of choriocarcinoma through synergistic apoptosis and ferroptosis strategy. Chem Eng J. 2023;472:144690.
130. Kaitu'u-Lino TJ, et al. Targeted nanoparticle delivery of doxorubicin into placental tissues to treat ectopic pregnancies. Endocrinology. 2013;154:911–9.
131. Bilinski A, Emanuel N. Fewer than 1% of United States clinical drug trials enroll pregnant participants. Am J Obstet Gynecol. 2025;232:e136–9.

Uterine Drug-Delivery Systems

Lauren E. Mehanna, Claire E. Rowlands, and Brittany E. Givens

Abstract Sustained and controlled release drug delivery systems (DDSs) are widely investigated for disease diagnosis and treatment. Advanced DDS provides critical advantages over traditional DDSs, particularly by bypassing systemic circulation and first-pass metabolism. This enhances the drug payload at the target site and reduces systemic side effects. Uterine drug delivery is already widely used with contraceptive intrauterine devices, but further explorations to treat uterine fibroids, uterine cancer, and endometriosis are still being developed. Advances in these systems will provide critical clinical enhancements over the current treatment options.

Keywords Drug delivery · Controlled drug delivery · Sustained drug delivery · Intrauterine devices · Polymeric drug delivery · Hydrogel scaffolds · Tissue regeneration · Receptor-mediated drug delivery · Uterine fibroids · Uterine cancer

1 Introduction

Advancing drug delivery strategies to target the uterus requires pushing the boundaries of engineering and pharmaceutical sciences to develop novel technology with translational potential. Drug delivery methods and approaches have improved over

L. E. Mehanna
Programs of Chemistry and Engineering, Centre College, Danville, KY, USA
e-mail: lauren.mehanna@centre.edu

C. E. Rowlands
Bluegrass Advanced Materials, Lexington, KY, USA
e-mail: crowlands@bgamaterials.com

B. E. Givens (✉)
Department of Chemical and Materials Engineering, Stanley and Karen Pigman College of Engineering, University of Kentucky, Lexington, KY, USA
e-mail: brittany.givens@uky.edu

S. G. Zambuto, M. L. Oyen (eds.), *Biomaterials for Women's Health Engineering*,
https://doi.org/10.1007/978-3-032-10745-9_19

time; however, targeted drug delivery to the uterus remains a critical challenge. For example, contraceptive delivery via intrauterine devices (IUDs) was first developed in the 1960s; however, there is no comparable drug delivery system (DDS) for treating disease [1, 2].

1.1 Endometriosis

Endometriosis is a condition in which the endometrium grows externally to the uterus [3]. This results in painful symptoms, scarring, and infertility [4, 5]. Currently, the available medications are only effective in treating endometriosis-related pain and do not treat the endometriosis growths [6]. Endometriosis impacts 1 in 10 females worldwide, and most are treated with medication [5]. In more severe cases, surgical removal of the tissue is also used. If fertility preservation is not a concern, hysterectomy is often recommended.

1.2 Asherman's Syndrome

Intrauterine adhesions (IUAs), also called Asherman's syndrome, are fibrous tissue that forms within the endometrium, and create partial or total occlusions within the uterine cavity [7]. IUAs are often caused by surgery, such as dilation and curettage, or injury to the endometrium, and the fibrous tissue that forms impairs the tissue's natural regenerative potential. IUAs can cause menstrual abnormalities, pelvic pain, contribute to miscarriages, and are one of the leading causes of infertility in women of childbearing age [8].

1.3 Uterine Fibroids

Uterine fibroids are growths in and around the uterus, originating from the myometrium [9]. Most uterine fibroids are noncancerous and may range in size from 1 mm to 20 cm. Fibroids impact as many as 80% of females between menarche and menopause. As with endometriosis, uterine fibroids can cause extreme pain and are typically removed via medication or surgery. Alternatively, uterine fibroids may be treated using uterine ablation. In uterine ablation, sometimes referred to as endometrial ablation, the uterine lining (endometrium) is destroyed to address problems associated with fibroids [10]. Traditionally, uterine ablation also significantly lowered female fertility; however, recent advances are focused on preserving fertility [11].

1.4 Uterine Cancer

The first-line treatment for uterine cancers is hysterectomy with or without bilateral salpingo-oophorectomy [12]. If the cancer is advanced or if the hysterectomy is undesired by the patient, chemotherapy may be used [13–15]. There are only two chemotherapeutic drugs that the US Food and Drug Administration (FDA) has approved to treat uterine cancer, and therefore, most chemotherapeutic methods are used off-label for ovarian cancer approvals [16, 17].

1.5 Uterine Anatomy

The human female reproductive system is distinguished between the "upper tract" and the "lower tract." The upper tract contains two bilateral ovaries that are connected to the uterine body via the fallopian tubes. At the base of the uterus, the cervix forms a barrier between the uterus and the vagina. Human implantation, placentation, and gestation then occur localized to the uterine body. When implantation occurs outside the uterus, this is considered an ectopic pregnancy. Ectopic pregnancies can be life-threatening. The uterus is comprised of three tissue layers: the endometrium, myometrium, and perimetrium. Large animals, such as sheep, have a uterine structure similar to that of humans. In fact, sheep represent the closest animal anatomy to the human uterus, and therefore, are a good model for vaginal DDS and vaginal prolapse, among others [18, 19].

Animals that have multiple live births, such as rodents, have a Y-shaped uterine structure, with uterine horns forming the "Y," which are the primary sites of implantation and gestation. Although pigs share close relationships with other human organs, such as skin, heart, and eyes, and are mammals that typically have multiple live births at a time, they also have a uterine horn structure [20, 21]. Unlike in rodents, the uterine horns in pigs have pleats that increase the available surface area (Fig. 1).

2 Contraceptive Delivery

2.1 Intrauterine Devices

IUDs are drug-eluting medical devices that are placed directly in the uterus and remain in place for 3–10 years. An IUD is placed by a doctor during an office visit. A medical provider uses a sounding device to determine the position of the uterus and then slides the IUD through the cervix and into the uterus. The IUD sits within the uterus, and the strings attached to the IUD protrude from the cervix into the vagina

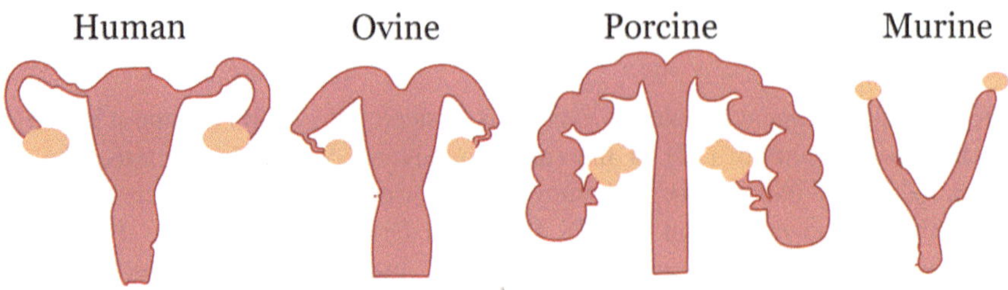

Fig. 1 Structural outlines of human, ovine, porcine, and murine uteruses. Uteruses are presented in descending order from similarity to the human uterus, with the ovine bearing the strongest resemblance. Porcine uteri share many structures with the human and ovine uteri; however, they also have uterine horns with a high surface area to accommodate multiple live births. Murine uteruses lack a uterine body and consist only of uterine tubes

Table 1 Current commercially available IUD products with FDA approval in the United States

Product	Type of IUD	Year of US FDA approval	Effective duration	In vivo drug release rate at the end of the effective duration (μg/day)	Parent company
ParaGard®	Copper	1988	10 years	200	Cooper Surgical, Inc. ®
Mirena®	Levonogestrel	2000	7 years	8.0	Bayer®
Liletta®	Levonogestrel	2015	6 years	8.6	AbbVie® and Medicines360®
Kyleena®	Levonogestrel	2016	5 years	7.4	Bayer®
Skyla®	Levonogestrel	2013	3 years	5.0	Bayer®

Adapted from Fanse et al. [1]

for removal. In rare cases (1 in 1000), uterine perforation occurs, in which the IUD either wholly or partially perforates through the uterus into the abdomen, bowels, or urinary tract [2].

Contraceptive IUDs are over 99% effective and offer sustained-release contraceptive delivery. Globally, approximately 19.4% of women use IUDs as a method of intrauterine contraception [22]. Most IUDs are polyethylene-based and between 28–36 mm long and 28–32 mm wide, and several have been US FDA-approved (Table 1). Non-hormonal IUDs contain copper, which is toxic to sperm cells, therefore preventing fertilization [23]. Copper IUDs were introduced in the 1960s, and ParaGard® was approved by the US FDA in 1988 [1, 2]. Copper IUDs are the longest-lasting IUDs with a lifetime of up to 10 years.

Copper IUDs undergo a burst-release of 100–296μg/day of Cu^{2+} ions followed by sustained-release of Cu^{2+} ions [24]. Copper concentrations above 80μM within the uterus are known to induce muscle contractions, which can then cause additional side effects such as heavier periods, increased cramping, and, in severe cases, evacuation of the device. Therefore, mitigation strategies have been investigated. Reducing the copper grain microstructure from a coarse-grained material to a fine-grained material reduces the burst release of copper to 146μg/day [23, 25]. Alternatively, copper alloys of copper–magnesium (Cu–0.4 Mg) [26], copper–zinc (Cu–38 Zn) [27], and copper–iron (Cu–5 Fe) [25] reduce the overall release of copper. Furthermore, these alloy materials are all biocompatible with the surrounding uterine tissue in the oxidized form.

Rather than changing the material, the shape and material of the IUD may also be altered to reduce copper ion release. For example, instead of a polyethylene frame, a nickel–titanium alloy frame used in VeraCept® may reduce side effects but only lasts for 5 years, compared to the 10-year ParaGard® currently on the market [28]. An intrauterine ball containing copper beads, Ballerine®, was developed in Australia and has been expanded to Europe, Africa, and the United States as an Investigational New Drug in 2023 [29, 30]. Ballerine® is also promising because it is much smaller than ParaGard®, therefore reducing the risk of uterine perforation or cervical expulsion.

Hormonal IUDs contain the synthetic form of the hormone progestin called levonorgestrel (LNG). Several hormonal IUDs are available in the United States, including Mirena®, Liletta®, Kyleena®, and Skyla®. Hormonal IUDs offer an advantage over copper IUDs because they can be used for treating heavy menstrual bleeding and as a hormone replacement therapy, in addition to providing contraception. LNG is locally released from the IUD into the uterus and suppresses endometrial growth during ovulation. The release of LNG thickens the cervical mucus, inhibiting the sperm motility to reach and fertilize the egg [1]. Additionally, LNG promotes thinning of the uterine lining, called the endometrium, making it more difficult for an egg to implant within the uterus and survive [1, 31, 32].

Hormonal IUDs have the same polyethylene frame; however, they also contain a drug-loaded poly(dimethylsiloxane) membrane. The drug reservoir is loaded with 13–52 mg of LNG, depending on the type and dosage, but it has a controlled release of only 6–18μg/day, gradually decreasing the release rate over time [1]. Similar to copper IUDs, hormonal IUDs have a burst effect where a higher concentration of LNG is released upon initial insertion, but then gradually decreases to a controlled release profile over time [33–35]. Although the general release profile has been studied, the mechanisms of LNG drug release from the drug reservoir are still not fully understood.

The first LNG-IUD under the name Mirena® was FDA-approved in 2000 for up to 8 years of use. Since then, three additional LNG-IUDs have gained approval—Skyla® in 2013 for up to 3 years of use, Liletta® in 2015 for up to 6 years of use, and Kyleena® in 2016 for up to 5 years of use. Although they are effective, hormonal IUDs create many side effects for patients, including irregularities in the menstrual cycle, such as cramping, breast tenderness, acne, headaches, and mood changes [36, 37].

3 Therapeutic Drug Delivery

3.1 Non-steroidal Anti-inflammatory Drugs

Pre-clinical development of treatment for uterine fibroids includes uterine artery embolization, a non-invasive technique by which particles are injected to treat uterine fibroids. Typically, this is followed by pain management using drugs, primarily non-steroidal anti-inflammatory drugs (NSAIDs).

A "T"-shaped fluidic system was used to investigate the release of ibuprofen-loaded poly(vinyl alcohol), hydrogel beads (IBU-BB) to reduce inflammation and pain following uterine artery embolization for the treatment of uterine fibroids [38]. Compared with release in a beaker under constant stirring, the T-shaped release system had a slower release profile. T-shaped diffusion with ketoprofen-loaded N-[tris (hydroxymethyl) methyl] acrylamide-gelatin microspheres followed a similar trend [39].

In non-pregnant adult Pre-Alpes female sheep artificially cycled to mimic human females with uterine fibroids, the plasma concentration of ibuprofen was lower in those that received an intrauterine injection of IBU-BB compared to those that received an IBU solution. A subsequent investigation quantified this difference as 70% lower in IBU-BB compared with IBU solution [40]. This indicates that the IBU-BB increases intrauterine retention of the IBU following injection and, therefore, may be a promising method of localized drug delivery for minimizing systemic toxicity. The inflammatory response was also quantified using inflammatory cells in sheep following embolization with either IBU-BB or BB [40]. IBU-BB had significantly lower quantities of cluster of differentiation 172a (CD172a), cluster of differentiation 11B (CD11B), major histocompatibility complex class II (MHC-II), cluster of differentiation 3 (CD3), cluster of differentation 44 (CD44), and von Willebrand factor (vWf) compared with BB 1 week following treatment. Further indicating that the IBU-BB exhibits positive anti-inflammatory effects following uterine fibroid embolization. However, after 3 weeks, the ibuprofen is completely released, and therefore, an inflammatory reaction around the beads returns [40, 41]. Specifically, researchers noted increased expression of Interleukin-6 (IL-6) and tumor necrosis factor-alpha (TNF-α) in the blood vessels and surrounding tissues after 3 weeks [42].

Stable resorbable microspheres (REMs) for embolization were developed to mitigate the inflammatory rebound observed with the IBU-BB [43]. These microspheres used poly(ethylene glycol) (PEG) as the hydrogel material and included the NSAIDs sodium diclofenac, flurbiprofen, niflumic acid, and ketoprofen. Niflumic acid had 3$\times$ higher loading compared with flurbiprofen and ketoprofen, and sodium diclofenac loading was unsuccessful. Therefore, all in vitro and ex vivo investigations were performed with niflumic acid-loaded REMs. Inflammation via prostaglandin synthesis was assessed in uterine explants from the uterine horns of New Zealand rabbits after 24-h incubation with niflumic acid-REMs. The results indicated that nuflumic acid-REMs significantly decreased prostaglandin synthesis, indicating positive anti-inflammatory effects.

3.2 *Receptor-Mediated Targeting*

Receptor-mediated targeting is used to enhance bioavailability and accumulation at a target site, using specific receptors for that target site. For example, CD44 is commonly overexpressed on endometrial cancer tumors and can be targeted with hyaluronic acid (HA). Ishikawa H cells were sorted according to their CD44 status, and HA uptake was higher in the CD44 high population compared with the CD44 low population of cells [44]. A zinc oxide-HA cocktail demonstrated enhanced cell death in the SCC-7 mouse squamous cell carcinoma and COS7 African green monkey kidney fibroblast-like cells and SCC-7 tumor-bearing mice [45]. HA may also be used to target the HA-binding proteins hyaluronan-binding protein 1 (HABP1) and hyaluronan-binding protein 2 (HABP2). HAPB1 plays a role in tumorigenesis, progression, invasion, and metastasis of tumors, as well as wound repair [46, 47]. HABP1 expression tends to be high in endometrial cancers with poor prognoses and is also overexpressed in malignant endometrial lesions compared with the benign endometrium [47, 48].

3.3 *Gene Targeting*

In gynecological cancers, including endometrial cancer, *PTEN* somatic mutations are common. Additionally, *PTEN* inactivation is present in endometriosis and endometrial hyperplasia [49]. *PTEN* is commonly targeted via the phosphoinositide 3-kinase (PI3K) pathway. For example, small interfering RNA knockdown of homeobox A11 (*HOXA11*) repressed apoptosis and promoted proliferation, migration, and invasion in Ishikawa endometrial cancer cells. This knockdown also increased platinum-resistance to cisplatin in the cells via the phosphatase and tension homologous (PTEN) / protein kinase B (AKT) pathway [50]. In contrast, microRNA upregulation of miR-135a, which influences the expression of PTEN and p-AKT, increased the proliferation, migration, and invasion of Ishikawa and HEC-1B cells following cisplatin treatment [51]. Thus, in addition to the oncogenic role of PTEN inactivation, it appears that the PTEN pathway also plays a role in platinum resistance, which comprises a critical amount of treatment failures in cancer therapeutics.

The tumor promoter gene 53 (*TP53*) is one of the most common genetic mutations in cancer, and in endometrial cancer, *TP53* mutations contribute to more aggressive cancers [52]. Bevacizumab (Avastin®) is a monoclonal antibody that blocks vascular endothelial growth factor (VEGF) and has been effective in treating many tumor types. Analysis of a randomized phase II study of advanced endometrial cancer concluded that cells with at least 80% p53 expression from immunohistochemistry analysis should be treated with bevacizumab in combination with chemotherapy upfront to enhance progression-free survival and overall survival [52]. In a pre-clinical investigation with a triple angiokinase molecular inhibitor, which inhibits tumor angiogenesis and therefore migration and invasion, Ebeid et al. demonstrated that there was a synergistic effect with paclitaxel in Ishikawa, Hec50Co, and KLE endometrial cancer cells in vitro and in tumor-bearing mice [53]. A separate pre-clinical investigation revealed that the MEK1/2 inhibitor PD98059, when also combined with paclitaxel, showed synergy to improve cell cycle arrest and apoptosis in Hec50co cells in vitro and in tumor-bearing mice. Specifically, the PD98059 was prepared in poly(amidoamine) (PAMAM)-coated poly(lactic-*co*-glycolic acid) (PLGA)-PEG nanoparticles and showed enhanced efficacy over soluble PD98059 [54].

3.4 Therapeutic IUDs

Drug-loaded implantable IUDs are under pre-clinical investigation for sustained-release devices. A crosslinked rod of poly(propylene fumarate) (PPF) and N-vinylpyrrolidone (NVP) was developed as a drug-eluting device to treat grade 1 endometrial cancer [55]. The NVP improves the hydrophilicity and drug encapsulation over PPF, and the IUD offers localized sustained-release delivery of everolimus, which, when delivered orally, results in adverse side effects, including immune suppression, anemia, fatigue, elevated blood glucose, and vomiting. The efficacy of this IUD was assessed using reduced liminal epithelial cell height and PI3K/AKT/mechanistic target of rapamycin (mTOR) pathway activity in rats for 21 days. Hot-melt extrusion was used to produce scaffolds that incorporated a poly (caprolactone) (PCL) backbone. Along with the PCL, cyclodextrin was loaded with either paclitaxel or carboplatin to treat uterine cancer [56]. In aqueous solution, both paclitaxel and carboplatin exhibited sustained-release, and in vitro cell studies with uterine cancer indicated great potential for these implants as cancer therapeutics.

Therapeutic IUDs are not limited to cancer, and other devices have been investigated pre-clinically for IUAs and endometriosis. Mifepristone to treat endometriosis was loaded into an implant inserted subcutaneously and provided sustained release for 1–3 months in rats [57]. These scaffolds were also made using a PCL backbone; however, it was a 90/10 (w/w%) mixture of PCL and Pluronic F68 as the emulsifier. Similarly, IUAs may be treated with the estrogen steroid hormone 17-β-estradiol (E2) to promote endometrial tissue regeneration. Oral delivery of E2 results in low uterine bioavailability; however, a silicone rubber stent resulted in 60-day delivery in rats [58]. Developing implantable devices using polymeric materials holds great promise in loading and releasing drug molecules for disease treatment for localized delivery and more effective outcomes.

4 Tissue Regeneration

The mechanisms that govern wound healing closely mimic the hallmarks of cancer [59]. Several mechanisms have been shown to improve the wound healing process, specifically in the uterus, including metallic nanoparticles and intrauterine antibacterial microneedle patches [60, 61]. Recent advancements in three-dimensional (3D) in vitro models for endometrial cancer have led to a more accurate representation of the tumor microenvironment compared to traditional 2D models or Matrigel [62, 63]. Notably, a novel hydrogel derived from decellularized endometrium demonstrated that incorporating extracellular matrix (ECM) components native to the endometrium increased the reproducibility of endometrial organoids compared to Matrigel [64]. Additionally, an innovative disintegration-controllable supramolecular gelatin hydrogel was used to develop a co-culture system of endometrial tumor spheroids and tumor-associated macrophages, shedding light on the interplay between M2 macrophages, ECM components, and endometrial cancer cells [65]. These studies underscore the importance of including endometrial cancer-specific ECM components in 3D models and using 3D models for high-throughput screening.

4.1 *Endometrium Regeneration*

The endometrium is one of the only tissues in mature adults capable of undergoing regeneration [66, 67]. Promoting endometrial regeneration through biomaterials combines the mechanical properties of the reproductive tissue with growth factors and other small molecules that mimic the native environment [68].

For IUAs treated with, or arising from, ablation, scar-free tissue regeneration is a critical concern [69]. Pre-clinical investigations to address this healing include hydrogel innovations to promote wound healing. For example, combining hydrogels with pharmacological therapeutics may promote surgery-free treatment of IUAs [70]. A common component in these systems to promote endometrial regeneration is platelet-rich plasma (PRP), which regulates the PI3K/AKT pathway, which regulates cell proliferation, growth, metabolism, and survival [71].

One such study investigated PEG methyl ether acrylate-based hydrogels containing L-serine, PRP, and allyl functionalized chitosan for an injectable treatment to IUAs [70]. In mice with IUAs, this injectable hydrogel resulted in localized drug release that promoted endometrial regeneration and a resumption of fertility in these mice. A similar investigation used PEG diacrylate, sodium alginate, L-serine, and PRP and reported comparable results for tissue regeneration and fertility restoration [72]. Using only naturally occurring polymers, hyaluronan and chitosan, with PRP and mouse adipose-derived stem cells (ADSCs), researchers confirmed endometrial regeneration and fertility restoration in mice [73]. These investigations indicate that numerous injectable biocompatible and biodegradable polymers can be used for treating IUAs.

4.2 Fetal Membrane Regeneration

To promote tissue regeneration, growth factor-releasing hydrogels were used following pre-term fetal membrane rupture [74]. Transglutaminase-PEG hydrogels were crosslinked and loaded with platelet-derived growth factor, shown to allow the infiltration of healing-associated cells, specifically human amniotic-derived mesenchymal cells in sheep. Furthermore, hydrogel stiffness was investigated as a variable, and stiff hydrogels exhibited lower cell infiltration compared with softer hydrogels. Additionally, softer hydrogels showed less swelling in the presence of amniotic fluid. This study demonstrated potential in using soft hydrogel materials for fetal membrane regeneration.

4.3 Hydrogel Scaffolds

Hydrogels are 3D hydrophilic polymer networks that are utilized in tissue engineering applications because they are able to retain water, have excellent elastic properties, and closely mimic the natural tissue ECM. These hydrogels are inserted as a scaffold at the injury site and integrate with the existing tissue. Hydrogel materials are biocompatible with native tissue and have low interfacial surface tension, which supports cell adhesion, proliferation, and differentiation for tissue integration and regeneration [75, 76]. Due to their biocompatible and often biodegradable properties, hydrogels are ideal for transporting cellular components and drug molecules to the site of injury. These cellular components can include growth factors, ECM proteins, and stem cells that promote tissue repair and lower immune rejection. Additionally, hydrogels are popular for their sol–gel transitions in response to environmental factors, such as temperature, pH, and light [77, 78]. There are numerous materials, including natural and synthetic polymers, that have been utilized to develop hydrogel scaffolds for tissue regeneration. By inducing natural tissue repair, hydrogel scaffolds are highly successful in treating endometrial diseases, preventing fibrous tissue formation, and improving fertility outcomes.

Recent advancements in 3D in vitro models for endometrial cancer have led to a more accurate representation of the tumor microenvironment compared to traditional 2D models or Matrigel [62, 63]. Notably, a novel hydrogel derived from decellularized endometrium demonstrated that incorporating ECM components native to the endometrium increased the reproducibility of endometrial organoids compared to Matrigel [64]. Additionally, an innovative disintegration-controllable supramolecular gelatin hydrogel was used to develop a co-culture system of endometrial tumor spheroids and tumor-associated macrophages, shedding light on the interplay between M2 macrophages, ECM components, and endometrial cancer cells [65]. These studies underscore the importance of including endometrial cancer-specific ECM components in 3D models and using 3D models for high-throughput screening. However, microvessel formation is a critical step in endometrial cancer progression, and these models did not include endothelial cells, which is a clear area for improvement addressed in our model. Additionally, the integration of these models with high-throughput screening remains a challenge, limiting their application to drug screening and large-scale mechanistic studies. Thus, an overarching goal of this paper was to develop a novel platform that captures 3D metastatic behavior and interfaces with standard high-throughput drug screening methods.

4.3.1 Natural Polymer Scaffolds

Natural polymers are developed from materials that can be created or extracted from nature. Hydrogels developed from natural polymers are common in tissue repair applications due to their high biocompatibility and low immune rejection response. However, natural polymers can have less desirable mechanical properties compared to synthetic polymers. Most hydrogels for uterine tissue repair combine natural polymer materials with cellular components for better integration at the tissue site and to deliver stem cells, commonly mesenchymal stem cells (MSCs), necessary for repair. These hydrogels can be delivered directly to the injured tissue through a solid scaffold or through an injectable viscous solution with thermoresponsive gelation properties.

Collagen

Collagen is the main structural protein in biological tissue. Collagen has many types, and collagen I provides the structural framework for new tissues. A collagen I hydrogel embedded with MSCs was used for direct uterine injection to promote tissue repair in rats [79]. MSC viability was assessed 48 h and 72 h post-encapsulation as well as via uterine retention in vivo. Ultimately, the collagen I hydrogel protected MSC viability and injections promoted endometrial vascularization, increased endometrial stromal cell (endoSC) proliferation, and improved myometrial thickness compared to the control.

Hyaluronic Acid

HA is another widely used hydrogel material in endometrial regeneration, as it is a natural polysaccharide beneficial in embryonic development for its biodegradable, anti-inflammatory, and antioxidant properties. HA plays a large role in endometrial proliferation, making it favorable as a scaffold material for drug delivery and endometrial regeneration of injured tissue. Wei et al. combined the properties of both collagen and HA to improve endometrial repair [80].

Type III collagen is a key ECM structural protein that is prominent in the endometrium and is capable of promoting cell proliferation, migration, and adhesion. Unlike type I collagen, type III collagen is downregulated after injury and may aid in tissue repair if replenished; however, collagen III in the form of recombinant human type III collagen (RHC) is water soluble and easily degraded at the injury site. Therefore, delivering RHC via an HA hydrogel provides the structural integrity and sustained release necessary for repair. The developed RHC-HA hydrogel improved endometrial cell proliferation, migration, and adhesion in vitro. It also enhanced angiogenesis and myometrial regeneration, while decreasing inflammatory factors associated with fibrosis in an in vivo murine model. Therefore, RHC was effectively being stabilized and released in a controlled manner in the HA hydrogel to promote endometrial regeneration.

Other uses of HA include encapsulating cells and cellular components, such as MSCs, similarly to collagen. Lin et al. developed an HA hydrogel loaded with human placenta-derived MSCs (HP-MSCs) to aid in the regeneration of thin endometrium in a rat model [81]. The hydrogel was injected at the site of an injured endometrium, and regeneration metrics were studied. The loaded hydrogel had a longer retention time, improved gland number and thickness, and decreased fibrotic tissue area in vivo compared to HP-MSCs alone. Additionally, the hydrogel promoted cell proliferation and angiogenesis among endometrial cells, while also facilitating the proliferation and migration of stromal and glandular cells.

Xin et al. used an HA hydrogel to encapsulate and deliver apoptotic bodies (ABs) derived from MSCs to damaged endometrial tissue from IUAs in a murine and rat model [82]. ABs are a form of extracellular vesicles that are released by dying cells undergoing apoptosis. ABs can include functional biomolecules, including microRNAs, mRNAs, DNA, lipids, and proteins [83]. These ABs, when released, can infiltrate surrounding tissue and induce cellular proliferation and wound healing [84]. MSCs can undergo apoptosis and release these ABs, being harnessed to improve endometrial regeneration. Embedding ABs into an HA hydrogel allowed for effective delivery of the ABs to damaged endometrial tissue.

Gelatin

Gelatin is derived from collagen via hydrolysis. As a collagen derivative, gelatin has similar biocompatibility and degradation to collagen. However, it also has a shorter amino acid sequence and fewer aromatic free radicals, making it less antigenic compared to collagen [85]. Furthermore, gelatin is limited by poor mechanical properties and thermal stability [86]. To combat these issues, gelatin is often physically or chemically crosslinked, such as with methacrylate groups to create gelatin methacrylate (GelMA). GelMA contains the same advantageous biocompatible properties of gelatin while improving the mechanical tunability and stability. GelMA has primarily been utilized to improve angiogenesis following injury or hormonal exposure.

Zambuto et al. developed a GelMA hydrogel to encourage endometrial angiogenesis and monitor trophoblast invasion [87]. Trophoblast invasion is important in enhancing blood flow to an embryo prior to placentation during pregnancy. The 3D hydrogel created encapsulated human umbilical vein endothelial cells (HUVECs) and human endoSCs co-cultures to mimic the endometrial perivasculature niche.

The GelMA hydrogel successfully encapsulated each cell type and, after 7 days, developed endothelial tube networks, important for angiogenesis. Endometrial epithelial cells (endoEpCs) also successfully adhered to the surface of the GelMA hydrogel within 6 h and remained adhered for 7 days, which was verified with cytokeratin 18 staining. Cytokeratin staining confirms that the epithelial cytoskeletal structure was anchored to the underlying basement membrane. Additionally, trophoblast invasion was observed for 7 days of GelMA spheroids with the encapsulated co-cultures, showing significant outgrowth over time.

Similarly, Pence et al. studied the impact of sex steroid hormones on endometrial-derived cell lines encapsulated in GelMA hydrogels for promoting angiogenesis [88]. Specifically, the hydrogels encapsulated endoEpCs or endoSCs. It was found that endoSCs can promote blood vessel formation in the presence of nonendometrial HUVECs. While it was shown that estradiol hormone supplementation enhanced proangiogenic gene expression in endoEpC-laden hydrogels, they did not form blood vessel networks in the presence of HUVECs. This work shows that there is a relationship between endometrial-derived cells and sex hormone exposure that needs to be accounted for in developing reliable GelMA proangiogenic hydrogel implants.

Sodium Alginate

Another hydrogel for encapsulating cells and cellular components is sodium alginate, which is a water-soluble, anionic polysaccharide. Shuai et al. used a sodium alginate hydrogel to deliver RHC and MSCs to endometrial tissue to improve endometrial thickness and fertility outcomes [89]. The hydrogels promoted cell stemness, proliferation, and migration in vitro. In vivo murine models revealed improved endometrial thickness, great recovery, angiogenesis, and maintained hormone homeostasis. Fang et al. also developed an alginate-based hydrogel crosslinked with RHC to promote endometrial regeneration [90]. In vitro testing revealed that the hydrogel had desired structural and biodegradable properties, allowed for endometrial cell proliferation, and improved stromal cell viability. In vivo testing in a murine model showed improved endometrial regeneration, downregulation of factors associated with fibrosis, and maintained hormonal homeostasis.

Chitosan

Chitosan is a naturally occurring cationic polysaccharide formed from the deacetylation of chitin. Chitin is one of the most abundant natural biopolymers, found within some fungi as well as in the exoskeleton of arthropods, such as crustaceans. Chitosan has better solubility and chemical reactivity compared to chitin, making it a promising material for hydrogel drug delivery [91]. Unlike other naturally occurring polymers, chitosan is the only cationic natural polymer due to the reactive amino groups within its structure [91]. Chitosan is typically used as a co-polymer in hydrogels [92].

Wenbo et al. developed a chitosan-heparin hydrogel to treat IUAs using stromal cell-derived factor-1α (SDF-1α) [92]. SDF-1α promotes the migration of endogenous cells to the injury site to promote tissue regeneration. In vitro testing showed successful hydrogel synthesis with good stability and effective loading and release of SDF-1α in aqueous solution. In vivo injections in rat uteruses promoted endometrial repair, reduced collagen deposition, and improved neovascularization. Additionally, the injured rat uterus showed no statistical differences from an uninjured uterus after 7 days post-treatment.

Zheng et al. developed an HA and chitosan hydrogel that encapsulated PRP and ADSCs to improve endometrial tissue repair of thin endometrium in a mouse model [73]. The PRPs and ADSCs encapsulated in the hydrogel were effectively released in aqueous solution and stimulated angiogenesis in endothelial cells in vitro. The hydrogel was then tested for endometrial repair in mice with a thin endometrium in vivo. The combination of both PRP and ADSCs within the hydrogel was necessary to improve uterine thickness, gland number, and proliferation of endometrial and MSCs. The hydrogel was also successful in restoring embryo implantation and pregnancy outcomes in mice with damage to their endometrium.

Decellularized ECM

Decellularized ECM (dECM) is a promising natural biomaterial used in hydrogel formation. Decellularization is the chemical, biological, or physical process of removing the cellular components, such as cells and their genetic material, from the tissue ECM to preserve the tissue's natural structure and mechanical properties. After decellularization, the tissue framework, consisting of ECM structural proteins and bioactive molecules, remains and serves as a guide for new tissue development. The dECM is often processed further to develop tissue-specific hydrogels that can be individualized and encourage tissue repair. Depending on the application, dECM hydrogels can also be crosslinked with a biocompatible polymer to specific properties.

López-Martínez et al. created a porcine endometrial dECM hydrogel supplemented with growth factors for endometrial repair in a murine model [93]. The developed hydrogel with growth factors improved endometrial regeneration in vivo after injury. There was an increase in the number of endometrial glands, endometrial area, a high cell proliferation index, promotion of angiogenesis, and reduction of fibrotic tissue. Li et al. developed an injectable hydrogel from human decellularized amniotic membranes to study endometrial tissue repair after IUA injury in a rat model [94]. The hydrogel was developed through the processes of decellularization, lyophilization, and enzyme digestion of tissue collected after c-section. The hydrogel was injected into injured rat uterine cavities in vivo and was successful in aiding the migration of epithelial endometrial cells into the wound area for repair, while preventing fibrosis from forming.

4.3.2 Synthetic Polymer Scaffolds

Synthetic polymers are produced through chemical processing in a laboratory or industrial setting. Synthetic polymers are attractive for their tunability of chemical and mechanical properties, which can improve their mechanical strength and stability [95, 96]. They are also less expensive and have better reproducibility compared to natural polymers [97]. Common synthetic polymers for scaffold formation include PCL, poly(lactic acid), poly(glycolic acid), PLGA, and poloxamers, among others. However, only a few of these materials, including PCL and poloxamers, have been utilized as nanofiber scaffolds in uterine applications. Similar to natural polymers, synthetic polymers can be delivered to injured tissue directly as a solid scaffold or through a liquid injection that gels based on thermoresponsive properties at the injury site.

Poly(caprolactone)

PCL is a desirable biodegradable and biocompatible synthetic polymer used for tissue repair. PCL has desirable viscoelastic properties compared to other biodegradable polymers and is therefore easy to synthesize into a variety of structures, such as particles, fibers, micelles, films, and so on [98]. Wang et al. utilized commercial bionanofiber gelatin/PCL membranes for endometrial tissue repair from IUAs in a rat model [99]. The gelatin/PCL membranes are an electrospun matrix with three layers consisting of gelatin-PCL-gelatin (Neo Modulus (Suzhou) Medical Sci-Tech Co., Ltd). It was found that implantation of these meshes after endometrial injury improved endometrial thickening, decreased collagen deposition, and increased cytokeratin staining that indicates epithelial cell recovery. Tissue repair using the gelatin/PCL membranes also improved fertility by increasing pregnancy rate and embryo implantation at the surgical site.

Additionally, PCL is desirable for smooth muscle engineering, such as the uterine myometrium. An intact and functional myometrium on the uterine wall is critical during pregnancy. Hanuman et al. demonstrate that electrospun PCL nanofibrous scaffolds are promising for uterine tissue regeneration [100]. Additionally, the disaccharide maltose was effectively conjugated to the PCL scaffolds to explore its role in ECM remodeling and improve compatibility with uterine cells on a synthetic scaffold material with desirable mechanical properties. The conjugated scaffolds increased hydrophilicity and improved human uterine fibroblast cell proliferation compared to unconjugated controls and tissue culture plastic. Therefore, maltose-conjugated PCL scaffolds are promising for future uterine tissue engineering applications.

Poloxamers

Poloxamers (also known under the trade name Pluronics®) are nonionic triblock copolymers that are utilized for their high solubility, low toxicity, temperature-dependent self-assembly, and thermo-reversible properties [101]. They can be synthesized as A-B-A or B-A-B triblock copolymers, where A is hydrophilic poly (ethylene oxide), and B is hydrophobic poly(propylene oxide). The thermoresponsive properties of poloxamers make them ideal for in situ delivery at an injury, as they are a liquid at room temperature, but gel at body temperature [102]. Additionally, poloxamers have the ability to form micelles at low concentrations and hydrogels at high concentrations that encapsulate drug molecules and cellular components for drug delivery and tissue repair. Poloxamer 407, also known as Pluronic® F-127, and Poloxamer 188, also known as Pluronic® F-68, are the only current FDA-approved poloxomers, making them the most widely studied for drug delivery [103].

Xu et al. developed a heparin-modified poloxamer hydrogel for the treatment of IUAs by improving the affinity and delivery of keratinocyte growth factor (KGF) to the injury site in a rat model [104]. KGF is a stromally derived, secreted peptide that acts as a mitogen for cultured cells and has been proven to facilitate wound healing and regeneration. Heparin incorporated into the hydrogel promotes stability for growth factors and cytokines through specific receptor binding, and when incorporated with a poloxamer hydrogel, can bind with the heparin-binding KGF. This hydrogel was successful in binding and releasing KGF in vitro with a sustained release profile. The hydrogel also improved the retention of KGF, functionality and fertility, endometrial epithelial cell proliferation, and angiogenesis in a rat model in vivo.

Zhou et al. encapsulated human umbilical cord MSCs (hUC-MSCs) within a poloxamer hydrogel using Pluronic® F-127 to improve regeneration of thin endometrial tissue in a rat model [105]. The poloxamer-hUC-MSC hydrogels increased the gland number, promoted endometrial tissue thickening, and improved angiogenesis in vivo. It was also found that IL-1β stimulates angiogenesis from the loaded hydrogels by promoting the release of pro-angiogenic factors from the hUC-MSCs at the injury site, proving a novel mechanism for how the thin endometrium is regenerated.

Wu et al. developed a pectin-Pluronic® F-127 hydrogel scaffold to deliver pectin-based E2-loaded microspheres and bone marrow-derived MSCs (BMSCs) to the endometrium for tissue repair in a murine model [106]. The microspheres encapsulating the estrogen steroid hormone 17β-estradiol (E2) were synthesized using a double emulsion (W/O/W) method. The microspheres and BMSCs were then mixed with a pectin and Pluronic® F-127 solution and formed into a scaffold at 37 °C based on the sol–gel transition of Pluronic® F-127. In vitro studies revealed that the hydrogel created a sufficient environment to maintain BMSC viability and that BMSCs and E2 microspheres were evenly loaded throughout the hydrogel. When injected in vivo, the loaded hydrogel promoted endometrial thickening, promoted angiogenesis, and reduced scar tissue formation, similar to the spontaneous regeneration. The hydrogels were also fully degraded by day 28. The thermoresponsive properties of Pluronic® F-127 allowed for controlled injection and gelation of the scaffold for successful therapeutic implantation.

Hybrid Materials

There are also examples of combining natural and synthetic materials to leverage the ideal properties of each. An example by Yao et al. highlights developing an aloe and poloxamer hybrid hydrogel using Pluronic F-127® to deliver E2 encapsulated in dellcellularized uterus nanoparticulates for IUA repair in a rate model [58]. This hybrid hydrogel was developed to improve the overall material's mechanical and release properties. Using pure poloxamer did not have sufficient biodegradable properties to prolong the release of E2 and increased toxicity. However, incorporating aloe vera, a naturally derived material, improved the biocompatibility, biodegradation, and temperature sensitivity of the hydrogel while decreasing toxicity. An in vivo model revealed that the hybrid aloe/poloxamer hydrogel successfully allowed for the successful release of E2 from the nanoparticulates in localized areas and promoted endometrial tissue regeneration after injury, as seen by morphological and functional metrics. The hybrid polymer also decreased fibrous tissue formation, therefore providing an effective preliminary approach for IUA treatment (Table 2).

5 Conclusion and Future Perspectives

This chapter set out to highlight investigations into localized uterine drug delivery and recent advances in biomaterials to treat diseases originating from uterine tissues. The chapter provides a brief background on endometriosis, IUAs or Asherman's syndrome, uterine fibroids, and uterine cancer. However, these introductions are brief, and interested readers are encouraged to seek additional sources elsewhere.

Localized delivery to the uterus offers key advantages for treating diseases, including endometriosis, IUAs, uterine fibroids, uterine cancer, and others. The goal of uterine drug delivery is to achieve a high drug payload within the uterus, avoiding first-pass metabolism and systemic circulation. To date, there have been significant clinical successes, primarily through IUDs for contraception. Contraceptive IUDs are over 99% effective and may deliver copper (non-hormonal) or LNG (hormonal) to prevent pregnancy. Numerous IUDs have been US FDA-approved for 3–10 years after placement. The T-shaped design for an IUD is almost exclusive for hormonal IUDs; however, other morphologies have also been approved for copper delivery.

The T-shaped design for an IUD has been adopted for intrauterine delivery of IUAs and uterine cancers. These devices are inserted into the uterus and release drugs slowly over time to provide localized drug delivery. In rats, these

Table 2 Overview of the properties of natural and synthetic polymers used as scaffolds in uterine applications

Name	Structure	Source	Applications in the uterus	Advantages	Disadvantages	Citation
Natural polymers						
Collagen	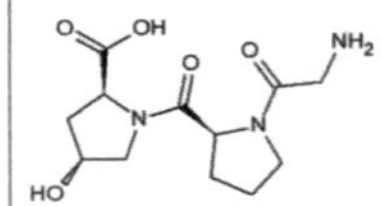	Main structural protein of the ECM	Thin endometrium	Improved biocompatibility due to being derived from biological sources Low toxicity for cells Improved incorporation, adhesion, and protection of cells and cellular components for delivery Faster degradation rate	Less stable Less tunable mechanical properties Less reliable reproducibility Difficult to scale Difficult to translate into multiple structures More expensive materials	[85, 89, 90, 93]
Gelatin	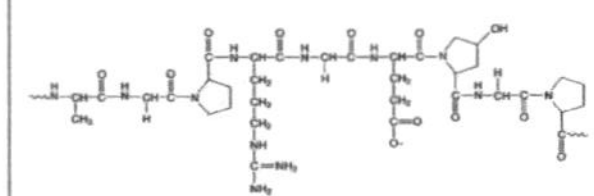	Collagen derivative obtained through hydrolysis	Promoting angiogenesis during pregnancy			[65, 85, 86, 99]
Hyaluronic Acid	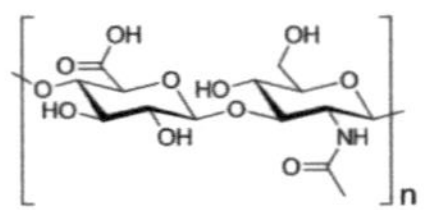	Anionic polysaccharide found in the ECM of mammalian tissues	IUAs Thin endometrium			[73, 81, 82]
Sodium alginate	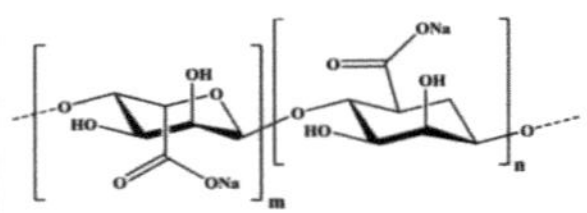	Anionic polysaccharide found in brown algae	Endometrial repair fertility			[72, 89, 90]
Chitosan	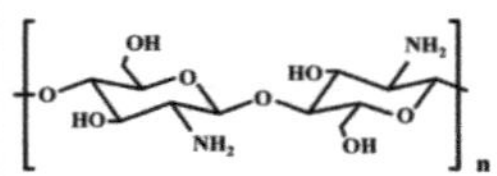	Derivative of chitin, found in some fungi and the exoskeleton of arthropods	IUAs Thin endometrium Fertility			[68, 70, 73, 92]
dECM	Composed of structural proteins and growth factors	Structural backbone of mammalian tissue with cellular and genetic components removed	Endometrial tissue repair			[58, 64, 93, 94]

Synthetic Polymers						
PCL	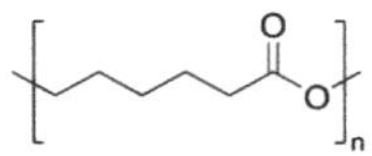	Ring-opening polymerization of caprolactone monomers; 5000–100,000 polymer molecular weight.	IUAs Uterine tissue repair	Synthesized easily into various structures (particles, fibers, micelles, films, etc.) Tunability of chemical and mechanical properties Easy reproducibility and scalability Less expensive than natural materials Potential biodegradable and biocompatible properties Better control of degradation rate	Generally lack the inherent biological cues to sustain cellular components Potential toxicity Slower degradation rate	[56, 98–100]

investigations were carried out for up to 3 months and showed enhanced efficacy compared with the existing delivery methods for the drugs of interest. In uterine drug delivery, many of the biomaterial carriers are focused on maintaining injectability. Therefore, many of the biomaterials are gel-based polymer systems that can be injected through a syringe and biodegrade once within the body. Using natural polymers for these applications often enhances biocompatibility compared with the synthetic polymers used for IUDs. Tissue regeneration is also under investigation with natural and gel-based biomaterials to promote wound healing and tissue regeneration. This may be a particularly useful avenue for treating scarring associated with IUAs for fertility preservation, among other applications.

Unfortunately, for many of the diseases mentioned, current treatment either focuses on the symptoms (endometriosis) or puts fertility at risk (IUAs and fibroids). These limitations highlight the need to advance treatment strategies for uterine conditions. Pre-clinical investigations are underway to treat critical diseases, including enhanced delivery of anti-inflammatory and chemotherapeutic agents. Significant advances remain necessary and are achievable by addressing the physical requirements of intrauterine drug delivery to meet clinical needs in uterine diseases. Translating pre-clinical investigations to the clinic can take up to 12 years, given the time required for efficacy and safety investigations prior to and including clinical trials. As such, any advances are slow-to-come. This is particularly true for many of the advances discussed in this chapter, as most date to 2020 or later. This would mean that the earliest projections for translation are 2032, if everything progressed perfectly.

References

1. Fanse S, Bao Q, Burgess DJ. Long-acting intrauterine systems: recent advances, current challenges, and future opportunities. Adv Drug Deliv Rev. 2022;191:114581. https://doi.org/10.1016/j.addr.2022.114581.
2. Rowlands S, Oloto E, Horwell DH. Intrauterine devices and risk of uterine perforation: current perspectives. Open Access J Contracept. 2016;7:19–32. https://doi.org/10.2147/OAJC.S85546.
3. Ulukus M, Cakmak H, Arici A. The role of endometrium in endometriosis. J Soc Gynecol Investig. 2006;13(7):467–76.
4. Elizur S, Mostafa J, Berkowitz E, Orvieto R. Endometriosis and infertility: pathophysiology, treatment strategies, and reproductive outcomes. Arch Gynecol Obstet. 2025;312(4):1037–48. https://doi.org/10.1007/s00404-025-08124-1.
5. Sridhar S, Gallant T, Brunn E. Overview of pathogenesis, symptoms, diagnosis, management, and prognosis of endometriosis and its role in infertility. J Gynecol Surg. 2022;38(1):3–6. https://doi.org/10.1089/gyn.2021.0160.
6. França PRC, Lontra ACP, Fernandes PD. Endometriosis: a disease with few direct treatment options. Molecules. 2022;27(13). https://doi.org/10.3390/molecules27134034.

7. Toma L, Socolov D, Matei D, Anton S, Balan R, Anton E, et al. Intrauterine adhesions and Asherman syndrome: a retrospective dive into predictive risk factors, diagnosis, and surgical perspectives. Diagnostics. 2025;15(8). https://doi.org/10.3390/diagnostics15080955.
8. Sun W, Xu W, Xiao M, Zhang X, Chen J, Zhang J, et al. Enhancing exosome stability and delivery with natural polymers to prevent intrauterine adhesions and promote endometrial regeneration: a review. J Nanobiotechnol. 2025;23(1):529. https://doi.org/10.1186/s12951-025-03603-8.
9. Düz SA, Mumcu A, Doğan B, Sarıdoğan E, Tuncay G, Onat T, et al. Metabolomics approach using HR-MAS NMR spectroscopy for the assessment of metabolic profiles of uterine fibroids. Anal Biochem. 2025;704:115885. https://doi.org/10.1016/j.ab.2025.115885.
10. Bofill Rodriguez M, Lethaby A, Grigore M, Brown J, Hickey M, Farquhar C. Endometrial resection and ablation techniques for heavy menstrual bleeding. Cochrane Database Syst Rev. 2019;1(1):CD001501. https://doi.org/10.1002/14651858.CD001501.pub5.
11. Zhang Q, Liang X, Chen Z. An updated review of thermal ablation technology for uterine fibroids and adenomyosis: focusing on protecting fertility. Int J Womens Health. 2024;16: 1551–63. https://doi.org/10.2147/ijwh.S473005.
12. Vrede SW, Kasius J, Bulten J, Teerenstra S, Huvila J, Colas E, et al. Relevance of molecular profiling in patients with low-grade endometrial cancer. JAMA Netw Open. 2022;5(12): e2247372. https://doi.org/10.1001/jamanetworkopen.2022.47372.
13. Khouri OR, Frey MK, Musa F, Muggia F, Lee J, Boyd L, et al. Neoadjuvant chemotherapy in patients with advanced endometrial cancer. Cancer Chemother Pharmacol. 2019;84(2):281–5. https://doi.org/10.1007/s00280-019-03838-x.
14. Matei D, Filiaci V, Randall ME, Mutch D, Steinhoff MM, DiSilvestro PA, et al. Adjuvant chemotherapy plus radiation for locally advanced endometrial cancer. N Engl J Med. 2019;380 (24):2317–26. https://doi.org/10.1056/NEJMoa1813181.
15. Nomura H, Aoki D, Michimae H, Mizuno M, Nakai H, Arai M, et al. Effect of taxane plus platinum regimens vs doxorubicin plus cisplatin as adjuvant chemotherapy for endometrial cancer at a high risk of progression: a randomized clinical trial. JAMA Oncol. 2019;5(6): 833–40. https://doi.org/10.1001/jamaoncol.2019.0001.
16. Bestvina CM, Fleming GF. Chemotherapy for endometrial cancer in adjuvant and advanced disease settings. Oncologist. 2016;21(10):1250–9. https://doi.org/10.1634/theoncologist.2016-0062.
17. Berezowitz JD, Givens BE. Nanocarrier drug delivery systems for gynecological cancer therapeutics. J Control Release. 2025;385:114028. https://doi.org/10.1016/j.jconrel.2025.114028.
18. Wang Y, Levate G, Rae MT, Duncan WC, Siemienowicz KJ. An ovine model shows that subcutaneous adipose tissue fibrosis occurs early in polycystic ovary syndrome (PCOS). J Mol Endocrinol. 2025;75(4). https://doi.org/10.1530/jme-25-0106.
19. McCracken JM, Calderon GA, Robinson AJ, Sullivan CN, Cosgriff-Hernandez E, Hakim JCE. Animal models and alternatives in vaginal research: a comparative review. Reprod Sci. 2021;28(6):1759–73. https://doi.org/10.1007/s43032-021-00529-y.
20. Dick I, Scott R. Pig ear skin as an in-vitro model for human skin permeability. J Pharm Pharmacol. 1992;44(8):640–5. https://doi.org/10.1111/j.2042-7158.1992.tb05485.x.
21. Han I, Bohrer L, Gibson-Corley K, Wiley L, Shrestha A, Harman B, et al. Biocompatibility of human induced pluripotent stem cell-derived retinal progenitor cell grafts in immunocompromised rats. Cell Transplant. 2022;31. https://doi.org/10.1177/09636897221104451.
22. Liu P, Meng J, Xiong Y, Wu Y, Xiao Y, Gao S. Contraception with levonorgestrel-releasing intrauterine system versus copper intrauterine device: a meta-analysis of randomized controlled trials. EClinicalMedicine. 2024;78:102926. https://doi.org/10.1016/j.eclinm.2024.102926.
23. Xu XX, Nie FL, Wang YB, Zhang JX, Zheng W, Li L, et al. Effective inhibition of the early copper ion burst release with ultra-fine grained copper and single crystal copper for intrauterine

device application. Acta Biomater. 2012;8(2):886–96. https://doi.org/10.1016/j.actbio.2011.10.018.

24. Alvarez F, Schilardi PL, de Mele MFL. Reduction of the "burst release" of copper ions from copper-based intrauterine devices by organic inhibitors. Contraception. 2012;85(1):91–8.
25. Yang L, Bao G, Yao C, Diao T, Su Z, Liu T, et al. Mitigating adverse effects of Cu-containing intrauterine devices using a highly biocompatible Cu5Fe alloy. Acta Biomater. 2024;189:651–67. https://doi.org/10.1016/j.actbio.2024.09.022.
26. Fan Q, Bao G, Ge D, Wang K, Sun M, Liu T, et al. Effective easing of the side effects of copper intrauterine devices using ultra-fine-grained Cu-0.4 Mg alloy. Acta Biomater. 2021;128:523–39.
27. Wang K, Bao G, Fan Q, Zhu L, Yang L, Liu T, et al. Feasibility evaluation of a Cu-38 Zn alloy for intrauterine devices: in vitro and in vivo studies. Acta Biomater. 2022;138:561–75. https://doi.org/10.1016/j.actbio.2021.11.006.
28. Turok DK, Nelson AL, Dart C, Schreiber CA, Peters K, Schreifels MJ, et al. Efficacy, safety, and tolerability of a new low-dose copper and nitinol intrauterine device: phase 2 data to 36 months. Obstet Gynecol. 2020;135(4):840–7. https://doi.org/10.1097/AOG.0000000000003756.
29. Barton BE, Erickson JA, Allred SI, Jeffries JM, Stephens KK, Hunter MI, et al. Reversible female contraceptives: historical, current, and future perspectivesdagger. Biol Reprod. 2024;110(1):14–32. https://doi.org/10.1093/biolre/ioad154.
30. Baram I, Weinstein A, Trussell J. The IUB, a newly invented IUD: a brief report. Contraception. 2014;89(2):139–41. https://doi.org/10.1016/j.contraception.2013.10.017.
31. Homminga I, Ter Meer AF, Groen H, Cantineau AEP, Hoek A. Thin endometrial lining: is it more prevalent in patients utilizing preimplantation genetic testing for monogenic disease (PGT-M) and related to prior hormonal contraceptive use? Hum Reprod. 2023;38(2):237–46. https://doi.org/10.1093/humrep/deac258.
32. Yu Y, Zhou Z, Wang L, Liu J. Effect of mirena intrauterine device on endometrial thickness, quality of life score, and curative effect in patients with perimenopausal abnormal uterine bleeding. Comput Math Methods Med. 2022;2022(1):5648918. https://doi.org/10.1155/2022/5648918.
33. Bao Q, Zou Y, Wang Y, Kozak D, Choi S, Burgess DJ. Drug release testing of long-acting intrauterine systems. J Control Release. 2019;316:349–58. https://doi.org/10.1016/j.jconrel.2019.11.015.
34. Bao Q, Fanse S, Lu XJ, Burgess DJ. Impact of drug loading on release from levonorgestrel intrauterine systems. Int J Pharm. 2023;631:122532. https://doi.org/10.1016/j.ijpharm.2022.122532.
35. Fanse S, Bao Q, Zou Y, Wang Y, Burgess DJ. Tailoring drug release from long-acting contraceptive levonorgestrel intrauterine systems. J Control Release. 2024;370:124–39. https://doi.org/10.1016/j.jconrel.2024.04.027.
36. Kerns JL, Keder LM, Cwiak CA, Westhoff CL, Creinin MD. Hormone-related side effects in new users of a levonorgestrel 52-mg intrauterine device. Am J Obstet Gynecol. 2024;231(6):628 e1–e10. https://doi.org/10.1016/j.ajog.2024.06.049.
37. Ewies AA. Levonorgestrel-releasing intrauterine system–the discontinuing story. Gynecol Endocrinol. 2009;25(10):668–73. https://doi.org/10.1080/09513590903159656.
38. Borovac T, Pelage JP, Kasselouri A, Prognon P, Guiffant G, Laurent A. Release of ibuprofen from beads for embolization: in vitro and in vivo studies. J Control Release. 2006;115(3):266–74. https://doi.org/10.1016/j.jconrel.2006.08.008.
39. Zhou C, Cui D, Zhang Y, Yuan H, Fan T. Preparation and characterization of ketoprofen-loaded microspheres for embolization. J Mater Sci Mater Med. 2012;23(2):409–18. https://doi.org/10.1007/s10856-011-4492-3.
40. Wassef M, Pelage JP, Velzenberger E, Namur J, Schwartz-Cornil I, Taylor RR, et al. Anti-inflammatory effect of ibuprofen-loaded embolization beads in sheep uterus. J Biomed Mater Res B Appl Biomater. 2008;86(1):63–73. https://doi.org/10.1002/jbm.b.30988.

41. Namur J, Wassef M, Pelage JP, Lewis A, Manfait M, Laurent A. Infrared microspectroscopy analysis of ibuprofen release from drug eluting beads in uterine tissue. J Control Release. 2009;135(3):198–202. https://doi.org/10.1016/j.jconrel.2008.12.017.
42. Verret V, Bevilacqua C, Schwartz-Cornil I, Pelage JP, Wassef M, Namur J, et al. IL6 and TNF expression in vessels and surrounding tissues after embolization with ibuprofen-loaded beads confirms diffusion of ibuprofen. Eur J Pharm Sci. 2011;42(5):489–95. https://doi.org/10.1016/j.ejps.2011.02.001.
43. Bedouet L, Moine L, Servais E, Beilvert A, Labarre D, Laurent A. Tunable delivery of niflumic acid from resorbable embolization microspheres for uterine fibroid embolization. Int J Pharm. 2016;511(1):253–61. https://doi.org/10.1016/j.ijpharm.2016.06.128.
44. Spadea A, Rios de la Rosa JM, Tirella A, Ashford MB, Williams KJ, Stratford IJ, et al. Evaluating the efficiency of hyaluronic acid for tumor targeting via CD44. Mol Pharm. 2019;16(6):2481–93. https://doi.org/10.1021/acs.molpharmaceut.9b00083.
45. Chen WH, Luo GF, Qiu WX, Lei Q, Hong S, Wang SB, et al. Programmed nanococktail for intracellular cascade reaction regulating self-synergistic tumor targeting therapy. Small. 2016;12(6):733–44. https://doi.org/10.1002/smll.201503280.
46. Schatz-Siemers N, Chen YT, Chen Z, Wang D, Ellenson LH, Du YN. Expression of the Receptor for Hyaluronic Acid-Mediated Motility (RHAMM) in endometrial cancer is associated with adverse histologic parameters and tumor progression. Appl Immunohistochem Mol Morphol. 2020;28(6):453–9. https://doi.org/10.1097/PAI.0000000000000763.
47. Hernandez JE, Gonzalez-Montiel A, Allos-Villalva JCC, Cantu D, Barquet S, Olivares-Mundo A, et al. Prognostic molecular biomarkers in endometrial cancer: a review. J Cancer Res Ther (Manch). 2019;7(3):17–28. https://doi.org/10.14312/2052-4994.2019-3.
48. Zhao J, Liu T, Yu G, Wang J. Overexpression of HABP1 correlated with clinicopathological characteristics and unfavorable prognosis in endometrial cancer. Tumour Biol. 2015;36(2):1299–306. https://doi.org/10.1007/s13277-014-2761-8.
49. Malentacchi F, Turrini I, Sorbi F, Projetto E, Castiglione F, Fambrini M, et al. Pilot investigation of the mutation profile of PIK3CA/PTEN genes (PI3K pathway) in grade 3 endometrial cancer. Oncol Rep. 2019;41(3):1560–74. https://doi.org/10.3892/or.2018.6939.
50. Kong C, Zhu Z, Li Y, Xue P, Chen L. Downregulation of HOXA11 enhances endometrial cancer malignancy and cisplatin resistance via activating PTEN/AKT signaling pathway. Clin Transl Oncol. 2021;23(7):1334–41. https://doi.org/10.1007/s12094-020-02520-6.
51. Wang J, Zhang L, Jiang W, Zhang R, Zhang B, Silayiding A, et al. MicroRNA-135a promotes proliferation, migration, invasion and induces chemoresistance of endometrial cancer cells. Eur J Obstet Gynecol Reprod Biol X. 2020;5:100103. https://doi.org/10.1016/j.eurox.2019.100103.
52. Thiel KW, Devor EJ, Filiaci VL, Mutch D, Moxley K, Alvarez Secord A, et al. TP53 sequencing and p53 immunohistochemistry predict outcomes when bevacizumab is added to frontline chemotherapy in endometrial cancer: an NRG Oncology/Gynecologic Oncology Group Study. J Clin Oncol. 2022;40(28):3289–300. https://doi.org/10.1200/JCO.21.02506.
53. Ebeid K, Meng X, Thiel KW, Do AV, Geary SM, Morris AS, et al. Synthetically lethal nanoparticles for treatment of endometrial cancer. Nat Nanotechnol. 2018;13(1):72–81. https://doi.org/10.1038/s41565-017-0009-7.
54. Wiwatchaitawee K, Mekkawy AI, Quarterman JC, Naguib YW, Ebeid K, Geary SM, et al. The MEK 1/2 inhibitor PD98059 exhibits synergistic anti-endometrial cancer activity with paclitaxel in vitro and enhanced tissue distribution in vivo when formulated into PAMAM-coated PLGA-PEG nanoparticles. Drug Deliv Transl Res. 2022;12(7):1684–96. https://doi.org/10.1007/s13346-021-01065-7.
55. Melendez B, Shah S, Jiang Y, Dottino J, Watson E, Pearce H, et al. Novel polymer-based system for intrauterine delivery of everolimus for anti-cancer applications. J Control Release. 2021;339:521–30. https://doi.org/10.1016/j.jconrel.2021.10.008.

56. Varan C, Aksut D, Sen M, Bilensoy E. Design and characterization of carboplatin and paclitaxel loaded PCL filaments for 3D printed controlled release intrauterine implants. Pharmaceutics. 2023;15(4):1154. https://doi.org/10.3390/pharmaceutics15041154.
57. Mei L, Bao J, Tang L, Zhang C, Wang H, Sun L, et al. A novel mifepristone-loaded implant for long-term treatment of endometriosis: in vitro and in vivo studies. Eur J Pharm Sci. 2010;39(5):421–7. https://doi.org/10.1016/j.ejps.2010.01.012.
58. Yao Q, Zheng YW, Lan QH, Wang LF, Huang ZW, Chen R, et al. Aloe/poloxamer hydrogel as an injectable beta-estradiol delivery scaffold with multi-therapeutic effects to promote endometrial regeneration for intrauterine adhesion treatment. Eur J Pharm Sci. 2020;148:105316. https://doi.org/10.1016/j.ejps.2020.105316.
59. MacCarthy-Morrogh L, Martin P. The hallmarks of cancer are also the hallmarks of wound healing. Sci Signal. 2020;13(648). https://doi.org/10.1126/scisignal.aay8690.
60. Toczek J, Sadlocha M, Major K, Stojko R. Benefit of silver and gold nanoparticles in wound healing process after endometrial cancer protocol. Biomedicine. 2022;10(3). https://doi.org/10.3390/biomedicines10030679.
61. Li S, Li Y, Yu F, Li N, Liu C, Mao J, et al. Human endometrium-derived adventitial cell spheroid-loaded antimicrobial microneedles for uterine regeneration. Small. 2022;18(31):e2201225. https://doi.org/10.1002/smll.202201225.
62. Chitcholtan K, Asselin E, Parent S, Sykes PH, Evans JJ. Differences in growth properties of endometrial cancer in three dimensional (3D) culture and 2D cell monolayer. Exp Cell Res. 2013;319(1):75–87. https://doi.org/10.1016/j.yexcr.2012.09.012.
63. Ahn J, Yoon MJ, Hong SH, Cha H, Lee D, Koo HS, et al. Three-dimensional microengineered vascularised endometrium-on-a-chip. Hum Reprod. 2021;36(10):2720–31. https://doi.org/10.1093/humrep/deab186.
64. Jamaluddin MFB, Ghosh A, Ingle A, Mohammed R, Ali A, Bahrami M, et al. Bovine and human endometrium-derived hydrogels support organoid culture from healthy and cancerous tissues. Proc Natl Acad Sci USA. 2022;119(44):e2208040119. https://doi.org/10.1073/pnas.2208040119.
65. Huang Y, Feng Q, Jiang H, Zhou W, Chen J, Gao J, et al. Mimicking the endometrial cancer tumor microenvironment to reprogram tumor-associated macrophages in disintegrable supramolecular gelatin hydrogel. Int J Nanomedicine. 2020;15:4625–37. https://doi.org/10.2147/IJN.S252074.
66. Salamonsen LA, Hutchison JC, Gargett CE. Cyclical endometrial repair and regeneration. Development. 2021;148(17). https://doi.org/10.1242/dev.199577.
67. Santamaria X, Isaacson K, Simón C. Asherman's syndrome: it may not be all our fault. Hum Reprod. 2018;33(8):1374–80.
68. Ghahremani-Nasab M, Babaie S, Bazdar S, Paiva-Santos AC, Del Bakhshayesh MR, Akbari-Gharalari N, et al. Infertility treatment using polysaccharides-based hydrogels: new strategies in tissue engineering and regenerative medicine. J Nanobiotechnol. 2025;23(1):162. https://doi.org/10.1186/s12951-025-03267-4.
69. Wang P-H, Yang S-T, Chang W-H, Liu C-H, Liu H-H, Lee W-L. Intrauterine adhesion. Taiwan J Obstet Gynecol. 2024;63(3):312–9. https://doi.org/10.1016/j.tjog.2024.02.004.
70. Lv H, Xu R, Xie X, Liang Q, Yuan W, Xia Y, et al. Injectable, degradable, and mechanically adaptive hydrogel induced by L-serine and allyl-functionalized chitosan with platelet-rich plasma for treating intrauterine adhesions. Acta Biomater. 2024;184:144–55. https://doi.org/10.1016/j.actbio.2024.06.043.
71. He Y, Sun MM, Zhang GG, Yang J, Chen KS, Xu WW, et al. Targeting PI3K/Akt signal transduction for cancer therapy. Signal Transduct Target Ther. 2021;6(1):425. https://doi.org/10.1038/s41392-021-00828-5.
72. Xie X, Ao X, Xu R, Lv H, Tan S, Wu J, et al. Injectable, stable, and biodegradable hydrogel with platelet-rich plasma induced by l-serine and sodium alginate for effective treatment of intrauterine adhesions. Int J Biol Macromol. 2024;270:132363. https://doi.org/10.1016/j.ijbiomac.2024.132363.

73. Zheng X, Huang R, Yin L, Yao M, Chu J, Yang F, et al. Injectable antioxidant hyaluronan/chitosan hydrogel as a platelet-rich plasma and stem cell carrier to promote endometrial regeneration and fertility restoration. Acta Biomater. 2025;195:201–15. https://doi.org/10.1016/j.actbio.2025.01.062.
74. Avilla-Royo E, Vonzun L, Seehusen F, Vallmajo-Martin Q, Famos F, Moser L, et al. Engineered platelet-derived growth factor-releasing hydrogels promote fetal membrane healing in vivo. Adv Funct Mater. 2023;33(9):2208910.
75. Lu P, Ruan D, Huang M, Tian M, Zhu K, Gan Z, et al. Harnessing the potential of hydrogels for advanced therapeutic applications: current achievements and future directions. Signal Transduct Target Ther. 2024;9(1):166. https://doi.org/10.1038/s41392-024-01852-x.
76. Guan X, Avci-Adali M, Alarcin E, Cheng H, Kashaf SS, Li Y, et al. Development of hydrogels for regenerative engineering. Biotechnol J. 2017;12(5):1600394. https://doi.org/10.1002/biot.201600394.
77. Wu F, Lei N, Yang S, Zhou J, Chen M, Chen C, et al. Treatment strategies for intrauterine adhesion: focus on the exosomes and hydrogels. Front Bioeng Biotechnol. 2023;11:1264006. https://doi.org/10.3389/fbioe.2023.1264006.
78. Xiao Y, Gu Y, Qin L, Chen L, Chen X, Cui W, et al. Injectable thermosensitive hydrogel-based drug delivery system for local cancer therapy. Colloids Surf B Biointerfaces. 2021;200:111581. https://doi.org/10.1016/j.colsurfb.2021.111581.
79. Wang J, Qin W, Zhong Y, Hu H, Yang J, Huang H, Huang N, Liu S, Li J, Zheng L, Qin A, Lu Z. Injectable collagen hydrogel combines human umbilical cord mesenchymal stem cells to promote endometrial regeneration in rats with thin endometrium. Int J Biol Macromol. 2024;254:127591. https://doi.org/10.1016/j.ijbiomac.2023.127591.
80. Wei S, Li Z, Xia H, Wang Z, Deng J, Li L, Huang R, Ye T, Huang Y, Yang Y. An endometrial biomimetic extracellular matrix (ECM) for enhanced endometrial regeneration using hyaluronic acid hydrogel containing recombinant human type III collagen. Int J Biol Macromol 2024;268:131723. https://doi.org/10.1016/j.ijbiomac.2024.131723.
81. Lin Y, Dong S, Ye X, Liu J, Li J, Zhang Y, et al. Synergistic regenerative therapy of thin endometrium by human placenta-derived mesenchymal stem cells encapsulated within hyaluronic acid hydrogels. Stem Cell Res Ther. 2022;13(1):66. https://doi.org/10.1186/s13287-022-02717-2.
82. Xin L, Wei C, Tong X, Dai Y, Huang D, Chen J, et al. In situ delivery of apoptotic bodies derived from mesenchymal stem cells via a hyaluronic acid hydrogel: a therapy for intrauterine adhesions. Bioact Mater. 2022;12:107–19. https://doi.org/10.1016/j.bioactmat.2021.10.025.
83. Xu X, Lai Y, Hua ZC. Apoptosis and apoptotic body: disease message and therapeutic target potentials. Biosci Rep. 2019;39(1):BSR20180992. https://doi.org/10.1042/BSR20180992.
84. Ryoo HD, Gorenc T, Steller H. Apoptotic cells can induce compensatory cell proliferation through the JNK and the Wingless signaling pathways. Dev Cell. 2004;7(4):491–501. https://doi.org/10.1016/j.devcel.2004.08.019.
85. Gorgieva S, Kokol V. Collagen-vs. gelatine-based biomaterials and their biocompatibility: review and perspectives. Biomaterials applications for nanomedicine. 2011;2(2011):17–52. https://doi.org/10.5772/1957.
86. Afewerki S, Sheikhi A, Kannan S, Ahadian S, Khademhosseini A. Gelatin-polysaccharide composite scaffolds for 3D cell culture and tissue engineering: towards natural therapeutics. Bioeng Transl Med. 2019;4(1):96–115. https://doi.org/10.1002/btm2.10124.
87. Zambuto SG, Clancy KB, Harley BA. A gelatin hydrogel to study endometrial angiogenesis and trophoblast invasion. Interface Focus. 2019;9(5):20190016.
88. Pence JC, Clancy KBH, Harley BAC. Proangiogenic activity of endometrial epithelial and stromal cells in response to estradiol in gelatin hydrogels. Adv Biosyst. 2017;1(9):1700056. https://doi.org/10.1002/adbi.201700056.
89. Shuai Q, Liang Y, Xu X, Halbiyat Z, Wang X, Cheng J, et al. Sodium alginate hydrogel integrated with type III collagen and mesenchymal stem cell to promote endometrium regeneration and fertility restoration. Int J Biol Macromol. 2023;253(Pt 6):127314. https://doi.org/10.1016/j.ijbiomac.2023.127314.

90. Fang Z, Lu C, Du W, Wang X, Yang H, Shi M, et al. Injectable self-assembled dual-crosslinked alginate/recombinant collagen-based hydrogel for endometrium regeneration. Int J Biol Macromol. 2023;236:123943. https://doi.org/10.1016/j.ijbiomac.2023.123943.
91. Yadav M, Kaushik B, Rao GK, Srivastava CM, Vaya D. Advances and challenges in the use of chitosan and its derivatives in biomedical fields: a review. Carbohydr Polym Technol Appl. 2023;5:100323. https://doi.org/10.1016/j.carpta.2023.100323.
92. Wenbo Q, Lijian X, Shuangdan Z, Jiahua Z, Yanpeng T, Xuejun Q, et al. Controlled releasing of SDF-1alpha in chitosan-heparin hydrogel for endometrium injury healing in rat model. Int J Biol Macromol. 2020;143:163–72. https://doi.org/10.1016/j.ijbiomac.2019.11.184.
93. Lopez-Martinez S, Rodriguez-Eguren A, de Miguel-Gomez L, Frances-Herrero E, Faus A, Diaz A, et al. Bioengineered endometrial hydrogels with growth factors promote tissue regeneration and restore fertility in murine models. Acta Biomater. 2021;135:113–25. https://doi.org/10.1016/j.actbio.2021.08.025.
94. Li X, Li P, Wang C, Shang T, Han H, Tong Y, et al. A thermo-sensitive and injectable hydrogel derived from a decellularized amniotic membrane to prevent intrauterine adhesion by accelerating endometrium regeneration. Biomater Sci. 2022;10(9):2275–86. https://doi.org/10.1039/d1bm01791h.
95. Thang NH, Chien TB, Cuong DX. Polymer-based hydrogels applied in drug delivery: an overview. Gels. 2023;9(7):523. https://doi.org/10.3390/gels9070523.
96. Reddy MSB, Ponnamma D, Choudhary R, Sadasivuni KK. A comparative review of natural and synthetic biopolymer composite scaffolds. Polymers (Basel). 2021;13(7):1105. https://doi.org/10.3390/polym13071105.
97. Sionkowska A. Current research on the blends of natural and synthetic polymers as new biomaterials: review. Prog Polym Sci. 2011;36(9):1254–76. https://doi.org/10.1016/j.progpolymsci.2011.05.003.
98. Christen MO, Vercesi F. Polycaprolactone: how a well-known and futuristic polymer has become an innovative collagen-stimulator in esthetics. Clin Cosmet Investig Dermatol. 2020;13:31–48. https://doi.org/10.2147/CCID.S229054.
99. Wang X, Yang CR, Zhao ZD, Liu DG, Li CZ. Gelatin/polycaprolactone membranes promote endometrial regeneration and restore fertility. Gynecol Endocrinol. 2024;40(1):2442728. https://doi.org/10.1080/09513590.2024.2442728.
100. Hanuman S, Nune M. Design and characterization of maltose-conjugated polycaprolactone nanofibrous scaffolds for uterine tissue engineering. Regen Eng Transl Med. 2022;8:334–44.
101. Zarrintaj P, Ramsey JD, Samadi A, Atoufi Z, Yazdi MK, Ganjali MR, et al. Poloxamer: a versatile tri-block copolymer for biomedical applications. Acta Biomater. 2020;110:37–67. https://doi.org/10.1016/j.actbio.2020.04.028.
102. Brambilla E, Locarno S, Gallo S, Orsini F, Pini C, Farronato M, et al. Poloxamer-based hydrogel as drug delivery system: how polymeric excipients influence the chemical-physical properties. Polymers (Basel). 2022;14(17):3624. https://doi.org/10.3390/polym14173624.
103. Khaliq NU, Lee J, Kim S, Sung D, Kim H. Pluronic F-68 and F-127 based nanomedicines for advancing combination cancer therapy. Pharmaceutics. 2023;15(8):2102. https://doi.org/10.3390/pharmaceutics15082102.
104. Xu HL, Xu J, Zhang SS, Zhu QY, Jin BH, ZhuGe DL, et al. Temperature-sensitive heparin-modified poloxamer hydrogel with affinity to KGF facilitate the morphologic and functional recovery of the injured rat uterus. Drug Deliv. 2017;24(1):867–81. https://doi.org/10.1080/10717544.2017.1333173.
105. Zhou S, Lei Y, Wang P, Chen J, Zeng L, Qu T, et al. Human umbilical cord mesenchymal stem cells encapsulated with Pluronic F-127 enhance the regeneration and angiogenesis of thin endometrium in rat via local IL-1beta stimulation. Stem Cells Int. 2022;2022(1):7819234. https://doi.org/10.1155/2022/7819234.
106. Wu Y, Gu S, Cobb JM, Dunn GH, Muth TA, Simchick CJ, et al. E2-loaded microcapsules and bone marrow-derived mesenchymal stem cells with injectable scaffolds for endometrial regeneration application. Tissue Eng Part A. 2024;30(3–4):115–30. https://doi.org/10.1089/ten.TEA.2023.0238.

Nanotechnological Approaches for Targeted Drug Delivery to Combat Breast and Ovarian Cancer

Vinitha Rani, Abdulla Obadat, Kyle Boyes, and Needa Brown

Abstract Breast and ovarian cancers are the leading causes of death in women globally. The current therapeutic strategies possess their pros and cons, often resulting in poor therapeutic outcomes. The current treatment modalities, while being effective to some extent, face major drawbacks such as fatigue, resistance development, hypertension, gastrointestinal issues, bleeding, and limited treatment options, significantly impacting the life span and survival in patients. Hence, there is a need to explore an alternative modality to combat these cons, thereby leading to a

V. Rani
Department of Materials Science and Engineering, University of Central Florida, Orlando, FL, USA
e-mail: vinitha.rani@ucf.edu

A. Obadat
Department of Materials Science and Engineering, University of Central Florida, Orlando, FL, USA

Department of Mechanical and Aerospace Engineering, University of Central Florida, Orlando, FL, USA
e-mail: abdulla.obadat@ucf.edu

K. Boyes
Department of Materials Science and Engineering, University of Central Florida, Orlando, FL, USA

Burnett School of Biomedical Sciences, University of Central Florida, Orlando, FL, USA
e-mail: ky650936@ucf.edu

N. Brown (✉)
Department of Materials Science and Engineering, University of Central Florida, Orlando, FL, USA

Department of Mechanical and Aerospace Engineering, University of Central Florida, Orlando, FL, USA

Burnett School of Biomedical Sciences, University of Central Florida, Orlando, FL, USA

Biionix Cluster, University of Central Florida, Orlando, FL, USA

NanoScience Technology Centre, University of Central Florida, Orlando, FL, USA
e-mail: needa.brown@ucf.edu

S. G. Zambuto, M. L. Oyen (eds.), *Biomaterials for Women's Health Engineering*,
https://doi.org/10.1007/978-3-032-10745-9_20

promising outcome benefiting the patients. Over the past few decades, researchers have been keen on exploring new routes to this, and thus, the emergence of nanotechnology in cancer therapy has become the most advanced domain of science that has paved the way toward diagnostics and targeted drug delivery in battling cancer. The nanocarriers or biomaterials, used in such applications, have been strategically designed to be an efficacious vehicle for drug delivery to target the mechanism of interest in tumor suppression. This book chapter deals with the applications of such nanomaterials/nanocarriers in delivering therapeutic agents, along with diving deeper into the therapeutic and diagnostic potential of these drug-loaded carriers to tackle breast and ovarian cancer.

Keywords Biomaterials · Breast cancer · Diagnostics · Drug delivery systems · Nanocarriers · Nanoformulation · Nanomedicine · Ovarian cancer · Nanotechnology · Therapy

1 Introduction to Breast and Ovarian Cancer

Cancer is considered to be one of the most devastating classes of human pathologies, causing millions of deaths every year across the globe. These groups of maladies contribute to over a hundred genetically diverse subtypes along with metabolic alterations. There is no clear understanding of the underlying causes for this, even though there are several studies out there trying to connect the missing pieces [1]. Among the different cancers identified, breast and ovarian cancer significantly impact women's health. Breast cancer is the most common cancer to affect women, while ovarian cancer is the leading cause of death from reproductive cancer in young women.

1.1 Overview of Breast Cancer

Breast cancer is defined as the uncontrolled division of malignant breast cells. Approximately one in eight women in the United States (13.1%) will be diagnosed with invasive breast cancer, and 1 in 43 (2.3%) are expected to die from this disease. In 2024, an estimated 310,720 new invasive breast cancer cases and 56,500 cases of ductal carcinoma were diagnosed in women. From the past decade (2012–2021), the breast cancer incidence has been increasing by an overall 1% annually, with a steep increase among women below the age of 50 years (1.4%), compared to those above 50 years (0.7%). Ethnicity also plays a vital role in determining the incidence rate. Black women tend to have 5% lower breast cancer incidence when compared to white women. The American Indian/Alaska native women have a 10% lower breast cancer incidence than white women [2, 3]. The mortality rate of breast cancer has decreased by 44% from approximately 33 deaths per 100,000 women in 1989 to 19 deaths per 100,000 in 2022. A modeling study sheds light on the reduction in mortality rate, stating that the reason behind this is the advancement in the therapeutic strategies for stages I–III (47%), metastatic disease (29%), and an additional 25% associated with early detection through screening procedures [4]. The future of cancer statistics is predicted to be 3.2 million new breast cancer cases and 1.1 million breast cancer-related deaths to occur by 2050 [5]. Young women, under 50 years, are most likely to develop breast cancer with aggressive biological features compared to older women, which includes larger tumor size, negative hormone receptor (HR) status, including progesterone, estrogen receptors (ERs), and overexpressed human epidermal growth factors that contribute to poor prognosis in young females [6].

1.2 Classification and Screening of Breast Tumors

Understanding the molecular subtypes and pathophysiology of breast cancer is crucial for understanding its progression and response to treatment. This understanding aids in strategizing personalized medicine and targeted therapies to improve the therapeutic outcome. According to the World Health Organization, breast cancer is classified into invasive breast carcinoma (70–75%) and lobular carcinoma (12–15%), based on pathological conditions. However, for prognostic and clinical evaluation, it has been classified into three subgroups based on immunohistochemical staining results for estrogen receptor (ER), progesterone receptor (PR), human epidermal growth factor receptor 2 (HER2), hormone receptor (HR)-positive, and triple-negative breast cancer (TNBC). In clinical practice, immunohistochemical results are often used to classify the four subtypes of breast cancer, namely, luminal A, luminal B, HER2-enriched, and TNBC. The luminal A subtype is characterized by the presence of high ER and PR, along with the overexpression of HER2 receptor and Ki67, which reflect slower cell growth, better response to hormone therapy, and better prognosis. On the other hand, luminal B subtypes are also HR-positive but can either be HER2– or HER2+. They show higher levels of Ki67, thus indicating faster cell growth, and can be treated either with chemotherapy or hormone therapy. In the third subtype of HER-2 enriched, these breast cancers are more aggressive and can benefit only from HER2-targeted therapies. While the TNBCs do not express ER, HER2, or PR, they have a higher risk of recurrence and poor prognosis [7, 8].

Breast cancer is also influenced by other internal factors such as increased age and sex hormone levels, early age of menarche, and late menopause. The most impactful external risk factors include alcohol consumption, obesity, and diabetes [9]. Breast cancer screening is done primarily through mammography, which is a form of low-dose X-ray screening. While mammograms reduce breast cancer deaths by approximately 20%, they are still a subject of controversy. Sometimes, mammogram screenings are prone to false positives and are not suitable for all tissue types. It can also result in significant radiation doses in high-risk patients who are screened frequently. Diagnostic procedures are performed on those who have suspected tumors from screening tests. Core-needle biopsy, fine-needle aspiration, and surgical excision are the most common collection methods. Tumor cells are then pathologically evaluated, usually with histological methods [10].

1.3 Current Treatment Strategies for Breast Cancer

Several therapeutic strategies are employed to treat breast cancer (Fig. 1). Surgical tumor removal is the standard procedure for non-metastatic tumors. Breast conservation surgery combined with radiotherapy is an effective treatment for early cancers and is preferred over radical mastectomy. While surgery is typically effective, it is often a first step in the treatment plan as it may not provide a complete solution for patients with metastasis and late stages of cancer [11]. Chemotherapy is another common treatment modality. It can be given preoperatively as part of a treatment plan (neoadjuvant chemotherapy) or as a specific treatment regimen independent of other treatments (adjuvant chemotherapy). Chemotherapeutic drugs such as doxorubicin, epirubicin, paclitaxel, docetaxel, cyclophosphamide, fluorouracil, and carboplatin have been shown to reduce the risk of breast cancer when used in

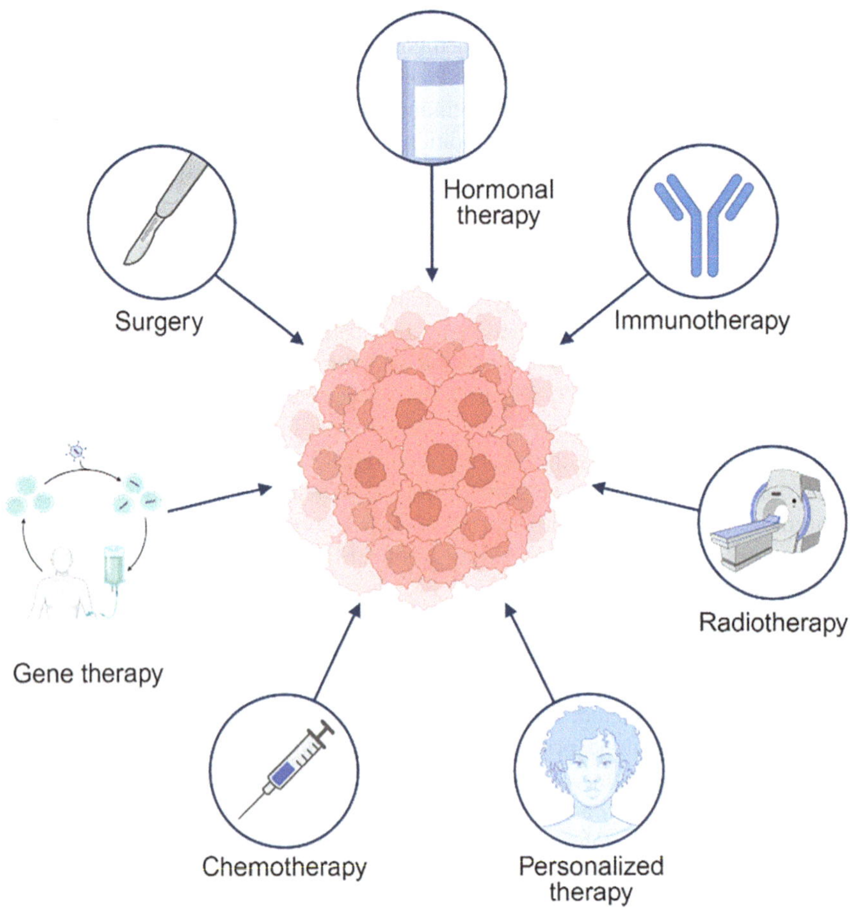

Fig. 1 Schematic diagram representing current therapeutic strategies in breast cancer management. (Created with BioRender.com)

combination. Taxane, sometimes in combination with anthracycline, makes up the standard chemotherapy regimen. High-risk patients, such as those with TNBC or HER2 positive subtypes, are recommended to receive the full chemotherapy regimen. Those with TNBC may also receive platinum-based agents. Chemotherapy is effective at reducing recurrence in high-risk patients but is not an absolute cure. Additionally, chemotherapy frequently produces severe side effects.

Radiotherapy is a very common treatment for breast cancer and is usually delivered via beam radiotherapy to either the whole breast or the local tumor site. Radiotherapy is frequently combined with other therapies and does not itself constitute a cure [10, 11]. Hormone therapy is given to most of the patients with HR-positive tumors. Tamoxifen is given to premenopausal patients, while postmenopausal patients are most frequently treated with aromatase inhibitors. Similarly, targeted therapy is given to those with HER2-positive cancer. Drugs such as Trastuzumab are effective at reducing recurrence risk in HER2-positive patients [10]. These treatments, however, leave a large gap in patients who will not benefit, as up to 30% of patients are HR and HER2 negative (TNBC), meaning that they will not benefit from hormone or targeted therapies [2]. Immunotherapy in breast cancer is varied, and its use depends on cancer subtype and specific cell markers. Among the most clinically relevant immunotherapies is the use of immune checkpoint inhibitors such as atezolizumab and paclitaxel in TNBC. These treatments are often combined with other treatment modalities, such as chemotherapy, and have been shown to be moderately effective. Gene therapy refers to a group of treatments that rely on targeting the genetic code, microRNA, and transcription factors of tumors, among other approaches. Gene therapy is a rapidly evolving and relatively novel field that currently lacks widespread clinical application [11].

1.4 Overview of Ovarian Cancer

Ovarian cancer is a malignant disease that pertains to the uncontrolled growth of cells in the ovaries of the female reproductive system. These rogue cells invade nearby tissues and organs, causing pathogenicity and leading to death if left untreated [12]. The highest incidence rates of ovarian cancer are consistent in Western countries such as the United States of America, Canada, France, Germany, and most of Europe. These higher incidences are due to longer life expectancies, larger populations, and increased risk exposures [13]. The estimated new cases for ovarian cancer in 2025 were 20,890, with an estimated death toll of 12,730 [14].

1.5 Classification and Screening of Ovarian Cancer

Even though certain studies state that genetic mutations are the main cause of ovarian cancer, the exact mechanisms underlying these genetic mutations need to be further explored. However, genetic predispositions found in heredity have been linked with 5–10% of ovarian cancer cases in women. Genetic mutations in the breast cancer genes 1 (BRCA 1) and breast cancer genes 2 (BRCA 2) have been linked with the development of ovarian cancer. BRCA 1 and BRCA 2 are the breast cancer genes that act as tumor suppressors, help repair damaged DNA, and prevent any buildup of genetic mutations. The mutations of these genes result in ineffective repair of double-stranded DNA, which leads to unstable cell growth. Individuals who inherit these mutated genes have a 15–60% lifetime risk of developing ovarian cancer [15, 16]. The two most common methods for ovarian cancer screening in early-stage development are cancer antigen 125 or carbohydrate antigen 125 (CA125) and ultrasound. At first, the patients are analyzed with the CA125 assay by measuring the amount of protein levels in the individual's blood. If more than 30 units/mL are found, then patients are screened through transvaginal ultrasound to locate the presence of any tumors. Since the early stage of ovarian carcinoma does not present any clear symptoms, an early diagnosis is rare. The early symptoms of ovarian cancer often include abdominal/pelvic pain and swelling, bloating, and gastrointestinal distress. These symptoms are often considered vague, and the patients are often misdiagnosed or diagnosed in the later stages, making them difficult to identify. However, with the later stages of the disease, increased symptoms of ascites and inflammation are more prone to appear [16]. However, for a complete diagnosis of any carcinomatous ovarian mass after increased symptoms, a laparotomy would be needed. This surgical procedure is performed by making an incision in the abdominal wall to examine the interior of the abdominal cavity through a laparoscopy [17].

1.6 Current Treatment Strategies for Ovarian Cancer

One of the treatment methods for ovarian cancer, debulking surgery, is often used in clinical scenarios. This method aims to reduce tumor sizes by surgically removing targeted carcinogenic masses. It has some supportive evidence leading to a persistent decrease in tumor growth and metastatic spread after surgery. However, this method of treatment is incredibly invasive and not 100% successful in preventing any future development of ovarian cancer post-surgery [18]. Other less invasive treatments for ovarian cancer include chemotherapeutic and intraperitoneal therapies. These treatments focus on delivering pharmaceutically developed drugs that target ovarian cancer cells in the body or specific regions, such as the intraperitoneal region [19]. They are effective in promoting anti-cancer environments and battling cancer cells gradually [20]. However, these treatments tend to have unwanted side effects and negative symptoms depending on the patients themselves.

Other therapeutic modalities include endocrine therapy, immunotherapy, and gene therapy. Endocrine therapy focuses on releasing steroid hormones (gonadotropins, estrogen, etc.) to inhibit or counter ovarian cancer growth/development [21]. Immunotherapy utilizes the body's natural defense (such as T cells containing tumor antigens) and infiltrating cancer tumor microenvironments, creating a difficult environment for the continued repair/development of those tumor cells. This form of immunoactivity is theorized to have great potential in combating ovarian tumor cells. Some commonly approved immunotherapies for ovarian cancers include pembrolizumab and dostarlimab [22, 23]. The final form of therapy for ovarian cancer is gene therapy which focuses on introducing genes that aim to promote immunotherapy and tumor suppression, especially correlating with the BRCA1 gene [24].

1.7 Shortcomings of the Current Standard of Care Therapy and the Application of Nanomedicine in Cancer Therapeutics

With the advancements in technologies related to cancer therapy, the standard of care (SOC) strategies have indeed made progress, decreased the mortality rates, and enabled patients to recover from cancer. However, the current therapeutic modalities still pose their shortcomings, along with causing a financial burden to the patients due to the treatment costs and multiple dose administration [25]. The drawbacks of the current treatment strategies are discussed below.

Therapeutic strategy varies as per the pathological state, and early detection will help in directing the right treatment option. The well-known primary therapy for breast and ovarian cancer, chemotherapy, still has potentially significant drawbacks. These agents lack tumor specificity, distribute within the disease site unevenly, and suppress the proliferation of normal cells along with cancer cells, resulting in non-tumor targets and inevitable adverse effects such as increased infection susceptibility, myelosuppression, alopecia, and so on. Another major drawback observed in chemotherapeutic agents is drug resistance, which leads to the reduced efficacy of the therapeutic strategy [26].

On the other hand, surgery, either mastectomy or lumpectomy, is the common procedure performed in breast cancer therapy. Apart from recurrence, the side effects include temporary numbness, scar tissue formation, seroma, and, in some cases, even nerve damage, thereby leading to discomfort in the armpit and lymph nodes. All these effects collectively can cause anatomical changes in the body [27]. The observed side effects of endocrine therapy include an increased risk of thromboembolic events, osteoporosis, hot flashes, and night sweats [28]. Immunotherapy for breast and ovarian cancer causes immune-related side effects that can lead to various adverse effects in the gastrointestinal region and skin, while radiotherapeutic procedures tend to cause cardiac and pulmonary injury, radiation dermatitis, lymphedema, radiation-induced malignancy, and so on [28, 29]. Antiangiogenic agents such as bevacizumab, cediranib, nintedanib, pazopanib, and Poly (ADP-ribose) polymerase (PARP) inhibitors such as olaparib, niraparib, and rucaparib are commonly used in treating breast and ovarian cancer. However, these drugs are said to be non-targeted to the tumor site, and multiple administrations lead to adverse effects, along with causing a financial burden on the patients [30]. The current therapies pose the above shortcomings, and hence, there is an urge to develop new targeted therapies to improve the patient's quality of life with minimal or no side effects.

2 Emerging Role of Nanomedicine in Breast and Ovarian Cancer

Nanomedicine is a term that integrates the application of nanotechnology in medicine, with an interest in enhancing diagnostic and therapeutic applications in treating diseases and disorders. Nanomedicine has already gained importance in a wide range of biomedical applications involving vaccine and drug discovery, nanosensor diagnostics, tissue engineering, and diagnostic imaging. Over the past decade, exploring and understanding the advancements in nanomaterials has grown in selectivity, affinity, and sensitivity, and it is anticipated that this emerging technology will play an increasing role in women's health [31].

The approach of nanomedicine in cancer therapy to achieve tumor-targeted drug delivery along with minimized adverse side effects and decreased administration dosage has been its ultimate goal. In the current decade, several nanoformulations and biomaterials are being designed and formulated for treating breast and ovarian cancer (Fig. 2), including active and passive targeting, stimuli-responsive, and thermo-responsive drug-loaded nanoformulations [32]. These novel nanocarriers and biomaterials, their applications, and shortcomings are discussed in the current section.

2.1 Role of Nanocarriers in Strategizing Cancer Treatment

Despite the advancements in medical science and technology, there is a hindrance in developing new strategies for cancer treatment [33]. Cancer progression and recurrence are the prominent contributors to this, and decoding the underlying mechanisms is yet a challenging task in research. Medical nanoscience deals with designing materials of nanoscale dimensions that range from 1 to 100 nm and are used to synthesize novel formulations or materials that can be used to diagnose or treat diseases and disorders [33–35].

In cancer therapeutics, nanoparticles are an excellent choice for targeted drug delivery. Their minute size and higher surface-to-volume ratio allow them to be the potential carriers to load any biological agent, drug, or gene and direct them toward the targeted site to render their mode of action. Different kinds of nanoparticles have been synthesized, which include graphene carbon nanoparticles, polymeric micelles, magnetic nanoparticles, liposomes, cubosomes, metallic nanoparticles, and so on. These nanocarriers have distinctive magnetic, physical, chemical, and optical

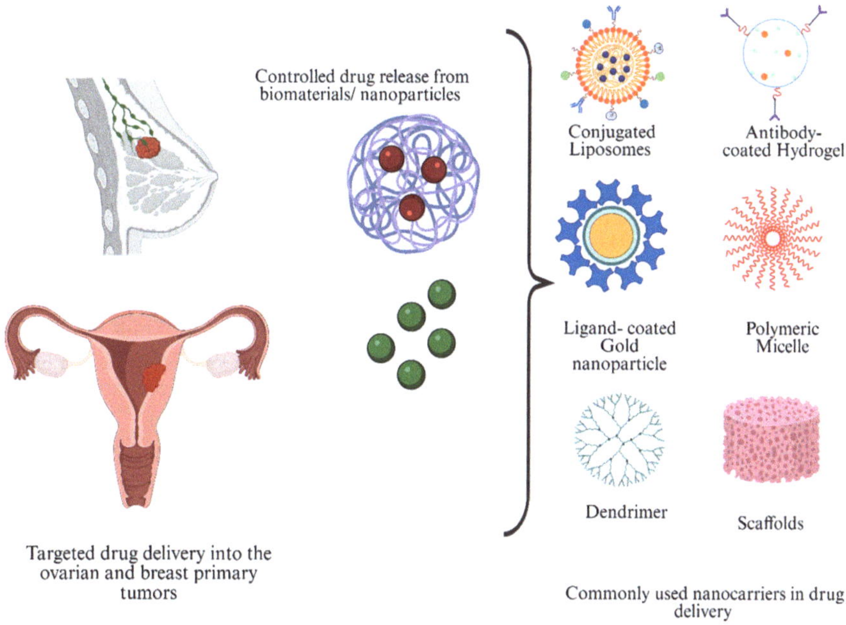

Fig. 2 Schematic diagram representing various drug delivery systems for targeted delivery in breast and ovarian cancer. (Created with BioRender.com)

properties, which could even be used for diagnostic purposes. On the other hand, nanomaterials have increased electrical conductivity and can be implanted at the tumor site [33, 36].

2.2 *Nanoparticle-Mediated Drug Delivery in Ovarian and Breast Cancer*

Chemotherapeutic agents, drugs, or small molecules can be encapsulated into carriers, which, when altered, can exploit the enhanced permeability retention (EPR) effect, an important strategy for improving targeted drug delivery by enhancing the bioavailability of the drug to the tumor site and minimizing the exposure to the healthy tissues. Layek et al., through their work, explain the role of mesenchymal stem cells (MSCs) as guideposts to target ovarian cancer. The team synthesized dibenzyl cyclooctyne (DBCO)-polyethylene glycol (PEG) functionalized paclitaxel-loaded nanoparticles using poly(D, L-lactide-co-glycolide) (PLGA). The team used MSCs as vehicles for tumor-specific accumulation of azide moieties, which could easily bind to DBCO in the tumor site. The functionalized drug-loaded nanoparticles were then used to target azide-bearing MSCs in ovarian tumors. The results of the study showed that when the tumors were labeled with azide-MSCs, the drug-loaded nanoparticles were well retained at the tumor site and also significantly reduced the tumor size when compared to the tumors that were not labeled with azide-MSCs [37]. Similarly, Ye et al. also reveal how the pH-responsive nanoparticles tend to enhance the chemodynamic therapy in ovarian cancer. The team synthesized an arsenic trioxide (ATO) drug delivery system (DDS) using arsenic-manganese nanoparticles, which could release the lethal arsenic ions (As^{3+}) and manganese ions (Mn^{2+}) to target ovarian human ovarian cancer cell line (SKOV3) cells via pH-responsive drug delivery. This nanoformulation not only ensured targeted drug delivery but also lowered the side effects on the vital organs, thus improving the efficacy of ATO for ovarian cancer treatment [38].

Chemoresistance is one of the drawbacks observed in ovarian cancer therapeutics. Hence, to overcome this, Liang et al. carried out a study to synthesize cyclic Arg-Gly-Asp (cRGD)-targeted heparin nanoparticles for the treatment of cisplatin-resistant ovarian cancer. The team synthesized a multifunctional cisplatin (DDP)-olaparib (Ola)-heparin (H)-cRGD (R) nanoparticle (DDP-Ola@HR) to deliver DDP and Ola. The heparin molecule suppressed the multidrug resistance-associated protein 2 and P-glycoprotein and thus promoted the intracellular drug delivery to the tumor site and downregulated the phosphatidylinositol 3-kinase/protein kinase B/mechanistic Target of Rapamycin (PI3K/Akt/mTOR) signaling pathway. This study paves the way for the use of a heparin-based drug-delivery system as an alternate approach to designing a multifunctional nanoplatform to tackle chemoresistance [39]. Babu and co-workers reveal the potency of chitosan-coated polylactic acid in the dual delivery of cisplatin-siRNA/plasmid DNA in tackling cisplatin-resistant human ovarian cancer cells. The team synthesized a multifunctional nanoparticle loaded with P62 siRNA, β5 plasmid DNA, and cisplatin and tested it against cisplatin-resistant 2008/C13 cells ovarian cancer cell lines. The results of the study showed that the cisplatin resistance index reduced from 4.62 to 3.62 after treatment, thereby proving the efficacy of the drug-loaded carriers as an efficient therapeutic modality against ovarian cancer [40].

Over the past decade, the monoclonal antibody-based therapeutic modality has gained a lot of importance for its promising outcomes. Dong et al. synthesized pH-responsive nanoparticles to deliver mRNA to tackle trastuzumab resistance in breast cancer. The nanocarriers were synthesized using a co-polymer methoxyl-poly (ethylene glycol)-*b*-poly (lactic-co-glycolic acid) conjugated with a pH-labile linker (Meo-PEG-$Dlink_m$-PLGA) along with cationic lipid (G0-C14) and then loaded with mRNA via electrostatic interaction. The synthesized nanoformulations were tested on an orthotopic tumor mouse model (female nude mice), which was subcutaneously injected with SKBR3-DR cells in the mammary fat pads. When the tumors reached the size of $\sim$100 mm^3, the animals were treated with nanoformulations and free mRNA. The results of the study state that the long-circulating mRNA could easily internalize into the tumor cells and upregulate the expression of Phosphatase and Tensin Homolog (PTEN), thus activating the PI3K/Akt signaling pathway that was blocked in the trastuzumab-resistant breast cancer cells, thereby suppressing tumor development [41]. Valcourt et al., in their study, worked on synthesizing nanoformulations loaded with a small-molecule drug called ABT-737 (poorly soluble in an aqueous medium), which can inhibit B-cell lymphoma 2 (Bcl-2) to reinstate the apoptotic signaling pathway and tend to be a strong, promising molecule for

TNBC therapy. The drug was encapsulated in poly (lactic acid-co-glycolic acid) nanoparticles functionalized with Notch-1 antibody and tested against TNBC cells. These drug-loaded nanoparticles can accumulate in the tumor region and reduce tumor burden to extend the survival period in the murine model [42].

Photodynamic therapy is another novel approach to treating breast cancer. Makhadmeh et al. reveal the potency of silica nanoparticles in enhancing the photodynamic therapy of breast cancer cells. The team made an effort to synthesize silica nanoparticles loaded with temoporfin to target MCF-7 cancer cells. The results of the study revealed that silica nanoparticles loaded with temoporfin irradiated with a laser beam significantly showed more effectiveness when compared to the bare drug temoporfin. This study shows us the dual role of silica nanoparticles in drug delivery along with photothermal therapy [43].

2.3 Commercially Available FDA-Approved Nanoformulations to Treat Breast and Ovarian Cancer

The United States Food and Drug Administration (U.S. FDA) belongs to the federal agency of the Department of Health and Human Services that works in the regulation and approval process of drugs for humans and animals [44]. Among the several nanocarriers, lipid-based formulations such as liposomes, solid-lipid nanoparticles, and micelles have gained a lot of importance in the commercial market due to their desirable properties.

Liposomes were the first drug-delivery system that was commercially available and, to date, are the most used nanoformulation to treat cancer. These lipid carriers have a similar composition to the biological membrane in humans and can incorporate both hydrophilic and lipophilic drugs. These liposomes can also be manipulated to provide a longer blood circulation time and extravasate through the leaky tumor vasculature via passive targeting. Apart from the above-mentioned (Table 1), some other commercially available nanomedicines include Caelyx, which are lipid-based nanoparticles with the active ingredient doxorubicin that is used in the treatment of ovarian and metastatic breast cancer. Protein–drug conjugates such as Pazenir, with the active ingredient paclitaxel, are used in the treatment of breast cancer. Kadcyla, with an active ingredient of DM1 (or Emtansine), is used in treating HER2+ breast cancer [46].

3 Role of Biomaterials in Drug Delivery in Targeting Ovarian and Breast Cancer

Biomaterials are considered to be specialized biocompatible materials that can be implanted (internally) or applied (externally) in the biological system. These are synthesized by the collaborative efforts of engineers, physicists, biologists, chemists, and clinicians and are used in advanced DDSs. Polymer and lipid biomaterials are

Table 1 Selected FDA-approved nanomedicines for cancer therapy

Drug name	Nanoparticle	Active drug	Cancer
Doxil	Liposome	Doxorubicin	Ovarian cancer, AIDS-related Kaposi's sarcoma (KS)/multiple myeloma
Myocet	Liposome	Doxorubicin	Metastatic breast cancer
Onivyde	Liposome	Irinotecan	Metastatic pancreatic cancer
Daunoxome	Liposome	Daunorubicin	HIV-associated KS
Vyxeos	Liposome	Daunorubicin and cytarabine	Acute myeloid leukemia
Ameluz	Liposome	5-Aminolaevulinic acid	Actinic keratoses
Abraxane	Polymeric	Paclitaxel	Breast cancer, non-small cell lung cancer, and pancreatic cancer
Genexol-PM	Polymeric	Paclitaxel	Breast cancer, non-small cell lung cancer and ovarian cancer
NKTR-102	Polymeric	Irinotecan	Breast cancer, ovarian cancer, colorectal cancer
Opaxio	Polymeric	Paclitaxel	Lung cancer, ovarian cancer, cervical cancer

Data adapted from Hristova-Panusheva et al. [45]

extensively used in drug delivery, and these are designed to release therapeutics for extended periods and can be modified to ensure targeted drug delivery [47, 48]. One of the drawbacks of conventional therapy is the repeated administration of the drug to the patients, and to overcome this issue, biomaterials for controlled drug release came into the picture, which could limit the dose administration. Researchers have been focusing on developing biomaterials as an alternative to pills and injections. The transdermal delivery systems have been using biomaterials science and microfabrication technology to synthesize drug-loaded biodegradable microneedle patches that can painlessly pierce the skin to enhance the drug permeability and thus leave no needle or biohazardous waste after use [47, 49]. The current focus is on synthesizing stimuli-responsive smart biomaterials that have been designed to respond to a wide range of environmental stimuli such as temperature, pH, enzymes, and pressure [47]. These biomaterials are widely used in strategizing treatment for breast and ovarian cancer. Yang et al. carried out a study for the sustained release of PARP inhibitor Talazoparib (TLZ) for treating BRCA-deficient ovarian cancer. TLZ-loaded PLGA implants were synthesized via the extrusion evaporation method. The in vivo efficacy of the drug-loaded implants was analyzed by injecting the implants into a murine $Brca2^{-/-}p53^{R172H/-}Pten^{-/-}$ genetically engineered peritoneally metastatic ovarian cancer (mOC) model. The results of the study state that the animals injected with TLZ implants showed double survival compared to the control animals, with no signs of organ toxicity in the intraperitoneal region, thereby suggesting sustained drug delivery to the targeted site [50].

Qiao and co-workers, through their study, explain the efficacy of magnesium implants in treating ovarian cancer. The degraded magnesium products from the biodegradable implants show great potential in antitumor activity. The team used an in vivo model by subcutaneously injecting SKOV3/Luc cells into female nude mice for tumor induction. After the tumor reached the desired size (5 mm), the animals were randomized into three groups: the control, titanium wire-implant, and magnesium wire-implant groups. The implants placed were about 0.8 mm in diameter and 5 mm in length. The results of the bioluminescence imaging revealed a significant decrease in the tumor volume of magnesium-treated mice when compared to that of the titanium-treated mice after 25 days of implantation [51].

Stephan et al., through their study, explained the role of biopolymer implants in enhancing the efficacy of adoptive T-cell therapy. The team synthesized a biopolymer implant that could efficiently deliver and expand tumor-reactive T cells to the tumor site, which was capable of getting rid of incompletely removed tumors. The 4T1 mouse breast tumor resection model was used for this study. The animals were injected with 4 T1 cells into the mammary glands, and after the growth, the tumors were resected, leaving less than 1% of the residue. The mice were randomized, and one of the groups was implanted with scaffolds that contained 7×10^6 tumor-reactive T cells directly into the resection cavity. Another two sets of animals received the adoptive T cells either intravenously or directly into the resection bed. The last set of animals was injected with pre-activated T cells containing IL-15 super agonist along with anti-CD28, anti-CD3, and anti-CD137 antibodies. The bioluminescence imaging suggested that the intravenously injected T cells and the control animals showed no changes in the relapse rate. The cells injected into the resection cavity showed a temporary reduction in the residual tumor growth. The cells pre-activated with the antibodies showed a prolonged relapse rate; however, they did not prevent the recurrence of the tumors. An interesting observation was noted in the animals receiving scaffold-delivered T cells, wherein none of the animals showed tumor relapse. This study paved the way for the usage of scaffolds as biomaterials to deliver T cells, as a therapeutic option for resected tumors, thereby reducing the metastatic relapse after surgery [52]. A few other common examples for clinical translation of biomaterials for immunotherapy in cancer include Abraxane, mRNA nanovaccine, and poly (lactic-co-glycolic acid) (e.g. engineered scaffold cancer vaccine system (WDVAX)) [53].

4 Limitations of DDSs and Strategies to Overcome Them

The DDS is considered to be one of the most efficient ways of delivering therapeutic agents to the targeted site with minimal or no side effects. The controlled release nanoformulations have gained importance due to their efficiency in releasing drugs at a predetermined rate for a specific period that can range from several days to months. It can also improve the target site accumulation, drug solubility, and pharmacological activity, and reduce toxicity with desirable pharmacokinetic properties [54]. However, in the case of aggressive solid tumors, the intratumoral environment may sometimes create a hurdle in drug delivery mechanisms.

Primarily, at the tumor site, drug resistance can occur due to the tumor-associated stromal extracellular matrix (ECM) or due to the ECM remodeling that can render a challenge for drug delivery. In some cases, during tumorigenesis, the increased deposition of collagen I and the relative fiber organization of the ECM can lead to low penetration of the nanoformulations. Lipid-based nanoformulations, which consist of a pH-sensitive release mechanism along with an MMP-2 cleavable PEG-peptide, may face challenges in their release mechanism that would hinder the cellular uptake following the shedding of the PEG moiety, thereby allowing the endosomal escape [55]. The other challenges in the biological system include the route of administration, which affects the bioavailability and biodistribution of the nanoformulations at the targeted site.

Even though most of the nanoformulations are biodegradable, controlling the biological fate of these carriers is hard, and the retention time and the half-life of these materials pose a risk to vital organ damage. A tricky challenge for these nanocarriers in the biological system is to bypass the biological barriers and avoid the mononuclear phagocytic system (MPS). In the body, the nanoparticles adsorb proteins to produce a protein corona, which directs the MPS in nanoparticle uptake. To bypass this uptake, the nanoparticles need to be coated with additional materials that prevent the adsorption of these carriers to the proteins. The overall challenges in DDS at a benchwork level involve the scale-up synthesis techniques, which involve the optimization and performance predictions that are very crucial in evaluating the therapeutic outcome in cancer treatment [57]. Despite the barriers, some nanoformulations have proven to show promising outcomes in clinical trials, as listed in Table 2.

Table 2 Summary of the nanoformulations in clinical trials for breast and ovarian cancer

Drug/sponsor	Active ingredient	Clinical trial	Cancer type
Topotecan liposomes injection (TLI) Spectrum Pharmaceuticals, Inc. (Henderson, NV, USA)	Topotecan	Phase 1 NCT00765973 Completed	Ovarian
LEP-ETU INSYS Therapeutics Inc (Phoenix, AZ, USA)	Paclitaxel	Phase 1 NCT00080418 Completed Phase 2 NCT01190982 Completed	Metastatic breast cancer
MM-302 Merrimack	Doxorubicin/anti-body fragment	Phase 1/2 terminated	Breast cancer
LiPlaCis Oncology venture	Cisplatin	Phase 1/2 NCT01861496	Metastatic breast cancer
SPI-77 NYU Langone Health	Cisplatin	Phase 2 NCT00004083 Completed	Ovarian cancer

Data adapted from Thi et al. [56]

Another limitation for the successful transition of the DDS from preclinical to clinical trial is the use of the most relevant animal model for breast/ovarian cancer. Researchers most commonly use rodent models to decode the underlying mechanism and study the influence of DDS in the biological system to develop innovative cancer therapeutics. Some of the most commonly used rodent models include the mouse intraductal model, used for studying cancer progression and the influence of DDS in the immunocompromised mice models. In this model, the human cancer cells are directly injected into the mouse mammary ducts, which allows the exact mimic and natural progression of the cancer cells in the mammary microenvironment. Once the tumors develop, the nanomaterials/biomaterials loaded with drugs are introduced at the tumor site, and their efficacy is studied. Cell-derived xenografts are performed in nude mice (deficient in T-cell function) or any other immunocompromised mice using aggressive cancer cell lines. This model makes it possible to induce various mammary/ovarian cancer cell lines into the animals in a short time and also represents a relatively homogenous mass, but unfortunately, it cannot mimic the immune system reaction and heterogeneity or the tumor microenvironment of the cancers from which these cell lines were derived. To overcome this limitation, the patient-derived xenograft is used. This model is generated by xenografting fresh human tumor biopsies from patients into immunocompromised mice that can recapitulate the diversity of breast cancer in host mice. This model retains the original tumor behavior and histopathology, and thus, the response of the DDS in these models could closely resemble that of the clinical trials, thereby rendering its successful translation. However, since the immunocompromised mice (deficient in T-cell, B-cell, and NK cell functions) are used to generate this model, it fails to understand the immune system reaction [58–60].

5 Summary and Conclusions

Breast and ovarian cancer are devastating cancers affecting most females around the globe. Even though there are several treatment procedures available in the market, they pose adverse effects and require multiple treatment doses. Nanoformulations/nanomaterials, an emerging field, tend to bypass the traditional methods, giving hope in improving the patient's quality of life. These nano-based DDS are considered to be next-generation medications, having the potency to extend the lifespan of patients by eradicating tumor recurrences. Despite the challenges in synthesis and delivery, these nano-based DDS are promising tools that aid in improving the therapeutic outcome. These are often used to design personalized medicines based on the needs, tumor stages, and heterogeneity in patients. These systems could also be functionalized or modified to target specific tumor microenvironments, proteins, or silence the tumor progression genes in breast and ovarian cancer. Several liposomal formulations are in ongoing clinical trials, and a few FDA-approved ones are also available in the market, which are actively recommended to breast and ovarian cancer patients. The potency of these targeted nanoformulations, as reported in many studies, encourages researchers and oncologists for the need to investigate more formulations that could serve as a building bridge between the bench and bedside formulations that can help serve mankind.

References

1. Upadhyay A. Cancer: an unknown territory; rethinking before going ahead. Genes Dis. 2021;8 (5):655–61.
2. American Cancer Society. Breast cancer facts and figures 2024–2025. Atlanta: American Cancer Society; 2024.
3. AACR Cancer Disparities progress Report 2024 Steering Committee, AACR cancer progress Report 2024 Steering Committee. Cancer in 2024. Cancer Discov. 2024;14(12):2324–31.
4. Giaquinto AN, Sung H, Newman LA, Freedman RA, Smith RA, Star J, Jemal A, Siegel RL. Breast cancer statistics 2024. CA Cancer J Clin. 2024;74(6):477–95.
5. Kim J, Harper A, McCormack V, Sung H, Houssami N, Morgan E, Mutebi M, Garvey G, Soerjomataram I, Fidler-Benaoudia MM. Global patterns and trends in breast cancer incidence and mortality across 185 countries. Nat Med. 2025;31:1154–62.
6. Xu S, Murtagh S, Han Y, Wan F, Toriola AT. Breast cancer incidence among US women aged 20 to 49 years by race, stage, and hormone receptor status. JAMA Netw Open. 2024;7(1): e2353331.
7. Fan L, Strasser-Weippl K, Li JJ, St Louis J, Finkelstein DM, Yu KD, Chen WQ, Shao ZM, Goss PE. Breast cancer in China. Lancet Oncol. 2014;15(7):e279–89.
8. Xiong X, Zheng LW, Ding Y, Chen YF, Cai YW, Wang LP, Huang L, Liu CC, Shao ZM, Yu KD. Breast cancer: pathogenesis and treatments. Signal Transduct Target Ther. 2025;10(1):49.
9. Loibl S, Poortmans P, Morrow M, Denkert C, Curigliano G. Epidemiology and risk factors. Breast Cancer Lancet. 2021;397:1750–69.
10. McDonald ES, Clark AS, Tchou J, Zhang P, Freedman GM. Clinical diagnosis and management of breast cancer. J Nucl Med. 2016;57(Supplement 1):9S–16S.
11. Wang J, Wu SG. Breast cancer: an overview of current therapeutic strategies, challenge, and perspectives. Breast Cancer: Targets Ther. 2023;31:721–30.
12. End-of-Life Care. End-of-life care - NCI. National Cancer Institute at the National Institutes of Health; 2021.
13. Hennessy BT, Coleman RL, Markman M. Ovarian cancer. Lancet. 2009;374(9698):1371–82.
14. SEER cancer stat facts: ovarian cancer. Bethesda: National Cancer Institute. https://seer.cancer.gov/statfacts/html/ovary.html.
15. Budiana IN, Angelina M, Pemayun TG. Ovarian cancer: pathogenesis and current recommendations for prophylactic surgery. J Türk-Ger Gynecol Assoc. 2019;20(1):47.
16. Colombo N, Van Gorp T, Parma G, Amant F, Gatta G, Sessa C, Vergote I. Ovarian cancer. Crit Rev Oncol Hematol. 2006;60(2):159–79.
17. Falcetta FS, Lawrie TA, Medeiros LR, da Rosa MI, Edelweiss MI, Stein AT, Zelmanowicz A, Moraes AB, Zanini RR, Rosa DD, Platt J. Laparoscopy versus laparotomy for FIGO stage I ovarian cancer. Cochrane Database Syst Rev. 2016;10:1465–858. John Wiley & Sons, Ltd, Laparoscopy, Laparotomy; Early Detection of Cancer.
18. Schorge JO, McCann C, Del Carmen MG. Surgical debulking of ovarian cancer: what difference does it make? Rev Obstet Gynecol. 2010;3(3):111.
19. Markman M. Intraperitoneal therapy of ovarian cancer. Oncologist. 1996;1(1–2):18–21. https://doi.org/10.1634/theoncologist.1-1-18.
20. Markman M, Reichman B, Hakes T, Curtin J, Jones W, Lewis JL Jr, Barakat R, Rubin S, Mychalczak B, Saigo P, Almadrones L. Intraperitoneal chemotherapy in the management of ovarian cancer. Cancer. 1993;71(S4):1565–70.

21. Li H, Liu Y, Wang Y, Zhao X, Qi X. Hormone therapy for ovarian cancer: emphasis on mechanisms and applications (review). Oncol Rep. 2021;46:223.
22. Odunsi K. Immunotherapy in ovarian cancer. Ann Oncol. 2017;28:viii1–7.
23. Prendecka-Wróbel M. Dostarlimab as a promising immunotherapy for endometrial cancer treatment–literature. J Pre-Clin Clin Res. 2023;17(3):186–94.
24. Tait DL, Obermiller PS, Jensen RA, Holt JT. Ovarian cancer gene therapy. Hematol Oncol Clin North Am. 1998;12(3):539–52.
25. Yang F, He Q, Dai X, Zhang X, Song D. The potential role of nanomedicine in the treatment of breast cancer to overcome the obstacles of current therapies. Front Pharmacol. 2023;14: 1143102.
26. Lee JJ, Saiful Yazan L, Che Abdullah CA. A review on current nanomaterials and their drug conjugate for targeted breast cancer treatment. Int J Nanomedicine. 2017;12:2373–84. https://doi.org/10.2147/IJN.S127329.
27. Lukasiewicz S, Czeczelewski M, Forma A, Baj J, Sitarz R, Stanislawek A. Breast cancer-epidemiology, risk factors, classification, prognostic markers, and current treatment strategies-an updated review. Cancers (Basel). 2021;13(17):4287. https://doi.org/10.3390/cancers13174287.
28. Lovelace DL, McDaniel LR, Golden D. Long-term effects of breast cancer surgery, treatment, and survivor care. J Midwifery Womens Health. 2019;64(6):713–24. https://doi.org/10.1111/jmwh.13012.
29. Garcia-Aranda M, Redondo M. Immunotherapy: a challenge of breast cancer treatment. Cancers (Basel). 2019;11(12):1822. https://doi.org/10.3390/cancers11121822.
30. Satora M, Kułak K, Zaremba B, Grunwald A, Świechowska-Starek P, Tarkowski R. New hopes and promises in the treatment of ovarian cancer focusing on targeted treatment—a narrative review. Front Pharmacol. 2024;15:1416555.
31. Lloyd-Parry O, Downing C, Aleisaei E, Jones C, Coward K. Nanomedicine applications in women's health: state of the art. Int J Nanomedicine. 2018;29:1963–83.
32. Thorat ND, Bauer J. Nanomedicine: next generation modality of breast cancer therapeutics. In: Nanomedicines for breast cancer theranostics. Elsevier; 2020. p. 3–16.
33. Lan H, Jamil M, Ke G, Dong N. The role of nanoparticles and nanomaterials in cancer diagnosis and treatment: a comprehensive review. Am J Cancer Res. 2023;13(12):5751.
34. Zhang W, Lu Y, Zang Y, Han J, Xiong Q, Xiong J. Photodynamic therapy and multi-modality imaging of up-conversion nanomaterial doped with AuNPs. Int J Mol Sci. 2022;23:1227. https://doi.org/10.3390/ijms23031227.
35. Cheng Z, Li M, Dey R, Chen Y. Nanomaterials for cancer therapy: current progress and perspectives. J Hematol Oncol. 2021;14:85. https://doi.org/10.1186/s13045-021-01096-0.
36. Yang J, Dai D, Zhang X, Teng L, Ma L, Yang YW. Multifunctional metal-organic framework (MOF)-based nanoplatforms for cancer therapy: from single to combination therapy. Theranostics. 2023;13:295–323. https://doi.org/10.7150/thno.80687.
37. Layek B, Shetty M, Nethi SK, Sehgal D, Starr TK, Prabha S. Mesenchymal stem cells as guideposts for nanoparticle-mediated targeted drug delivery in ovarian cancer. Cancer. 2020;12 (4):965.
38. Ye M, Ye R, Wang Y, Guo M, Zhu M, Yin F, Wang Y, Lai X, Wang Y, Qi Z, Wang J. Targeted pH-responsive biomimetic nanoparticle-mediated starvation-enhanced chemodynamic therapy combined with chemotherapy for ovarian cancer treatment. Int J Pharm. 2024;661:124426.
39. Liang X, Yang Y, Huang C, Ye Z, Lai W, Luo J, Li X, Yi X, Fan JB, Wang Y, Wang Y. cRGD-targeted heparin nanoparticles for effective dual drug treatment of cisplatin-resistant ovarian cancer. J Control Release. 2023;356:691–701.
40. Babu A, Wang Q, Muralidharan R, Shanker M, Munshi A, Ramesh R. Chitosan coated polylactic acid nanoparticle-mediated combinatorial delivery of cisplatin and siRNA/plasmid DNA chemosensitizes cisplatin-resistant human ovarian cancer cells. Mol Pharm. 2014;11(8): 2720–33.

41. Dong Z, Huang Z, Li S, Wang Y, Yao Y, Yang X, Xu X. Nanoparticles (NPs)-mediated systemic mRNA delivery to reverse trastuzumab resistance for effective breast cancer therapy. Acta Pharm Sin B. 2023;13(3):955–66.
42. Valcourt DM, Dang MN, Scully MA, Day ES. Nanoparticle-mediated co-delivery of Notch-1 antibodies and ABT-737 as a potent treatment strategy for triple-negative breast cancer. ACS Nano. 2020;14(3):3378–88.
43. Makhadmeh GN, AlZoubi T, Aljarrah AM, Al Alami JH, Zyoud SH. Enhancing photodynamic therapy efficacy through silica nanoparticle-mediated delivery of temoporfin for targeted in vitro breast cancer treatment. Photodiagn Photodyn Ther. 2024;46:104034.
44. Chaurasia M, Singh R, Sur S, Flora SJ. A review of FDA approved drugs and their formulations for the treatment of breast cancer. Front Pharmacol. 2023;14:1184472.
45. Hristova-Panusheva K, Xenodochidis C, Georgieva M, Krasteva N. Nanoparticle-mediated drug delivery systems for precision targeting in oncology. Pharmaceuticals. 2024;17(6):677.
46. Rodríguez F, Caruana P, De la Fuente N, Español P, Gamez M, Balart J, Llurba E, Rovira R, Ruiz R, Martín-Lorente C, Corchero JL. Nano-based approved pharmaceuticals for cancer treatment: present and future challenges. Biomolecules. 2022;12(6):784.
47. Fenton OS, Olafson KN, Pillai PS, Mitchell MJ, Langer R. Advances in biomaterials for drug delivery. Adv Mater. 2018;30(29):1705328.
48. Bangham AD, Horne RW. Negative staining of phospholipids and their structural modification by surface-active agents as observed in the electron microscope. J Mol Biol. 1964;8(5):660–IN10.
49. Farokhzad OC, Langer R. Impact of nanotechnology on drug delivery. ACS Nano. 2009;3(1): 16–20.
50. Yang S, Green A, Brown N, Robinson A, Senat M, Testino B, Dinulescu DM, Sridhar S. Sustained delivery of PARP inhibitor Talazoparib for the treatment of BRCA-deficient ovarian cancer. Front Oncol. 2023;13:1175617.
51. Qiao S, Wang Y, Zan R, Wu H, Sun Y, Peng H, Zhang R, Song Y, Ni J, Zhang S, Zhang X. Biodegradable Mg implants suppress the growth of ovarian tumor. ACS Biomater Sci Eng. 2020;6(3):1755–63.
52. Stephan SB, Taber AM, Jileaeva I, Pegues EP, Sentman CL, Stephan MT. Biopolymer implants enhance the efficacy of adoptive T-cell therapy. Nat Biotechnol. 2015;33(1):97–101.
53. Shi Y. Clinical translation of nanomedicine and biomaterials for cancer immunotherapy: progress and perspectives. Adv Ther. 2020;3(9):1900215.
54. Ezike TC, Okpala US, Onoja UL, Nwike CP, Ezeako EC, Okpara OJ, Okoroafor CC, Eze SC, Kalu OL, Odoh EC, Nwadike UG. Advances in drug delivery systems, challenges and future directions. Heliyon. 2023;9(6):e17488.
55. Cukierman E, Khan DR. The benefits and challenges associated with the use of drug delivery systems in cancer therapy. Biochem Pharmacol. 2010;80(5):762–70.
56. Thi TT, Suys EJ, Lee JS, Nguyen DH, Park KD, Truong NP. Lipid-based nanoparticles in the clinic and clinical trials: from cancer nanomedicine to COVID-19 vaccines. Vaccine. 2021;9(4): 359.
57. Gavas S, Quazi S, Karpiński TM. Nanoparticles for cancer therapy: current progress and challenges. Nanoscale Res Lett. 2021;16(1):173.
58. Liu C, Wu P, Zhang A, Mao X. Advances in rodent models for breast cancer formation, progression, and therapeutic testing. Front Oncol. 2021;11:593337.
59. Harlan BA, Nikitin AY. A quest for better mouse models of breast and ovarian cancers. EBioMedicine. 2015;2(10):1268–9.
60. Paschall AV, Liu K. An orthotopic mouse model of spontaneous breast cancer metastasis. J Vis Exp. 2016;114:54040.

Therapeutic Applications of Exosomes for Women's Reproductive Health

Alexandra M. Harrison, Yuanxin Xu, Adelyn A. Fisher, and Christina M. Bailey-Hytholt

Abstract Treating gynecological and reproductive health conditions requires a multifaceted approach, and the use of biologics is increasingly being explored. More specifically, exosomes isolated from mesenchymal stem cells derived from relevant biological sources (e.g., bone marrow, menstrual blood, etc.) have shown advantageous properties for gynecological conditions. In this chapter, we first introduce the biological role of exosomes in women's reproductive health. Next, we summarize the current state of exosome use as a therapeutic for the following reproductive health conditions: endometriosis, polycystic ovary syndrome, infertility due to implantation failure and primary ovarian insufficiency, preeclampsia, and pelvic floor dysfunction. Exosomes in clinical trials for reproductive health applications are then highlighted. This chapter concludes with perspectives and opportunities of using exosomes as a therapeutic for disorders and complications facing women's reproductive health. Overall, the use of exosomes to treat conditions influencing reproductive health is in an early stage, with most studies taking place within the past 5 years. With much left to be explored in the field, the advantages and challenges of exosome-based therapeutics are still being realized. The studies discussed throughout the chapter highlight the potential for transformative medicine for a range of women's health applications.

Keywords Exosomes · Mesenchymal stem cells (MSCs) · microRNA · Women's reproductive health · Endometriosis · Polycystic ovary syndrome (PCOS) · Infertility · Preeclampsia · Pelvic floor dysfunction (PFD)

Abbreviations

EV	Extracellular vesicle
HESCs	Human endometrial stromal cells

A. M. Harrison · Y. Xu · A. A. Fisher · C. M. Bailey-Hytholt (✉)
Department of Chemical Engineering, Worcester Polytechnic Institute, Worcester, MA, USA
e-mail: amharrison@wpi.edu; yxu13@wpi.edu; aafisher@wpi.edu; cmbailey@wpi.edu

S. G. Zambuto, M. L. Oyen (eds.), *Biomaterials for Women's Health Engineering*,
https://doi.org/10.1007/978-3-032-10745-9_21

miRNA	microRNA
MMP-2	Matrix metalloproteinase-2
MSCs	Mesenchymal stem cells
PCOS	Polycystic ovary syndrome
PFD	Pelvic floor dysfunction
POI	Primary/premature ovarian insufficiency
POP	Pelvic organ prolapse
SUI	Stress urinary incontinence
TNF-α	Tumor necrosis factor-α
USCs	Urinary-derived stem cells

1 Exosomes and Their Biological Role in Women's Reproductive Health

Exosomes, an extracellular vesicle (EV) natively secreted by cells for communication, are increasingly being explored for their therapeutic capacity and biocompatibility, with recent studies demonstrating their potential to advance reproductive health [1]. Exosomes serve important roles universal to all cell and tissue types, including the facilitation of cell-to-cell communication and regulation of metabolic activity and immune responses [2, 3]. More specifically, exosomes are important in gynecological health to mediate cell signaling between reproductive tissues and regulate hormone production. The biological role and function of exosomes have sparked interest in their use to diagnose and treat disorders that predominantly influence women's reproductive health, such as endometriosis, polycystic ovary syndrome (PCOS), preeclampsia, and so on. This chapter focuses on recent studies that have demonstrated the potential of exosomes as therapeutic agents to improve women's reproductive health.

EVs originate from late-stage endosomes through inward budding of multicellular vesicles [2, 3]. They are released into the extracellular space through the exocytosis of the multicellular vesicles with the plasma membrane of the cell [2, 3]. Exosomes, a specialized class of EVs, contain a variety of bioactive molecules such as proteins (e.g., CD63 or CD81 [3]) and nucleic acids (e.g., microRNA (miRNA), messenger RNA (mRNA), DNA, circular RNA, long non-coding RNA, etc. [4]), encapsulated by a lipid bilayer [5]. The specific composition of these spherical or cup-shaped vesicles, ranging in size from 30 to 150 nm, is dependent on the secreting cell type and environment [2, 6–9]. After release into the extracellular space, exosomes travel to both neighboring and distant cells [7].

Exosome communication is vital to overall gynecological health, and improper signaling can lead to a variety of gynecological disorders discussed throughout this chapter [10]. For example, it has been shown that there are specific proteins only expressed in peritoneal fluid-derived exosomes from endometriosis patients, including peroxiredoxin-1 (PRDX1), histone H2A type2-C, annex A2 (ANXA2), inter-alpha-trypsin inhibitor heavy chain 4 (ITIH4), and tubulin chain-α [11]. While the pathogenesis of endometriosis is not completely understood, cargo from endometriosis patient-derived exosomes influences inflammatory cytokine presence, angiogenesis, cell migration and invasion, and disruption of the immune state, which all contribute to the creation of endometriotic lesions [11, 12]. Protein expression in exosomes varies between endometriosis patients compared to their healthy counterparts [12]. PCOS patients have differing exosome contents (e.g., miRNAs, piwi-interacting RNA, transfer RNAs, etc.) compared to healthy patients [10]. The miRNA content of exosomes derived from PCOS patients is particularly important, as the miRNAs can influence an increase in inflammation and alter metabolic and insulin states, which progress PCOS pathogenesis [10].

Precise cell communication is necessary to ensure a healthy pregnancy. The first heightened concentration of exosomes in maternal blood is triggered by exposure to the hypoxic and hyperglycemic environment of early pregnancy [3, 7, 13]. Exosomes produced by the early trophectoderm influence trophoblast cells to proliferate and invade to remodel and dilate the spiral arteries to allow adequate blood exchange between the mother and fetus [7]. Previous work has shown that the concentration of exosomes derived from the placenta in maternal blood increases with increased gestational age [3, 7]. Placental exosomes can be identified by proteins such as placental alkaline phosphatase, as well as specific miRNA including miRNA-127, miRNA-134, and chromosome 19 miRNA cluster (C19MC) miRNAs [14, 15]. An important role of placental trophoblast cells is to ensure that the fetus, considered a foreign tissue to the immune system, is accepted [3, 7, 16]. Placental exosomes deliver a variety of immunosuppressive molecules and miRNA to suppress the activity of immune natural killer and T cells [7]. Slight deviations in exosome contents or exosome concentration can signal a variety of complications, including preeclampsia or pre-term birth [3, 7].

Interest in the therapeutic potential of exosomes has increased in recent years as exosomes have been investigated for applications in drug delivery, cancer and gene therapy, and regenerative medicine [17–20]. Exosomes are readily accepted by other cells in the body as a native lipid vesicle, making them an ideal natural carrier of therapeutic material for drug delivery [21]. In clinical trials, exosomes have shown promising results in the treatment of COVID-19, cancer, cardiovascular diseases, and neurological disorders [22]. In reproductive health, several studies have investigated their role in cell communication, with brief examples noted in this section above. More recently, exosomes are being explored as diagnostic and therapeutic tools for women's reproductive health [23, 24].

This chapter summarizes progress on the characterization and application of exosomes for therapeutic use in reproductive health. This chapter will discuss studies examining exosome therapies for endometriosis, PCOS, infertility due to implantation failure and primary ovarian insufficiency (POI), preeclampsia, and pelvic floor dysfunction (PFD). Exosome therapeutics will be considered for their characteristics and ability to influence cell and tissue behavior.

2 Therapeutic Applications of Exosomes for Women's Reproductive Health

Exosome research has focused on elucidating the mechanisms of cell-to-cell communication and has begun to utilize these particles as diagnostic and therapeutic tools. In the studies discussed below, exosomes are commonly harvested from the cell culture supernatant of mesenchymal stem cells (MSCs) derived from various biological sources. Exosomes are isolated from these sources through cascading centrifugal and ultracentrifugal runs [25, 26]. After isolation, exosomes are stored in a neutral buffer, often phosphate-buffered saline, for characterization and subsequent use [27, 28]. Exosomes contain a range of biological contents, including miRNA, mRNA, DNA, lipids, and various proteins and hormones (Fig. 1a) [4]. In the studies highlighted throughout this chapter, researchers investigated the use of exosomes as a therapy for a range of gynecological conditions (Fig. 1b). Exosome therapeutics for reproductive health are in an early stage, and studies have so far focused on conditions including endometriosis, PCOS, infertility-related conditions, including implantation failure and POI, preeclampsia, and PFD, which are the main conditions discussed in this chapter. While each of these conditions is crucial to treat due to its impact on women's health, and we focus on them individually, it is important to note that there are also relationships between them. For example, endometriosis and PCOS can often influence infertility and pregnancy-related challenges, and pregnancy itself impacts pelvic floor function [29, 30]. Exosomes, as a therapeutic, offer an approach to combat underlying mechanisms contributing to each of these conditions and complications. The following sections explore the early stages of exosome therapeutic development for women's reproductive health. We review recent investigations using exosomes toward treating endometriosis, PCOS, and infertility conditions such as POI, preeclampsia, and PFD.

2.1 Endometriosis

Endometriosis, a chronic inflammatory disease affecting ~10% of women globally, is caused by the growth of endometrial-like tissue outside of the uterus, resulting in severe pelvic pain and increased infertility rate [12, 31]. The cause of endometriosis is being investigated, but genetic and environmental factors are thought to play a significant role [32, 33]. EVs, and particularly exosomes, have the potential to be a reliable therapeutic for endometriosis due to their targeted disruption of endometriosis pathogenesis [21]. Exosome therapies for the treatment of endometriosis focus on the reduction of inflammatory markers, notably through the use or restriction of mechanisms linked to macrophage activity.

Endometriosis is typically associated with chronic inflammation, development into fibrosis, and the formation of scar tissue present in endometriotic lesions [34]. Endometriosis has been linked to an increased expression of fibrotic markers

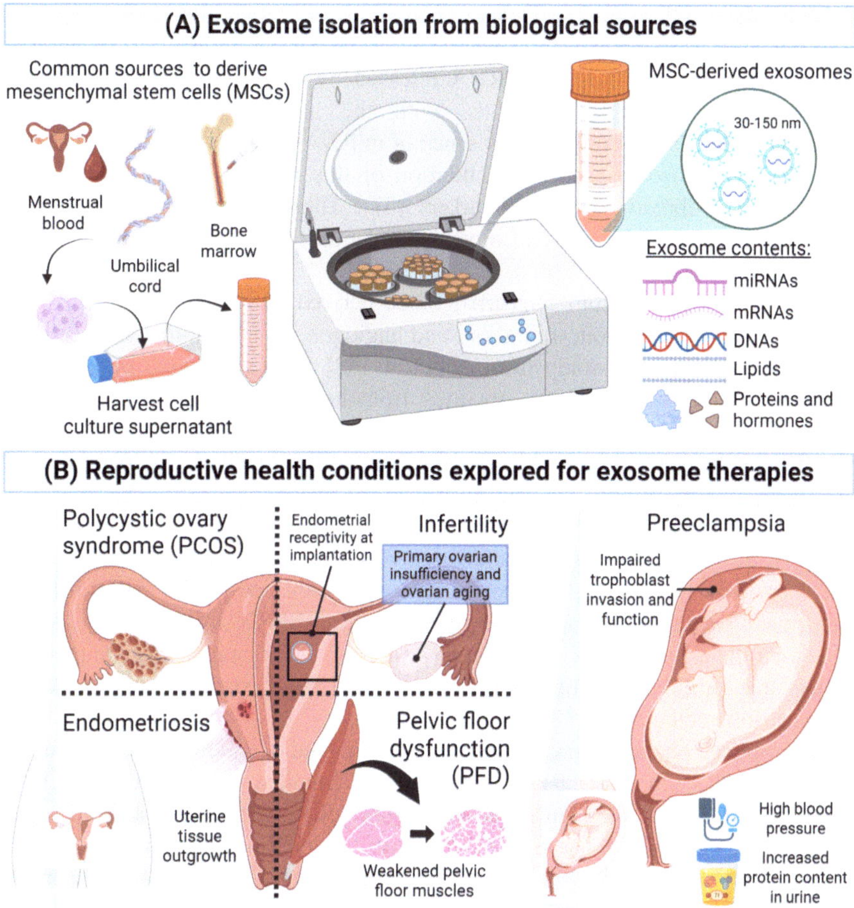

Fig. 1 Cartoon schematic of exosome isolation and their therapeutic applications for reproductive and gynecological health. (**a**) Isolation of exosomes from menstrual blood-, umbilical cord-, and bone marrow-derived MSCs. (**b**) Depiction of various women's reproductive health conditions that have shown potential to benefit from exosome-based therapies

and decreased levels of miRNA-214 [35]. This knowledge was leveraged by Wu et al. in a 2018 study to investigate the effects of miRNA-214-enriched exosomes isolated from ectopic endometrial stromal cells on murine endometriosis models [36]. Exosomes containing miRNA-214 mimics were used to treat endometriosis mouse models, where the exosomes significantly reduced the amount of endometriotic lesions and fibrosis compared to no treatment and treatment with control exosomes without miRNA-214 enrichment [36]. In 2024, Song et al. revealed the effect of umbilical cord MSC-derived exosomes on endometrial fibrosis [37]. Human endometrial stromal cells (HESCs) were used to test the function of the umbilical cord MSC-derived exosomes on transforming growth factor-beta

(TGF-β)-induced fibrosis [37]. The gene expression of fibrosis biomarkers decreased after treatment with the exosomes compared to the control groups [37]. Song et al. found that miRNA-140-3p, a miRNA released by umbilical cord MSC-derived exosomes, was strongly associated with the anti-fibrotic effects observed [37]. Their studies confirmed the presence of miRNA-140-3p in the umbilical cord MSC-derived exosomes and that inhibition of this miRNA influenced the gene expression of fibrosis-related biomarkers [37]. These results demonstrated that umbilical cord MSC-derived exosomes have therapeutic potential for anti-fibrosis on HESCs.

Exosomes isolated from menstrual blood-derived MSCs reduced markers of inflammation, proliferation, migration, and angiogenesis in endometriotic cells, as demonstrated in a 2023 study from Asl et al. [38]. Exosomes were isolated from menstrual blood-derived MSCs obtained from healthy women between 27 and 35 years of age who had regular menstrual cycles, successfully delivered at least one healthy full-term infant without requiring fertility treatments, experienced no pregnancy complications, and had no history of miscarriage [38]. The exosomes were used to treat endometriotic cells isolated from women diagnosed with endometriosis through laparoscopic examination who presented with symptoms of irregular menstrual cycles alongside pelvic pain or a suspected pelvic mass [38]. The exosomes isolated from menstrual blood-derived MSCs from healthy donors decreased the expression of interleukin-1β (IL-1β), an inflammatory gene that promotes the proliferation of endometriotic cells and simultaneously reduces endometriotic cell growth [38].

Macrophage phagocytosis is thought to be impaired in endometriosis, leading to overgrowth of endometrial tissue and a reduced immune response to this ectopic tissue growth [31, 39]. Huang et al. investigated the effects of exosomes isolated from ectopic endometrial tissue of patients with endometriosis and miRNA-301a-3p on THP-1 human monocytic cell-derived macrophage phagocytosis and polarization [40]. In previous studies, miRNA-301a-3p-rich exosomes increased polarization of macrophages and subsequent malignant behavior in pancreatic cancer cells [41]. In the study from Huang et al., THP-1-derived macrophages were treated with ectopic tissue-derived exosomes, and a significant reduction in phagocytic activity was observed. This reduction in phagocytotic activity demonstrated that ectopic tissues influence the behavior of neighboring tissues, which results in tissue growth outside of the uterus as commonly seen in endometriosis patients [40]. Through the same dosing process, Huang et al. measured the polarization of these initial THP-1-derived M1 macrophages and found that after treatment with exosomes, the number of anti-inflammatory, tissue repair M2 macrophages increased significantly, indicating a switch from the abundance of pro-inflammatory M1 macrophages [40]. Similarly, in a 2021 study, Li et al. discovered that nanovesicles derived from THP-1-derived macrophages reduce the capacity of eutopic endometrial stromal cells isolated from endometriosis patient samples to form endometrial lesions [42].

Peritoneal fluid, which fills the space between the wall of the abdomen and the encased organs, can play a crucial role in the progression of endometriosis due to its contents and contributions to the local immune environment [43]. Liu et al.

employed exosomes isolated from macrophages derived from peritoneal fluid patient samples to reveal that long non-coding cell adhesion molecule L1-like antisense RNA 1 (CHL1-AS1) promotes the progression of endometriosis through the upregulation of miRNA-610, a finding that has led to subsequent discussion of the molecule [44, 45]. When treated with peritoneal macrophage-derived exosomes, ectopic endometrial stromal cells showed significantly increased migration, invasion, and expression of long non-coding RNA CHL1-AS1 [44]. To further understand the role of this RNA, Liu et al. transfected peritoneal macrophages with a short interfering RNA that interfered with the long non-coding RNA CHL1-AS1, followed by exosome isolation [44]. Treatment with these interfering exosomes reversed the once heightened invasive behavior of endometrial cells and reduced their proliferation [44]. These results were further observed in murine models, where the volume and weight of endometrial lesions increased with normal peritoneal macrophage exosomes and decreased with interfering exosomes [44].

2.2 *Polycystic Ovary Syndrome*

PCOS is the most common endocrine disorder, affecting approximately 15–18% of women of reproductive age [46]. In individuals with PCOS, high levels of androgen and testosterone are produced by the ovaries and can lead to symptoms including irregular menstrual cycles, acne and excess hair growth, weight gain, and infertility [10, 47]. Current treatments for PCOS focus on lifestyle changes, treating individual symptoms, or hormone therapies such as birth control or ovulation promoters [48]. Exosome therapies can expand on current treatment strategies and offer a new approach to regulate hormonal abnormalities and inflammatory response in PCOS patients [49].

Exosomes isolated from human umbilical cord MSCs were demonstrated by Park et al. in 2023 as a promising therapy to treat PCOS-related dysfunctions, including deregulating pathogenic gene expression and regulating metabolism through androgen-producing in vitro cell studies and PCOS in vivo mouse model studies. Park et al. treated H295R, a human-ovarian-theca-like cell line, immortalized adrenocortical steroid-producing cells with MSC-derived exosomes to regulate androgen production [50]. Park et al. found a significant reduction in gene expression of cytochrome P450 (Cyp) 17a1, Cyp11a1, and DENN domain (DENND) 1a, important genes that generate androgen, in both MSC-derived conditioned media and MSC-derived exosome-treated H295R cells [50]. Further, MSC-derived exosomes were found to reverse metabolism, restore ovarian function, and restore fertility in a mouse model of PCOS [50].

In women of childbearing age, PCOS is the most common endocrine and metabolic disorder [51]. Due to the metabolic nature of the syndrome, Cao et al. used exosomes produced by adipose MSCs, which secrete regulatory factors for metabolism, to restore ovarian structure in PCOS mouse models and establish adipose MSC-derived exosomes as a potential therapeutic for PCOS [52]. By injecting these exosomes into a PCOS mouse model, Cao et al. observed significant improvement in blood glucose levels, number of corpus lutea, and testosterone levels, which were comparable to the unaltered control mice [52]. In this experiment, the exosomes were found in abundance in the liver, enhancing the uptake of glucose by liver cells and stimulating the phosphorylation of AKT, a kinase involved in cell survival, growth, and metabolism [52].

In studying granulosa cells isolated from samples from PCOS patients, Zhao et al. observed significant inflammatory responses compared to healthy patient controls and linked this finding to the nuclear factor kappa-B (NF-κB) inflammation regulation signaling pathway [53]. Treatment with human umbilical cord MSCs alleviated this inflammation in PCOS granulosa cells, measured through differential expression of inflammatory markers tumor necrosis factor alpha (TNF-α) and interferon gamma (INF-γ) [53]. When healthy cells were dosed with the same exosomes, no differences in expression of TNF-α and INF-γ were observed [53]. Additionally, treatment with human umbilical cord MSC-derived exosomes promoted the production of progesterone in PCOS granulosa cell culture and reduced cell apoptosis [53].

Building from the knowledge that PCOS is related to metabolic abnormalities and that cumulus cells are responsible for secreting growth hormones, Zhao et al. employed metabolically regulating adipose MSC-derived exosomes containing miRNA-323-3p to decrease symptoms of PCOS in patient-sampled cumulus cell cultures and PCOS mouse models [54]. Unmodified exosomes and exosomes modified with an increased concentration of miRNA-323-3p were tested with PCOS patient cumulus cells in vitro [54]. Experiments with modified exosomes showed significant upregulation of miRNA-323-3p and reduction in the expression of programmed cell death protein 4 [54]. The same result was observed in a PCOS mouse model induced by letrozole treatment, confirming the inverse relationship between miRNA-323-3p and programmed cell death protein 4 [54]. This relationship may be leveraged to decrease cumulus cell death in PCOS patients to increase the availability of healthy oocytes.

2.3 *Infertility*

Infertility is classified by the medical community as the inability to conceive a child after frequent unprotected sex for at least 1 year, or 6 months if the woman is over 35 years of age [55]. Affecting roughly 13% of women aged 18–49 years old [56], infertility can be due to lifestyle and environmental factors, physical reproductive organ abnormalities, or specific conditions such as ovulatory disorders (PCOS and POI), endometriosis, or hyperprolactinemia [57]. Exosome therapeutics are being explored to alleviate major drivers of infertility: implantation failure and POI, also referred to as premature ovarian failure.

A key mechanism for a successful pregnancy is the implantation of the embryo into the decidualized endometrium [58]. Clinically, unsuccessful implantation is the leading cause of infertility and is a common cause of failure in assistive reproductive procedures, such as in vitro fertilization, where roughly 75% of embryos do not successfully implant per cycle [59–61]. This can be due to physical reproductive organ abnormalities, endometrial receptivity, thrombophilia, or embryonic genetic factors, among other causes [62]. Any of these factors, especially when combined, can interfere with the biological crosstalk that leads to apposition between the blastocyst and endometrium and disrupt implantation [62].

Endometrial receptivity is essential to successful implantation and a healthy pregnancy [63]. A study performed by Tan et al. in 2021 revealed miRNA-100-5p to be instrumental in the influence that EVs from two epithelial endometrial adenocarcinoma cell lines had on trophoblast cells [64]. miRNA-100-5p is found to be upregulated during pregnancy in the placental villi and serum from the mother [65]. In Transwell invasion and cell proliferation assays, EVs isolated from receptive Ishikawa cells increased HTR-8/SVneo extravillous trophoblast cell migration and invasion, while EVs isolated from nonreceptive HEC-1-A cells significantly decreased these cell behaviors [64]. Tan et al. found expression of miRNA-100-5p to be 20× higher in receptive cell EVs than those from nonreceptive cells [64].

POI is defined as the loss of normal ovarian function before the age of 40 years, regardless of cause [66]. This can also be classified within ovarian aging, which includes reproductive decline due to age [67]. Since the first report of the effects of chemotherapy on female reproduction in the 1970s, there have been several studies conducted that conclude a definitive tie between chemotherapy treatment and the depletion of ovarian reserves, a prime example of fertility loss due to external factors encompassed by POI [68, 69]. A 2023 study conducted by Xiao et al. found exosomes isolated from human umbilical cord MSCs to be able to prevent and recover ovarian damage in mouse tissue and mouse models after treatment with a chemotherapeutic frequently used in the treatment of ovarian, breast, and lung cancer [69]. While ovaries grown in vitro with *cis*-diamminechloroplatinum (II) exhibited reduced volume compared to the control group, a combined treatment with both the chemotherapeutic and human umbilical cord MSC-derived exosomes prevented this reduction with no significant difference compared to the control group [69]. Additionally, treatment with the human umbilical cord MSC-derived exosomes prevented DNA breakage and follicle death that was seen in the treatment group that only received the chemotherapeutic [69]. In mice that received 10 days of treatment with *cis*-diamminechloroplatinum (II) followed by injection with human umbilical cord MSC-derived exosomes, fertility and follicle function were restored compared to the mice that only received the chemotherapeutic [69]. In culture with mouse granulosa cells, human umbilical cord MSC-derived exosomes protected against *cis*-diamminechloroplatinum (II) damage and reduced key inflammatory factors [69].

In 2024, Liu et al. identified that exosomes derived from follicular fluid, which contained miRNA-320a-3p-mediated, inhibited Forkhead Box Q1 (FOXQ1) expression, resulting in the prevention of ovarian aging [27]. Exosomes isolated from follicular fluid samples from "young" under 30-year-old and "old" over 38-year-old patients showed no differences in size, particle concentration, or protein markers [27]. In further experiments, exosomes were isolated from follicular fluid obtained from "young" mice and granulosa cells isolated from the ovaries of "old" mice

[27]. Young exosomes decreased old granulosa cell apoptosis at a dose of 5 μg/mL [27]. In 40-week-old mice given local injections of fluorescently labeled young exosomes, fluorescence was observed throughout the liver, kidneys, and ovaries, showing the highest intensity in both ovaries [27]. The ovaries of treated mice were significantly larger in volume and weight, indicating partial rescue from age-related ovarian dysfunction [27]. This was identified to be the result of miRNA-320-3p within the exosomes, confirmed by further plasmid transfection experiments [27].

2.4 Preeclampsia

Preeclampsia is a pregnancy-related complication characterized by hypertension and insufficient blood flow to the fetus that affects ~15% of pregnancies and is typically diagnosed around 20 weeks of gestation or later [70]. Currently, treatment strategies consist of symptom management, and the only cure for preeclampsia is giving birth [70]. Early detection strategies have become a focal point of the field [71]. While early diagnoses could prevent the onset of symptoms, it is critical to develop therapeutics for cases that cannot be managed with current treatment options.

One major cause of preeclampsia is thought to be due to insufficient invasion and remodeling of maternal spiral arteries by extravillous trophoblast cells [72]. As a result, exosome therapeutics have focused on methods to increase trophoblast migration and proliferation. Li et al. employed exosomes isolated from chorionic villous-derived MSCs and revealed a significant increase in the invasive behaviors of extravillous trophoblasts [72]. Using JEG-3 immortalized hyper-triploid placental carcinoma and HTR-8/SVneo immortalized extravillous trophoblast cells, Li et al. observed that chorionic villous MSC-derived exosomes promoted migration and proliferation of the trophoblast cells [72]. RNA sequencing revealed that the upregulation of Tripartite Motif Containing 72 and downregulation of Tumor Protein P53 due to exosome treatment were drivers of the observed migration and proliferation changes [72].

To further understand the previously established knowledge that miRNA-18b and Notch2 regulate trophoblast cell invasion and migration and trophoblast proliferation and invasion, respectively, Yang et al. treated primary placental cells from healthy and preeclamptic donors with exosomes isolated from umbilical cord blood MSCs [28, 73, 74]. In preeclamptic samples of placental tissue and their exosomes, the relative expression of miRNA-18b is downregulated [28]. Across characteristic assessments, in vitro cell studies, and in vivo rat models of preeclampsia, exosomes derived from umbilical cord blood MSCs inhibited preeclamptic symptoms of high systolic pressure and urinary protein concentration [28].

A study performed by Liu et al. to investigate the invasion and migration of trophoblast cells revealed the positive effects of miRNA-139-5b, which was previously reported to promote the proliferation and invasion of trophoblast cells [75, 76]. Exosomes isolated from human umbilical cord MSCs were incubated with HTR-8/SVneo extravillous trophoblast cells, resulting in a significant increase in the expression of miRNA-139-5b and activating the extracellular signal-regulated kinase (ERK)/matrix metalloproteinase-2 (MMP-2) pathway [75]. For in vivo rat experiments, exosomes from human umbilical cord MSCs were harvested, and preeclampsia rat models were dosed with the exosomes to determine the effects of miRNA-139-5b on preeclampsia symptoms [75]. When treated with miRNA-139-5b containing exosomes, preeclampsia rat models exhibited reduced blood pressure values and proteinuria, two common symptoms in preeclampsia [75].

Exosomes containing miRNA-101 have been shown to improve placental trophoblast proliferation and migration, which is essential for healthy placenta development, which has potential for preeclampsia treatment [77]. Cui et al. leveraged this knowledge to test the influence of miRNA-101-laden EVs isolated from human umbilical cord MSCs [78]. Through in silico analyses, the downstream target genes for miRNA-101 were identified to contain the BRD4 complex, a protein that is often implicated in preeclampsia due to its contributions in controlling inflammation and anti-angiogenic factors [78, 79]. HTR-8/SVneo cells that were transfected with exosomes containing miRNA-101 showed reduced expression of BRD4 and increased cell proliferation and migration [78]. The human umbilical cord MSCs were infected with lentiviral vectors containing miRNA-101, and their exosomes were harvested for injection into preeclampsia rat models [78]. Exosomes with increased levels of miRNA-101 ameliorated the conditions of preeclampsia in rat models and reduced the expression of BRD4 [78].

2.5 *Pelvic Floor Dysfunction*

The pelvic floor is a set of muscles that span the bottom of the pelvis, supporting the bladder, uterus, colon, and reproductive organs [80]. Patients with PFD can have weakened, over-tight, or improperly coordinated pelvic floor muscles. This could cause urination difficulty, constipation, pelvic pain, and sexual dysfunction [81]. Pelvic organ prolapse (POP) occurs when female pelvic organs shift downward from their normal position and push against the vaginal walls, which can cause the vagina, uterus, or both to protrude from the pelvic floor [82]. Conservative therapeutic approaches focus on targeted muscle exercises and treatments for mild PFD symptom relief, while surgery is considered for patients whose symptoms persist after conservative management [83].

Degradation of elastic fibers in pelvic floor musculature is a result of the stretching of the vagina during childbirth [84]. This degradation of elastic fiber has been linked to pelvic floor disorders and can lead to stress urinary incontinence (SUI) and POP [85]. Recently, exosomes derived from MSCs have been considered as a new therapy to treat PFD by their various therapeutic properties, including self-renewal and proliferation, multipotency, immunoregulation, inflammation reduction, and tissue repair [86, 87]. Exosomes isolated from MSCs have been shown to reduce cell apoptosis and promote cellular proliferation, which can be beneficial for patients with PFD to help restore cell and nerve fiber density [87].

Exosomes isolated from bone marrow MSCs treated with or without TNF-α have been studied in a rat model of PFD [88]. Both exosomes derived from MSCs treated with and without TNF-α successfully restored void volume and bladder void pressure, but the TNF-α exosomes did so at a higher level than exosomes without TNF-α treatment [88]. Additionally, for multiple proteins and inflammatory cytokines tested, including Elastin, Collagen I, Collagen III, IL-1, TNF-α, and MMP-2, exosomes derived from MSCs treated with TNF-α outperformed exosomes from MSCs not treated with TNF-α in restoring protein levels in the anterior vaginal wall of PFD rats back to those observed in the control rat group [88].

SUI is one of the most prevalent issues related to PFD that is caused by weakened pelvic floor muscles, nerve damage, and extracellular matrix degradation, leading to urinary leakage and void dysfunction [89, 90]. The dual immunomodulatory effect of exosomes derived from bone marrow MSCs, which reduces pro-inflammatory cytokines, TNF-α, and IL-1β, while simultaneously promoting anti-inflammatory cytokines, IL-10, and TGF-β, jointly repairs tissue damage in SUI [90–92]. Additionally, bone marrow MSC-derived exosomes stimulate the generation of new muscle fibers by increasing the expression of myogenic markers, such as paired box 7 transcription factor and myogenic differentiation factor [90, 93]. Moreover, exosomal miRNA-126 and miRNA-210 have been shown to help stimulate the formation of new blood vessels and enhance cells' ability to withstand oxidative stress, which may support better blood circulation and aid in the repair of tissues in the urethral sphincter and pelvic floor muscles [90].

3 Exosomes in the Clinic for Women's Reproductive Health

A small number of ongoing clinical trials use exosomes as both biomarkers and therapeutic agents for a range of reproductive health conditions (Table 1). The three clinical trials using exosomes for therapeutic applications are for infertility-related conditions. A clinical trial conducted in 2024 sponsored by Biotech Fertility C.A. applied exosomes from the patient's platelets or non-exosomal activated platelet factors via intraovarian injection performed over the course of 4 months [94]. A clinical trial sponsored by Tang-Du Hospital in China is recruiting volunteers to test the efficacy of autologous platelet-rich plasma, umbilical cord MSC-derived exosomes, or mechanically engineered umbilical cord MSC-derived exosomes in treating thin endometrium and severe intrauterine adhesions [95]. To measure the impact of patient-sampled adipose-derived stem cells or their exosomes on ovarian regeneration following premature ovarian failure, the Jumeirah American Clinic is recruiting volunteers to undergo intraovarian injections with regular observational follow-ups over the course of 1 year [96].

The diagnostic applications in current clinical trials include diseases such as ovarian cancer and preeclampsia. While the chapter did not focus on diagnostic applications, it is important to note that in order to treat these conditions with

Table 1 Clinical trials investigating exosomes as biomarkers and therapeutics for women's reproductive health conditions

Condition	Year of initiation	Application	Sponsor	Status	Clinical trial number
Preeclampsia	2016	Diagnostic	Cairo University	Completed	NCT03562715
Ovarian cancer	2018	Diagnostic	Lei Li	Unknown	NCT03738319
Preeclampsia	2019	Diagnostic	University of Alabama at Birmingham	Recruiting	NCT04154332
Oocyte maturation	2021	Diagnostic	Chinese University of Hong Kong	Recruiting	NCT04382872
Premature ovarian insufficiency, diminished ovarian reserve	2023	Diagnostic	Vitti Labs, LLC	Suspended	NCT06072794
Female infertility, assisted reproductive techniques	2024	Therapeutic	Biotech Fertility C.A.	Completed	NCT06773572
Ovarian cancer	2024	Diagnostic	Lei Li	Not yet recruiting	NCT06558019
Female infertility, intrauterine adhesions, thin endometrial lining	2025	Therapeutic	Tang-Du Hospital	Recruiting	NCT06896747
Gonadal dysfunction, gonadal failure	2025	Therapeutic	Jumeriah American Clinic	Recruiting	NCT06841328
Ovarian cancer	2025	Diagnostic	Fudan University	Not yet recruiting	NCT06925126

A search on clinicaltrials.gov was conducted using the keyword "reproductive health" as the condition/disease and "exosome" as the intervention/treatment. These filters were used together or separately to yield 10 records of studies where exosomes were used as either a diagnostic (7/10) or therapeutic (3/10) tool

appropriate therapeutics, it is critical to be able to accurately diagnose reproductive health issues, and exosomes are demonstrating potential in this area as well.

4 Future Perspectives and Opportunities

Exosome therapeutics show promise for reproductive health applications, yet it is early in the transition from fundamental exosome research to clinical application, which means their advantages and drawbacks yet to be fully realized. Fundamental studies on the role of exosomes in cell communication and disease progression are influencing their applications in both therapeutics and diagnostics. Overcoming the hurdles of sample purity, yield, variability, and stability in the application of exosomes is crucial for their transition from fundamental research to the clinic. The efforts toward further developing exosome isolation, standardization, and storage have sparked an increased interest in combining natural exosome properties with the advantages of customizable biomaterials to control exosome composition. In this section, we provide perspective, questions, and suggestions that researchers can consider.

Innovations in Diagnostic Applications, Isolation, and Composition
Exosomes as a therapeutic agent currently lag behind their use as a diagnostic. There have been several studies demonstrating the use of exosomes to aid in diagnosing the gynecological conditions discussed throughout this chapter. A few recent highlights on diagnostic studies within the past 5 years include a study by Liu et al., focused on the diagnosis of premature ovarian failure [97]. Liu et al. discovered that exosomes derived from patients with premature ovarian failure showed a distinct difference in levels of Yy2 mRNAs, which play key roles in regulating gene expression and were linked to ameliorating conditions of premature ovarian failure in aged granulosa cells [97–99]. Munoz et al. characterized exosomes as a diagnostic for placenta accreta, a pregnancy complication where the placenta improperly attaches to the uterine wall, preventing normal detachment after birth, which can result in severe blood loss and often necessitates early delivery [100]. Exosomes isolated from the plasma of mothers with placenta accreta were found in tenfold abundance and showed higher expression of miRNAs-92, -103, and -192 than those from the plasma of a normal pregnancy [100]. Endometriosis is commonly misdiagnosed due to the wide range of symptoms and the lack of non-invasive diagnostics [101]. In an effort to combat this, Jiang et al. isolated exosomes from samples of endometrial fluid from the uterine cavity and identified several key miRNAs that were significantly upregulated in samples from patients with endometriosis: miRNA-210-30, miRNA-20b-5p, miRNA-625-5p, and miRNA-342-5p [102]. Beyond recent literature, Table 1 demonstrates that 7 of the 10 clinical trials using exosomes for reproductive health applications are for diagnostic purposes. While therapeutic applications almost exclusively use exosomes derived from MSCs, exosomes for diagnostic applications originate from the specific tissue involved in the complication.

Over the past few decades, MSCs have received attention for their use in regenerative medicine [103]. MSCs have been sourced from several biological fluids, including adipose MSCs, bone marrow MSCs, umbilical cord MSCs, menstrual blood MSCs, and gingival MSCs [104, 105]. More recently, studies have observed that the soluble paracrine factors, including exosomes, that MSCs secrete play an important role in their therapeutic effect [106]. Using exosomes from MSCs as opposed to the live cells themselves minimizes some challenges faced with cell delivery, with exosome advantages including non-immunogenicity, stability, and ease of handling compared to cell therapies [107]. This has led to a rapid increase in the number of studies in the past decade pursuing MSC-derived exosomes for a wide range of therapies, including those discussed throughout this chapter.

While exosomes help alleviate some of the challenges that come with delivering whole, live cells, new challenges need to be addressed [108]. The low yield of pure exosomes from a given biological source can be a bottleneck for clinical translation [109]. While exosomes are typically more stable in solution than MSCs, advancements in cryopreservation are still being investigated to improve shelf-life. Standardization of characterizing and purifying exosomes is needed within the field. Finally, since exosomes are a heterogeneous population of vesicles, there is an increased variability between samples compared to the use of synthetic vesicles to deliver the target therapeutic payload.

The method to load a specific cargo within exosomes is another area that is being optimized [110]. Endogenous methods are more common in the studies presented in this chapter, where the therapeutic agent, such as a miRNA, is either natively found in the MSC-derived exosomes, introduced to the MSCs via a plasmid transfection to produce exosomes containing that molecule, or a combination where native miRNA is enhanced within the exosomes. While most studies, including those in this chapter, have focused on the nucleic acid, often a miRNA, present in the exosomes, exosomes have several additional components that can be considered for therapeutic efficacy, including the loaded proteins and lipid composition. Future studies may consider engineering this composition, and in this case, methods to load nucleic acids in exosomes post-isolation can also be investigated.

Biomaterials for Modification of Exosome Composition and Performance

There is both an opportunity and a need to investigate exosome-biomaterial composites for the treatment of reproductive health conditions, and it is a natural next step that can be explored in the field. Inspiration can be drawn from other applications that have begun investigating exosome-biomaterial composites. For example, in the treatment of inflammatory diseases (osteoarthritis, multiple sclerosis), exosome therapeutics are employed to regulate immune cell function and facilitate skin repair with enhanced stability, targeting, and retention through combined use with biomaterials such as hydrogels, nanoparticles, or engineered scaffolds [111, 112]. In new therapeutic strategies to treat multiple sclerosis, engineered exosomes with functionalized surfaces and enriched payloads are created for the combined natural vesicle benefits of biocompatibility and biodegradability with synthetic advantages in decreasing host immune responses and freedom of modification [112]. A study conducted in 2022 investigated the effects of culturing bone marrow MSCs on biphasic calcium phosphate, a synthetic bone material, on the polarized state of their secreted EVs to maximize bone regeneration in the case of maxillofacial bone defects [112, 113]. Rana et al. showed that EVs released from biomaterial-cultured cells contained fewer pro-inflammatory cytokines and produced more anti-inflammatory cytokines, believing this process to load the EVs with content that is more pro-bone-regenerative [112, 113]. Biomaterials can be used to enhance existing exosome structures or to manipulate the production of exosomes to exhibit desired characteristics for the system in question.

Biomaterials have been explored for their potential to ameliorate the gynecological conditions discussed in this chapter [114]. For infertility applications, polymeric scaffolds have been created to engineer uterine and ovarian tissue [114, 115]. With the inclusion of exosome therapeutics, these engineered scaffolds could have a greater effect on the longevity of sustained uterine and ovarian tissue. In PFD, researchers and clinicians have applied synthetic meshes, tissue-engineered scaffolds, and injectable therapy biomaterials to strengthen the pelvic floor and regenerate muscle loss [83]. Maintaining muscle integrity is imperative to improving the condition of patients with PFD to allow for other courses of treatment, such as physical therapy and lifestyle changes [81]. Exosome therapeutics have been reported to reduce cell apoptosis and promote cell proliferation—when combined with a biomaterial scaffold, this hybrid therapeutic has the potential to further promote rebuilding and restructuring of the pelvic floor. Similar to biomaterial approaches pursued to treat PFD, endometriosis treatments seek to repair damaged tissue and deliver therapeutic agents [116, 117]. A number of studies have shown the potential of hybrid exosome-liposomes to combine the unique benefits of both natural and synthetic particles for targeted drug and gene delivery [118, 119]. This also has the potential to target treatments during pregnancy, through combining the natural vesicle's ability to direct delivery to placental cells and the synthetic particle's stability and reduced inflammatory effects.

Advancing isolation, standardization, storage, and composition of exosomes as described above is important for any application using exosomes as a therapeutic. More specifically for reproductive and gynecological health, the use of exosomes is in a nascent stage, and there are other conditions poised to benefit from exosome therapeutics, such as ovarian cancer, gestational diabetes, uterine fibroids, and more. The prospective approach to treating reproductive and gynecological health with hybrid exosome-biomaterials has the potential to greatly advance the field. Engineering approaches to advance exosome cargo, isolation, and delivery will continue to expand their use for women's health applications.

Acknowledgments The authors acknowledge support from the National Science Foundation (NSF) Building Research Capacity of New Faculty in Biology (BRC-BIO) program (Award #2334660) and NSF EArly-Concept Grants for Exploratory Research (EAGER) program (Award #2433264). Any opinions, findings, and conclusions or recommendations expressed in this material are those of the author(s) and do not necessarily reflect the views of the NSF. Figures were created with Biorender.com.

References

1. Keshtkar S, Asvar Z, Najafi H, Heidari M, Kaviani M, Sarvestani FS, Tamaddon AM, Sadati MS, Hamidizadeh N, Azarpira N. Exosomes as natural vectors for therapeutic delivery of bioactive compounds in skin diseases. Front Pharmacol. 2025;16:1485769.
2. Kalluri R, LeBleu VS. The biology, function, and biomedical applications of exosomes. Science. 2020;367:6478.
3. Mitchell MD, Peiris HN, Kobayashi M, Koh YQ, Duncombe G, Illanes SE, Rice GE, Salomon C. Placental exosomes in normal and complicated pregnancy. Am J Obstet Gynecol. 2015;213 (4):S173–81.

4. Xie D, Qian B, Li X. Nucleic acids and proteins carried by exosomes from various sources: potential role in liver diseases. Front Physiol. 2022;13:957036.
5. Gurung S, Perocheau D, Touramanidou L, Baruteau J. The exosome journey: from biogenesis to uptake and intracellular signalling. Cell Commun Signal. 2021;19(1):47.
6. Isola AL, Chen S. Exosomes: the messengers of health and disease. Curr Neuropharmacol. 2017;15(1):157–65.
7. Czernek L, Düchler M. Exosomes as messengers between mother and fetus in pregnancy. Int J Mol Sci. 2020;21(12):4264.
8. Dilsiz N. Hallmarks of exosomes. Future Sci OA. 2022;8(1):FSO764.
9. Liang L, Wang N, Li X, Zhang Z, Zhu Z, Zhuo Y, Jiang X, Wang J, Guo C, Guo S, Zhou P, Zhu Y, Gan Y, Yu M. Shape engineering of exosomes for endoplasmic reticulum-targeted delivery and amplified anticancer efficacy. Nano Today. 2024;57:102377.
10. Hadidi M, Karimabadi K, Ghanbari E, Rezakhani L, Khazaei M. Stem cells and exosomes: as biological agents in the diagnosis and treatment of polycystic ovary syndrome (PCOS). Front Endocrinol (Lausanne). 2023;14:1269266.
11. Nazri HM, Imran M, Fischer R, Heilig R, Manek S, Dragovic RA, Kessler BM, Zondervan KT, Tapmeier TT, Becker CM. Characterization of exosomes in peritoneal fluid of endometriosis patients. Fertil Steril. 2020;113(2):364–373.e2.
12. Chu X, Hou M, Li Y, Zhang Q, Wang S, Ma J. Extracellular vesicles in endometriosis: role and potential. Front Endocrinol. 2024;15:1365327.
13. Salomon C, Kobayashi M, Ashman K, Sobrevia L, Mitchell MD, Rice GE. Hypoxia-induced changes in the bioactivity of cytotrophoblast-derived exosomes. Oudejans C, editor. PLoS One. 2011;8(11):e79636.
14. Burkova EE, Sedykh SE, Nevinsky GA. Human placenta exosomes: biogenesis, isolation, composition, and prospects for use in diagnostics. IJMS. 2021;22(4):2158.
15. Ouyang Y, Mouillet JF, Coyne CB, Sadovsky Y. Review: placenta-specific microRNAs in exosomes - good things come in nano-packages. Placenta. 2014;35(Suppl):S69–73.
16. Harrison AM, Bailey-Hytholt CM. Recent progress in 2D, 3D, and on-a-chip models of the placenta. Cells Tissues Organs. 2025;214(6):477–511.
17. Inamdar S, Nitiyanandan R, Rege K. Emerging applications of exosomes in cancer therapeutics and diagnostics. Bioeng Transl Med. 2017;2(1):70–80.
18. Gaglani S, Gonzalez-Kozlova E, Lundon DJ, Tewari AK, Dogra N, Kyprianou N. Exosomes as a next-generation diagnostic and therapeutic tool in prostate cancer. Int J Mol Sci. 2021;22(18):10131.
19. Jangam TC, Desai SA, Patel VP, Pagare NB, Raut ND. Exosomes as therapeutic and diagnostic tools: advances, challenges, and future directions. Cell Biochem Biophys. 2025;83:2805.
20. Gao P, Li X, Du X, Liu S, Xu Y. Diagnostic and therapeutic potential of exosomes in neurodegenerative diseases. Front Aging Neurosci. 2021;13:790863.
21. Peruzzi JA, Gunnels TF, Edelstein HI, Lu P, Baker D, Leonard JN, Kamat NP. Enhancing extracellular vesicle cargo loading and functional delivery by engineering protein-lipid interactions. Nat Commun. 2024;15(1):5618.
22. Rezaie J, Feghhi M, Etemadi T. A review on exosomes application in clinical trials: perspective, questions, and challenges. Cell Commun Signal. 2022;20(1):145.
23. Kumar MA, Baba SK, Sadida HQ, Marzooqi SA, Jerobin J, Altemani FH, Algehainy N, Alanazi MA, Abou-Samra AB, Kumar R, Al-Shabeeb Akil AS, Macha MA, Mir R, Bhat AA. Extracellular vesicles as tools and targets in therapy for diseases. Sig Transduct Target Ther. 2024;9(1):1–41.
24. Wang Y, Ma H, Zhang X, Xiao X, Yang Z. The increasing diagnostic role of exosomes in inflammatory diseases to leverage the therapeutic biomarkers. J Inflamm Res. 2024;25(17):5005–24.

25. Wang D, Na Q, Song GY, Wang L. Human umbilical cord mesenchymal stem cell-derived exosome-mediated transfer of microRNA-133b boosts trophoblast cell proliferation, migration and invasion in preeclampsia by restricting SGK1. Cell Cycle. 2020;19(15):1869–83.
26. Yang C, Lim W, Park J, Park S, You S, Song G. Anti-inflammatory effects of mesenchymal stem cell-derived exosomal microRNA-146a-5p and microRNA-548e-5p on human trophoblast cells. Mol Hum Reprod. 2019;25(11):755–71.
27. Liu Y, Mu H, Chen Y, Li K, Mei Q, Wang L, Tang T, Shen Q, Li H, Zhang L, Li J, Xiang W. Follicular fluid-derived exosomes rejuvenate ovarian aging through miR-320a-3p-mediated FOXQ1 inhibition. Life Med. 2024;3(1):lnae013.
28. Yang Z, Shan N, Deng Q, Wang Y, Hou Y, Mei J, Wu Z. Extracellular vesicle-derived microRNA-18b ameliorates preeclampsia by enhancing trophoblast proliferation and migration via Notch2/TIM3/mTORC1 axis. J Cell Mol Med. 2021;25(10):4583–95.
29. Vannuccini S, Clifton VL, Fraser IS, Taylor HS, Critchley H, Giudice LC, Petraglia F. Infertility and reproductive disorders: impact of hormonal and inflammatory mechanisms on pregnancy outcome. Hum Reprod Update. 2016;22(1):104–15.
30. Baruch Y, Manodoro S, Barba M, Cola A, Re I, Frigerio M. Prevalence and severity of pelvic floor disorders during pregnancy: does the trimester make a difference? Healthcare (Basel). 2023;11(8):1096.
31. Scheck S, Paterson ESJ, Henry CE. A promising future for endometriosis diagnosis and therapy: extracellular vesicles - a systematic review. Reprod Biol Endocrinol. 2022;20:174.
32. Chen Z, Wang X. The role and application of exosomes and their cargos in reproductive diseases: a systematic review. Vet Sci. 2022;9(12):706.
33. Chiorean DM, Mitranovici MI, Toru HS, Cotoi TC, Tomuţ AN, Turdean SG, Cotoi OS. New insights into genetics of endometriosis—a comprehensive literature review. Diagnostics. 2023;13(13):2265.
34. Vissers G, Giacomozzi M, Verdurmen W, Peek R, Nap A. The role of fibrosis in endometriosis: a systematic review. Hum Reprod Update. 2024;30(6):706–50.
35. Abe W, Nasu K, Nakada C, Kawano Y, Moriyama M, Narahara H. miR-196b targets c-myc and Bcl-2 expression, inhibits proliferation and induces apoptosis in endometriotic stromal cells. Hum Reprod. 2013;28(3):750–61.
36. Wu D, Lu P, Mi X, Miao J. Exosomal miR-214 from endometrial stromal cells inhibits endometriosis fibrosis. Mol Hum Reprod. 2018;24(7):357–65.
37. Song M, Ma L, Zhu Y, Gao H, Hu R. Umbilical cord mesenchymal stem cell-derived exosomes inhibits fibrosis in human endometrial stromal cells via miR-140-3p/FOXP1/Smad axis. Sci Rep. 2024;14(1):8321.
38. Davoodi Asl F, Sahraei SS, Kalhor N, Fazaeli H, Sheykhhasan M, Soleimani Moud S, Naserpour L, Sheikholeslami A. Promising effects of exosomes from menstrual blood-derived mesenchymal stem cells on endometriosis. Reprod Biol. 2023;23(3):100788.
39. Liu YY, Liu YK, Hu WT, Tang LL, Sheng YR, Wei CY, Li MQ, Zhu XY. Elevated heme impairs macrophage phagocytosis in endometriosis. Reproduction. 2019;158(3):257–66.
40. Huang Y, Zhu L, Li H, Ye J, Lin N, Chen M, Pan D, Chen Z. Endometriosis derived exosomal miR-301a-3p mediates macrophage polarization via regulating PTEN-PI3K axis. Biomed Pharmacother. 2022;147:112680.
41. Wang X, Luo G, Zhang K, Cao J, Huang C, Jiang T, Liu B, Su L, Qiu Z. Hypoxic tumor-derived Exosomal miR-301a mediates M2 macrophage polarization via PTEN/PI3Kγ to promote pancreatic cancer metastasis. Cancer Res. 2018;78(16):4586–98.
42. Li Q, Yuan M, Jiao X, Huang Y, Li J, Li D, Ji M, Wang G. M1 macrophage-derived nanovesicles repolarize M2 macrophages for inhibiting the development of endometriosis. Front Immunol. 2021;12:707784.
43. Oral E, Olive D, Arici A. The peritoneal environment in endometriosis. Hum Reprod Update. 1996;2(5):385–98.

44. Liu T, Liu M, Zheng C, Zhang D, Li M, Zhang L. Exosomal lncRNA CHL1-AS1 derived from peritoneal macrophages promotes the progression of endometriosis via the miR-610/MDM2 Axis. Int J Nanomed. 2021;16:5451–64.
45. Bahramy A, Zafari N, Izadi P, Soleymani F, Kavousi S, Noruzinia M. The role of miRNAs 340-5p, 92a-3p, and 381-3p in patients with endometriosis: a plasma and mesenchymal stem-like cell study. Biomed Res Int. 2021;2021:5298006.
46. Teede HJ, Misso ML, Costello MF, Dokras A, Laven J, Moran L, Piltonen T, Norman RJ, International PCOS Network. Recommendations from the international evidence-based guideline for the assessment and management of polycystic ovary syndrome. Fertil Steril. 2018;110 (3):364–79.
47. Teede H, Deeks A, Moran L. Polycystic ovary syndrome: a complex condition with psychological, reproductive and metabolic manifestations that impacts on health across the lifespan. BMC Med. 2010;8:41.
48. Stańczak NA, Grywalska E, Dudzińska E. The latest reports and treatment methods on polycystic ovary syndrome. Ann Med. 2024;56(1):2357737.
49. Zhang Z, Shi C, Wang Z. The physiological functions and therapeutic potential of exosomes during the development and treatment of polycystic ovary syndrome. Front Physiol. 2023;14: 1279469.
50. Park HS, Cetin E, Siblini H, Seok J, Alkelani H, Alkhrait S, Liakath Ali F, Mousaei Ghasroldasht M, Beckman A, Al-Hendy A. Therapeutic potential of mesenchymal stem cell-derived extracellular vesicles to treat PCOS. Int J Mol Sci. 2023;24(13):11151.
51. Goodarzi MO, Dumesic DA, Chazenbalk G, Azziz R. Polycystic ovary syndrome: etiology, pathogenesis and diagnosis. Nat Rev Endocrinol. 2011;7(4):219–31.
52. Cao M, Zhao Y, Chen T, Zhao Z, Zhang B, Yuan C, Wang X, Chen L, Wang N, Li C, Zhou X. Adipose mesenchymal stem cell–derived exosomal microRNAs ameliorate polycystic ovary syndrome by protecting against metabolic disturbances. Biomaterials. 2022;288: 121739.
53. Zhao Y, Pan S, Wu X. Human umbilical cord mesenchymal stem cell-derived exosomes inhibit ovarian granulosa cells inflammatory response through inhibition of NF-κB signaling in polycystic ovary syndrome. J Reprod Immunol. 2022;152:103638.
54. Zhao Y, Tao, Mei, Wei, Meiling D, Shengye W, Hongping, Wang X. Mesenchymal stem cells derived exosomal miR-323-3p promotes proliferation and inhibits apoptosis of cumulus cells in polycystic ovary syndrome (PCOS). Artif Cells Nanomed Biotechnol. 2019;47(1):3804–13.
55. Gnoth C, Godehardt E, Frank-Herrmann P, Friol K, Tiffes J, Freundl G. Definition and prevalence of subfertility and infertility. Hum Reprod. 2005;20:1144–7.
56. Anyalechi GE, Hong J, Kreisel K, Torrone E, Boulet S, Gorwitz R, Kirkcaldy RD, Bernstein K. Self-reported infertility and associated pelvic inflammatory disease among women of reproductive age — National Health and Nutrition Examination Survey, United States, 2013–2016. Sex Transm Dis. 2019;46(7):446–51.
57. Walker MH, Tobler KJ. Female infertility. In: StatPearls. Treasure Island: StatPearls Publishing; 2025.
58. Cha J, Sun X, Dey SK. Mechanisms of implantation: strategies for successful pregnancy. Nat Med. 2012;18(12):1754–67.
59. Ma J, Gao W, Li D. Recurrent implantation failure: a comprehensive summary from etiology to treatment. Front Endocrinol (Lausanne). 2023;13:1061766.
60. Ferraretti AP, Goossens V, de Mouzon J, Bhattacharya S, Castilla JA, Korsak V, Kupka M, Nygren KG, Nyboe Andersen A. European IVF-monitoring (EIM), Consortium for European Society of Human Reproduction and Embryology (ESHRE). Assisted reproductive technology in Europe, 2008: results generated from European registers by ESHRE. Hum Reprod. 2012;27(9):2571–84.
61. Edwards RG. Human implantation: the last barrier in assisted reproduction technologies? Reprod Biomed Online. 2006;13(6):887–904.

62. Simon A, Laufer N. Assessment and treatment of repeated implantation failure (RIF). J Assist Reprod Genet. 2012;29(11):1227–39.
63. Blanco-Breindel MF, Singh M, Kahn J. Endometrial receptivity. In: StatPearls [Internet]. Treasure Island: StatPearls Publishing; 2025.
64. Tan Q, Shi S, Liang J, Cao D, Wang S, Wang Z. Endometrial cell-derived small extracellular vesicle miR-100-5p promotes functions of trophoblast during embryo implantation. Mol Ther Nucleic Acids. 2021;23:217–31.
65. Yang Q, Gu WW, Gu Y, Yan NN, Mao YY, Zhen XX, Wang JM, Yang J, Shi HJ, Zhang X, Wang J. Association of the peripheral blood levels of circulating microRNAs with both recurrent miscarriage and the outcomes of embryo transfer in an in vitro fertilization process. J Transl Med. 2018;16(1):186.
66. Touraine P, Chabbert-Buffet N, Plu-Bureau G, Duranteau L, Sinclair AH, Tucker EJ. Premature ovarian insufficiency. Nat Rev Dis Primers. 2024;10(1):1–21.
67. Wu J, Liu Y, Song Y, Wang L, Ai J, Li K. Aging conundrum: a perspective for ovarian aging. Front Endocrinol. 2022;13:952471.
68. Miller JJ, Williams GF, Leissring JC. Multiple late complications of therapy with cyclophosphamide, including ovarian destruction. Am J Med. 1971;50(4):530–5.
69. Xiao Y, Peng Y, Zhang C, Liu W, Wang K, Li J. hucMSC-derived exosomes protect ovarian reserve and restore ovarian function in cisplatin treated mice. J Biomed Res. 2023;5:382–93.
70. Fox R, Kitt J, Leeson P, Aye CYL, Lewandowski AJ. Preeclampsia: risk factors, diagnosis, management, and the cardiovascular impact on the offspring. J Clin Med. 2019;8(10):1625.
71. Ng KW, Chaturvedi N, Coté GL, Fisher SA, Mabbott S. Biomarkers and point of care screening approaches for the management of preeclampsia. Commun Med. 2024;1:1–15.
72. Li Y, Wang C, Xi H m, Li W t, Liu Y j, Feng S, Chu Y j, Wang Y h. Chorionic villus-derived mesenchymal stem cells induce E3 ligase TRIM72 expression and regulate cell behaviors through ubiquitination of p53 in trophoblasts. FASEB J. 2021;35(12):e22005.
73. Wang S, Wang X, Weng Z, Zhang S, Ning H, Li B. Expression and role of microRNA 18b and hypoxia inducible factor-1α in placental tissues of preeclampsia patients. Exp Ther Med. 2017;14(5):4554–60.
74. Zhao WX, Wu ZM, Liu W, Lin JH. Notch2 and Notch3 suppress the proliferation and mediate invasion of trophoblast cell lines. Biol Open. 2017;6(8):1123–9.
75. Liu H, Wang F, Zhang Y, Xing Y, Wang Q. Exosomal microRNA-139-5p from mesenchymal stem cells accelerates trophoblast cell invasion and migration by motivation of the ERK/MMP-2 pathway via downregulation of protein tyrosine phosphatase. J Obstet Gynaecol Res. 2020;46(12):2561–72.
76. Huang J, Zheng L, Kong H, Wang F, Su Y, Xin H. miR-139-5p promotes the proliferation and invasion of trophoblast cells by targeting sFlt-1 in preeclampsia. Placenta. 2020;92:37–43.
77. Zou Y, Jiang Z, Yu X, Zhang Y, Sun M, Wang W, Ge Z, De W, Sun L. MiR-101 regulates apoptosis of trophoblast HTR-8/SVneo cells by targeting endoplasmic reticulum (ER) protein 44 during preeclampsia. J Hum Hypertens. 2014;28(10):610–6.
78. Cui J, Chen X, Lin S, Li L, Fan J, Hou H, Li P. MiR-101-containing extracellular vesicles bind to BRD4 and enhance proliferation and migration of trophoblasts in preeclampsia. Stem Cell Res Ther. 2020;11:231.
79. Liong S, Barker G, Lappas M. Bromodomain protein BRD4 is increased in human placentas from women with early-onset preeclampsia. Reproduction. 2018;155(6):573–82.
80. Good MM, Solomon ER. Pelvic floor disorders. Obstet Gynecol Clin N Am. 2019;46(3):527–40.
81. Quaghebeur J, Petros P, Wyndaele JJ, Wachter SD. Pelvic-floor function, dysfunction, and treatment. Eur J Obstet Gynecol Reprod Biol. 2021;265:143–9.
82. Jelovsek JE, Maher C, Barber MD. Pelvic organ prolapse. Lancet. 2007;369(9566):1027–38.
83. Lin M, Lu Y, Chen J. Tissue-engineered repair material for pelvic floor dysfunction. Front Bioeng Biotechnol. 2022;10:968482.

84. Liu X, Zhao Y, Pawlyk B, Damaser M, Li T. Failure of elastic fiber homeostasis leads to pelvic floor disorders. Am J Pathol. 2006;168(2):519–28.
85. Downing K. Chapter 8: Biochemistry and ultrastructure of pelvic floor tissues and organs. In: Hoyte L, Damaser M, editors. Biomechanics of the female pelvic floor. Academic Press; 2016. p. 181–208.
86. Han Y, Li X, Zhang Y, Han Y, Chang F, Ding J. Mesenchymal stem cells for regenerative medicine. Cells. 2019;8(8):886.
87. Xu L, Sima Y, Xiao C, Chen Y. Exosomes derived from mesenchymal stromal cells: a promising treatment for pelvic floor dysfunction. Hum Cell. 2023;36(3):937–49.
88. Zhou C, Wu Y, Wan S, Lou L, Gu S, Peng J, Zhao S, Hua X. Exosomes isolated from TNF-α-treated bone marrow mesenchymal stem cells ameliorate pelvic floor dysfunction in rats. J Cell Mol Med. 2024;28(12):e18451.
89. Kalata U, Pomian A, Jarkiewicz M, Kondratskyi V, Lippki K, Barcz E. Influence of stress urinary incontinence and pelvic organ prolapse on depression, anxiety, and insomnia-a comparative observational study. J Clin Med. 2023;13(1):185.
90. Nasrollahzadeh Saravi M, Mohseni M, Menbari Oskouie I, Razavi J, Delgado Cidranes E, Majidi ZM. Exosome therapy in stress urinary incontinence: a comprehensive literature review. Biomedicine. 2025;13(5):1229.
91. Luo Z, Lin J, Sun Y, Wang C, Chen J. Bone marrow stromal cell-derived exosomes promote muscle healing following contusion through macrophage polarization. Stem Cells Dev. 2021;30(3):135–48.
92. Luo ZW, Sun YY, Lin JR, Qi BJ, Chen JW. Exosomes derived from inflammatory myoblasts promote M1 polarization and break the balance of myoblast proliferation/differentiation. World J Stem Cells. 2021;13(11):1762–82.
93. Rolland TJ, Peterson TE, Singh RD, Rizzo SA, Boroumand S, Shi A, Witt TA, Nagel M, Kisby CK, Park S, Rowe LA, Paradise CR, Becher LRE, Paradise BD, Stalboerger PG, Trabuco EC, Behfar A. Exosome biopotentiated hydrogel restores damaged skeletal muscle in a porcine model of stress urinary incontinence. npj Regener Med. 2022;7(1):58.
94. Navarro C. Efficacy of autologous exosomes vs platelet-derived growth factors for ovarian regeneration in women with ovarian insufficiency and infertility: observational, prospective, randomized, comparative, double-blind, analytical, prospective clinicaltrialsgov; 2025. Report no.: NCT06773572.
95. Zhangwanlin. Evaluation of the therapeutic effects of mechanically engineered umbilical cord-derived stem cell exosomes on endometrial injury: a prospective, non-randomized, parallel-controlled clinical study. clinicaltrialsgov; 2025. Report no.: NCT06896747.
96. Ramasamy R. Fertility enhancement through regenerative treatment in ovaries and testes: (FERTILE): prospective observational study evaluating safety and efficacy. clinicaltrials.gov; 2025. Report no.: NCT06841328.
97. Liu T, Jing F, Huang P, Geng Z, Xu J, Li J, Chen D, Zhu Y, Wang Z, Huang W, Chen C. Thymopentin alleviates premature ovarian failure in mice by activating YY2/Lin28A and inhibiting the expression of let-7 family microRNAs. Cell Prolif. 2021;54(8):e13089.
98. Li L, Li Y, Timothy Sembiring Meliala I, Kasim V, Wu S. Biological roles of Yin Yang 2: its implications in physiological and pathological events. J Cell Mol Med. 2020;24(22): 12886–99.
99. Parvin A, Erabi G, Mohammadpour D, Maleki-Kakelar H, Sadeghpour S, Pashaei MR, Taheri-Anganeh M, Ghasemnejad-Berenji H. Infertility: focus on the therapeutic potential of extracellular vesicles. Reprod Biol. 2024;24(3):100925.
100. Munoz JL, Einerson BD, Silver RM, Mulampurath S, Sherman LS, Rameshwar P, Prewit EB, Ramsey PS. Serum exosomal microRNA pathway activation in placenta accreta spectrum: pathophysiology and detection. AJOG Glob Rep. 2024;4(1):100319.
101. Bontempo AC, Mikesell L. Patient perceptions of misdiagnosis of endometriosis: results from an online national survey. Diagnosis (Berl). 2020;7(2):97–106.

102. Jiang Y, Chai X, Chen S, Chen Z, Tian H, Liu M, Wu X. Exosomes from the uterine cavity mediate immune dysregulation via inhibiting the JNK signal pathway in endometriosis. Biomedicine. 2022;10(12):3110.
103. Pittenger MF, Discher DE, Péault BM, Phinney DG, Hare JM, Caplan AI. Mesenchymal stem cell perspective: cell biology to clinical progress. npj Regener Med. 2019;4(1):1–15.
104. Tang Y, Zhou Y, Li HJ. Advances in mesenchymal stem cell exosomes: a review. Stem Cell Res Ther. 2021;12(1):71.
105. Sima Y, Chen Y. MSC-based therapy in female pelvic floor disorders. Cell Biosci. 2020;10: 104.
106. Nikfarjam S, Rezaie J, Zolbanin NM, Jafari R. Mesenchymal stem cell derived-exosomes: a modern approach in translational medicine. J Transl Med. 2020;18(1):449.
107. Tan F, Li X, Wang Z, Li J, Shahzad K, Zheng J. Clinical applications of stem cell-derived exosomes. Sig Transduct Target Ther. 2024;9(1):1–31.
108. Tzng E, Bayardo N, Yang PC. Current challenges surrounding exosome treatments. Extracell Vesicles. 2023;2:100023.
109. Perocheau D, Touramanidou L, Gurung S, Gissen P, Baruteau J. Clinical applications for exosomes: are we there yet? Br J Pharmacol. 2021;178(12):2375–92.
110. Antimisiaris SG, Mourtas S, Marazioti A. Exosomes and exosome-inspired vesicles for targeted drug delivery. Pharmaceutics. 2018;10(4):218.
111. Saleem M, Shahzad KA, Marryum M, Singh S, Zhou Q, Du S, Wang S, Shao C, Shaikh II. Exosome-based therapies for inflammatory disorders: a review of recent advances. Stem Cell Res Ther. 2024;15(1):477.
112. Ojeda-Hernández DD, Hernández-Sapiéns MA, Reza-Zaldívar EE, Canales-Aguirre A, Matías-Guiu JA, Matías-Guiu J, Mateos-Díaz JC, Gómez-Pinedo U, Sancho-Bielsa F. Exosomes and biomaterials: in search of a new therapeutic strategy for multiple sclerosis. Life (Basel). 2022;12(9):1417.
113. Rana N, Suliman S, Al-Sharabi N, Mustafa K. Extracellular vesicles derived from primed mesenchymal stromal cells loaded on biphasic calcium phosphate biomaterial exhibit enhanced macrophage polarization. Cells. 2022;11(3):470.
114. Wang X, Wu D, Li W, Yang L. Emerging biomaterials for reproductive medicine. Eng Regen. 2021;2:230–45.
115. Sadr SZ, Fatehi R, Maroufizadeh S, Amorim CA, Ebrahimi B. Utilizing fibrin-alginate and Matrigel-alginate for mouse follicle development in three-dimensional culture systems. Biopreserv Biobank. 2018;16(2):120–7.
116. Sahni M, Day ES. Nanotechnologies for the detection and treatment of endometriosis. Front Biomater Sci. 2023;2:1279358.
117. Dai W, Liang J, Guo R, Zhao Z, Na Z, Xu D, Li D. Bioengineering approaches for the endometrial research and application. Mater Today Bio. 2024;26:101045.
118. Lin Y, Wu J, Gu W, Huang Y, Tong Z, Huang L, Tan J. Exosome–liposome hybrid nanoparticles deliver CRISPR/Cas9 system in MSCs. Adv Sci (Weinh). 2018;5(4):1700611.
119. Liu A, Yang G, Liu Y, Liu T. Research progress in membrane fusion-based hybrid exosomes for drug delivery systems. Front Bioeng Biotechnol. 2022;10:939441.

Engineering Technology for Women's Health

Organ-on-Chip Technology for Women's Health Engineering

Cristina I. Bonilla Carrillo and Samantha G. Zambuto

Abstract Organ-on-chip (OoC) technology has emerged as a transformative platform for modeling human physiology with enhanced biological relevance compared to traditional in vitro and animal models. By integrating microfluidics, tissue engineering, and biomaterials, OoC systems enable precise control of cellular microenvironments, mechanical cues, and biochemical signaling. This chapter provides an overview of the principles underlying OoC technology and highlights its growing impact on women's health research, a field historically limited by underrepresentation in clinical trials and inadequate preclinical models. We discuss recent regulatory advances, including the Food and Drug Administration Modernization Act 2.0 and the adoption of New Approach Methodologies, which support the use of human-relevant nonclinical systems. Key applications in drug delivery, diagnostics, tissue engineering, and disease modeling of the female reproductive system are reviewed, with emphasis on ovarian, endometrial, placental, and vaginal OoC platforms. Additionally, the role of biomaterials in enhancing physiological fidelity and enabling dynamic tissue remodeling is examined. Finally, future directions are explored, including multi-organ integration, precision medicine, patient-specific modeling, and positioning OoC technology as a critical tool for advancing translational research and improving outcomes in women's health.

Keywords Women's health · Organ-on-chip · Biomimicking · Microfluidic · Tissue engineering · Biomaterials · Precision medicine · Modeling · Microphysiological systems · Engineering technology

---

C. I. Bonilla Carrillo · S. G. Zambuto (✉)
Department of Mechanical and Aerospace Engineering, University of Kentucky, Lexington, KY, USA
e-mail: cristina.bonilla@uky.edu; samantha.zambuto@uky.edu

S. G. Zambuto, M. L. Oyen (eds.), *Biomaterials for Women's Health Engineering*,
https://doi.org/10.1007/978-3-032-10745-9_22

1 Introduction to Organ-on-Chip Technology

A team of researchers at the Wyss Institute for Biologically Inspired Engineering at Harvard University adapted computer microchip manufacturing methods to create "Organs-on-Chips." Organ-on-Chip (OoC) technology consists of microfluidic devices designed to recapitulate the complex structures and functions of living human organs (Fig. 1). These platforms are typically fabricated from clear flexible polymers and contain microfluidic channels lined with living human cells, enabling the recreation of a three-dimensional microenvironment that closely mimics in vivo organ conditions. Consequently, OoC systems provide a highly controlled platform for applications such as drug delivery, disease modeling, and personalized medicine, without involving humans or animals [1].

The conceptual foundation of OoC can be traced back to 2007, when Dr. Donald Ingber, Founding Director of the Wyss Institute, encountered an early demonstration of a "lung-on-a-chip" device that incorporated microfluidic channels but lacked living cells. Although this initial prototype did not achieve functional success, it laid the groundwork for subsequent innovation. The student who developed the original device later joined Ingber's laboratory, where, following extensive iterative experimentation, the team succeeded. This breakthrough culminated in the

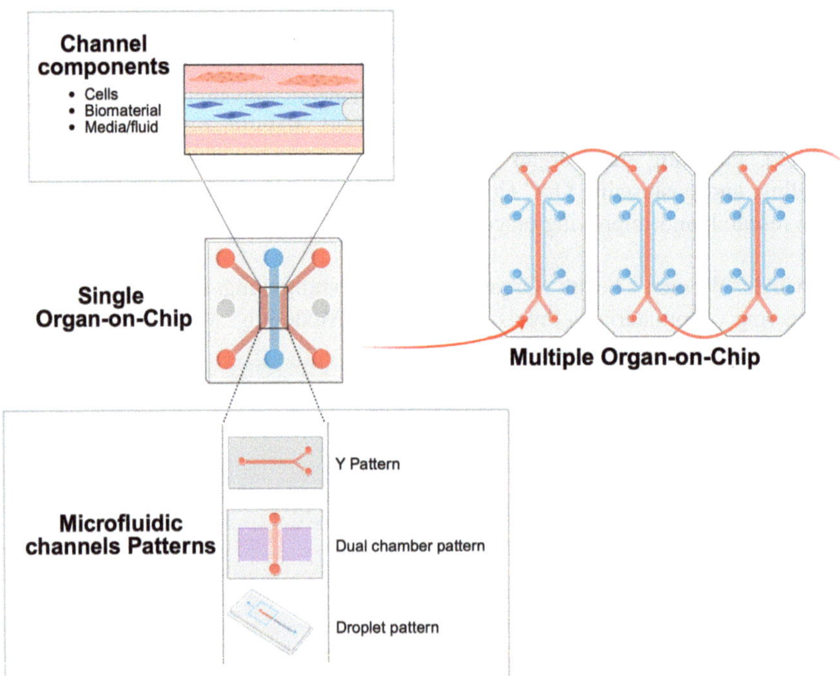

Fig. 1 Example microfluidic channel patterns and architecture for organ-on-chip technology

development of the first functional human lung-on-a-chip, which was reported in the landmark 2010 Science publication, "Reconstituting Organ-Level Lung Functions on a Chip" [1].

Parallel to these developments, significant contributions emerged from the Massachusetts Institute of Technology. In 2005, Roger Kamm's laboratory developed a microfluidic prototype to study angiogenesis, introducing a pivotal design that utilized minute posts to contain hydrogels via surface tension. This engineering solution prevented material leakage before solidification, a technique that proved essential for creating stable three-dimensional cell cultures. By the early 2010s, this technology enabled the high-resolution visualization of breast cancer cell extravasation and the role of macrophages in tumor progression, capturing biological processes with a level of detail unattainable in vivo models [2].

The widespread adoption of these standardized platforms has catalyzed a shift in how biological experiments are designed. Since this breakthrough, OoC technology has significantly advanced the fields of tissue engineering and microfabrication. Conventional cell culture models have evolved from simple two-dimensional monocultures into complex three-dimensional co-culture systems that more accurately reproduce native cellular microenvironments and tissue architecture. These developments have enabled improved control over cell polarization, direct cell-cell interactions, and the propagation of chemical and electrical signaling [3].

From an engineering perspective, the design of OoC systems relies on microsystems technology, which encompasses fabrication techniques for creating planar devices with microscale and nanoscale features. OoC platforms typically integrate microfluidic channels with electrical or non-electrical components, fabricated using lithographic, injection molding, or bioprinting methods [3] (Fig. 1). Depending on their intended application and functionality, OoC devices may model a single organ or incorporate multiple tissues representative of entire organ systems, capturing biological processes with a level of detail unattainable in vivo models. The success of these research applications led to the commercial translation of the technology through the launch of the AIM Biotech Company, which enabled researchers worldwide to implement high-resolution 3D co-cultures with increased reproducibility via commercial availability. Since this breakthrough, the market has expanded with specialized companies like ibidi, which focuses on standardized imaging-compatible slides, and Emulate, a spin-off from the Wyss Institute that has pioneered the mass manufacturing of organ chips to meet industrial and academic demands.

Based on tissue organization and physiological function, OoC architecture can be broadly categorized into two main categories. The first category comprises solid organ chips, which are cultured as three-dimensional tissue constructs that enable extensive cell–cell and cell–matrix interactions within a tightly controlled microenvironment. These systems often employ micro-pillar or micro-well-based designs and are widely used to model organs and tissues, such as liver, tumors, cardiac tissue, and adipose tissue, where bulk tissue function and metabolic activity are central (Fig. 2). The second category includes barrier tissue chips, which are specifically engineered to recreate natural biological barriers between distinct fluidic compartments, they support the formation of functional epithelial interfaces, allowing

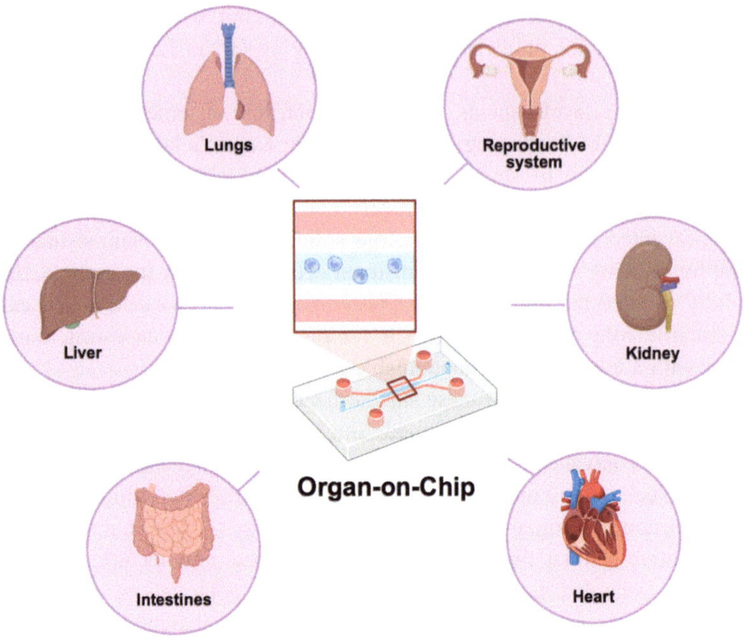

Fig. 2 Example organs modeled using organ-on-chip (OoC) technology

investigation of selective transport, permeability, and barrier integrity under dynamic flow conditions, and this category is commonly applied to models of the gut, lung, and skin, where regulated exchange between compartments is essential to physiological function [3].

The selection of materials, fabrication methods, and biological components in an OoC system is strongly dictated by the purpose of the experiment and the type of tissue architecture required. This selection process involves three critical that must be coordinated: first, biological considerations are fundamental as they allow for the definition of cell source, such as primary cells, stem cells, and cell lines; second, fabrication strategies are crucial to achieve the necessary microstructural complexity and resolution for the precise patterning of microfluidic channels; and finally, material selection is vital to guarantee the system's success (Fig. 3) [3].

There is no experimental model more physiologically relevant than the human body itself, and OoC technology represents a powerful step toward recreating human biology outside the body. Over the past decade, OoC systems have enabled unprecedented capabilities to engineer living physiological tissues and to simulate human-specific conditions with increased precision, reliability, and reproducibility. Traditional biomedical research often relies on lengthy validation pipelines and extensive animal testing, many of which fail to translate successfully to humans due to fundamental biological differences. OoC addresses this limitation by providing human-relevant experimental environments that were previously unattainable. A fundamental element in achieving this high level of biomimicry is the versatile use of scaffolds. Depending on the tissue's complexity, these platforms can function effectively with or without the inclusion of biomaterials. This strategic choice allows

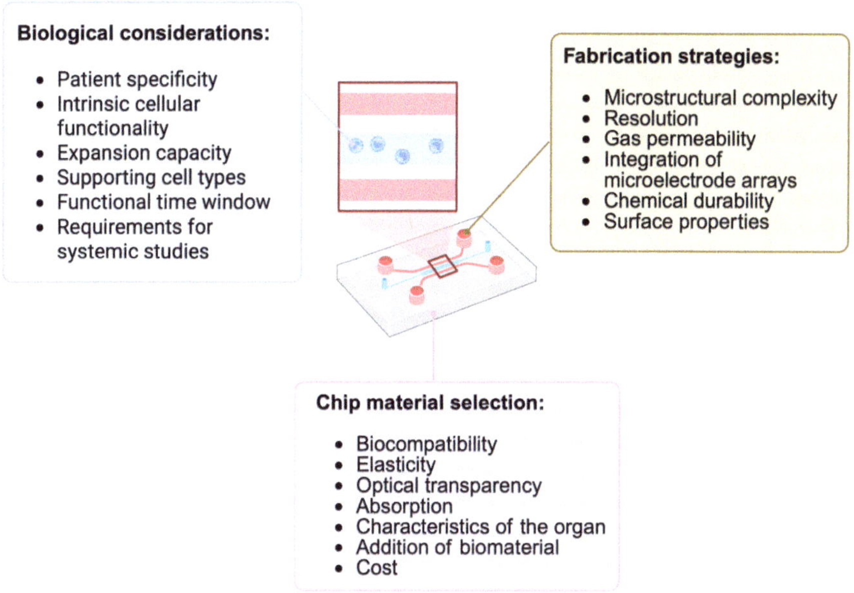

Fig. 3 Integration of biological requirements, material selection, and fabrication strategies for design and fabrication of organ-on-chip (OoC) systems

researchers to tailor the microenvironment to specific research needs, a topic we will discuss later in the chapter when exploring the different approaches for incorporating biomaterials into these systems.

As articulated by Dr. Donald Ingber, OoC "opens an entire palette to paint with" in terms of discovery, therapeutic intervention, and diagnostics. By enabling the investigation of complex physiological processes in controlled, human-based systems, OoC platforms offer a transformative opportunity to advance biomedical research, particularly in areas such as women's health [4, 5]. This transformative potential is especially critical given that, until the early 1990s, women were systematically excluded from most clinical trials. Consequently, many aspects continue to rely on data derived predominantly from male populations or animal models that fail to adequately reflect female physiology (Fig. 4) [6]. OoC models achieve the creation of valuable discoveries for the women's health system.

2 Applications for on-Chip Technology

Advances in OoC technologies align closely with the newest Food and Drug Administration (FDA) regulations about New Approach Methodologies (NAMs) and, at the same time, offer powerful tools to improve targeted drug delivery, disease modeling, and tissue engineering. Collectively, this innovative technology holds hope for addressing big improvements and challenging scientific issues, especially in women's health.

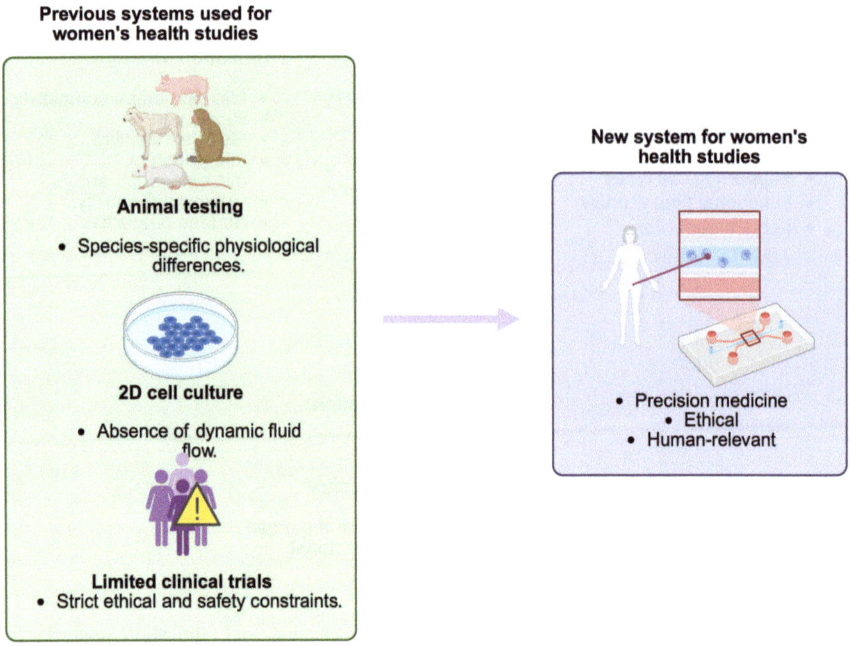

Fig. 4 Comparison between standard and novel systems used for women's health studies

2.1 NAMs-FDA Mod. Act 2.0

The U.S FDA is the federal agency responsible for safeguarding public health by ensuring the safety, efficacy, and quality of drugs, biological products, medical devices, food, and other regulated products [7]. In 2022, the FDA Modernization Act 2.0 was passed, which is a new law that amends the federal Food, Drug, and Cosmetic Act by replacing the phrase "preclinical tests" with "nonclinical tests." Nonclinical tests are defined as tests "conducted in vitro, in silico, or in chemical, or a non-human in vivo test that occurs before or during the clinical trial phase of the investigation of the safety and effectiveness of a drug, and may include animal tests, or non-animal or human biology-based test methods, such as cell-based assays, microphysiological systems (MPSs), or bio-printed or computer models" [8].

By changing this legal terminology, the Act authorizes the FDA to accept data from NAMs, a broad category of experimental and computational tools that are developed, validated, and refined to reduce, replace, or refine animal use in research. NAMs aim to decrease the number of animals required for testing, improve experimental design when animal models are still necessary, and replace animal studies whenever scientifically feasible. These objectives align closely with the development and implementation of organoids and the OoC system, which, as discussed previously, represent powerful human-based laboratory models that offer substantially higher physiological relevance [8].

Despite progress in biomedical research, women have been historically underrepresented in clinical trials and basic science studies. Over the past three decades, only a limited number of drugs have been approved for use in pregnancy, such as Atobisan for preterm labor and Makena (later revoked) for reducing the risk of preterm birth [9], leaving a vast therapeutic gap in women's health. Globally, approximately 830 women die every day from preventable causes related to pregnancy and childbirth. This critical health crisis is a central focus of the United Nations Sustainable Development Goal (SDG) 3, which aims to ensure healthy lives and promote well-being for all. More specifically, SDG Target 3.1 establishes a global mandate to reduce the maternal mortality ratio to less than 70 per 100,000 live births by 2030 [10].

Together, the FDA authorization of the use of human-relevant nonclinical models and the UN's goals act as a unified front to promote a safer, more inclusive era of medical research. This legal and political alignment empowers bioengineered systems to finally provide the human-specific precision required to eliminate preventable maternal mortality and bridge the gap in women's health.

Bioengineered on-chip systems offer a unique opportunity to address these gaps, helping to incorporate diverse reproductive cell types, physiologically relevant extracellular matrix (ECM) components, and tightly controlled biochemical and mechanical cues. Parameters such as matrix composition, stiffness, three-dimensional architecture, and dynamic signaling can be precisely tuned, enabling the study of complex processes including hormonal regulation, menstrual cycle, pregnancy, placental function, and reproductive disorders [11]. In the sections below, we highlight several important applications within women's health that directly benefit from the implementation of OoC technology.

2.2 *Drug Delivery*

Drug delivery refers to the methods and technologies used to administer pharmaceutical compounds to achieve the desired therapeutic effect. Conventional drug administration routes often face significant limitations, including poor targeting, systemic side effects, and suboptimal bioavailability. In response, sustained research and investment have driven the development of advanced drug delivery strategies designed to improve therapeutic precision and efficacy [12].

The traditional drug development pipeline remains costly, time-intensive, and characterized by low clinical success rates. A key contributor to these challenges is the limited predictive power of animal models and conventional two-dimensional cell cultures, which often fail to capture the complexity of human tissue microenvironments and can lead to misleading efficacy or toxicity data. That is why targeted drug delivery systems represent a major advancement in this field; they enable the selective transport of therapeutic agents to specific tissues or disease sites while minimizing exposure to healthy organs [12]. These systems can modulate pharmacokinetics and biodistribution, prolong circulation time, and enhance drug stability and bioavailability.

OoC technologies address many of these limitations by providing dynamic, three-dimensional models that better reflect in vivo physiology. Microfluidic systems allow precise manipulation of microliter-scale fluid volumes, enabling controlled delivery of nutrients, drugs, and signaling molecules while supporting real-time cell–cell and tissue–tissue interaction. The geometry and architecture of these devices recreate physiological length scales, concentration gradients, and fluid-induced mechanical forces, important conditions to aim a realistic cellular behavior. Making them values for studies important conditions on drug delivery, such as the pharmacokinetics (absorption, distribution, metabolism, and excretion of the drug in the body) and pharmacodynamics (impact over time and across concentrations of the drugs in the body) [13]. When integrated with OoC, these parameters can enhance predictions of drug interactions, toxicity, and variability due to age, genetics, disease, or formulation [14].

The treatment of conditions related to women's reproductive health and pregnancy presents unique challenges due to highly specialized biological barriers and microenvironments, such as the vaginal mucosa and the placenta. These complexities have hindered drug development; in the last few decades, only two new medications have been specifically approved for use during pregnancy. This therapeutic gap is a direct consequence of the "Shadows of Thalidomide," where animal testing failed to predict devastating teratogenic risks, leading to a decades-long exclusion of pregnant women from clinical research [15]. Furthermore, the lack of sex-specific nonclinical models has resulted in dangerous pharmacological oversights, such as with Zolpidem, where it was discovered years after its release that women metabolize the drug 35% slower than men, requiring a mandatory 50% dosage reduction [16]. To address these gaps, OoC platforms offer a transformative opportunity to study drug transport and toxicity in human-relevant, female-specific environments, providing the precision necessary to avoid the historical tragedies of the past [17].

This therapeutic gap is largely due to the ethical and physiological risks of traditional testing. However, these challenges can be effectively addressed by OoC models, which support the development of new strategies for non-pregnant women, reproductive tract disorders, and pregnancy research. By mimicking the human-specific transport and metabolism at the placental and mucosal barriers, these human-relevant nonclinical systems provide a safe, controlled environment to validate new treatments, finally moving beyond the stagnation of the past 30 years (Fig. 5).

2.3 Diagnostics

These new technologies have appeared as powerful tools for modeling complex human diseases, including rare genetic disorders, infectious pathologies, and conditions influenced by host–microbiome interactions, letting simulated the communication inter-organ and whole-body like physiological responses, allowing researchers to reproduce human-specific reactions to drugs, radiation, toxins, and pathogens with a high level of accuracy difficult to achieve with vitro models or

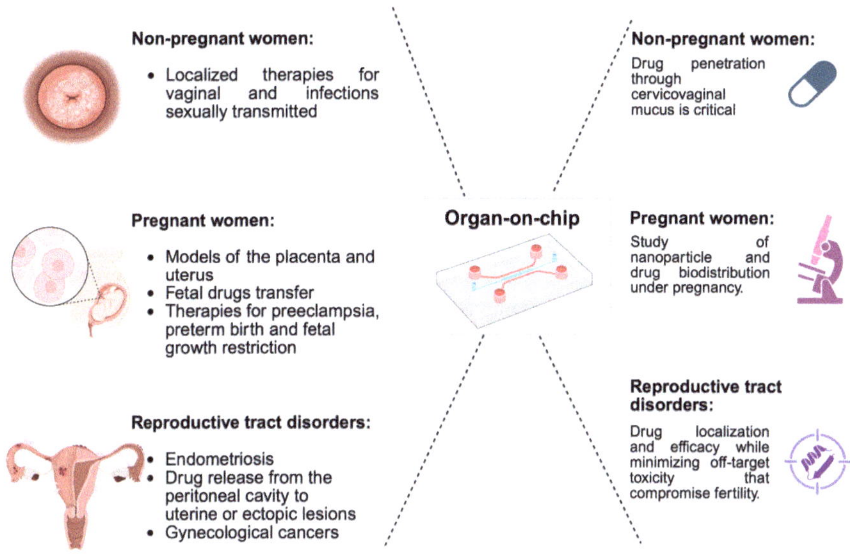

Fig. 5 Considerations for targeted drug delivery modeling across non-pregnant, pregnant, and pathological tissues

animal studies [18]. A clear advantage of OoC platforms is the ability to recreate organ-level architecture while simultaneously incorporating biomechanical cues (shear stress, cyclic strain, and pressure gradients) important to maintaining physiological tissue function [19].

OoC systems allow the opportunity of integrating advanced genetic engineering tools, including CRISPR-based editing, transposase systems, and RNA interference. These approaches enable the development of isogenic disease models (patient-derived cells or organoids compared to healthy counterparts), facilitating the identification of pathological phenotypes, disease-specific biomarkers, and potential regenerative or reparative mechanisms. It is a bridge to eventually reach patient-specific research [20].

These systems have therefore emerged as transformative platforms for studying reproductive pathologies, offering opportunities to investigate disease mechanisms, evaluate therapeutic responses, and move toward personalized diagnostic and treatment strategies. To date, OoC research in this domain has primarily focused on key anatomical components, including the ovary, fallopian tube, endometrium, placenta, and vaginal tissue [5].

2.4 Tissue Engineering

OoC technology draws its conceptual foundation from two complementary fields: tissue engineering and microfluidics. From tissue engineering, OoC adopts the principle of biomimicry, which seeks to reproduce in vitro the physical, chemical, and biological conditions that cells experience within the human body. This biomimetic strategy is traditionally implemented through the seeding of cells into tailored scaffolds, combined with biochemical signals, physical stimuli, and supported by controlled culture bioreactor environments. Microfluidics, in turn, provides the technological framework that enables this mimicry to be realized within miniaturized devices where spatial organization and dynamic control can be precisely regulated [21].

This field represents the convergence of advances in tissue engineering, microfabrication, and microsystems technology, enabling the miniaturization of human organ functions onto compact devices. Biomechanical, biophysical, and multicellular cues are integrated in a spatiotemporally controlled manner [21].

The traditional tissue engineering pipeline focuses on combining patient-derived donor cells with biomaterial and biological stimuli to recreate native tissue microenvironments. However, scaling such constructs to clinically relevant sizes presents persistent challenges, particularly with respect to oxygen delivery, nutrient transport, and the establishment of fully functional vascular networks. OoC platforms address these limitations by applying similar cell culture strategies at the microscale, enabling the creation of highly reproducible micrometer-sized tissues within miniaturized bioreactors (Fig. 6) [21].

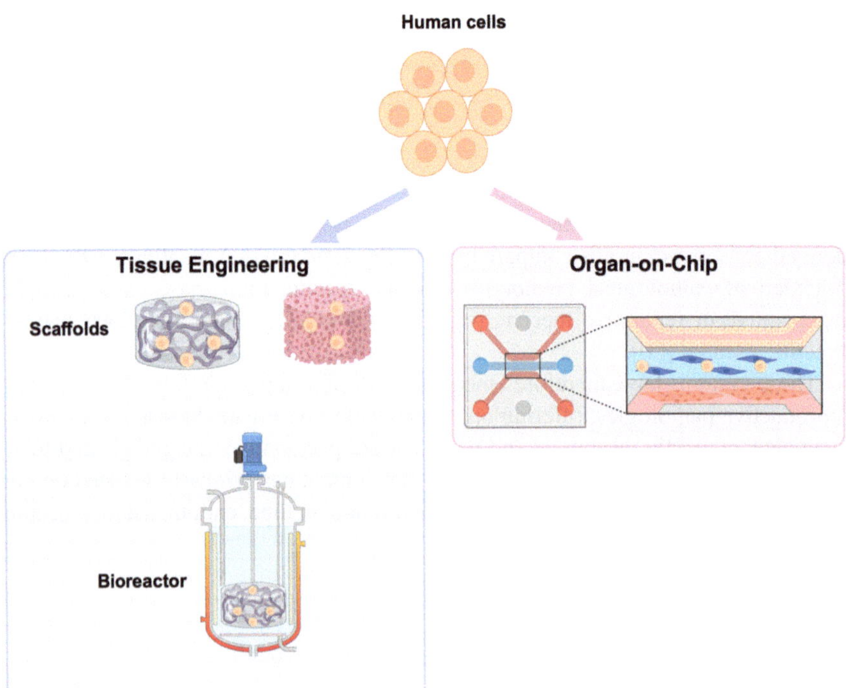

Fig. 6 Synergy between tissue engineering and organ-on-chip (OoC) technologies for biomimetic tissue recreation

3 Role of Biomaterials in on-a-Chip Tech

Materials play a central role in the development and performance of microfluidic and OoC platforms, as they constitute the physical substrates that support cell culture, tissue formation, and device functionality [22]. Currently, OoC systems are primarily constructed from inorganic materials, elastomers, and thermoplastics, chosen for their optical transparency, mechanical flexibility, and ease of fabrication (Table 1).

However, structural materials alone cannot fully replicate the biological complexity of the human body. To create truly human-relevant devices, the integration of biomaterials is essential. Biomaterials enable the recreation of biomimetic environments by providing mechanical support, biochemical signaling, and defined physical

Table 1 Material selection and examples for microfluidic devices [22]

Material type	Material	Key characteristics	Advantages
Inorganic materials	Glass	Optically transparent Low adsorption of hydrophobic molecules Non-gas permeable	Excellent imaging quality Chemical stability
Elastomers	Polydimethylsiloxane (PDMS)	Elastic, gas-permeable, optically transparent Low Young's modulus	Easy prototyping Supports complex 3D microstructures Mimics soft tissues
	Thermoset polyester (TPE), Polyurethane methacrylate (PUMA), Norland adhesive 81 (NOA81)	Higher rigidity. Improved solvent resistance	Reduced small-molecule absorption Rapid prototyping
Biodegradable polymers	Poly(octamethylene maleate(anhydride) citrate) (POMaC), Poly(lactic-co-glycolic) acid (PLGA)	Tunable degradation and mechanical properties Biocompatible	Controlled degradation Suitable for dynamic tissue remodeling
Thermoplastics	Poly(methyl methacrylate) (PMMA), Polycarbonate (PC), Polystyrene (PS), Cyclic olefin polymer (COP), Cyclic olefin copolymer (COC)	Rigid Optically transparent Low gas permeability	Scalable manufacturing Low autofluorescence Chemical resistance
Paper-based materials	Cellulose paper	Easy fabrication Supports metabolic sensing	Low-cost diagnostics, high-throughput assays

Table 2 Biomaterial and scaffold examples for enhanced physiological mimicry [23]

Material type		Material	Key characteristics	Advantages
Hydrogels	Natural	Collagen, alginate, gelatin, fibrin	ECM mimicry Promotes cell adhesion and differentiation	ECM mimicry Promotes cell adhesion and differentiation
	Synthetic	Polyethylene glycol (PEG), Polyethylene glycol diacrylate PEG-DA	Controlled stiffness and degradation Reproducibility	Controlled stiffness and degradation Reproducibility
	Hybrid	Natural–synthetic blends	Reduced batch variability Tunable properties	Reduced batch variability Tunable properties
Basement membrane extracts		Matrigel®	ECM-rich Biologically complex	ECM-rich Biologically complex

architectures that regulate cell adhesion, proliferation, differentiation, and overall function. By combining the structural integrity of synthetic polymers with the biological cues of the ECM, researchers can more accurately simulate dynamic physiological conditions [23].

Components such as hydrogels (collagen, fibronectin, and hyaluronic acid) and basement membrane extracts (Matrigel®) are vital for creating organ-specific microenvironments. These materials could incorporate growth factors and bioactive molecules that guide tissue formation and promote desired cellular behavior (Table 2). The strategic alignment of a material's mechanical properties with the biocompatibility of organic scaffolds provides the versatility needed for advanced biomedical applications [23].

4 Literature Review

A literature review was conducted to summarize human-relevant nonclinical platforms within the specific context of women's health. By evaluating existing research, we aim to identify critical gaps in the engineering of reproductive tissues, assess the maturity of current OoC technologies, and highlight the most promising applications for clinical translation.

The literature review was conducted by searching four major electronic databases: Scopus, Nature, IEEE Xplore, and PubMed (Fig. 7). Articles from the past 5 years (2020–2025) were identified to highlight the most recent advancements in the field. Our search terms covered topics related to identifying advancements in MPSs and OoC technologies applied to female reproductive health. To achieve this, complex search queries each database using different research formulas according to the idea (Table 3).

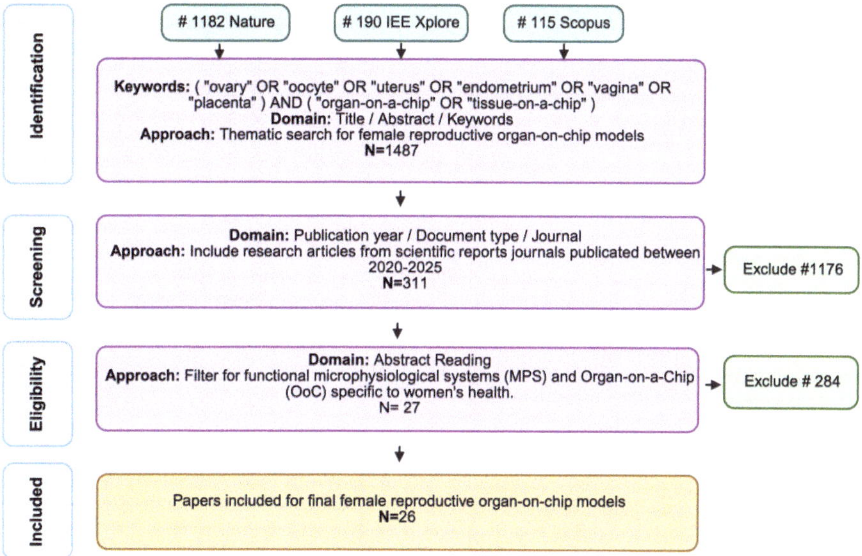

Fig. 7 Search methodology for literature review

5 Future Opportunities

5.1 Women-on-a-Chip

Over the past decade, significant progress has been made in advancing the fundamental understanding of the human reproductive system. However, research and technological development focused on the female reproductive system remain comparatively underdeveloped. As discussed throughout this chapter, OoC technology is an inherently interdisciplinary field that provides a powerful framework for reconstructing the complexity of human organs and their physiological and pathophysiological processes, offering a unique opportunity to model the intricate dynamics of the female reproductive system with higher biological relevance than traditional in vitro approaches.

Future advances in OoC systems should prioritize increasing model complexity through the integration of multi-organ platforms, the incorporation of immune cells to simulate systemic immune responses, and the development of more sophisticated vascular networks and tissue architectures. Additionally, addressing the challenges associated with long-term dynamic studies is critical, particularly through the incorporation of an actuator capable of reproducing physiological mechanical stimuli such as blood flow, cyclic strain, and contractility. Equally important is the need to overcome limitations related to standardization, reproducibility, and scalability across different OoC platforms, including harmonized methods for data acquisition, processing, and analysis, as well as the implementation of robust quality control frameworks. Collectively, these advancements are essential for the successful translation of OoC technologies into clinical and translational research [50].

Table 3 Summary of selected literature on female reproductive OoC models

References	Target organ	Year	Title	Biomaterial	Device material	Cell type
[24]	Cervix	2024	Mucus production, host-microbiome interactions, hormone sensitivity, and innate immune responses modeled in human cervix chips	Collagen Type I and Fibronectin	PDMS microfluidic chips	Primary human cervical epithelial cells
[25]	Cervix	2023	Validation of an on-chip p16ink4a/Ki-67 dual immunostaining cervical cytology system using microfluidic device technology	–	Indium tin oxide (ITO) electrode and a PDMS fluidic channel	Fixed cervical cells
[26]	Cervix	2021	OoC of the cervical epithelial layer: A platform to study normal and pathological cellular remodeling of the cervix	Matrigel	PDMS and Glass substance	Immortalized cervical epithelial cells
[27]	Endometrium	2025	Developing an endometrium-on-a-Chip model to explore biological mechanisms in the Peri-implantation period of pregnancy	Cultrex Hydrogel	PDMS and glass with O2	Bovine endometrial cells (stromal, luminal epithelial, and glandular epithelial cells)
[28]	Endometrium	2025	Microengineered patient-derived endometrium-on-a-chip for the evaluation of endometrial receptivity and personalized translational medicine	Fibrogen	PDMS	Primary epithelial organoids, stromal cells, and human umbilical vein endothelial cells (HUVECs)
[29]	Endometrium	2025	An engineered human placental organoid MPS in a vascular niche to model viral infection	Matrigel gelation	Customized insert-based organ chip (MPS) with a polyethylene terephthalate porous membrane	Human trophoblast stem cells (hTSCs) and vascular endothelial cells

[30]	Endometrium	2024	Establishment of a three-dimensional microengineered vascularized endometrium-on-a-chip for personalized medicine	Fibrinogen and aprotinin	–	Mice and human stromal cells and HUVECs
[31]	Endometrium	2021	Three-dimensional microengineered vascularized endometrium-on-a-chip	Fibrinogen	PDMS	Endometrial stromal fibroblasts, endometrial epithelial cells, and HUVECs
[32]	Implantation	2025	Type I interferon exposure of an implantation-on-a-chip device alters invasive extravillous trophoblast (EVT) function	Collagen type-I and Matrigel	PDMS	EVTs and maternal endothelial cells
[33]	Implantation	2022	A microphysiological model of human trophoblast invasion during implantation	Collagen type-I and Matrigel	PDMS	Primary human EVTs and decidualization stromal cells
[34]	Implantation	2021	A 3-dimensional microfluidic platform for modeling human EVT invasion and toxicological screening	Fibronectin	PDMS	Human EVTs and endothelial cells
[35]	Multi-organ	2025	Development of a novel dual reproductive organ on a chip: recapitulating bidirectional endocrine crosstalk between the uterine endometrium and the ovary	Hyaluronic acid, collagen, and agarose	PDMS	Human endometrial stem cells and human ovarian granulosa and theca cells
[36]	Multi-organ	2024	Functional, patient-derived 3D tri-culture models of the uterine wall in a microfluidic array	Matrigel	PDMS	Primary endometrial tissue samples and myometrial smooth muscle cells (SMCs)
[37]	Multi-organ	2023	Microfluidic technology and simulation models in studying pharmacokinetics during pregnancy	Type IV collagen Matrigel	PDMS	Primary human maternal and fetal cells

(continued)

Table 3 (continued)

References	Target organ	Year	Title	Biomaterial	Device material	Cell type
[38]	Diseases	2025	Fetal response to maternal exposures of environmental chemicals: Utility of a four-cell human feto-maternal interface OoC	Matrigel	PDMS with glass substrate	Human maternal decidua cells, chorion trophoblast cells, amnion mesenchymal cells, and amnion epithelial cells
[39]	Diseases	2021	A reconfigurable microfluidic building block platform for high throughput nonhormonal contraceptive screening	–	PDMS with dragon skin	Oocyte mice cells
[40]	Diseases	2020	OvCa-Chip microsystem recreates vascular endothelium-mediated platelet extravasation in ovarian cancer	Collagen-fibronectine membrane	PDMS	Ovarian cancer cells, HUVECs, and platelets
[41]	Oocyte	2025	Dynamic microdevice culture during bovine oocyte maturation decreases lipid accumulation and improves blastocyst cell numbers	–	PMMA laminated with $PDMS_{LAM}$ and Pluronic F-127	Bovine cumulus–oocyte complexes
[42]	Oocyte	2023	Characterization of oocyte hardening using a microfluidic aspiration-assisted electrical impedance spectroscopy system	–	PDMS and SUEX® dry film	Mouse oocytes
[43]	Placenta	2025	3D-bioprinted placenta-on-a-chip platform for modeling the human maternal–fetal barrier	Gelatin methacryloyl	Poly(ethylene glycol) diacrylate and PDMS	Human trophoblast stem cells, primary placenta-derived stromal fibroblasts, and human umbilical vein endothelial cells
[44]	Placenta	2023	Self-assembled human placental model from trophoblast stem cells in a dynamic OoC system	Collagen I	PDMS mixed with monomer and curing agent	hTSCs, HUVECs
[45]	Placenta	2023	Healthy and diseased placental barrier on-a-chip models suitable for standardized studies	–	OrganoPlate 3-lane	Human choriocarcinoma cell line BeWo b30 clone and HUVECs

[46]	Placenta	2022	Fluidic flow enhances the differentiation of placental trophoblast-like 3D tissue from human pluripotent stem cell (hiPSC) maintenance in a perfused macrofluidic device	Matrigel	PMMA and PDMS	hiPSCs
[47]	Placenta	2020	Development of an OoC device for study of placental pathologies	Type I collagen	PDMS and polycarbonate membrane	Human trophoblast cell line (BeWo cells) and HUVECs
[48]	Vagina	2024	Modeling healthy and dysbiotic vaginal microenvironments in a human vagina-on-a-chip	Collagen type IV	PDMS	Human uterine fibroblast cells, human vaginal epithelial cells
[49]	Vagina	2022	Vaginal microbiome–host interactions modeled in a human vagina-on-a-chip	Collagen type IV	PDMS	Primary human vaginal cells, primary human uterine fibroblasts

In the context of women's health, OoC systems offer promising opportunities for the integration of advanced analytical techniques, such as mass spectrometry, to detect metabolites, proteins, peptides, and other biomolecules in biological samples. This integration can facilitate the identification of cancer-related biomarkers, enabling earlier diagnosis and improved prognostic evaluation. OoC platforms can also be applied to toxicological studies of the female reproductive system, drug transport analysis, and the assessment of drug efficacy, analyze DNA and RNA sequences, and incorporate biosensors to convert biological signals into measurable electrical outputs, enhancing the diagnostic and monitoring capabilities of the systems [50].

The successful implementation of OoC technology in female reproductive health depends on the strategic integration of specialized features that go beyond simple cell culture (Table 4). These do not represent static existing technologies, but rather a roadmap for future development. By focusing on these primary applications, including personalized drug screening, maternal-fetal transport analysis, and microbiome interactions, researchers can develop more robust tools for clinical translation and the study of complex disorders.

Table 4 Future directions and recommended features for female reproductive OoC models [5]

OoC model	Target tissue	Primary applications
Ovarian organ chip	Ovary	Study of ovarian cancer progression Assessment of chemotherapeutic toxicity and efficacy Analysis of tumor invasion, platelet-mediated interactions, and endothelial transmigration Early detection and molecular stratification of ovarian cancer using patient-derived samples
Fallopian tube OoC	Fallopian tube epithelium	Investigation of early initiation and progression of high-grade serous ovarian carcinoma Modeling precursor lesions and early tumorigenesis
Endometrial OoC	Endometrium	Study of menstrual cycle regulation, endometriosis, embryo implantation timing, and endometrial cancer
Placental OoC	Placental barrier	Modeling of pre-eclampsia Analysis of placental dysfunction, barrier integrity, hormone secretion, and maternal–fetal transport
Amniotic membrane OoC	Amniotic epithelium and mesenchyme	Investigation of preterm birth, maternal–fetal communication, and inflammatory or infectious responses
Vaginal OoC	Vaginal mucosa and microbiota	Study of bacterial vaginosis, vaginal microbiome dynamics, sperm migration, and reproductive health
Integrated vaginal–cervical OoC models	Vaginal–cervical interface	Investigation of viral and bacterial transmission mechanisms, including human papillomavirus Diagnostic and preventive applications

5.2 Sex Differences

Reproductive health has largely focused on maternal health and human immunodeficiency virus infection, particularly in low- and middle-income countries. Although these efforts have yielded important improvements, they have also contributed to a narrow conceptualization of women's health that overlooks many non-reproductive conditions [51].

Sex-specific biological differences, combined with gender-related demographic trends, further complicate women's health outcomes. Women generally have longer life expectancies than men, which results in a higher burden of chronic illness and age-related conditions [51]. OoC provides a transformative opportunity to develop experimental systems that move beyond pregnancy- and menstruation-centered models to address health conditions specific to different stages of the female life cycle, including puberty, menopause, and aging, and start to exhibit sex-dependent mechanisms, such as breast cancer and hormone-related disorders.

5.3 Precision Medicine

Precision medicine aims to tailor prevention strategies, diagnostic tools, and therapeutic interventions to individual patients based on their unique biological characteristics, disease subtypes, and treatment responses. OoC technology plays a central role in advancing precision medicine by enabling the use of patient-derived cells and tissues to create physiologically relevant, individualized disease models. These platforms allow for the evaluation of drug efficacy, toxicity, and therapeutic response in a controlled environment that closely mimics human physiology, thereby reducing reliance on animal models and improving translational accuracy [52].

Personalization is achieved by selecting patient-derived or stem cell-derived tissues, tailoring culture media through the addition of specific chemical compounds or recombinant biomarkers, and adjusting microfluidic flow parameters to reproduce patient-specific physiological environments. By systematically integrating personal health data (genetic information, environmental and toxicant exposure, circulating biomarker profiles, and lifestyle-related factors) into OoC platforms, these systems enable more accurate modeling of disease progression, facilitate biomarker discovery, and support the evaluation of individualized therapeutic responses, thereby strengthening the connection between in vitro experimentation and personalized clinical decision-making [53].

Acknowledgments Figures were created in BioRender. Zambuto, S. (2026) https://BioRender.com/c50ieuj. This publication was supported by the National Center for Research Resources and the National Center for Advancing Translational Sciences, National Institutes of Health, through Grant KL2TR001996 (S.G.Z.). The content is solely the responsibility of the authors and does not necessarily represent the official views of the NIH. Assistance in technical paraphrasing was provided by Google Gemini. (Google, 2024). https://gemini.google.com/. All text was written and edited by the authors.

References

1. Ingber D. Human organs-on-chips. 2010. https://wyss.harvard.edu/technology/human-organs-on-chips/
2. Matheson R. Capturing cell growth in 3-D Spinout's microfluidics device better models how cancer and other cells interact in the body. 2015. https://news.mit.edu/2015/cancer-cell-growth-3-d-microfluidics-0814
3. Leung CM, et al. A guide to the organ-on-a-chip. Nat Rev Methods Primers. 2022;2 https://doi.org/10.1038/s43586-022-00118-6.
4. Kedar S, editor. Innovate and elevate. Sharon Kedar, MBA, CFA, Youtube; 2025.
5. Pan M, Chen H, Deng K, Xiao K. Organ-on-a-chip models of the female reproductive system: current progress and future perspectives. Micromachines. 2025;16:1125. https://doi.org/10.3390/mi16101125.
6. Regensteiner JG, et al. Barriers and solutions in women's health research and clinical care: a call to action. Lancet Reg Health Am. 2025;44:101037. https://doi.org/10.1016/j.lana.2025.101037.
7. U.S. Food and Drug Administration. What we do. 2023. https://www.fda.gov/about-fda/what-we-do
8. U.S. Food and Drug Administration. New Approach Methods (NAMs). 2024. https://www.fda.gov/food/toxicology-research/new-approach-methods-nams
9. Souza JP, et al. A global analysis of the determinants of maternal health and transitions in maternal mortality. Lancet Glob Health. 2024;12:e306–16. https://doi.org/10.1016/s2214-109x(23)00468-0.
10. Women U. SDG 3: Ensure healthy lives and promote well-being for all at all ages. https://www.unwomen.org/en/news/in-focus/women-and-the-sdgs/sdg-3-good-health-well-being
11. Zambuto SG, Scott AK, Oyen ML. FDA modernization act 2.0 and reproductive research. Nat Rev Bioeng. 2024;2:984–6. https://doi.org/10.1038/s44222-024-00252-8.
12. Srivastava A, Ahmad A, Siddiqui S, Islam A. Innovations in targeted drug delivery: from nanotechnology to clinical applications. Next Nanotechnol. 2026;9:100336. https://doi.org/10.1016/j.nxnano.2025.100336.
13. Li Z, Hui J, Yang P, Mao H. Microfluidic organ-on-a-chip system for disease modeling and drug development. Biosensors. 2022;12:370. https://doi.org/10.3390/bios12060370.
14. Rowland M, Peck C, Tucker G. Physiologically-based pharmacokinetics in drug development and regulatory science. Annu Rev Pharmacol Toxicol. 2011;51:45–73. https://doi.org/10.1146/annurev-pharmtox-010510-100540.
15. Kaplan RM, Song S, Majeti N, Nikolov MC. Sex distribution of clinical trial participants: how often are women excluded? J Gen Intern Med. 2025;40:3267–8. https://doi.org/10.1007/s11606-025-09428-3.
16. Mudge L. The gender health gap: 10 times medicine failed women. 2023. https://www.livescience.com/gender-health-gap-times-medicine-failed-women
17. Swingle KL, Ricciardi AS, Peranteau WH, Mitchell MJ. Delivery technologies for women's health applications. Nat Rev Bioeng. 2023;1:408–25. https://doi.org/10.1038/s44222-023-00040-w.
18. Ingber DE. Human organs-on-chips for disease modelling, drug development and personalized medicine. Nat Rev Genet. 2022;23:467–91. https://doi.org/10.1038/s41576-022-00466-9.
19. Zommiti M, et al. Organs-on-chips platforms are everywhere: a zoom on biomedical investigation. Bioengineering. 2022;9:646. https://doi.org/10.3390/bioengineering9110646.
20. Celotti M, et al. Protocol to create isogenic disease models from adult stem cell-derived organoids using next-generation CRISPR tools. STAR Protocols. 2024;5:103189. https://doi.org/10.1016/j.xpro.2024.103189.
21. Zhao Y, Wang EY, Lai FBL, Cheung K, Radisic M. Organs-on-a-chip: a union of tissue engineering and microfabrication. Trends Biotechnol. 2023;41:410–24. https://doi.org/10.1016/j.tibtech.2022.12.018.

22. Ding C, Chen X, Kang Q, Yan X. Biomedical application of functional materials in organ-on-a-chip. Front Bioeng Biotechnol. 2020;8 https://doi.org/10.3389/fbioe.2020.00823.
23. Ramírez-González GA, Consumi-Tubito C, Vargas-Méndez E, Centeno-Cerdas C. Advancing organ-on-a-chip systems: the role of scaffold materials and coatings in engineering cell microenvironment. Polymers. 2025;17:1263. https://doi.org/10.3390/polym17091263.
24. Izadifar Z, et al. Mucus production, host-microbiome interactions, hormone sensitivity, and innate immune responses modeled in human cervix chips. Nat Commun. 2024;15 https://doi.org/10.1038/s41467-024-48910-0.
25. Hashimoto K, et al. Validation of an on-chip p16ink4a/Ki-67 dual immunostaining cervical cytology system using microfluidic device technology. Sci Rep. 2023;13 https://doi.org/10.1038/s41598-023-44273-6.
26. Tantengco OAG, Richardson LS, Medina PMB, Han A, Menon R. Organ-on-chip of the cervical epithelial layer: a platform to study normal and pathological cellular remodeling of the cervix. FASEB J. 2021;35 https://doi.org/10.1096/fj.202002590rrr.
27. Kpeglo D., et al. 1–7 (IEEE, PDMS and glass-based microfluidic devices).
28. Lee G, et al. Microengineered patient-derived endometrium-on-a-chip for the evaluation of endometrial receptivity and personalised translational medicine. Nat Commun. 2025;16 https://doi.org/10.1038/s41467-025-65406-7.
29. Wang Y, et al. An engineered human placental organoid microphysiological system in a vascular niche to model viral infection. Commun Biol. 2025;8 https://doi.org/10.1038/s42003-025-08057-0.
30. Lee G, Ahn J. 41–46 (IEEE, PDMS and glass-based microfluidic devices).
31. Ahn J, et al. Three-dimensional microengineered vascularised endometrium-on-a-chip. Hum Reprod. 2021;36:2720–31. https://doi.org/10.1093/humrep/deab186.
32. Simoni MK, et al. Type I interferon exposure of an implantation-on-a-chip device alters invasive extravillous trophoblast function. Cell Rep Med. 2025;6:101991. https://doi.org/10.1016/j.xcrm.2025.101991.
33. Park JY, et al. A microphysiological model of human trophoblast invasion during implantation. Nat Commun. 2022;13 https://doi.org/10.1038/s41467-022-28663-4.
34. Pu Y, Gingrich J, Veiga-Lopez A. A 3-dimensional microfluidic platform for modeling human extravillous trophoblast invasion and toxicological screening. Lab Chip. 2021;21:546–57. https://doi.org/10.1039/d0lc01013h.
35. Park S-R, et al. Development of a novel dual reproductive organ on a chip: recapitulating bidirectional endocrine crosstalk between the uterine endometrium and the ovary. Biofabrication. 2021;13:015001. https://doi.org/10.1088/1758-5090/abbd29.
36. Busch C, et al. Functional, patient-derived 3D tri-culture models of the uterine wall in a microfluidic array. Hum Reprod. 2024;39:2537–50. https://doi.org/10.1093/humrep/deae214.
37. Kammala AK, Richardson LS, Radnaa E, Han A, Menon R. Microfluidic technology and simulation models in studying pharmacokinetics during pregnancy. Front Pharmacol. 2023;14 https://doi.org/10.3389/fphar.2023.1241815.
38. Moyer HL, et al. Fetal response to maternal exposures of environmental chemicals: utility of a four-cell human feto-maternal interface organ-on-chip. Chem Biol Interact. 2025;421:111782. https://doi.org/10.1016/j.cbi.2025.111782.
39. Lee J-H, Van Der Linden C, Diaz FJ, Wong PK. 72–75 (IEEE, Reconfigurable elastomer blocks with integrated membrane filters).
40. Saha B, et al. OvCa-Chip microsystem recreates vascular endothelium–mediated platelet extravasation in ovarian cancer. Blood Adv. 2020;4:3329–42. https://doi.org/10.1182/bloodadvances.2020001632.
41. Vit FF, et al. Dynamic microdevice culture during bovine oocyte maturation decreases lipid accumulation and improve blastocyst cell numbers. Sci Rep. 2025; https://doi.org/10.1038/s41598-025-29435-y.
42. Cao Y, Floehr J, Schnakenberg U. (IEEE, PDMS chip with glass-integrated aspiration orifice).

43. Cao R, et al. Assessment of nanotoxicity in a human placenta-on-a-chip from trophoblast stem cells. Ecotoxicol Environ Saf. 2024;285:117051. https://doi.org/10.1016/j.ecoenv.2024.117051.
44. Cao R, Wang Y, Liu J, Rong L, Qin J. Self-assembled human placental model from trophoblast stem cells in a dynamic organ-on-a-chip system. Cell Prolif. 2023;56 https://doi.org/10.1111/cpr.13469.
45. Rabussier G, et al. Healthy and diseased placental barrier on-a-chip models suitable for standardized studies. Acta Biomater. 2023;164:363–76. https://doi.org/10.1016/j.actbio.2023.04.033.
46. Deng P, et al. Fluidic flow enhances the differentiation of placental trophoblast-like 3D tissue from hiPSCs in a perfused macrofluidic device. Front Bioeng Biotechnol. 2022;10 https://doi.org/10.3389/fbioe.2022.907104.
47. Mosavati B, Oleinikov AV, Du E. Development of an organ-on-a-chip-device for study of placental pathologies. Int J Mol Sci. 2020;21:8755. https://doi.org/10.3390/ijms21228755.
48. Gulati A, Jorgenson A, Junaid A, Ingber DE. Modeling healthy and Dysbiotic vaginal microenvironments in a human vagina-on-a-chip. J Vis Exp. 2024; https://doi.org/10.3791/66486.
49. Mahajan G, et al. Vaginal microbiome-host interactions modeled in a human vagina-on-a-chip. Microbiome. 2022;10 https://doi.org/10.1186/s40168-022-01400-1.
50. Deng Z-M, et al. Organ-on-a-chip: future of female reproductive pathophysiological models. J Nanobiotechnol. 2024;22 https://doi.org/10.1186/s12951-024-02651-w.
51. Bustreo FK, Bhadelia F, Afsan Beard J, Araujo de Carvalho I. Women's health beyond reproduction: meeting the challenges. Bull World Health Organ. 2012;90:478. https://doi.org/10.2471/blt.12.103549.
52. Emulate. Using organ-on-a-chip technology to unlock patient-derived precision medicine. 2025. https://emulatebio.com/using-organ-on-a-chip-technology-to-unlock-patient-derived-precision-medicine/
53. Van Den Berg A, Mummery CL, Passier R, Van Der Meer AD. Personalised organs-on-chips: functional testing for precision medicine. Lab Chip. 2019;19:198–205. https://doi.org/10.1039/c8lc00827b.

Advancing Reproductive Tissue Engineering with Bioprinting

Pei Wen Xiao and Kayla J. Wolf

Abstract Reproductive tissue engineering is a powerful approach for developing advanced in vitro research platforms and regenerative therapies. Yet, replicating native tissue structure and function remains a major challenge, as it requires integrating complex architectures and biophysical cues that are difficult to produce with manual fabrication methods. Bioprinting comprises a variety of technologies to direct tissue assembly, enabling control over the tissue architecture and cellular microenvironment. Here, we review recent bioprinting applications in reproductive tissue engineering, which are still early stage and focused on constructing implantable regenerative scaffolds or modeling tumor progression in vitro. We also highlight opportunities to bioprint architecturally complex, functional tissues to serve as next-generation in vitro models and cell-based therapies. Coupled with innovations in organoids and biomaterials, bioprinting can accelerate reproductive tissue engineering and broaden both experimental and therapeutic applications.

Keywords Bioprinting · Biomanufacturing · Tissue engineering · In vitro models · Regenerative medicine

1 Introduction

Remarkable progress in bioprinting tissues, including heart [1], liver [2], and cartilage [3], has led to the development of new regenerative therapies and in vitro research platforms. However, bioprinting innovations have seldom been applied to reproductive tissue engineering despite substantial opportunities for the field. Tissue engineering is already indispensable to biomedical research in other organ systems, enabling breakthroughs in disease modeling, drug screening, and regenerative medicine [4, 5]. Regulatory bodies are increasingly accepting "clinical trials in a dish" to refine or minimize animal testing [6], and several cell-based therapeutics have

P. W. Xiao · K. J. Wolf (✉)
Nancy E. and Peter C. Meinig School of Biomedical Engineering, Cornell University, Ithaca, NY, USA
e-mail: px63@cornell.edu; kaylawolf@cornell.edu

S. G. Zambuto, M. L. Oyen (eds.), *Biomaterials for Women's Health Engineering*,
https://doi.org/10.1007/978-3-032-10745-9_23

already reached the market [7]. Simultaneously, bioprinting technologies enable complex tissue fabrication comprising spatially organized multicellular architectures with perfusable networks that mimic essential structures and functions of native tissues [3, 8]. Leveraging bioprinting to engineer reproductive tissues as regenerative therapies and physiologically relevant model systems would profoundly impact gynecological care while addressing long-standing research inequities in women's health [9].

Reproductive tissue function is critically dependent on biophysical cues originating from tissue architecture and composition [10–12]. Although reproductive tissues, including the uterus, ovaries, vagina, fallopian tubes, and breast, are functionally diverse, they share key structural traits. For example, polarized glandular tubules embedded within supportive stroma constitute the endometrium and much of breast tissue [13, 14]. The absence of critical biophysical cues in vitro impairs tissue function; early studies of epithelial cells derived from the endometrium and cultured on 2D tissue culture plastic did not remain hormonally responsive [15, 16]. In contrast, Kirk et al. demonstrated that endometrial glandular fragments cultured as 3D vesicles in suspension maintained a more hormonally responsive phenotype relative to 2D monolayers [17]. Over the last several decades, additional features, including extracellular matrix (ECM) incorporation, co-culture of multiple cell types, and stratification of epithelial and stromal cell layers, have been recapitulated in vitro [18–20]. Reproductive tissues-on-chip have modeled structural cues and cell organization to study uterine stromal-endothelial cell crosstalk [21], trophoblast invasion toward endothelialized vessels [22], and vaginal tissue–microbe interactions [23]. Collectively, these models reinforce the value of incorporating critical architecture and cellular complexity to recapitulate function. Still, the architectures that can be practically fabricated are limited with manual fabrication methods.

Bioprinting encompasses an evolving technological toolkit for manufacturing tissues with architectural and compositional complexity, which is poised to transform reproductive tissue engineering. Two key applications currently of interest are (i) the high-throughput assembly of advanced tissue models to investigate molecular mechanisms and identify potential therapeutics and (ii) the development of bioprinted constructs as regenerative scaffolds or cell-based therapies. Specific applications vary by tissue type (Fig. 1). Importantly, integrating cutting-edge bioprinting tools with recent progress in biomaterials and organoid technologies could significantly accelerate the development of functional reproductive tissues. Here, we summarize the current state of bioprinting in reproductive tissue engineering and highlight opportunities to integrate recent technological innovations to ultimately improve clinical care.

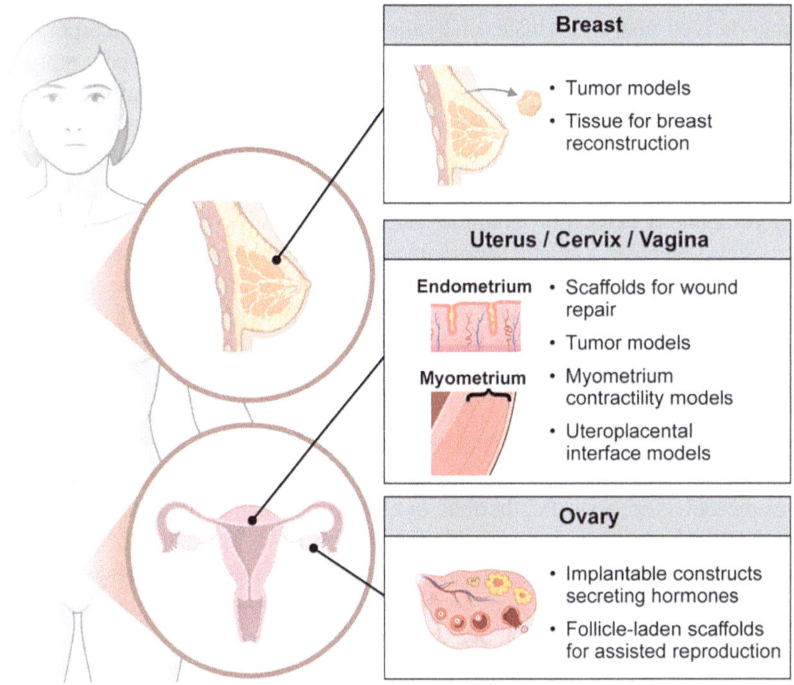

Fig. 1 Current applications of bioprinted tissues and scaffolds relevant to specific reproductive tissues. In breast tissue, bioprinting methods are developing to automate tumor model fabrication for high-throughput drug testing and to engineer implantable constructs for post-mastectomy reconstruction. In the uterus, cervix, and vagina, in which applications often overlap, research has centered on developing regenerative scaffolds and in vitro tumor models. Less explored applications include modeling myometrial contractility and the uteroplacental interface. In the ovary, bioprinting efforts have focused on creating bioprosthetic constructs to restore hormonal and reproductive function

2 Current Bioprinting Applications in Female Reproductive Tissues

Bioprinting technologies can be categorized into extrusion-based, droplet-based, or light-based techniques, each of which been extensively reviewed elsewhere [24, 25]. In extrusion-based bioprinting, used widely in tissue engineering, continuous or discrete filaments are dispensed by pneumatic or mechanical actuation [25]. Extrusion-based printing can be further classified as direct ink writing (DIW) or embedded printing, in which inks are extruded onto a free-standing surface or into a 3D support bath, respectively [26]. DIW requires shear-thinning inks that exhibit a yield stress, facilitating ink flow during nozzle translation while stabilizing free-standing structures after ink deposition [25, 26]. Gelatin and gelatin methacrylate (GelMa) are commonly used, which support cell adhesion and exhibit thermally-tunable viscoelastic properties [24–26]. Other materials, including decellularized tissue-derived matrix, alginate, or hyaluronic acid (HA), can be incorporated with gelatin to enhance mechanical properties or bioactivity [24–26]. Many reproductive tissue bioprinting studies leverage DIW to fabricate grid-like scaffolds laden with cells or bioactive factors that can enhance tissue regeneration or reduce scarring upon implantation into an injury site [27–35]. In contrast, embedded printing consists of extruding shear-thinning ink into a shear-thinning support bath composed of hydrogels or cells. For example, freeform reversible embedding of suspended hydrogels leverages a gelatin sacrificial support bath that can be dissolved or melted to release the printed structure after fabrication [36]. Alternatively, sacrificial writing into functional tissue consists of printing sacrificial inks into baths of cellular aggregates, leaving perfusable vascular networks in cell-dense tissues [37]. While resolution is limited by ink and bath properties, embedded printing facilitates complex architecture formation with soft materials.

Relative to extrusion-based printing, droplet-based and light-based bioprinting offer higher resolution but with limited applications. Droplet-based printing leverages piezoelectric, acoustic, thermal, or electrostatic actuation to deposit small (e.g., nanoliter) ink droplets onto a surface layer by layer, resulting in high-resolution prints [38]. However, droplet-based systems typically require low viscosity inks with low cell density to permit droplet formation without clogging nozzles [38]. Resulting tissue constructs typically do not exhibit sufficient mechanical integrity to maintain their structure at larger scales, hindering use for large tissue fabrication. Droplet-based bioprinting has been used to automate high-throughput fabrication of a spatially controlled 3D ovarian cancer cell and fibroblast coculture model [39]. Light-based bioprinting can produce large constructs with higher resolution than most extrusion-based methods [25]. Light is projected layer by layer into a photocurable ink bath along one axis, resulting in a 3D object. Volumetric bioprinting drastically reduces build times of traditional light-based methods by leveraging a rotating bath to enable near-instantaneous light-based bioprinting [40, 41]. Although light-based printing is generally faster and higher resolution than extrusion-based printing, inks must be photocurable yet non-cytotoxic, and light exposure must be minimized to avoid damaging cells. Additionally, inks cannot contain high cell densities because cellular structures refract light and limit light penetration. Although these requirements limit the application space, vascularized adipose tissue for breast reconstruction has been fabricated using light-based multi-material printing [42].

Reproductive tissue bioprinting studies mainly consist of (i) the development of regenerative tissue scaffolds and (ii) fabrication of tissue models for investigating pathophysiological processes, namely, cancer progression, to identify promising therapeutics (Fig. 2) [43]. These studies established the feasibility of various bioinks for regenerative medicine and tissue model fabrication relevant to the reproductive system (Table 1). We note that 3D printing to create anatomical models for clinical training and education has been a significant focus in reproductive health literature, but these methods are distinct from bioprinting as they do not contain living cells or biomaterials intended for implantation or cell culture. These anatomical models are

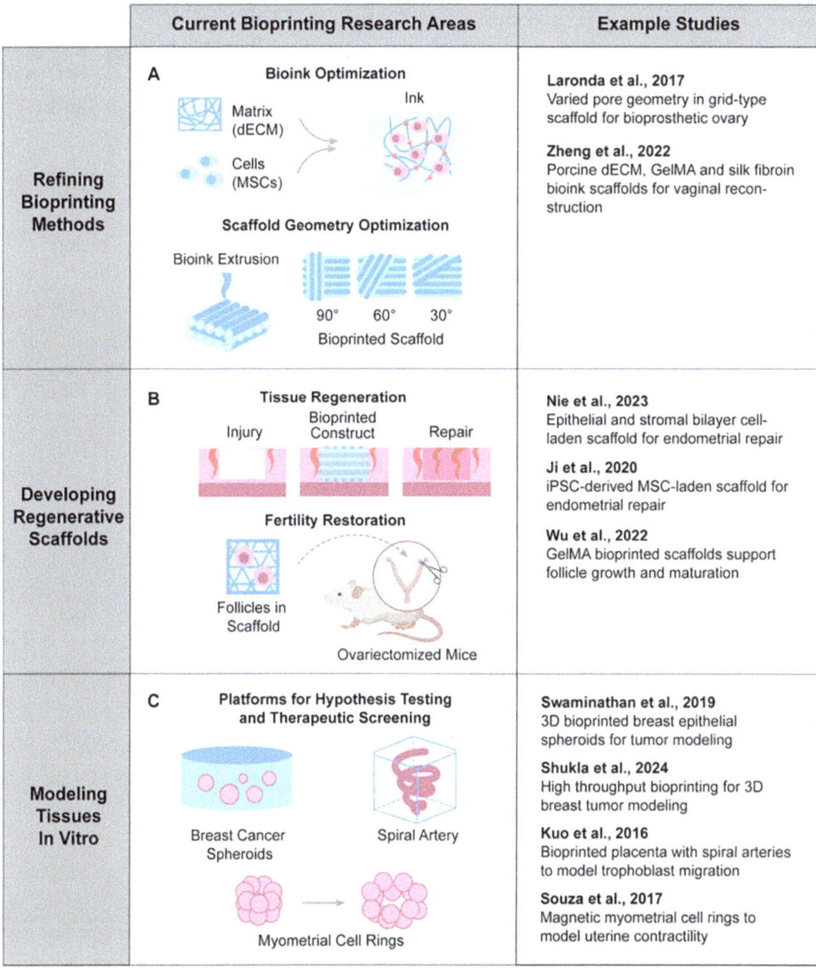

Fig. 2 Current bioprinting research efforts and representative studies in reproductive tissue engineering. (**a**) Efforts to refine bioprinting focus on optimizing bioinks by adjusting matrix composition (e.g., with dECM) and adding various cell types, such as MSCs, as well as fine-tuning scaffold geometry to influence tissue architecture and function. (**b**) Bioprinted constructs are being developed for tissue regeneration (e.g., endometrial repair) and fertility restoration by supporting follicle growth and function in vivo. (**c**) Bioprinting is used to automate the fabrication of engineered tissue research platforms that mimic physiological and pathological conditions for hypothesis testing and therapeutic screening. Example models include breast tumor spheroids in 3D matrices, embedded spiral arteries, and contractile myometrial rings

produced by translating medical images into printed physical replicas to inform patients about their healthcare and allow surgical residents to practice complex, patient-specific surgeries [44–47]. This review focuses on bioprinting living, functional tissues and biomaterial-based regenerative scaffolds. We review recent tissue-specific applications in the following subsections.

Table 1 Summary of biomaterials used in 3D bioprinting of reproductive systems

	Bioink			Bioprinting	
	Matrix	Cell types	Additives	Method	Reference
Gelatin/ alginate	Gelatin, alginate	Human-induced mesenchymal stem cells	–	Extrusion (scaffold)	[29]
	Gelatin, alginate	–	G-CSF, PLGA	Extrusion (scaffold)	[30]
	Gelatin, alginate	–	–	Extrusion	[64]
	Gelatin, alginate, fibrinogen	HeLa	–	Extrusion (scaffold)	[65]
	Gelatin, alginate, Matrigel	HeLa	–	Extrusion	[66]
	Matrigel, gelatin–alginate, collagen–alginate	Breast epithelial cell lines	–	Extrusion	[70]
Gelatin	Gelatin	Murine follicles	–	Extrusion (scaffold)	[35]
	GelMA, ColMA	Human amnion mesenchymal stem cell	–	Extrusion (scaffold)	[54]
	GelMA	BeWo human placental cell line	–	Extrusion	[57]
	GelMA	Human umbilical vein endothelial cells, HTR8 extravillous trophoblast	–	Extrusion	[58]
	GelMA, methacrylated HA	Human adipose-derived stem cells, dermal fibroblasts, umbilical vein endothelial cells	–	Light-based	[42]
Gelatin/ dECM	Decellularized porcine vaginal tissue, gelatin, alginate	Bone marrow mesenchymal stem cells	–	Extrusion (scaffold)	[33]
	Decellularized porcine vaginal tissue, GelMA	Bone marrow mesenchymal stem cells	SF	Stereolithography	[34]
	Decellularized swine ovarian tissue, gelatin, alginate	Primary ovarian cells	–	Extrusion (scaffold)	[69]

(continued)

Table 1 (continued)

	Bioink			Bioprinting Method	Reference
	Matrix	Cell types	Additives		
dECM	Decellularized caprine adipose tissue	Human breast cancer cells	–	Extrusion	[73]
	Decellularized porcine breast tissue	Primary human breast fibroblasts, human breast cancer cell lines	–	Extrusion	[72]
Non-gelatin	Alginate	Endometrial epithelial cells, endometrial stromal cells	HA	Extrusion (scaffold)	[31]
	Allyl-functionalized poly(glycidol)	Human adipose-derived stromal cells, human breast cancer cell lines	HA	Extrusion	[71]

ColMA methacrylated collagen, *dECM* decellularized extracellular matrix, *G-CSF* granulocyte colony-stimulating factor, *GelMA* methacrylated gelatin, *HA* hyaluronic acid, *PLGA* polylactic-coglycolic acid, *SF* silk fibroin

2.1 Uterus: Endometrium and Myometrium

Multiple studies have investigated bioprinted tissue scaffolds as a potential therapeutic strategy to promote endometrium regeneration. The native endometrium is a highly vascularized, glandular tissue critical for embryo implantation and growth [14]. In the absence of implantation, the endometrium is shed and regenerated during normal menstruation [48]. However, damage from infection or surgical procedures can lead to various pathologies, including Asherman's syndrome, a condition characterized by extensive scar tissue formation that results in infertility and abnormal menstrual cycles [49]. Even without prior injury, infertility patients may present with a thin endometrium (<7 mm), where the endometrial lining fails to reach the normal thickness during the menstrual cycle [50]. Tissue scaffolds have successfully promoted tissue growth and regeneration in skin, bone, cartilage, and other tissues [51], motivating application to endometrial regeneration. These scaffolds are often laden with stem cells, which may promote regeneration via paracrine signaling [51]. In normal menstrual cycles, bone marrow-derived progenitor cells contribute directly to endometrial regeneration [52]. Furthermore, a pilot clinical study reported putative benefits from stem cell therapy [53]. In this study, 18 patients with Asherman's syndrome or endometrial atrophy were treated with patient-specific bone marrow-derived stem cells injected into spiral arterioles by catheterization, resulting in a ~2 mm increase in endometrium thickness after treatment. However, this study lacked a control group and was limited in sample size. Nevertheless, these studies collectively motivated mesenchymal stem cell (MSC)-laden regenerative scaffold bioprinting to promote regeneration after scaffold implantation [29, 31, 32, 54, 55].

To improve regeneration, Ji et al. designed a porous, grid-type bioprinted scaffold composed of a gelatin–alginate hydrogel laden with human-induced pluripotent stem cell-derived MSCs (hiMSCs) [29]. In rat models of endometrial injury, treatment with hiMSC-laden scaffolds increased regenerated tissue thickness and gland density relative to hiMSCs or empty scaffolds alone [29]. Furthermore, mice models of endometrial injury treated with the bioprinted hiMSC-laden scaffolds exhibited improved pregnancy outcomes, including increased pregnancy rate and embryo number compared to controls [29]. However, complete restoration of normal function and structure of endometrial lining was not achieved, as the number of glands and regenerated endometrium thickness was significantly less than in the sham group [29]. Wen et al. transplanted 3D bioprinted gelatin–alginate scaffolds containing granulocyte colony-stimulating factor (G-CSF)-laden microspheres into rat models of intrauterine adhesions (IUAs) and observed endometrial repair over 28 days [30]. The bioprinted G-CSF microsphere scaffolds improved endometrial regeneration, suppressed fibrosis, and improved pregnancy outcomes relative to microsphere-laden monolithic gels and microspheres alone [30]. These studies suggest that scaffolds promote regeneration and functional recovery of injured endometrium but do not achieve full restoration.

Grid-type regenerative scaffolds have been fabricated with bioink compositions tailored to increase regenerative effect. To improve the physical properties and biocompatibility of GelMA inks, Feng et al. generated a composite ink composed of methacrylated gelatin and collagen (GelMA-ColMA) mixed with human amniotic mesenchymal stem cells (haMSCs) and crosslinked with blue light [54]. Scaffolds printed with GelMA-ColMA exhibited a dense, interconnected microporous structure with enhanced mechanical strength compared to GelMA hydrogel alone [54]. In rat models of endometrial injury, GelMA-ColMA scaffolds laden with haMSCs supported endometrial regeneration [54]. Given the important role of HA in promoting tissue regeneration [56], Nie et al. used a sodium alginate-HA ink mixed with endometrial epithelial cells and stromal cells for endometrial regeneration [31]. The scaffold promoted partial restoration of the endometrium thickness and significantly improved pregnancy outcomes in rat IUA models relative to the injury group and the group treated with a non-printed graft [31]. These studies indicate the importance of both bioink composition and scaffold architecture in improving therapeutic outcomes.

Bioprinted constructs have also been used to model uteroplacental interactions in pregnancy. Kuo et al. patterned trophoblasts and microenvironmental cues using GelMA-based inks to model trophoblast migration in preeclampsia, a condition characterized by failed vascular remodeling at the uteroplacental interface [57]. Using the bioprinted model, the authors observed a positive correlation between epidermal growth factor (EGF) concentration and trophoblast migration rates. The authors also demonstrated that bioprinting could recapitulate some architectural features of spiral arteries. Although EGF is already a well-established chemoattractant, and the influence of the spiral architecture on migration was not investigated, this study highlights the opportunity to recreate complex tissue architectures using bioprinting. In a later study, the authors fabricated a similar model with a perfusable, endothelialized lumen [58].

Despite the critical role of myometrial contractility in reproductive health [59, 60], few studies have leveraged bioprinting for myometrium engineering. Souza et al. used magnetic bioprinting to fabricate contractile myometrial rings by loading cells with magnetic particles and applying a magnetic field to spatially organize cells [61]. These rings were fabricated in 384-well plates, enabling high-throughput testing of multiple small molecules on contractility across cells from three different patients. Contractility response to indomethacin and nifedipine, typically administered to suppress uterine contractions, was dose-dependent and patient-specific. This work highlights the potential of automated bioprinting for tissue fabrication to enable high-throughput screening while leveraging contractility as a functional readout.

2.2 *Cervix and Vagina*

The cervix and vagina are critical for the mechanical function of the female reproductive system, but can be severely injured by childbirth or physical trauma [62]. In some cases, these tissues may be absent due to congenital defects [63]. The uterus, vagina, and cervix exhibit nonlinear, dynamic mechanical properties to accommodate pregnancy and labor [11, 59]. Regenerative scaffolds must ultimately rescue these critical mechanical properties to promote normal tissue function. To this end, several groups incorporated tissue-specific, decellularized ECM (dECM) into bioinks to support cell growth and function with limited success. For example, Hou et al. printed 3D scaffolds composed of gelatin and alginate bioinks containing porcine vaginal dECM and bone marrow-derived MSCs [33]. Upon transplantation into rats, scaffolds containing the encapsulated MSCs supported vascularization and epithelization of the printed vaginal construct [33]. While promising, the regenerated epithelium was immature. In another study, Zheng et al. used porcine vaginal dECM, GelMa, and silk fibroin (SF) bioink to print a vaginal scaffold laden with bone marrow-derived MSCs for vaginal reconstruction [34]. The authors posited that SF addition would increase construct stiffness and strength while maintaining low immunogenicity. When implanted into rats with complete vaginectomy and rabbits with partial vaginectomy, SF-containing scaffolds loaded with bone marrow-derived MSCs supported stem cell viability. Scaffolds also supported angiogenesis, rapid epithelialization, muscle regeneration, glycogen secretion, and nerve repair during tissue regeneration [34]. These studies did not explicitly test the effect of incorporating dECM into the scaffold on tissue regeneration, and dECM presents regulatory and manufacturing challenges to clinical translation.

Bioprinted vaginal scaffolds have also been designed to modulate inflammation or deliver probiotics. To address vaginal wall repair in pelvic floor prolapse, Paul et al. bioprinted endometrial mesenchymal stem/stromal cells in hydrogel inks onto electrospun polycaprolactone meshes and demonstrated an anti-inflammatory response after scaffold implantation in vivo [28]. To address bacterial vaginosis, Kyser et al. bioprinted gelatin–alginate scaffolds containing *Lactobacillus crispatus* and achieved sustained probiotic release in vitro over 28 days [64]. These studies highlight the multifunctional potential of bioprinted scaffolds beyond tissue repair.

Bioprinting has also been leveraged to model cervical cancer. Zhao et al. bioprinted HeLa cells mixed with gelatin–alginate–fibrinogen into grid-type scaffolds to investigate tumor growth within controlled 3D architectures [65]. Printed HeLa cells assumed a spheroid morphology within 5 days and exhibited increased proliferation and matrix metalloproteinase protein expression compared to cells cultured on 2D plastic. Cells in 3D bioprinted scaffolds also exhibited increased chemoresistance compared to cells in 2D cultures, highlighting the role of the microenvironment in driving cancer progression and treatment response. Using a similar approach, Pang et al. recapitulated epithelial-mesenchymal transition by treating bioprinted models with transforming growth factor beta (TGF-β) [66]. Although the same benefits could likely be achieved by manual embedding into monolithic gels, bioprinting enables automated fabrication of high-throughput screening platforms.

2.3 *Ovary*

Ovarian function is central to reproductive health, regulating pubertal development and menstrual cycles from menarche to menopause through coordinated folliculogenesis and hormone production [67]. Ovarian bioprinting has focused on recapitulating follicle maturation within scaffolds for assisted reproduction technologies [35, 55, 68]. Aiming to restore fertility in pediatric cancer patients, Laronda et al. demonstrated the feasibility of using implantable bioprinted scaffolds embedded with ovarian follicles to restore fertility [35]. They seeded mouse follicles into 3D printed grid-type scaffolds with extruded lines angled at either 30°, 60°, or 90° between printed layers [35]. Upon implantation into surgically sterilized mice, the 30° and 60° scaffolds provided optimal support for follicles, enhancing vascularization and ovarian function relative to mice treated with the 90° scaffolds or those lacking implanted scaffolds [35]. The sterilized mice treated with scaffolds became pregnant from natural mating and gave birth to live pups. The optimal performance of the 30° and 60° scaffolds may be attributed to the pore geometry, which prevented follicles from overspreading and losing shape [35]. Similarly, Zheng et al. demonstrated that bioprinted scaffolds laden with porcine dECM and primary ovarian cells support hormone secretion and neovascularization in a mouse model of ovarian failure [69]. These studies indicate potential for printed ovarian constructs to restore function and fertility.

2.4 Breast

Several groups have automated breast tumor model fabrication with bioprinting [70–72]. Swaminathan et al. bioprinted preformed 3D breast epithelial spheroids in alginate-based bioinks containing collagen or gelatin, which maintained structure, polarization, and function over 96 h post-printing [70]. When treated with paclitaxel, the pre-formed spheroids embedded in bioink exhibited greater resistance compared to single cells mixed with bioink [70]. Similarly, Horder et al. 3D-printed human adipose-derived stromal cell spheroids in HA-based hydrogels to investigate breast tumor cell–adipocyte interactions [71]. The bioprinted HA hydrogel supported adipocyte function and differentiation, enabling the study of tumor-adipose crosstalk in a 3D microenvironment. In this model, adipocytes promoted tumor cell proliferation and migration, and tumor cells induced lipolysis in adipocytes [71]. González-Callejo used a dECM-based bioink to pattern a stromal compartment surrounding a tumor core, mimicking the spatial organization and microenvironment of breast carcinomas for high-throughput drug testing [72]. Similarly, Shukla et al. developed bioink containing tumor cells and dECM from adipose tissue to bioprint in vitro models [73], underscoring the potential for bioprinting to automate tissue model fabrication.

In addition to cancer modeling, bioprinted breast tissue may serve as an implantable living material for post-mastectomy breast reconstruction. To this end, Hedemann et al. used multi-layer stereolithographic bioprinting to produce vascularized adipose tissue [42]. This design consists of a layer of methacrylated HA (HAMa) patterned with a star-shaped channel system embedded between GelMA/HAMa layers containing human adipose stem cells and dermal fibroblasts. The bioprinted adipose tissue demonstrated sustained cell viability and proliferation over 21 days. Moreover, the system supported adipogenesis in 3D culture, demonstrated by an increase in the number of fat vesicles along with adiponectin and leptin levels. Perfusion of endothelialized channels supported long-term culture and growth by increasing nutrient delivery and metabolic waste removal. Endothelial cells within channels self-organized into microvascular-like vessels that extended into the adjacent adipose tissue after 2 weeks. Although they would require substantial development and validation, bioprinted patient-specific grafts could eventually replace synthetic implants.

3 Future Challenges and Opportunities for Bioprinting Reproductive Tissues

Recent studies showcase potential applications of bioprinted constructs in reproductive tissue engineering, including serving as regenerative scaffolds [28–33, 35, 54, 64, 68, 69] and therapeutic testing platforms [39, 57, 58, 61, 65, 66, 70–73]. However, the tissues and scaffolds produced in these studies are simplistic compared to what is achievable with current bioprinting technologies. Regenerative scaffold fabrication has been dominated by extrusion of grid-type structures, even while the clinical efficacy of this strategy remains inconclusive. Bioprinted models for high-throughput screening have similarly relied on limited fabrication strategies, often leaving key architectural features such as tissue layer stratification and anisotropy unaddressed. Integrating state-of-the-art bioprinting technologies with organoids and tailored biomaterials will accelerate the development of physiologically relevant models and effective regenerative therapies. Additionally, designing these fabrication strategies with respect to the tissue life cycle (e.g., menstrual phase, pregnancy stage, and menopause status) will deepen fundamental understanding and enhance clinical translation. Here, we describe these opportunities to advance reproductive tissue bioprinting (Fig. 3).

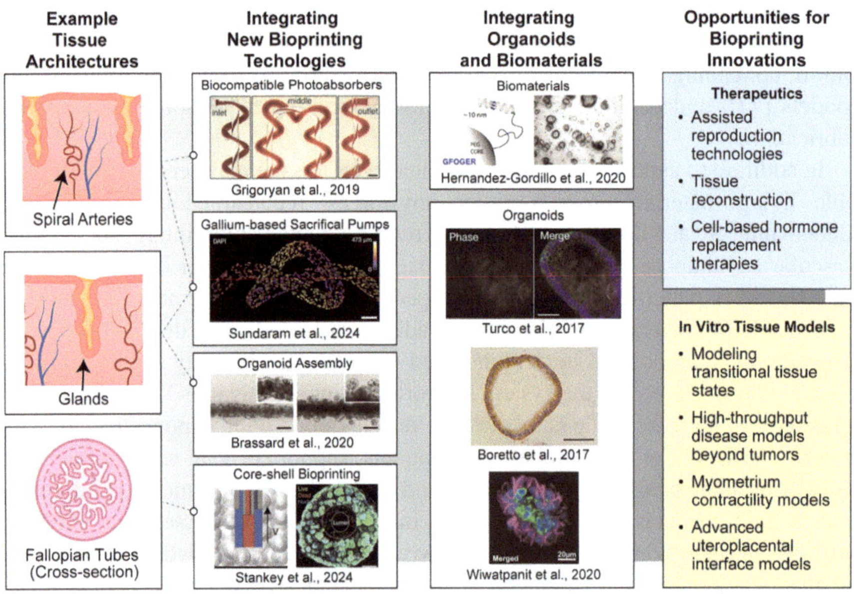

Fig. 3 Future opportunities for integrating bioprinting technologies with reproductive tissue engineering to address clinical and research needs. Left: Example tissue architectures, such as spiral arteries, endometrial glands, and the fallopian tube stratification, illustrate structural targets for engineered models. Center: Innovations in bioprinting, including biocompatible photoabsorbers [84], gallium-based sacrificial pumps [85], organoid extrusion/self-assembly [86], and core–shell bioprinting [90], enable precise control over tissue geometry and perfusion. Right: The integration of biomaterials conducive to organoid growth [83] with patient-derived organoids [74–76] offers new potential for constructing physiologically relevant reproductive tissues. These advances open opportunities for therapeutic applications (e.g., assisted reproduction, tissue reconstruction, and hormone therapies) and in vitro models for studying tissues in transition, disease mechanisms, myometrium contractility, and uteroplacental interactions

3.1 Bioprinting Organoids and Tailored Biomaterials

Recent advances in organoid culture protocols present opportunities to develop organoid-based cellular bioinks by integrating cells and optimized media into bioprinting workflows [74–76]. Multiple protocols for generating and expanding patient-derived endometrial organoids have recently been developed. Building on earlier success in generating gut organoids from adult stem cells [77, 78], Boretto et al. and Turco et al. generated endometrial organoids by embedding single adult endometrial cells in Matrigel and expanding the cells in defined medium [74, 75]. Resulting organoids were dominated by epithelial cells that secreted glycogens and responded to hormone treatment. Wiwatpanit generated scaffold-free endometrial organoids by aggregating epithelial and stromal cells at pre-determined ratios in suspension [76]. After 2 weeks in culture with exogenous hormones, organoids exhibited a core–shell structure in which epithelial cells coated a stromal aggregate. Organoids cultured with excess androgens (characteristic of polycystic ovarian syndrome) exhibited hyperproliferation and dysregulated gene expression relative to controls treated with normal hormonal cues. Endometrial organoids can also be generated from shed cells in menstrual effluent, sharing the same morphology, hormone responsiveness, and transcriptomic signature as biopsy-derived organoids [79]. Although current protocols do not fully recapitulate all endometrial cell types, they are a valuable tool for sourcing patient-specific cells that could be leveraged in bioprinting.

Protocols for directly differentiating reproductive tissue cell types from hiPSCs are also emerging. Miyazaki et al. established a protocol for differentiating hiPSCs to endometrial fibroblasts, which express endometrial markers, including progesterone receptor [80]. Prolonged hormonal treatment of the hiPSC-derived fibroblasts induced expression of decidualization markers [80]. Ovarian granulosa-like cells have also been differentiated from hiPSCs via transcription factor overexpression and recapitulate follicle formation and steroidogenesis [81]. Ovarian tissues derived from hiPSCs could be implanted as cell-based therapies for conditions involving impaired hormone or oocyte production, with bioprinting offering a scalable approach to generate implantable constructs.

Recent advances in organoid protocols are paralleled by biomaterial innovations that support organoid expansion and maintenance. Epithelial organoids typically require basement membrane-derived matrices such as Matrigel or Geltrex to support epithelial morphology and function. However, these materials are limited by batch-to-batch variability, undefined composition, animal origin, and the presence of exogenous growth factors [82]. In contrast, synthetic alternatives offer precisely tunable physical and biochemical properties with modular functional groups that enable independent control over properties including stiffness, degradability, and adhesivity [82]. For example, Hernandez-Gordillo et al. developed synthetic matrices with tunable biophysical properties by combining 8-arm polyethylene glycol macromers with various combinations of ECM- and integrin-binding peptides [83]. Hydrogels functionalized with the $\alpha 2\beta 1$ integrin-binding peptide enhanced differentiation, function, and proliferation in human endometrial organoids, as well as duodenal and colonic enteroids, compared to matrices incorporating alternative peptides. Although this material lacks the shear-thinning properties needed for direct extrusion bioprinting, it can be incorporated into bioprinting workflows by processing as fragments or microparticles for embedded bioprinting baths. Alternatively, existing printable ink formulations could be functionalized with the adhesive peptide to optimize the cell microenvironment in printed constructs.

3.2 Recapitulating Complex Tissue Architectures

Bioprinting technology has rarely been used to recapitulate native architectures in engineered reproductive tissues. Several structural motifs, including vasculature and epithelial glands, could be reproduced with existing technologies. Bioprinted spiral artery models are already in the early stages of development to facilitate studies of pregnancy and preeclampsia [57] and could be improved with high-resolution light-based printing [84] or printed gallium-based engineered sacrificial capillary pumps [85]. Likewise, gland architectures in the endometrium could be replicated by leveraging extrusion and self-organization previously used in gut epithelium [86]. The breast presents a unique challenge due to its adipose-rich microenvironment and hierarchical glandular structures [13]. Still, reconstructing this architecture could support more accurate modeling of breast cancer and lactation, while also informing the design of implantable tissues for post-mastectomy reconstruction.

Beyond vasculature and glands, larger-scale structural and mechanical features could be replicated with bioprinting to impart mechanical function. Recapitulating smooth muscle alignment in the myometrium with strategies used in skeletal muscle and cardiac tissues would enhance studies of uterine contractility and promote the development of regenerative patches for surgical repair [87]. Spatial gradients in biophysical properties are also critical for the function of reproductive organs and could be patterned. For example, the cervix exhibits a stiffness gradient from the inner to the outer region during mid to late pregnancy, which likely contributes to its load-bearing function as the uterus expands [59, 88]. The ovary also exhibits a gradient in mechanical stiffness in which the soft medulla is surrounded by the relatively stiffer cortex; this gradient may support folliculogenesis and is often disrupted in polycystic ovarian syndrome [10]. Gradients could be recapitulated using mixing nozzles that control cell, matrix, and crosslinker concentrations in bioink during printing [89]. For generating therapeutic tissues consisting of concentric layers, such as the fallopian tube, core–shell bioprinting offers a promising strategy [90]. Finally, regenerative scaffolds beyond traditional grid geometries could be designed by incorporating aligned linear channels or other guidance cues that direct tissue expansion and organization. While fabricating a fully functional uterus for transplantation remains out of reach, advances in uterus-on-a-chip models are paving the way for increasingly sophisticated tissues that may eventually facilitate whole organ engineering. These examples highlight untapped opportunities for leveraging bioprinting technologies to generate desired architectures in engineered reproductive tissues.

3.3 Bioprinting Dynamic, Integrated Tissue Systems

Leveraging bioprinting to model transitional tissue states (e.g., early development, puberty, pregnancy, lactation, and menopause) is an exciting frontier in reproductive tissue engineering. These life stages involve profound shifts in hormone levels, tissue architecture, and organ function that affect reproductive and overall health, yet remain poorly understood due in part to a lack of models. Critical species-specific differences significantly limit the validity of animal models, while ethical and practical constraints preclude detailed mechanistic investigation in human subjects [91]. One striking example is the menstrual cycle, which features cyclical remodeling of the endometrium. While organoid models mimic cellular response to decidualization cues, they lack the architectural complexity needed to study tissue breakdown and repair. Beyond enabling the incorporation of glandular and vascular features, bioprinting can help recreate stratified tissue representing different cycle phases. Endometrial cells from patients of various ages or menstrual stages can be incorporated to capture population-based or patient-specific remodeling. Automated tissue manufacturing via bioprinting also facilitates high-throughput model generation to accelerate discovery. Going forward, tissues could be printed in isolation or in integrated multi-tissue fluidic chips, which have previously been used with ex vivo human and mouse tissues to recapitulate hormonal crosstalk over the 28-day menstrual cycle [92]. Furthermore, these tissues could be incorporated into multi-organ chip platforms to investigate systemic crosstalk [93], providing valuable insights into conditions affecting multiple organs such as preeclampsia or menopause.

4 Conclusion

Bioprinting is a powerful technology for constructing complex, tissue-like architectures that closely mimic native tissues. Most applications in reproductive tissues have focused on extrusion-based fabrication of regenerative scaffolds and automated production of in vitro models for therapeutic testing. Increased integration of state-of-the-art bioprinting technologies with organoids and tailored bioinks promises to advance reproductive tissue engineering for both research and clinical applications. For example, endometrial models featuring polarized glands and perfusable vasculature could enable physiologically relevant studies of menstruation, implantation, and menopause. Such studies are often difficult or impossible to perform in animal models or human subjects due to species differences and ethical constraints. Beyond modeling, bioprinting also facilitates therapeutic scaffold and tissue fabrication. Advanced regenerative scaffolds could enhance surgical and wound recovery, while engineered tissue could be implanted for reconstruction. Looking further ahead, bioprinted ovarian tissues could directly treat a variety of conditions, including infertility and menopause symptoms. By serving as in vitro models and regenerative therapies, bioprinted reproductive tissues promise to address longstanding gaps in both research and healthcare.

Acknowledgments This work was funded by NIH grant 3U54CA267738-03S1, which was prematurely terminated.

References

1. Jafari A, et al. Latest advances in 3D bioprinting of cardiac tissues. Adv Mater Technol. 2022;7: 2101636.
2. Ma L, et al. Current advances on 3D-bioprinted liver tissue models. Adv Healthc Mater. 2020;9: 2001517.
3. Murphy SV, Coppi P, Atala A. Opportunities and challenges of translational 3D bioprinting. Nat Biomed Eng. 2020;4:370–80.
4. Shafiee A, Atala A. Tissue engineering: toward a new era of medicine. Annu Rev Med. 2017;68:29–40.
5. Loewa A, Feng JJ, Hedtrich S. Human disease models in drug development. Nat Rev Bioeng. 2023;1:545–59.
6. Ahmed SM, Ahmed SM, Shivnaraine RV, Wu JC. FDA modernization act 2.0 paves the way to computational biology and clinical trials in a dish. Circulation. 2023;148:309–11.
7. Bashor CJ, Hilton IB, Bandukwala H, Smith DM, Veiseh O. Engineering the next generation of cell-based therapeutics. Nat Rev Drug Discov. 2022;21:655–75.
8. Wolf KJ, Weiss JD, Uzel SGM, Skylar-Scott MA, Lewis JA. Biomanufacturing human tissues via organ building blocks. Cell Stem Cell. 2022;29:667–77.
9. Mirin AA. Gender disparity in the funding of diseases by the U.S. National Institutes of Health. J Women's Health. 2021;30:956–63.
10. Matsuzaki S. Mechanobiology of the female reproductive system. Reprod Med Biol. 2021;20: 371–401.
11. Baah-Dwomoh A, McGuire J, Tan T, De Vita R. Mechanical properties of female reproductive organs and supporting connective tissues: a review of the current state of knowledge. Appl Mech Rev. 2016;68:060801.
12. Cadena I, Chen A, Arvidson A, Fogg KC. Biomaterial strategies to replicate gynecological tissue. Biomater Sci. 2021;9:1117–34.
13. Guinebretière JM, Menet E, Tardivon A, Cherel P, Vanel D. Normal and pathological breast, the histological basis. Eur J Radiol. 2005;54:6–14.
14. Yamaguchi M, et al. Three-dimensional understanding of the morphological complexity of the human uterine endometrium. iScience. 2021;24:102258.
15. Kirk D, King RJB, Peachey L, Taylor AWT. Normal human endometrium in cell culture. In Vitro. 1978;14:651–62.
16. Liszczak TM, Richardson GS, MacLaughlin DT, Kornblith PL. Ultrastructure of human endometrial epithelium in monolayer culture with and without steroid hormones. In Vitro. 1977;13:344–56.
17. Kirk D, Alvarez RB. Morphologically stable epithelium vesicles cultured from normal human endometrium in defined media. In Vitro Cell Dev Biol. 1986;22:604–14.
18. Arnold JT, Kaufman DG, Seppälä M, Lessey BA. Endometrial stromal cells regulate epithelial cell growth in vitro: a new co-culture model. Hum Reprod. 2001;16:836–45.

19. Wang H, et al. A novel model of human implantation: 3D endometrium-like culture system to study attachment of human trophoblast (Jar) cell spheroids. Mol Hum Reprod. 2012;18:33–43.
20. Bentin-Ley U, et al. Isolation and culture of human endometrial cells in a three-dimensional culture system. J Reprod Fertil. 1994;101:327–32.
21. Gnecco JS, et al. Compartmentalized culture of perivascular stroma and endothelial cells in a microfluidic model of the human endometrium. Ann Biomed Eng. 2017;45:1758–69.
22. Park JY, et al. A microphysiological model of human trophoblast invasion during implantation. Nat Commun. 2022;13:1252.
23. Mahajan G, et al. Vaginal microbiome-host interactions modeled in a human vagina-on-a-chip. Microbiome. 2022;10:201.
24. Murphy SV, Atala A. 3D bioprinting of tissues and organs. Nat Biotechnol. 2014;32:773–85.
25. Matai I, Kaur G, Seyedsalehi A, McClinton A, Laurencin CT. Progress in 3D bioprinting technology for tissue/organ regenerative engineering. Biomaterials. 2020;226:119536.
26. Zhang YS, et al. 3D extrusion bioprinting. Nat Rev Methods Primer. 2021;1:1–20.
27. Sun H, et al. Partial regeneration of uterine horns in rats through adipose-derived stem cell sheets†. Biol Reprod. 2018;99:1057–69.
28. Paul K, et al. 3D bioprinted endometrial stem cells on melt electrospun poly ε-caprolactone mesh for pelvic floor application promote anti-inflammatory responses in mice. Acta Biomater. 2019;97:162–76.
29. Ji W, et al. 3D bioprinting a human iPSC-derived MSC-loaded scaffold for repair of the uterine endometrium. Acta Biomater. 2020;116:268–84.
30. Wen J, et al. 3D-printed hydrogel scaffold-loaded granulocyte colony-stimulating factor sustained-release microspheres and their effect on endometrial regeneration. Biomater Sci. 2022;10:3346–58.
31. Nie N, et al. 3D bio-printed endometrial construct restores the full-thickness morphology and fertility of injured uterine endometrium. Acta Biomater. 2023;157:187–99.
32. Chen S, Tan S, Zheng L, Wang M. Multilayered shape-morphing scaffolds with a hierarchical structure for uterine tissue regeneration. ACS Appl Mater Interfaces. 2024;16:6772–88.
33. Hou C, et al. Printing 3D vagina tissue analogues with vagina decellularized extracellular matrix bioink. Int J Biol Macromol. 2021;180:177–86.
34. Zheng J, et al. Enhancing vaginal reconstruction through 3D bioprinted scaffolds using a novel vECM-GelMA-SF bioink. Biofabrication. 2024;17:015030.
35. Laronda MM, et al. A bioprosthetic ovary created using 3D printed microporous scaffolds restores ovarian function in sterilized mice. Nat Commun. 2017;8:15261.
36. Hinton T, et al. Three-dimensional printing of complex biological structures by freeform reversible embedding of suspended hydrogels. Sci Adv. 2015;1:e1500758.
37. Skylar-Scott MA, et al. Biomanufacturing of organ-specific tissues with high cellular density and embedded vascular channels. Sci Adv. 2019;5:eaaw2459.
38. Gupta D, Derman ID, Xu C, Huang Y, Ozbolat IT. Droplet-based bioprinting. Nat Rev Methods Primer. 2025;5:1–26.
39. Xu F, et al. A three-dimensional in vitro ovarian cancer coculture model using a high-throughput cell patterning platform. Biotechnol J. 2011;6:204–12.
40. Kelly BE, et al. Volumetric additive manufacturing via tomographic reconstruction. Science. 2019;363:1075–9.
41. Bernal PN, et al. Volumetric bioprinting of complex living-tissue constructs within seconds. Adv Mater. 2019;31:1904209.
42. Hedemann N, et al. Light-based multi-material bioprinting of vascularised adipose tissue for breast fatty tissue engineering. Biofabrication. 2025;17:025034.
43. Chen S, et al. 3D bioprinting technology innovation in female reproductive system. Mater Today Bio. 2025;31:101551.
44. Mackey A, et al. Three-dimensional–printed uterine model for surgical planning of a cesarean delivery complicated by multiple Myomas. Obstet Gynecol. 2019;133:720.

45. Li P, et al. The 3D reconstructions of female pelvic autonomic nerves and their related organs based on MRI: a first step towards neuronavigation during nerve-sparing radical hysterectomy. Eur Radiol. 2018;28:4561–9.
46. Sayed Aluwee SAZB, et al. Evaluation of pre-surgical models for uterine surgery by use of three-dimensional printing and mold casting. Radiol Phys Technol. 2017;10:279–85.
47. Towner MN, et al. Creation and piloting of a model for simulating a minimally invasive myomectomy. Cureus. 2019;11:e4223.
48. Critchley HOD, Maybin JA, Armstrong GM, Williams ARW. Physiology of the endometrium and regulation of menstruation. Physiol Rev. 2020;100:1149–79.
49. Conforti A, Alviggi C, Mollo A, De Placido G, Magos A. The management of Asherman syndrome: a review of literature. Reprod Biol Endocrinol. 2013;11:118.
50. Wang Y, Tang Z, Teng X. New advances in the treatment of thin endometrium. Front Endocrinol. 2024;15:1269382.
51. Liu N, Zhang X, Guo Q, Wu T, Wang Y. 3D bioprinted scaffolds for tissue repair and regeneration. Front Mater. 2022;9:925321.
52. Tal R, et al. Adult bone marrow progenitors become decidual cells and contribute to embryo implantation and pregnancy. PLoS Biol. 2019;17:e3000421.
53. Santamaria X, et al. Autologous cell therapy with CD133+ bone marrow-derived stem cells for refractory Asherman's syndrome and endometrial atrophy: a pilot cohort study. Hum Reprod. 2016;31:1087–96.
54. Feng M, et al. Bioprinting of a blue light-cross-linked biodegradable hydrogel encapsulating amniotic mesenchymal stem cells for intrauterine adhesion prevention. ACS Omega. 2021;6: 23067–75.
55. Guo J, et al. 3D printed controllable microporous scaffolds support embryonic development in vitro. J Cell Physiol. 2022;237:3408–20.
56. Wolf KJ, Kumar S. Hyaluronic acid: incorporating the bio into the material. ACS Biomater Sci Eng. 2019;5:3753–65.
57. Kuo CY, et al. Development of a 3D printed, bioengineered placenta model to evaluate the role of trophoblast migration in preeclampsia. ACS Biomater Sci Eng. 2016;2:1817–26.
58. Kuo C-Y, et al. Trophoblast–endothelium signaling involves angiogenesis and apoptosis in a dynamic bioprinted placenta model. Biotechnol Bioeng. 2019;116:181–92.
59. Myers KM, Elad D. Biomechanics of the human uterus. Wiley Interdiscip Rev Syst Biol Med. 2017;9:1–20.
60. Koutras A, et al. Physiology and pathology of contractility of the myometrium. In Vivo. 2021;35:1401–8.
61. Souza GR, et al. Magnetically bioprinted human myometrial 3D cell rings as a model for uterine contractility. Int J Mol Sci. 2017;18:683.
62. Lopez HN, Focseneanu MA, Merritt DF. Genital injuries acute evaluation and management. Best Pract Res Clin Obstet Gynaecol. 2018;48:28–39.
63. Cunha GR, et al. Development of the human female reproductive tract. Differentiation. 2018;103:46–65.
64. Kyser AJ, et al. Fabrication and characterization of bioprints with Lactobacillus crispatus for vaginal application. J Control Release. 2023;357:545–60.
65. Zhao Y, et al. Three-dimensional printing of Hela cells for cervical tumor model in vitro. Biofabrication. 2014;6:035001.
66. Pang Y, et al. TGF-β induced epithelial–mesenchymal transition in an advanced cervical tumor model by 3D printing. Biofabrication. 2018;10:044102.
67. Oktem O, Oktay K. The ovary: anatomy and function throughout human life. Ann N Y Acad Sci. 2008;1127:1–9.
68. Wu T, et al. Three-dimensional bioprinting of artificial ovaries by an extrusion-based method using gelatin-methacryloyl bioink. Climacteric. 2022;25:170–8.
69. Zheng J, et al. Ovary-derived decellularized extracellular matrix-based bioink for fabricating 3D primary ovarian cells-laden structures for mouse ovarian failure correction. Int J Bioprinting. 2022;8:597.

70. Swaminathan S, Hamid Q, Sun W, Clyne AM. Bioprinting of 3D breast epithelial spheroids for human cancer models. Biofabrication. 2019;11:025003.
71. Horder H, et al. Bioprinting and differentiation of adipose-derived stromal cell spheroids for a 3D breast cancer-adipose tissue model. Cells. 2021;10:803.
72. González-Callejo P, et al. 3D bioprinted breast tumor-stroma models for pre-clinical drug testing. Mater Today Bio. 2023;23:100826.
73. Shukla P, Bera AK, Yeleswarapu S, Pati F. High throughput bioprinting using decellularized adipose tissue-based hydrogels for 3D breast cancer modeling. Macromol Biosci. 2024;24: 2400035.
74. Turco MY, et al. Long-term, hormone-responsive organoid cultures of human endometrium in a chemically defined medium. Nat Cell Biol. 2017;19:568–77.
75. Boretto M, et al. Development of organoids from mouse and human endometrium showing endometrial epithelium physiology and long-term expandability. Dev Camb. 2017;144:1775–86.
76. Wiwatpanit T, et al. Scaffold-free endometrial organoids respond to excess androgens associated with polycystic ovarian syndrome. J Clin Endocrinol Metab. 2020;105:769–80.
77. Sato T, et al. Single Lgr5 stem cells build crypt-villus structures in vitro without a mesenchymal niche. Nature. 2009;459:262–5.
78. Sato T, et al. Long-term expansion of epithelial organoids from human colon, adenoma, adenocarcinoma, and Barrett's epithelium. Gastroenterology. 2011;141:1762–72.
79. Cindrova-Davies T, et al. Menstrual flow as a non-invasive source of endometrial organoids. Commun Biol. 2021;4:651.
80. Miyazaki K, et al. Generation of progesterone-responsive endometrial stromal fibroblasts from human induced pluripotent stem cells: role of the WNT/CTNNB1 pathway. Stem Cell Rep. 2018;11:1136–55.
81. Pierson Smela MD, et al. Directed differentiation of human iPSCs to functional ovarian granulosa-like cells via transcription factor overexpression. eLife. 2023;12:e83291.
82. Aisenbrey EA, Murphy WL. Synthetic alternatives to Matrigel. Nat Rev Mater. 2020;5:539–51.
83. Hernandez-Gordillo V, et al. Fully synthetic matrices for in vitro culture of primary human intestinal enteroids and endometrial organoids. Biomaterials. 2020;254:120125.
84. Grigoryan B, et al. Multivascular networks and functional intravascular topologies within biocompatible hydrogels. Science. 2019;464:458–64.
85. Sundaram S, et al. Sacrificial capillary pumps to engineer multiscalar biological forms. Nature. 2024;636:361–7.
86. Brassard JA, Nikolaev M, Hübscher T, Hofer M, Lutolf MP. Recapitulating macro-scale tissue self-organization through organoid bioprinting. Nat Mater. 2021;20:22–9.
87. Heidari Kani M, et al. 3D cell culturing and possibilities for myometrial tissue engineering. Ann Biomed Eng. 2017;45:1746–57.
88. Duan H, et al. Shear-wave sonoelastographic assessment of cervix in pregnancy. Acta Obstet Gynecol Scand. 2020;99:1458–68.
89. Weiss JD, et al. A low-cost, open-source 3D printer for multimaterial and high-throughput direct ink writing of soft and living materials. Adv Mater. 2025;37:2414971.
90. Stankey PP, et al. Embedding biomimetic vascular networks via coaxial sacrificial writing into functional tissue. Adv Mater. 2024;36:2401528.
91. Critchley HOD, et al. Menstruation: science and society. Am J Obstet Gynecol. 2020;223:624–64.
92. Xiao S, et al. A microfluidic culture model of the human reproductive tract and 28-day menstrual cycle. Nat Commun. 2017;8:14584.
93. Ronaldson-Bouchard K, et al. A multi-organ chip with matured tissue niches linked by vascular flow. Nat Biomed Eng. 2022;6:351–71.

Other Engineering Technologies: Systems Biology Approaches for Understanding Maternal–Neonatal Immunology

Caitlin M. Sullivan and Sepideh Dolatshahi

Abstract Pregnancy is a dynamic, multidimensional process requiring precise coordination between maternal, fetal, and placental systems. Traditional reductionist approaches, while valuable, cannot capture the complexity of maternal–neonatal immunology. Systems biology provides a framework to integrate multi-scale data, build predictive models, and design interventions. This chapter introduces systems biology concepts, outlines modeling strategies, and highlights successful applications that include case studies of placental antibody transfer and systems immunology at the maternal–fetal interface.

Keywords Systems biology · Integrative approaches · Maternal–fetal immunology · Computational immunology · Digital twin of a woman · Precision maternal care · Pregnancy modeling · Mechanistic modeling · Data-driven modeling · Transplacental antibody transfer · Biomaterials-systems biology integration · Population heterogeneity · New approach methodologies · Women's health immunoengineering

1 Introduction

Pregnancy presents an immunological paradox. It requires maternal immune tolerance to a semi-allogeneic fetus while maintaining robust defense against infection. This balancing act unfolds dynamically across biological scales—from molecular signaling networks to whole-body adaptations—over the course of gestation. Traditional, reductionist approaches have uncovered many individual mechanisms but fall short of capturing the integrated, systems-level nature of pregnancy immunology.

C. M. Sullivan · S. Dolatshahi (✉)
Department of Biomedical Engineering, University of Virginia, Charlottesville, VA, USA
e-mail: sbq8wb@virginia.edu; sdolatshahi@virginia.edu

S. G. Zambuto, M. L. Oyen (eds.), *Biomaterials for Women's Health Engineering*,
https://doi.org/10.1007/978-3-032-10745-9_24

1.1 Introducing Systems Immunology as a Nascent Discipline

We argue that advancing women's health generally, and particularly at the maternal–fetal interface, requires embracing *systems biology*: a nascent discipline that unites biology, engineering, and computational modeling to understand and predict immune function holistically. Specifically, when dealing with the immune system, with all of its diverse cellular and molecular players, it becomes necessary to take a systems approach. In this chapter, we present not just a set of tools, but a framework for thinking that reflects the future of immunology-informed women's health research.

1.2 Vision and Learning Objectives

Our perspective is shaped by teaching and research at the intersection of immunology and computation. Inspired by the next generation of scientists and engineers, we envision a field where researchers:

1. Explain immune processes at multiple scales and synthesize their integration to produce function.
2. Abstract complex immune biology into quantitative frameworks for holistic, unbiased problem solving.
3. Apply data-driven and mechanistic models to generate actionable insights and design inclusive, personalized solutions.
4. Collaborate confidently across disciplines to design rational, testable interventions.
5. Communicate findings effectively across technical and clinical audiences.

1.3 How This Chapter Delivers on This Vision

This chapter delivers on this vision by using pregnancy and early life immunology as a running example. We show why systems biology is essential for women's health. Beginning with an overview of pregnancy's multi-dimensional biology (Section 2, 3), we then outline the axes of integration that necessitate computational approaches (Section 4, 5) and present a modeling framework that formalizes systems thinking (Section 6). Through case studies of maternal–fetal immunity (Section 7), we demonstrate how data-driven and mechanistic models advance understanding and inform interventions. Finally, we look ahead to future opportunities (Section 8), calling for collaborative, bilingual problem-solvers, who speak in systems biology and immunology languages, to define this evolving discipline.

2 Women's Health and Pregnancy: Dynamic and Multi-Dimensional

Pregnancy is one of the most complex and dynamic physiological states in human biology. It demands immune tolerance to a semi-allogeneic fetus while maintaining effective defense against pathogens, ensuring maternal health, and supporting fetal development. This balancing act unfolds across multiple biological scales—molecular signaling, cellular interactions, tissue remodeling, and systemic hormonal regulation—and follows a precisely orchestrated temporal trajectory.

Traditional biomedical research has approached pregnancy and women's health through reductionist methods, focusing on individual cells, pathways, or molecules in isolation. While these approaches have generated important foundational knowledge, they fall short of capturing the integrated, adaptive nature of maternal–fetal physiology, nor can they capture the broader complexities of women's health.

Women's biology is inherently multi-factorial, shaped by:

- *Hormonal rhythms* that fluctuate during the menstrual cycle and shift dramatically during pregnancy and menopause;
- *Genetic and epigenetic diversity*, including variations in sex chromosomes (e.g., XXY, XYY, and Turner syndrome) and mosaicism that cause differences between tissues, often neglected in large-scale studies;
- *Environmental and behavioral factors*, such as nutritional status, stress, and exposure to endocrine-disrupting chemicals, all of which modulate reproductive milestones and immune function.

As illustrated in Fig. 1, female hormonal profiles are highly dynamic, showing cyclic changes during menstruation and sharp rises in estrogen and progesterone during pregnancy, followed by declines postpartum and later in menopause. Genetics also plays a role in hormonal timing—mothers and daughters often share similar ages of menarche—while lifestyle can delay or accelerate reproductive milestones [14]. For example, elite athletes or women with low body fat may experience delayed onset or secondary amenorrhea, whereas chronic stress and environmental exposures are linked to earlier menarche [27, 29, 42].

These biological complexities translate into sex-specific immune differences. A recent longitudinal systems-level study published in *Nature* [23] demonstrated that testosterone therapy in individuals assigned female at birth attenuates Type I interferon (IFN-I) and, therefore, tumor necrosis factor alpha (TNF-α) responses. Interestingly, it has been reported that men experience more severe SARS-CoV-2 infections due to weaker IFN-I activity and aberrant inflammation characterized by excessive TNF-α [43]. Similarly, women with polycystic ovary syndrome, characterized by androgen excess, also show elevated serum TNF-α [15] and heightened infection risk [11]. In contrast, estrogens have been implicated in autoimmunity, a disease category that disproportionately affects women—approximately 63% of autoimmune disease diagnoses in the United States occur in females [1]. Although

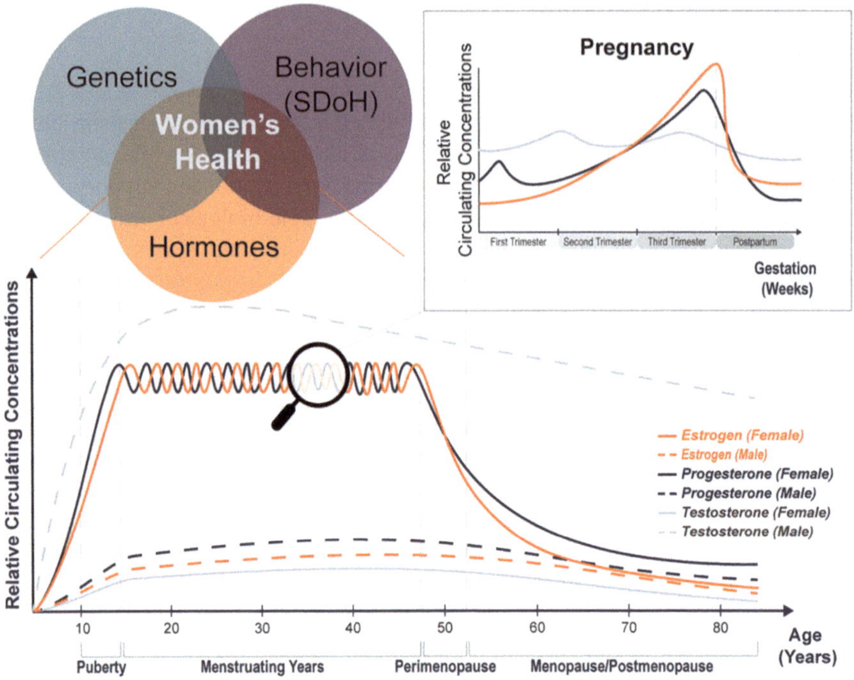

Fig. 1 Women's health as a dynamic interplay of genetics, hormones, and behavior across the lifespan. This schematic illustrates how women's biology is shaped by genetic factors, fluctuating hormone levels, and behavioral and social determinants of health (SDoH). The main graph shows circulating estrogen, progesterone, and testosterone levels in females and males from puberty through menopause (cartoon showing averaged trends across the population), highlighting the cyclic hormonal patterns unique to women. The inset zooms in on pregnancy, where hormone levels rise dramatically to support fetal development and immune adaptation. Together, these factors create a complex, individualized landscape for women's health, underscoring the need for systems-level approaches to study immunity and reproductive biology

mechanisms remain incompletely understood, hormonal regulation is thought to play a critical role in this predisposition [17, 32].

Despite these profound biological differences, female reproductive health remains understudied. In pregnancy, research is particularly challenging: maternal immunity undergoes unique adaptations to support the fetus, and the human placenta's specialized antibody transfer mechanisms cannot be accurately modeled in animals.

This dynamic, multi-dimensional landscape requires tools that can integrate information across molecular, cellular, and physiological scales, capture temporal dynamics that evolve over hours, days, or trimesters, and account for variability between individuals and populations rather than relying on one-size-fits-all assumptions.

Systems biology provides such a framework. By combining experimental data, computational modeling, and engineering principles, systems approaches allow us to study women's health and pregnancy as complex, adaptive systems. In this chapter, we argue that advancing maternal and neonatal health depends on embracing this holistic perspective—an emerging discipline we term *systems immunology*—and demonstrate through case studies how it works synergistically with traditional experimental approaches to address critical gaps in reproductive health.

3 Human Pregnancy is Immunologically Unique

The intricate balance between immune tolerance and defense against pathogens is achieved through *systemic and local immune remodeling*, tightly regulated by placental signals, hormonal changes, and genetic factors. These adaptations unfold dynamically across trimesters, enabling successful implantation, fetal growth, and eventual parturition [2, 5].

3.1 Dynamic Immune Shifts Across Trimesters

Human placentation is exceptional among mammals, characterized by deep trophoblast invasion and prolonged maternal–fetal contact. This anatomical and functional distinctiveness drives complex immune dynamics:

- *Early pregnancy*: Enhanced innate immune activity supports implantation and placental development. Natural killer (NK) cells and monocytes/macrophages dominate the decidual tissue, coordinating vascular remodeling and trophoblast invasion. A controlled pro-inflammatory milieu facilitates endometrial breakdown and embryo implantation.
- *Mid-pregnancy*: Immune function transitions to a tolerogenic state. Placental hormones, particularly progesterone and estrogen, promote the expansion of regulatory T cells (Tregs), suppress effector T cell activity, and skew helper T cell responses toward Th2 dominance. This immune shift coincides with pregnancy-associated remission in several autoimmune diseases, including rheumatoid arthritis and multiple sclerosis.
- *Late pregnancy*: A return to pro-inflammatory signaling prepares the body for labor. Increased cytokine production and innate immune activation drive cervical ripening, membrane rupture, and uterinecontractions [2].

Recent studies using systems-level and machine learning approaches have identified key signaling pathways underpinning these phenotypic switches, offering a holistic view of maternal immune adaptation and enabling the prediction of gestational age [5]. Interestingly, the authors used deep longitudinal immune signaling measurements from a cohort of mothers who delivered at term to build a computational model that could predict gestational age at the time of measurement.

These trimester-specific adaptations are conserved among humans but occur with different timing and depth in other species due to shorter gestations, shallower decidualization, and less invasive placentation. Notably, deep trophoblast invasion in humans enables maternal antibody transfer, a key evolutionary advantage absent in many mammals.

3.2 Systemic Remodeling: Innate and Adaptive Immunity

Pregnancy-associated immune adaptation is not a uniform suppression, but rather a reprogramming of both innate and adaptive immunity:

- *Innate immunity*: Maternal blood during pregnancy contains increased levels of monocytes and neutrophils with enhanced phagocytic activity and complement sensitivity compared to non-pregnant individuals. These changes allow rapid clearance of pathogens, minimizing prolonged inflammation that could endanger the fetus [2].
- *Adaptive immunity*: Regulatory T and B cells expand, while overall circulating T, B, and NK cell frequencies decrease. T lymphocytes exhibit altered signaling profiles, shifting toward tolerance-promoting phenotypes [20].
- *Antibody remodeling*: Pregnancy-induced characteristic changes in immunoglobulin G (IgG) glycosylation, favoring galactosylated and sialylated forms associated with anti-inflammatory activity. These changes may contribute to autoimmune disease remission and modulate vaccine responsiveness [31, 34].

3.3 Microchimerism and Immune Memory

Pregnancy has long-lasting effects on maternal immunity. Fetal microchimerism—the persistence of fetal cells in maternal tissues—alters immune cell composition and may influence future immune responses [28]. These changes suggest that pregnancy shapes maternal immune memory, potentially affecting responses in subsequent pregnancies and long-term maternal health.

3.4 Clinical Implications and Evolutionary Context

Immune remodeling during pregnancy influences both disease susceptibility and maternal–fetal immunity:

- Increased risk of infections such as influenza and listeriosis due to modified adaptive responses.
- Modulation of autoimmune diseases, with some improving (e.g., rheumatoid arthritis) and others worsening for some patients (e.g., systemic lupus erythematosus).
- Optimized maternal-to-fetal antibody transfer, providing passive neonatal protection.

From an evolutionary perspective, these adaptations support fetal tolerance while preserving sufficient immune defense. They also limit the applicability of animal models, making human-centered approaches—including in silico and systems immunology studies—essential for understanding pregnancy immunology.

4 Systems Biology: Foundations and Needs in Women's Health

4.1 What Is Systems Biology?

Systems biology is an integrative research discipline that combines experimental data with computational and mathematical modeling to understand biological processes holistically. Unlike traditional reductionist approaches that focus on single molecules or pathways in isolation, systems biology emphasizes context and interconnectedness, capturing how components of biological systems interact dynamically across multiple scales of time, space, and complexity (Integr Biol, 2012).

Core principles of systems biology include:

- *Multi-scale integration*: Bridging molecular, cellular, tissue, organ, and population-level processes;
- *Network thinking*: Recognizing feedback loops and interdependent signaling pathways;
- *Prediction and hypothesis generation*: Using computational models to simulate outcomes and guide experiments.

This approach complements in vitro and in vivo methods, offering a systemic understanding of physiology and disease. Douglas Lauffenburger and Peter Sorger have described systems biology as analysis along multiple *axes of integration* [24], which we adapt and modify here to the context of women's health (Fig. 2).

4.2 Axes of Integration

Systems biology operates along three major axes of integration that are particularly relevant for reproductive and maternal–fetal health.

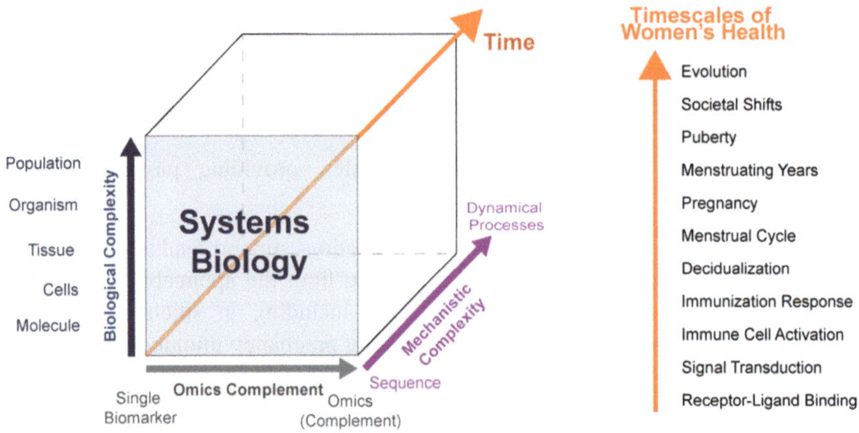

Fig. 2 Axes of integration and timescales relevant to women's health. The left panel illustrates the multi-dimensional nature of systems biology, integrating biological complexity (from molecules to populations), omics complement (from single biomarkers to multi-omics datasets), and mechanistic complexity (from static measurements to dynamic processes evolving over time). This is adapted from: Lauffenburger [24]. The right panel highlights key hormonal, biological, and mechanistic timescales shaping women's health—from rapid molecular signaling events to pregnancy-associated immune adaptations and long-term evolutionary changes. Together, these axes and timescales underscore the need for multi-scale, systems-level approaches to study female physiology and immunity

4.2.1 Holistic Complexity

Holistic complexity (horizontal axis in Fig. 2) refers to the progression from analyzing a single molecule target (gene, transcript, protein) all the way to high-dimensional datasets consisting of the collection of all possible targets (genomics, transcriptomics, proteomics, metabolomics, compendium of clinical data, etc.).

- At lower holistic complexity, research might focus on a single biomarker (e.g., estrogen receptor expression in placental tissue).
- At higher complexity, systems biology leverages entire datasets to uncover emergent relationships (e.g., integrating maternal blood transcriptomics, placental proteomics, and neonatal immune phenotyping to characterize pregnancy complications).

When analyzing "omics" datasets, you can look at single targets of interest or perform differential expression analysis, but the complexity of the data enables more dynamic, high-dimensional analyses. With increasing holistic complexity, you can transition from asking whether a target is expressed to investigating the relationships between targets using methods such as correlation network construction or multivariate regression analysis, where univariate statistical analyses will give way to multivariate statistical learning approaches. Through the comparison of samples from controls and experimental perturbations, unsupervised clustering can help uncover groups of targets in an unbiased manner, and pathway analysis can find whether targets belonging to known biological pathways are perturbed or up- or downregulated in a concerted way.

This axis enables data-driven discovery, revealing patterns and regulatory networks that cannot be inferred from single-target studies. For example, systems serology approaches have uncovered antibody glycosylation features that govern selective maternal-to-fetal IgG transfer—features overlooked by traditional immunology assays focused solely on antibody titer or neutralization. Another example of this is discussed later in this chapter, Case Study 3 (Sect. 7).

4.2.2 Biological Complexity

Biological complexity (Vertical axis in Fig. 2) represents the hierarchical organization of biology—from individual molecules to cells, tissues, organs, and populations. Investigating physiological phenomena and pathologies at various scales allows researchers to gain complementary insights that cannot be captured when studying a single scale in isolation. This integration can involve:

- *Cell-level behavior* driven by molecular properties (e.g., hormone receptor signaling shaping immune cell responses);
- *Tissue and organ-level behavior* emerging from cell properties (e.g., how trophoblast cell invasion remodels uterine vasculature during implantation);
- *Organism-level behavior* dependent on tissue and organ properties (e.g., maternal systemic immune adaptations influenced by placental signaling);
- *Population-level behavior* determined by organismal properties (e.g., variability in pregnancy outcomes shaped by genetic, hormonal, and environmental diversity).

Bridging these spatiotemporal scales is a central goal of systems biology. By coupling multi-scale experimental data with computational modeling, researchers can capture cross-level dependencies and predict emergent behaviors—a rapidly growing field known as multi-scale modeling.

In women's health, this approach is particularly valuable. For example, understanding preterm birth risk requires linking molecular inflammatory signals in uterine tissues, cellular responses of immune populations, organ-level changes in the cervix and placenta, maternal physiological adaptations, and population-level epidemiological patterns. Without integrating these scales, isolated studies may miss critical interactions driving disease susceptibility or treatment response.

4.2.3 Mechanistic Complexity

Mechanistic complexity (Depth axis in Fig. 2) captures the level of detail and dynamical understanding with which biological systems are studied and modeled.

Lauffenburger and Sorger described this axis as spanning from basic information about molecular sequence and structure, through thermodynamic and biochemical interactions, to kinetic and transport processes, and ultimately toward comprehensive models that describe the dynamic operation of entire biological systems [24].

In the context of immunology and women's health, mechanistic complexity also reflects the ability to account for:

- *Cellular origin and maturation*: For example, tracing how regulatory T cells develop in the thymus and adapt during pregnancy;
- *Spatial dynamics*: Modeling how immune cells traffic between the bone marrow, blood, decidua, and placenta to regulate maternal–fetal tolerance;
- *Multi-layered signaling and feedback*: Capturing receptor–ligand binding, cytokine gradients, and intracellular pathways that coordinate responses over time;
- *Systems-level immune dynamics*: Integrating these mechanisms into predictive models that simulate maternal immune adaptations or fetal antibody acquisition across gestation.

Progression along this axis transforms static, descriptive snapshots into quantitative, dynamic representations of biological processes. For instance, understanding maternal vaccine efficacy requires more than knowing which antibody subclasses are produced—it demands mechanistic models that capture the kinetics of B cell activation, transport across placental barriers, and competition for Fc receptor binding, ultimately predicting antibody transfer to the fetus.

Mechanistic complexity is therefore essential to translate immune biology into actionable interventions, providing a systems-level view of how cellular and molecular mechanisms collectively shape maternal and neonatal health.

All of these axes have the concept of temporal dynamics intertwined (red arrow). Naturally, complexity increases as we look over a longer period of time. This is illustrated by hormonal dynamics (Fig. 1), where changes are occurring on various timescales guided by the menstrual cycle, pregnancy, and reproductive capability (e.g., puberty and menopause). More broadly, we can think about complexity as a function of time in the context of molecular half-life (seconds–weeks), duration of cell–cell interactions (milliseconds–days), tissue and organ system mechanisms and processes (minutes–months), phenotypic changes (seconds–years), and evolutionary changes (decades–millenniums) (Fig. 1, right).

Together, these axes of integration provide the multidimensional lens required to understand the interplay of hormones, immunity, genetics, and environment in women's health.

4.3 Why Women's Health Needs Systems Approaches

Historically, women have been underrepresented in biomedical research, and datasets that capture pregnancy dynamics holistically are sparse. Complex feedback between maternal immune responses, endocrine regulation, and fetal development cannot be fully explained by reductionist studies or by animal models that fail to replicate human-specific features.

Human pregnancy itself is a compelling case study for systems approaches.

- A healthy pregnancy requires precisely timed immune and hormonal adaptations, where local immune tolerance coexists with systemic defense mechanisms.
- Reductionist models have struggled to explain multifactorial outcomes such as preterm birth or altered vaccine responses in pregnancy.
- Past tragedies, such as the thalidomide crisis, highlight how traditional preclinical models failed to predict teratogenic effects in humans due to species differences in placental biology and fetal development [22, 38].

Systems biology offers a solution:

- Virtual clinical studies can safely explore drug effects and immunization strategies in protected populations such as pregnant women.
- Computational models can account for temporal and inter-individual variability, integrating clinical, omics, and imaging data.
- Predictive, system-level analyses can inform personalized interventions, such as optimal timing of maternal vaccination or drug dosing.

While traditional experimental methods remain indispensable, they naturally complement systems approaches. When integrated across axes of holistic, biological, and mechanistic complexity, systems biology provides the framework needed to address multifactorial, dynamic challenges in women's health and pregnancy.

5 Technological Advances Enabling Systems Biology

To some extent, we have all been systems biologists in our thinking; we might have marveled at the interconnected nature of ecological systems in the world and how the extinction or introduction of a single species can have major consequences on the overall ecosystem. We have wondered about homeostasis in biology and how feedback systems might enable it. We might have discovered that changing the abundance of a single molecule might totally change our understanding of the system from not being sensitive to that molecule (due to being saturated) to now being directly modulated by it. In our scientific pursuits about biology, traditional reductionist experiments have been essential for identifying precise components and mechanisms within biological systems. However, they often lack the ability to contextualize these components, capturing their downstream and upstream signaling effects and the system-wide consequences of their interactions. Systems biology has emerged as a discipline precisely to bridge this gap, enabled by technological advances and interdisciplinary innovation that allow researchers to interrogate biology at unprecedented depth and scale.

5.1 Scientific Frontiers Enabling Systems Approaches

In *A First Course in Systems Biology*, Eberhard O. Voit describes the "confluence and synergism of three scientific frontiers" as the driving force behind the emergence of systems biology [37].

5.1.1 Frontier 1: Data Explosion Across Biological Scales

- Landmark achievements such as the *Human Genome Project (2003), Human Microbiome Project (2013)*, and ongoing initiatives like the *Human Cell Atlas* and *Human Protein Atlas* have generated vast reference datasets.
- Advances in *next-generation sequencing* revolutionized genomics and transcriptomics, allowing for high-throughput, parallel analysis of RNA and DNA.
- Today, researchers can probe epigenetics, chromatin accessibility, and spatial transcriptomics at *single-cell and even single-nucleus resolution*, capturing unprecedented detail on gene regulation and cell–cell communication.

5.1.2 Frontier 2: Interdisciplinary Technological Innovation

- Instrumentation and experimental platforms now enable multi-modal profiling of biological systems.
- High-throughput omics technologies—genomics, proteomics, metabolomics, and epigenomics—deliver multidimensional datasets essential for systems-level analysis.
- Single-cell technologies and spatial omics (e.g., multiplexed imaging and spatially resolved RNA sequencing) reveal cellular heterogeneity and tissue organization in complex sites like the placenta and decidua.
- Advanced biomaterials and organ-on-chip models allow controlled studies of maternal–fetal interfaces, overcoming limitations of traditional cell culture and animal models.
- Imaging and biosensors enable longitudinal monitoring, capturing dynamic processes over time.

5.1.3 Frontier 3: Computational and Statistical Methods

- The deluge of high-dimensional data necessitates robust computational methods for integration and interpretation.
- Coding languages such as Python, R, and MATLAB have evolved to support bioinformatics and systems biology, offering specialized tools such as:

  - *Seurat* for single-cell data analysis;
  - *Gene Set Enrichment Analysis* for pathway discovery;
  - *Bioinformatics Toolbox* in MATLAB for large-scale omics workflows.
- Machine learning and mechanistic modeling techniques enable hypothesis generation, feature selection, and predictive simulations that would be infeasible with traditional statistical tools alone.

5.2 *Implications for Women's Health*

Hormonal regulation, genetic diversity, and environmental factors profoundly shape female physiology, yet these relationships remain vastly understudied. Technological advances now allow unbiased, exploratory, hypothesis-generating analyses that can directly address these gaps.

A prime example is the application of spatially resolved single-cell transcriptomics to study placenta accreta spectrum (PAS) disorder [4], revealing localized molecular disruptions that traditional histology and bulk transcriptomics could not detect.

By combining rich, multi-scale datasets, advanced experimental platforms, and powerful computational models, systems biology provides the necessary toolkit to dissect women's health and pregnancy as complex, adaptive systems, paving the way for precision medicine and safer maternal interventions.

6 Computational Modeling in Systems Immunology in a Nutshell

Understanding complex biological systems like maternal–fetal immunity requires tools that can integrate diverse data types, reveal hidden patterns, and predict system behavior under different conditions. Computational modeling serves this role, bridging experimental observations and mechanistic understanding.

Modeling typically begins with a clear biological or clinical question: Which maternal immune factors predict neonatal outcomes? How do hormones and immune signals interact dynamically during pregnancy? Which interventions—such as maternal vaccines—can most effectively protect newborns? When is the optimal time to administer vaccines with the goal of maximizing the total antibody transferred to the newborn?

Answering these questions is the goal of the modeling effort and involves selecting the right data types and structure. Longitudinal studies track changes across trimesters; cross-sectional datasets provide snapshots of immune or hormonal states.

Bulk assays capture averaged signals, whereas single-cell and spatial technologies uncover heterogeneity at the maternal–fetal interface. Incorporating clinical metadata such as maternal age, stress, or comorbidities enriches modeling by capturing population-level variability.

The next step is choosing a modeling strategy. Broadly, computational models fall into two complementary categories or "flavors," which often work synergistically to characterize and quantify biological processes (Fig. 3).

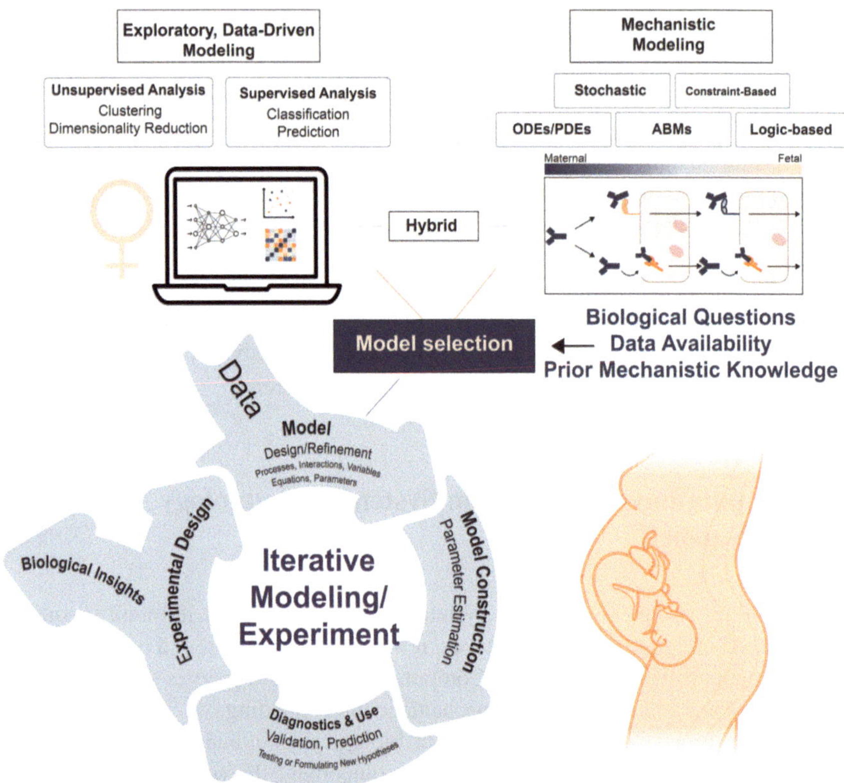

Fig. 3 How computational models help us understand pregnancy and immunity. Scientists can study complex processes like maternal–fetal immunity using two main types of computational models. Data-driven exploratory models (left) search for patterns in large datasets, helping predict outcomes such as preterm birth or vaccine response. Mechanistic models (right) use biological knowledge to simulate how immune cells and antibodies behave over time, exploring "what if" scenarios that are difficult to test experimentally. Choosing between these approaches depends on the questions asked, the data available, and how much is already known about the biology. Both modeling styles feed into an iterative cycle (bottom left, adapted from Chou et al. [7]) where experiments and simulations inform each other, gradually refining our understanding and leading to better ways to protect maternal and newborn health

6.1 Exploratory, Data-Driven Modeling

Exploratory models uncover patterns in high-dimensional datasets without assuming prior mechanistic knowledge. These approaches are particularly powerful for analyzing high-dimensional datasets typical in immunology, such as flow cytometry, single-cell RNA sequencing (scRNA-seq), or multiplex antibody profiling.

- *Statistical learning techniques*—such as clustering, principal component analysis (PCA), partial least squares regression (PLSR), and network inference—are primarily used for hypothesis generation and biological interpretation. These methods can identify immune cell subsets or signaling pathways associated with pregnancy outcomes.
- *Machine learning approaches*—including random forests, gradient boosting, support vector machines, and deep neural networks—excel at predictive tasks, finding non-linear relationships that are difficult to capture with classical statistics. For example, machine learning models can integrate omics data, clinical measurements, and imaging to predict preterm birth risk or response to vaccination.
- *Emerging artificial intelligence (AI) and large language models (LLMs)*—Recent advances in AI, particularly transformer-based models and foundation models trained on large biomedical datasets, offer new ways to analyze complex biological information. LLMs can synthesize heterogeneous data sources (literature, omics, imaging, and clinical notes), support automated hypothesis generation, and even assist in model selection or parameter estimation. While still in early stages for maternal–fetal research, these tools hold promise for accelerating discovery and enabling more adaptive, real-time computational modeling.

An alternative way to categorize these methods is to group them into supervised and unsupervised methods. Supervised methods (e.g., logistic regression, support vector machines, decision trees, random forests, and neural networks) predict outcomes from labeled data—such as classifying preterm versus full-term deliveries from maternal serology. Regression-based methods predict continuous variables, for example, estimating gestational age from clinical and immunological features. Unsupervised methods (e.g., clustering algorithms like k-means, dimensionality reduction techniques such as PCA) uncover structure in unlabeled data. In maternal–fetal immunology, unsupervised analyses have revealed progressive antibody profile shifts during pregnancy, which were then refined using supervised discriminant analyses to pinpoint drivers of altered neonatal immunity.

These approaches are particularly useful for identifying candidate biomarkers and generating hypotheses that can later be tested experimentally or formalized in mechanistic models.

6.2 Mechanistic Modeling

Mechanistic models are built on established biological knowledge, using mathematical representations of components and interactions. These models are particularly suited for studying immunology, where dynamic, multi-compartment processes (e.g., immune cell trafficking, cytokine signaling, and antibody transfer) are key to understanding outcomes. These models explicitly represent biological processes using mathematical formulations.

Different classes of mechanistic models are used depending on the question:

- *Ordinary differential equations (ODEs)* capture temporal dynamics (e.g., B cell maturation and IgG placental transfer).
- *Partial differential equations* incorporate both time and spatial gradients (e.g., modeling inflammation spreading through placental tissue).
- *Agent-based models (ABMs)* simulate discrete behaviors of interacting cells, such as germinal center dynamics.
- *Boolean or logic-based models* describe gene regulatory networks using on/off rules.
- *Stochastic models* account for randomness, particularly important in systems with low molecular counts or probabilistic cell decisions.
- *Constraint-based models* map metabolic pathways under biochemical constraints.

Hybrid approaches combine these frameworks—for instance, an ODE model of antibody kinetics coupled with an ABM of immune cell interactions. This combination can yield both quantitative predictions (amount of antibody transferred) and qualitative classifications (good vs. poor transfer) based on how antibodies elicit antibody-mediated effector function in fetal immune cells.

Mechanistic models offer unique predictive power. They allow researchers to test virtual interventions, such as changing vaccination timing or altering receptor expression, which cannot be readily studied in humans. This is particularly valuable in pregnancy research, where ethical and logistical constraints limit experimental approaches.

A landmark example of mechanistic modeling in maternal–fetal immunity is the transplacental IgG transfer model developed by our group [39]. Built from ODEs, this model describes receptor-mediated transport of IgG subclasses through placental syncytiotrophoblasts and endothelial cells and is further described in Case Study 2.

6.3 From Data to Insight: The Iterative Modeling Cycle

Regardless of approach, computational modeling is an iterative process. It begins with a well-defined biological or clinical question and available data. Models are designed to match the system's scale and complexity—simple Boolean models may suffice for signaling networks, while multi-compartment ODEs better capture pharmacokinetics or immune responses.

Model calibration uses experimental or clinical datasets to estimate parameters. Cross-validation and sensitivity analyses then test robustness and highlight which parameters most strongly influence outcomes. New hypotheses generated by the model guide further experiments, which, in turn, refine and validate the model. This cycle—*data* → *model* → *hypothesis* → *experiment/clinical study* → *new data*—enables continuous learning about complex biological systems.

6.4 Complementarity of Approaches

In practice, data-driven and mechanistic modeling are not separate silos. Exploratory analysis of high-dimensional immune data can identify key regulators or pathways driving biological responses, which are then incorporated into mechanistic models, providing a testbed for hypothesis testing and prediction. Conversely, mechanistic simulations generate synthetic data that guide machine learning feature selection or inform personalized predictions.

In maternal–fetal immunology, combining these approaches is particularly powerful. Data-driven clustering can stratify patients by immune profiles linked to preterm birth, while mechanistic models simulate how altering cytokine signaling or vaccine timing could shift these profiles. Together, they offer a systems-level toolkit to understand and eventually engineer immune responses during pregnancy.

7 Case Studies: Systems Immunology for Maternal–Fetal Health

In this section, we present three case studies (Fig. 4) that collectively illustrate how systems approaches reshape our understanding of maternal–fetal immunity and inform actionable strategies for women's health.

- *Case Study 1* uses systems serology and data-driven modeling to uncover molecular determinants of selective antibody transfer from mother to fetus.
- *Case Study 2* builds on these discoveries with a mechanistic computational model that predicts neonatal antibody levels and informs vaccination strategies.
- *Case Study 3* showcases how single-cell and spatial transcriptomics reveal localized drivers of placental disorders, challenging decades-old hypotheses.

Together, these studies demonstrate an iterative, integrative process central to systems immunology: exploratory data-driven analyses identify key features, mechanistic models explain and predict biological dynamics, and multi-scale high-resolution data capture spatial and temporal heterogeneity and, in turn, reveal additional

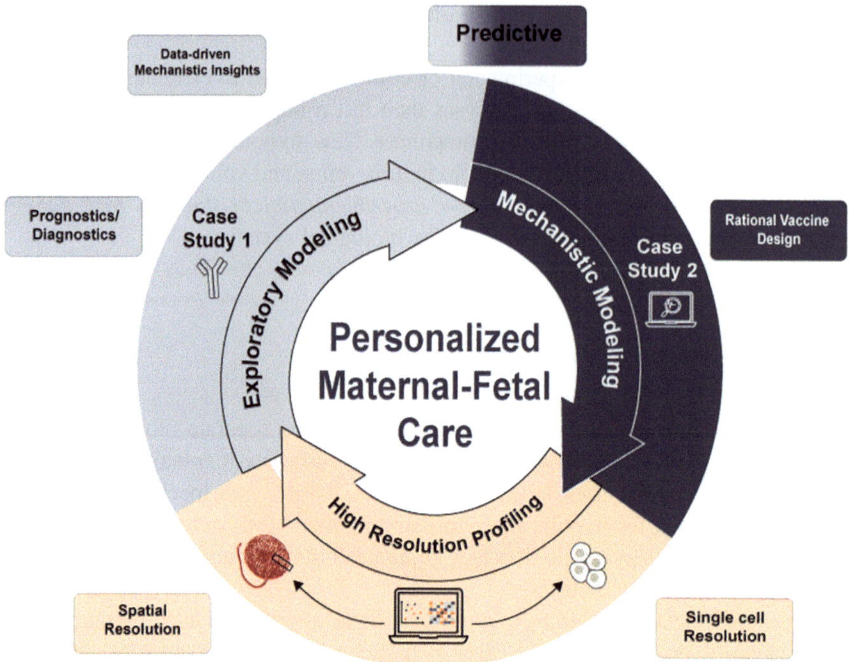

Fig. 4 Synergistic modeling approaches enabling personalized maternal–fetal care. This framework illustrates how three case studies—exploratory data-driven modeling (Case Study 1), mechanistic modeling (Case Study 2), and high-resolution spatial and single-cell profiling (Case Study 3)—inform each other to advance predictive and personalized maternal–fetal care. High-dimensional profiling supports biomarker discovery and diagnostics, data-driven analyses generate mechanistic hypotheses, and mechanistic models guide experimental design and rational intervention strategies such as vaccine optimization

mechanistic insights afforded by single-cell resolution. This approach lays the foundation for rational design of interventions, predictive diagnostics, and ultimately, a digital twin of pregnancy for personalized maternal–fetal care. Eventually, adaptive digital twins of women would allow the integration of various sex-specific hormonal, genetic, and behavioral insights at various scales from molecular-cellular to women-specific organs to population levels.

7.1 Unbiased Analysis of Snapshot Data—Systems Serology Reveals Selective Antibody Transfer

Infants face heightened vulnerability to infections during early life due to an immature adaptive immune system and limited vaccine responsiveness. Transplacental IgG transfer provides crucial passive immunity during this period and underpins the rationale for maternal immunization strategies. Current centers for disease control and prevention (CDC) guidelines recommend Tdap and influenza vaccination in the third trimester to boost maternal antibodies for neonatal protection, and similar strategies have been explored for COVID-19, seasonal flu, RSV, and other pathogens.

For decades, these guidelines, as well as general vaccine development efforts (for non-pregnant populations), were informed by simple titer measurements and neutralization function of antibodies as measured in maternal and fetal blood at birth. Systems serology provided a transformative, data-driven lens to reveal these determinants [3, 8]. By profiling high-dimensional antibody features—antigen specificity, Fc receptor binding, glycosylation states, and effector functions—systems serology enabled an unbiased analysis of maternal–fetal antibody transfer followed by data-driven computational analysis to identify patterns and develop data-driven hypotheses about the mechanisms of transplacental antibody transfer.

In a landmark study [19], with the objective of defining features that promote or impede transfer, paired maternal and cord blood samples from Tdap-vaccinated women were analyzed with multi-level partial least squares discriminant analysis, revealing that antibodies with enhanced NK cell activation and neutrophil phagocytosis were preferentially transferred, whereas those mediating monocyte phagocytosis were largely retained in maternal circulation. We used orthogonalized PLSR (OPLSR) and identified Fc glycosylation as a major driver of transfer efficiency, with digalactosylated IgG enriched in cord blood, while agalactosylated species were retained in maternal blood.

Subsequent work by our group extended these findings to special populations:

- *Maternal HIV infection* alters antibody Fc profiles and selectively impairs transfer efficiency [12].
- *Preterm birth* reduces overall IgG transfer, disproportionately affecting certain antibody functions [13].

Together, these studies showed that placental antibody transfer is not a simple bulk filtration process but a selective, functionally tuned mechanism. This case study exemplifies a core tenet of systems immunology: exploratory, unbiased modeling identifies hidden molecular determinants. However, in these studies, the understanding of antibody transfer was based on static comparisons of maternal and cord blood antibody titers at delivery. While foundational, this approach could not capture the nuanced selectivity of IgG transport across the placenta. As we summarized in our recent review [40], the placental transfer process is influenced by multiple dynamically changing placental and maternal regulators. Data-driven exploratory modeling based on systems serology laid the foundation for mechanistic frameworks by identifying the features—Fc glycan profiles, Fc receptor affinities, and effector functions—that should be incorporated into predictive models of antibody transfer (Case Study 2).

Mechanistic predictive modeling—informed by data-driven hypotheses resulting from exploratory analyses—can capture temporal dynamics, test hypotheses about molecular regulators, and provide a predictive framework for optimizing maternal vaccine strategies.

7.2 *Make Room for In Silico Modeling: Predicting Dynamics and Personalizing Maternal Immunization*

While systems serology uncovered key molecular determinants of placental IgG transfer (Case Study 1), these insights were derived from static, cross-sectional measurements at birth. A mechanistic, time-resolved understanding of transfer dynamics remained elusive, largely because experimental approaches to study this process throughout pregnancy are limited. The barriers to experimental studies in this space include inter-species differences, ethical and logistical constraints, and the vast inter-person variability across the human population:

- *Species differences*: Common animal models diverge significantly from human pregnancy. Mice transfer most IgG postnatally through breastmilk, and even non-human primates lack deep trophoblast invasion and human-specific Fc receptor expression. More generally and related to women's health, while humans have a menstrual cycle, mice have an estrous cycle, and rather than menstruate, they reabsorb their endometrial lining if conception does not occur [6, 30].
- *Ethical and logistical constraints*: Direct longitudinal sampling of fetal blood in pregnant women is rare, with most dynamic data coming from older cordocentesis studies.
- *Clinical variability*: Human pregnancies differ widely in placental architecture, Fc receptor expression, and maternal immune status, complicating generalized empirical conclusions.

These limitations underscore the need for human-centric, predictive computational approaches to predict how maternal vaccination and biological variability influence antibody transfer.

To address this gap, we developed the first quantitative mechanistic model of human placental IgG transfer [39]. The model encodes known biology into a system of ODEs describing IgG subclass transport across the placental barrier. In addition to the established role of the neonatal Fc receptor (FcRn) in antibody transfer, other non-canonical antibody Fc-binding receptors, namely, Fc gamma receptors (FcγRs), were included in this model. The model consisted of three compartments: syncytiotrophoblast (STB) layer that modeled FcRn-mediated IgG binding and transcytosis, the Interstitial stroma that accounted for diffusion between STB and fetal endothelium, and the endothelial cell (EC) layer, which incorporated FcγRIIb-mediated transcytosis, whose contribution to subclass selectivity was previously unclear. This model also captured competition among IgG1–4 for receptor-mediated transport.

Model parameters were estimated from cordocentesis data [25] and published receptor binding kinetic parameters. Iterative calibration using CaliPro [21] refined parameter ranges to fit these data, while sensitivity analysis using Latin hypercube sampling and OPLSR identified the most influential regulators of transfer in terms of quantity and diversity.

An important feature of mechanistic modeling is to further refine our mechanistic understanding by revealing new mechanisms or narrowing down the set of mechanistic hypotheses that were previously thought to be plausible. Here, among the most notable findings of the model, FcγRIIb was identified as a key regulator of transplacental antibody transfer. The model reproduced the known IgG subclass transfer hierarchy (IgG1 > IgG3 > = IgG4 > IgG2) [9], which could not be explained by FcRn alone due to the similar affinity of FcRn to all subclasses. In silico knockout of the FcRn in ECs showed that even in the absence of FcRn, the well-documented IgG transfer hierarchy can be captured. The role of this low-affinity FcR was previously observed but thought to be minor in comparison with FcRn [18].

Another key finding afforded by the mechanistic modeling process was the observation that IgG subclasses compete for shared Fc receptor binding sites, affecting transfer efficiency. This model-driven hypothesis can have important implications when thinking about the maternal pool of antibodies that have accumulated due to their lifelong exposures and vaccination history, culminating in the IgG subclass proportions present during their pregnancy. These proportions vary from mother to mother and affect the transfer of antibodies to their newborns and can be considered when designing personalized prenatal vaccines.

In vitro validation for this subclass competition phenomenon was performed in parallel using human umbilical vein endothelial cells. These experiments confirmed that subclass-specific transfer efficiency is modulated not only by abundance but also by FcR expression and affinity, particularly in instances where FcRs are limited.

In addition to identifying molecular regulators of transfer, mechanistic modeling can be used as an in silico testbed to translate these mechanistic insights into actionable strategies by testing therapeutic interventions and vaccines. To that end, we augmented the IgG transfer model of the placenta with a representation of maternal immune kinetics post-vaccination, adapted from established plasma cell activation and IgG secretion models [10, 41] that were fitted to TDAP vaccination data [35]. Simulations of maternal immunization at 10, 20, and 30 weeks of gestation showed that second-trimester vaccination (~25 weeks) achieved higher fetal IgG levels at birth than the current third-trimester CDC recommendation.

Our model revealed additional actionable insights, such as personalized vaccination strategies by incorporating other sources of inter-patient variability besides gestational length. These include, and are not limited to, the relative role of variability in placental FcR expression and maternal IgG Fc glycosylation in transfer. In addition to timing, vaccination dosing and formulation, which could, in turn, modulate the IgG titer and affinity through modifying Fc glycosylation, can be tested with this in silico framework. As the mechanistic model matures with respect to the mechanistic accuracy and complexity, these insights can be further relied upon for rational vaccine design strategies and in silico clinical trials.

This work illustrates how mechanistic models complement exploratory systems serology. Data-driven analyses (Case Study 1) identified molecular features that influence transfer. Mechanistic ODE models (Case Study 2) integrated these features into a dynamic, predictive framework. Together, they provide a foundation for rational maternal vaccine design, enabling safe exploration of personalized immunization strategies that account for gestational timing, receptor expression heterogeneity, and population-level variability. This human-centered, computational approach embodies the essence of systems immunology: leveraging mathematical models to safely accelerate therapeutic innovation where traditional experimentation is limited.

Having said that, antibody transfer and maternal–fetal immunity involve more than circulating molecules and receptor-mediated transport. Placental function and pregnancy disorders such as PAS are influenced by cellular heterogeneity, tissue microenvironments, and spatial organization—layers of complexity not captured by bulk serology or compartmental models alone.

Recent advances in *single-cell and spatially resolved transcriptomics* have opened a new frontier: the ability to profile cellular ecosystems at the maternal–fetal interface with unprecedented resolution. In the next case study (Case Study 3), we highlight how these technologies and computational analysis have redefined our understanding of PAS disorder pathogenesis, illustrating the future of multi-scale, systems-level approaches to women's reproductive immunology.

7.3 Heterogeneity Matters: High-Resolution Profiling Unveils Local Drivers of Pathology

PAS disorders, characterized by abnormal placental adherence and invasion, are a leading cause of maternal morbidity and mortality. Traditionally, PAS has been attributed to excessive trophoblast invasion, a view shaped by histological observations and limited bulk assays. However, this reductionist perspective has failed to explain why PAS incidence continues to rise or why clinical severity varies so markedly between patients.

From Single-Cell Resolution to Spatial Context: A paradigm shift began with single-cell transcriptomic profiling of healthy human placentation. The foundational atlas by Vento-Tormo and colleagues [36] revealed unexpected complexity at the maternal–fetal interface: diverse trophoblast, decidual, and immune cell subsets dynamically interacting to support implantation and tolerance. This high-resolution view laid the groundwork for interrogating pathological states like PAS.

Afshar et al. [4] advanced this approach by combining scRNA-seq and spatially resolved transcriptomics to profile placental tissues from PAS patients and controls [4]. Computational pipelines (Seurat, Harmony, UMAP clustering) characterized cellular composition and transcriptional states, while gene set enrichment analyses identified pathway-level dysregulation. Analysis and synthesis of these data revealed that decidual and endothelial cells in PAS lesions had altered expression of genes related to angiogenesis, cytoskeletal remodeling, and adhesion. Spatial mapping revealed localized matrix changes, including collagen (COL3A1) deposition and focal EGFL6 expression, suggesting microenvironmental remodeling rather than global trophoblast over-invasion. Pathway enrichments varied site-specifically, indicating regional vascular signaling disruptions that influence abnormal placental attachment.

These findings highlight intra- and inter-patient heterogeneity as a central feature of PAS pathophysiology. Such variability may explain differing clinical presentations and inform why uniform treatment strategies often fall short.

This work showcases how technological advances—single-cell resolution, spatially resolved transcriptomics, and integrative computational pipelines—enable systems-level insights into pregnancy disorders. Specifically, computational analysis of spatial and single-cell data enabled the mechanistic hypothesis that localized vascular and stromal signaling shifts drive adhesion defects. Cross-scale integration in this work connected molecular and cellular phenotypes to population-level obstetric risk factors. Future predictive modeling can inform precision interventions by identifying region-specific targets for diagnostics or localized therapies to mitigate PAS severity.

As multi-omics data grows richer and more accessible, data-driven and mechanistic modeling can be fused, linking molecular and cellular heterogeneity, tissue microenvironmental structure, and whole-pregnancy outcomes across diverse populations.

Such multi-scale integration embodies the next frontier of systems immunology, extending beyond molecular transport models (Case Study 2) to cellular ecosystems and spatial tissue dynamics that underlie complex pregnancy disorders.

Together, these examples highlight the core principles of systems immunology:

- Integration of multi-dimensional data;
- Iterative synergy between data-driven discovery and mechanistic modeling;
- Cross-scale reasoning that connects molecules, cells, tissues, and whole-pregnancy outcomes;
- A human-centered approach that accounts for variability across individuals and populations.

By uniting these approaches, systems immunology provides a quantitative, holistic, and predictive framework for understanding pregnancy and advancing women's health. This discipline bridges gaps left by traditional experimental models, accelerates therapeutic design, and moves us closer to a future where personalized maternal care—including digital twins of pregnancy—is not only possible but routine.

8 Bluesky: Bridging the Gaps and Unmet Needs

8.1 Immunoengineering to the Rescue: Advancing Women's Health with Systems Biology

Women's health is chronically underfunded and historically overlooked, resulting in persistent knowledge gaps in reproductive health and pregnancy research. As of 2020, only 5% of global research and development funding was allocated to women's health, with a mere 4% focused on conditions unrelated to fertility or cancer [26].

In the aftermath of the thalidomide crisis, the Food and Drug Administration (FDA) issued guidance that effectively excluded most premenopausal women from clinical trials for decades. This policy, aimed at protecting fetal safety, unintentionally created a massive data void. Even after the 1993 mandate requiring women's inclusion in clinical trials, inequities persist. A 2022 Harvard Medical School study reported that women remain underrepresented in trials for cardiovascular disease, mental health disorders, and cancer, which are the leading causes of morbidity in women [33].

This underrepresentation is compounded by insufficient diversity in datasets, which often fail to capture critical variables such as sex, race, and hormonal status (e.g., perimenopausal, pregnant, and postmenopausal). For pregnancy specifically, the lack of longitudinal maternal–fetal datasets has slowed the development of effective, evidence-based interventions.

Despite growing recognition of sex-based biological differences, much of biomedical research remains grounded in male physiology. For example, immune responses to vaccines may vary with menstrual cycle phase [16], yet this phenomenon remains poorly studied and rarely incorporated into immunization strategies.

8.2 *Precision Medicine and the Promise of Digital Twins*

The emerging field of precision medicine aims to tailor healthcare based on a person's genetics, hormonal milieu, environmental exposures, and SDoH. This approach could dramatically benefit women's health, particularly in reproductive medicine.

Systems biology, with its ability to integrate high-dimensional, multi-scale data, offers the analytical framework needed to develop predictive models for personalized care. For instance, combining genomics, immunoprofiling, hormone dynamics, and clinical metadata could guide individualized preventive screening schedules or optimal maternal vaccination timing.

Convergence with AI and digital twin technologies amplifies this potential. A *digital twin of a woman* (Fig. 5)—a computational model that dynamically simulates an individual's physiology, taking into account the woman-specific hormonal, genetic, and social and environmental determinants of health—can enable:

- In silico experimentation to explore interventions safely;
- Risk stratification and real-time monitoring during pregnancy;
- Personalized clinical decision-making, for example, dosing for immunotherapies or contraceptives.

This approach could transform the diagnosis and treatment of conditions like endometriosis, which currently require invasive exploratory surgery for confirmation, or help predict adverse pregnancy outcomes early enough for clinical intervention.

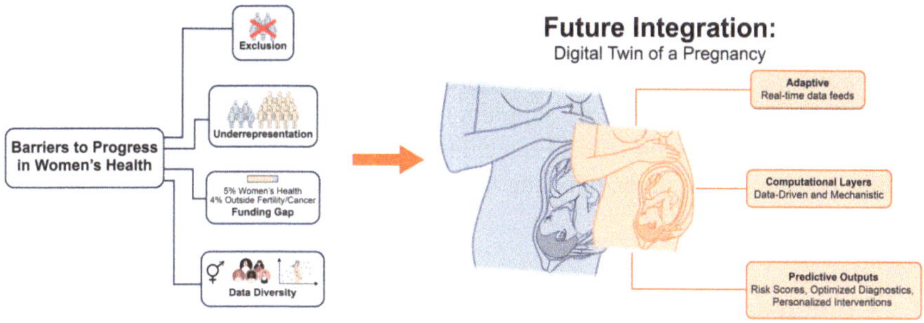

Fig. 5 Vision for a digital twin of pregnancy. Overcoming systemic barriers in women's health research—exclusion, underrepresentation, funding gaps, and limited data diversity—opens the door to a future where real-time data streams feed into advanced computational models, enabling adaptive digital twins that predict risk, guide diagnostics, and deliver personalized interventions for every pregnancy

8.3 Systems Biology and Biomaterials—A Convergent Frontier

Systems biology is primed to address complexity and the interplay of genetics, hormones, and behavior in women's health. Similarly, biomaterials research naturally demands integration across biological, mechanistic, and time scales to capture in vivo relevance. Earlier in the year, the FDA announced phasing out mandatory animal testing for certain monoclonal antibodies, and the National Institutes of Health announced that it would no longer fund studies with animal models only. Both committed more focus and funding for the development of new approach methodologies (NAMs): organoids, organ-on-a-chip, and computational models. While biomaterials and systems biology approaches still need much work to better recapitulate the in vivo context, the convergence of systems biology and biomaterials research offers an exciting frontier for accelerating discovery and therapeutic innovation. While biomaterials provide the physical scaffolds or delivery vehicles for intervention, systems biology supplies the computational and multi-omic frameworks to rationally guide their design, predict biological responses, and optimize outcomes.

Mechanistic and data-driven models can narrow down the immune pathways or tissue signals to target, revealing critical spatiotemporal cues needed for immune modulation during pregnancy. For example, insights from models of maternal Fc receptor-mediated antibody transfer or combinatorial cytokine signaling that influence the transfer of immunity from mothers to infants can shape the release kinetics of Fc-bearing nanoparticles or tunable release of immunomodulators in nanoparticle or hydrogel platforms. Conversely, biomaterials themselves can be used as sensors or perturbation tools—delivering barcoded payloads or capturing longitudinal biosignals—to generate the high-dimensional datasets required for robust modeling.

As next-generation in vitro platforms (e.g., placenta-on-chip) and maternal–fetal digital twins gain traction, integrating these tools into coherent, predictive frameworks to *iterate* on therapeutic interventions before human clinical trials holds grand potential. Together, this synergy supports the design of more physiologically relevant models, facilitates preclinical screening of biomaterial-based therapeutics, and enables precision immunoengineering tailored to maternal and neonatal needs.

9 Conclusion

The study of maternal–fetal immunology sits at the intersection of complexity and consequence. The immune system in pregnancy should balance tolerating the semi-allogeneic fetus while defending against pathogens to preserve maternal health. The inherent dynamic, multiscale, and deeply context-dependent complexity of reproductive health requires the integrative power of systems biology. This chapter introduced the principles and applications of systems biology, emphasizing that it is both a mindset and a toolkit that thrives on integration, inter-personal heterogeneity, and an iterative experimental-computational process. Through case studies, we illustrated how computational models can predict antibody transfer, reveal heterogeneity in the maternal–fetal interface, and guide interventions such as maternal vaccination.

Looking ahead, synergies between systems biology and biomaterials represent a powerful frontier. Mechanistic models and multi-scale simulations can inform the rational design of biomaterials by predicting how cells and tissues respond to topography, stiffness, or cytokine release over time. Conversely, engineered biomaterials can serve as structured platforms for generating high-quality, longitudinal data that calibrate and validate these models. For example, pregnancy-on-a-chip systems could simulate the maternal–fetal interface under different immunological or hormonal conditions, offering a testbed for in silico and experimental co-discovery. In this way, the relatively young disciplines of modeling and materials can co-evolve in the pursuit of predictive, personalized maternal care.

References

1. Abend AH, He I, Bahroos N, Christianakis S, Crew AB, Wise LM, Lipori GP, He X, Murphy SN, Herrick CD, Avasarala J, Weiner MG, Zelko JS, Matute-Arcos E, Abajian M, Payne PRO, Lai AM, Davis HA, Hoberg AA, Fairweather D. Estimation of prevalence of autoimmune diseases in the United States using electronic health record data. J Clin Invest. 2025;135(4) https://doi.org/10.1172/JCI178722.
2. Abu-Raya B, Michalski C, Sadarangani M, Lavoie PM. Maternal immunological adaptation during normal pregnancy. Front Immunol. 2020;11:575197. https://doi.org/10.3389/fimmu.2020.575197. PMID: 33133091; PMCID: PMC7579415.

3. Ackerman ME, Barouch DH, Alter G. Systems serology for evaluation of HIV vaccine trials. Immunol Rev. 2017;275(1):262–70. https://doi.org/10.1111/imr.12503.
4. Afshar Y, Yin O, Jeong A, Martinez G, Kim J, Ma F, Jang C, Tabatabaei S, You S, Tseng HR, Zhu Y, Krakow D. Placenta accreta spectrum disorder at single-cell resolution: a loss of boundary limits in the decidua and endothelium. Am J Obstet Gynecol. 2024;230(4):443.e1–443.e18. https://doi.org/10.1016/j.ajog.2023.10.001. Epub 2024 Jan 30. PMID: 38296740.
5. Aghaeepour N, Ganio EA, Mcilwain D, Tsai AS, Tingle M, Van Gassen S, Gaudilliere DK, Baca Q, McNeil L, Okada R, Ghaemi MS, Furman D, Wong RJ, Winn VD, Druzin ML, El-Sayed YY, Quaintance C, Gibbs R, Darmstadt GL, Shaw GM, Stevenson DK, Tibshirani R, Nolan GP, Lewis DB, Angst MS, Gaudilliere B. An immune clock of human pregnancy. Sci Immunol. 2017;2(15):eaan2946. https://doi.org/10.1126/sciimmunol.aan2946. PMID: 28864494; PMCID: PMC5701281.
6. Caligioni C. Assessing reproductive status/stages in mice. Curr Protocols Neurosci/Editorial Board, Jacqueline N. Crawley ... [et Al.], APPENDIX, Appendix-4I. 2009; https://doi.org/10.1002/0471142301.nsa04is48.
7. Chou IC, Voit EO. Recent developments in parameter estimation and structure identification of biochemical and genomic systems. Math Biosci. 2009;219(2):57–83. https://doi.org/10.1016/j.mbs.2009.03.002. Epub 2009 Mar 25. PMID: 19327372; PMCID: PMC2693292.
8. Chung AW, Kumar MP, Arnold KB, Yu WH, Schoen MK, Dunphy LJ, Suscovich TJ, Frahm N, Linde C, Mahan AE, Hoffner M, Streeck H, Ackerman ME, McElrath MJ, Schuitemaker H, Pau MG, Baden LR, Kim JH, Michael NL, Alter G. Dissecting polyclonal vaccine-induced humoral immunity against HIV using systems serology. Cell. 2015;163(4):988–98. https://doi.org/10.1016/j.cell.2015.10.027.
9. Clements T, Rice TF, Vamvakas G, Barnett S, Barnes M, Donaldson B, Jones CE, Kampmann B, Holder B. Update on transplacental transfer of IgG subclasses: impact of maternal and fetal factors. Front Immunol. 2020;11 https://doi.org/10.3389/fimmu.2020.01920.
10. Dari A, Boulton M, Neyens M, Le Gars M, Valenzuela B, Shukarev G, Cárdenas V, Ruiz-Guiñazú J, Sadoff J, Hoetelmans RMW, Ruixo JJP. Quantifying antibody persistence after a single dose of COVID-19 vaccine Ad26.COV2.S in humans using a mechanistic modeling and simulation approach. Clin Pharmacol Ther. 2023;113(2):380–9. https://doi.org/10.1002/cpt.2796.
11. de Medeiros SF, Yamamoto MMW, de Medeiros MAS, Yamamoto AKLW, Barbosa BB. Polycystic ovary syndrome and risks for COVID-19 infection: a comprehensive review: PCOS and COVID-19 relationship. Rev Endocr Metab Disord. 2022;23(2):251–64. https://doi.org/10.1007/s11154-022-09715-y.
12. Dolatshahi S, Butler AL, Siedner MJ, Ngonzi J, Edlow AG, Adong J, Jennewein MF, Atyeo C, Bassett IV, Roberts DJ, Lauffenburger DA, Alter G, Bebell LM. Altered maternal antibody profiles in women with human immunodeficiency virus drive changes in transplacental antibody transfer. Clin Infect Dis. 2022;75(8):1359–69. https://doi.org/10.1093/cid/ciac156. PMID: 35245365; PMCID: PMC9555842.
13. Dolatshahi S, Butler AL, Pou C, Henckel E, Bernhardsson AK, Gustafsson A, Bohlin K, Shin SA, Lauffenburger DA, Brodin P, Alter G. Selective transfer of maternal antibodies in preterm and fullterm children. Sci Rep. 2022;12(1):14937. https://doi.org/10.1038/s41598-022-18973-4. PMID: 36056073; PMCID: PMC9440225.
14. Gajdos ZKZ, Henderson KD, Hirschhorn JN, Palmert MR. Genetic determinants of pubertal timing in the general population. Mol Cell Endocrinol. 2010;324(1–2):21–9. https://doi.org/10.1016/j.mce.2010.01.038.
15. Gao L, Gu Y, Yin X. High serum tumor necrosis factor-alpha levels in women with polycystic ovary syndrome: a meta-analysis. PLoS One. 2016;11(10):e0164021. https://doi.org/10.1371/journal.pone.0164021.
16. Gibson EA, Li H, Fruh V, Gabra M, Asokan G, Jukic AMZ, Baird DD, Curry CL, Fischer-Colbrie T, Onnela J-P, Williams MA, Hauser R, Coull BA, Mahalingaiah S. Covid-19 vaccination and menstrual cycle length in the apple women's health study. Npj Digit Med. 2022;5(1):165. https://doi.org/10.1038/s41746-022-00711-9.

17. Grimaldi CM, Cleary J, Dagtas AS, Moussai D, Diamond B. Estrogen alters thresholds for B cell apoptosis and activation. J Clin Invest. 2002;109(12):1625–33. https://doi.org/10.1172/JCI14873.
18. Ishikawa T, Takizawa T, Iwaki J, Mishima T, Ui-Tei K, Takeshita T, Matsubara S, Takizawa T. Fc gamma receptor IIb participates in maternal IgG trafficking of human placental endothelial cells. Int J Mol Med. 2015;35(5):1273–89. https://doi.org/10.3892/ijmm.2015.2141.
19. Jennewein MF, Goldfarb I, Dolatshahi S, Cosgrove C, Noelette FJ, Krykbaeva M, Das J, Sarkar A, Gorman MJ, Fischinger S, Boudreau CM, Brown J, Cooperrider JH, Aneja J, Suscovich TJ, Graham BS, Lauer GM, Goetghebuer T, Marchant A, Lauffenburger D, Kim AY, Riley LE, Alter G. Fc Glycan-mediated regulation of placental antibody transfer. Cell. 2019;178(1):202–215.e14. https://doi.org/10.1016/j.cell.2019.05.044. Epub 2019 Jun 13. PMID: 31204102; PMCID: PMC6741440.
20. Jiang W, Tang Y, Yang R, Long Y, Sun C, Han T, Wei W. Maternal smoking, nutritional factors at different life stage, and the risk of incident type 2 diabetes: a prospective study of the UK Biobank. BMC Med. 2024;22(1):50. https://doi.org/10.1186/s12916-024-03256-8. PMID: 38302923; PMCID: PMC10835913.
21. Joslyn LR, Kirschner DE, Linderman JJ. CaliPro: a calibration protocol that utilizes parameter density estimation to explore parameter space and calibrate complex biological models. Cell Mol Bioeng. 2021;14(1):31–47. https://doi.org/10.1007/s12195-020-00650-z.
22. Kim JH, Scialli AR. Thalidomide: the tragedy of birth defects and the effective treatment of disease. Toxicol Sci. 2011;122(1):1–6. https://doi.org/10.1093/toxsci/kfr088. Epub 2011 Apr 19. Erratum in: Toxicol Sci. 2012;125(2):613. PMID: 21507989.
23. Lakshmikanth T, Consiglio C, Sardh F, Forlin R, Wang J, Tan Z, Barcenilla H, Rodriguez L, Sugrue J, Noori P, Ivanchenko M, Piñero Páez L, Gonzalez L, Habimana Mugabo C, Johnsson A, Ryberg H, Hallgren Å, Pou C, Chen Y, Brodin P. Immune system adaptation during gender-affirming testosterone treatment. Nature. 2024;633(8028):155–64. https://doi.org/10.1038/s41586-024-07789-z.
24. Lauffenburger DA. The multiple dimensions of Integrative Biology. Integr Biol. 2012;4(1):9–9. https://doi.org/10.1039/c1ib90041b.
25. Malek A, Sager R, Kuhn P, Nicolaides KH, Schneider H. Evolution of maternofetal transport of immunoglobulins during human pregnancy. Am J Reprod Immunol. 1996;36(5):248–55. https://doi.org/10.1111/j.1600-0897.1996.tb00172.x. PMID: 8955500.
26. Moley K. Closing the gender health gap is a $1 trillion opportunity. Biopharma Dealmakers. 2024; https://doi.org/10.1038/d43747-024-00021-x.
27. Papadimitriou A, Papadimitriou DT. Endocrine-disrupting chemicals and early puberty in girls. Children. 2021;8(6):492. https://doi.org/10.3390/children8060492.
28. Pham G, Shao T-Y, Kinder JM, Peng Y, Turner LH, Way SS. Pregnancy induced displacement of preexisting microchimeric cells in the absence of maternal B and T cells. Front Immunol. 2024;15:1478465. https://doi.org/10.3389/fimmu.2024.1478465.
29. Ramezani Tehrani F, Mirmiran P, Gholami R, Moslehi N, Azizi F. Factors influencing Menarcheal age: results from the Cohort of Tehran Lipid And Glucose Study. Int J Endocrinol Metab. 2014;12(3):e16130. https://doi.org/10.5812/ijem.16130.
30. Rudolph M, Döcke W-D, Müller A, Menning A, Röse L, Zollner TM, Gashaw I. Induction of overt menstruation in intact mice. PLoS One. 2012;7(3):e32922. https://doi.org/10.1371/journal.pone.0032922.
31. Schlaudecker EP, Ambroggio L, McNeal MM, Finkelman FD, Way SS. Declining responsiveness to influenza vaccination with progression of human pregnancy. Vaccine. 2018;36(31):4734–41. https://doi.org/10.1016/j.vaccine.2018.05.117. Epub 2018 Jun 22. PMID: 29941326; PMCID: PMC6295331.
32. Seillet C, Laffont S, Trémollières F, Rouquié N, Ribot C, Arnal J-F, Douin-Echinard V, Gourdy P, Guéry J-C. The TLR-mediated response of plasmacytoid dendritic cells is positively regulated by estradiol in vivo through cell-intrinsic estrogen receptor α signaling. Blood. 2012;119(2):454–64. https://doi.org/10.1182/blood-2011-08-371831.

33. Sosinsky AZ, Rich-Edwards JW, Wiley A, Wright K, Spagnolo PA, Joffe H. Enrollment of female participants in United States drug and device phase 1-3 clinical trials between 2016 and 2019. Contemp Clin Trials. 2022;115:106718. https://doi.org/10.1016/j.cct.2022.106718.
34. Taton M, Willems F, Widomski C, Martin C, Jiang Y, Renard K, Cogan A, Necsoi C, Ackerman ME, Marchant A, Dauby N. Impact of pregnancy on polyfunctional IgG and memory B cell responses to Tdap immunization. Vaccine. 2023;41(27):4009–18. https://doi.org/10.1016/j.vaccine.2023.05.035. Epub 2023 May 25. PMID: 37244810.
35. van der Lee S, van Rooijen DM, de Zeeuw-Brouwer M-L, Bogaard MJM, van Gageldonk PGM, Marinovic AB, Sanders EAM, Berbers GAM, Buisman A-M. Robust humoral and cellular immune responses to pertussis in adults after a first acellular booster vaccination. Front Immunol. 2018;9 https://doi.org/10.3389/fimmu.2018.00681.
36. Vento-Tormo R, Efremova M, Botting RA, Turco MY, Vento-Tormo M, Meyer KB, Park J-E, Stephenson E, Polański K, Goncalves A, Gardner L, Holmqvist S, Henriksson J, Zou A, Sharkey AM, Millar B, Innes B, Wood L, Wilbrey-Clark A, Teichmann SA. Single-cell reconstruction of the early maternal–fetal interface in humans. Nature. 2018;563(7731):347–53. https://doi.org/10.1038/s41586-018-0698-6.
37. Voit EO. A first course in systems biology. 2nd ed. Garland Science; 2017. https://doi.org/10.4324/9780203702260.
38. Warkany J. Why I doubted that thalidomide was the cause of the epidemic of limb defects of 1959 to 1961. Teratology. 1988;38:217–9.
39. Wessel RE, Dolatshahi S. Quantitative mechanistic model reveals key determinants of placental IgG transfer and informs prenatal immunization strategies. PLoS Comput Biol. 2023;19(11): e1011109. https://doi.org/10.1371/journal.pcbi.1011109. PMID: 37934786; PMCID: PMC10656024.
40. Wessel RE, Dolatshahi S. Regulators of placental antibody transfer through a modeling lens. Nat Immunol. 2024;25(11):2024–2036. https://doi.org/10.1038/s41590-024-01971-1. Epub 2024 Oct 8. PMID: 39379658; PMCID: PMC12306195.
41. White MT, Griffin JT, Akpogheneta O, Conway DJ, Koram KA, Riley EM, Ghani AC. Dynamics of the antibody response to plasmodium falciparum infection in African children. J Infect Dis. 2014;210(7):1115–22. https://doi.org/10.1093/infdis/jiu219.
42. Yu EJ, Choe S-A, Yun J-W, Son M. Association of early menarche with adolescent health in the setting of rapidly decreasing age at menarche. J Pediatr Adolesc Gynecol. 2020;33(3):264–70. https://doi.org/10.1016/j.jpag.2019.12.006.
43. Zhang H, Tang Y, Tao J. Sex-related overactivation of NLRP3 inflammasome increases lethality of the male COVID-19 patients. Front Mol Biosci. 2021;8 https://doi.org/10.3389/fmolb.2021.671363.

Index

A

Adipose tissue-derived stem cells (ASCs), 291
Aging, 8, 37, 45, 72, 122, 129–132, 136–137, 151, 169, 186, 349, 366, 372, 373, 377–379, 412, 434, 438–446, 539, 573
Amnion, 186, 187, 324–340, 344–346, 348–350, 570, 582
Angiogenesis, 93–96, 103, 127, 130, 207, 238, 239, 283, 287, 290, 295, 297, 330, 331, 335, 338, 343, 344, 368, 376, 396, 419, 436, 437, 442–445, 494, 498–500, 502, 504, 536, 557, 585, 618

B

Biodistribution, 469–475, 526, 561
Biofabrication, 223, 450
Biological barriers, 469, 470, 526, 557, 562
Biologic grafts, 24, 73, 99–105
Biomaterials, 7, 36, 60, 73, 137, 151, 195, 219, 235, 261, 279, 313, 324, 366, 403, 411, 446, 462, 495, 520, 544, 558, 578, 608
Biomaterials science, 64, 524
Biomechanics, 3–31, 67, 149–169, 185, 210, 267, 313
Biomimicking, 315
Bioprinting, 64, 219, 223, 270, 316, 448, 450, 557, 577–592
Bone, 5, 84, 182, 233, 281, 330, 366, 394, 410, 436, 502, 535, 582, 606
Bone formation, 345, 367–370, 376, 379, 398, 418
Bone injury, 365, 366, 374–376
Bone regeneration, 102, 336, 342, 343, 369, 379, 380, 416, 420, 424, 545
Breast cancer, 420, 422, 513–528, 557, 573, 583, 590

C

Calcific aortic valve disease (CAVD), 434–452
Cervix, 5, 36, 61, 121, 149, 185, 210, 270, 489, 568, 579, 605
Chorion, 186, 324–330, 332, 334–341, 344–346, 348–350, 570
Collagen, 5, 38, 62, 82, 123, 150, 186, 214, 242, 263, 286, 310, 325, 367, 396, 418, 434, 497, 526, 542, 566, 582, 618
Computational immunology, 598, 609–613
Computational models, 30, 106, 310, 318–319, 603, 607, 609, 610, 613, 620–622
Controlled drug delivery, 491
Controlled hormone release, 416

D

Data-driven modeling, 611, 613, 614
Diagnostic devices, 12–20
Diagnostics, 3–31, 165, 166, 234, 444–446, 452, 465, 515, 520, 521, 533, 534, 542–545, 559, 562–563, 565, 572, 573, 614, 619, 621
Diffusion, 38, 242, 261, 269, 283, 318, 319, 443, 492, 616
Digital twin of a woman, 614, 620, 621

S. G. Zambuto, M. L. Oyen (eds.), *Biomaterials for Women's Health Engineering*, https://doi.org/10.1007/978-3-032-10745-9

Drug delivery, 38, 66, 107, 316, 416, 419, 461–481, 487, 488, 492–494, 497, 499, 502, 503, 506, 513–528, 533, 556, 559, 561–563
Drug delivery systems (DDS), 466, 471, 487–506, 521–523, 525–527, 561

E
ECM remodeling, 42–46, 185–187, 194, 263, 326, 436, 437, 440, 444, 445, 449, 501, 526
Elastic fibers, 38–41, 43–45, 194, 441, 442, 541
Endometriosis, 164, 209, 232, 467, 488, 532, 572, 620
Endothelial cells (ECs), 124, 134, 165, 188, 207, 238, 239, 244, 261, 269, 289, 291–293, 295, 296, 310, 327, 330, 331, 338, 339, 341, 434–438, 442, 469, 476, 497, 500, 568, 570, 578, 612, 616–618
Endothelial dysfunction, 440, 442
Engineering technology, 555–573
Estrogen, 6, 42, 76, 127, 206, 232, 306, 367, 396, 410, 437, 494, 515, 599
Estrogen (17β-estradiol, E2), 412, 416, 502
Exosomes, 325, 531–546
Extensibility, 8, 12, 20, 152, 155, 156, 158–159, 162
Extracellular matrix (ECM), 35, 62, 91, 124, 150, 182, 207, 241, 261, 285, 310, 326, 372, 411, 434, 495, 526, 561, 578

F
FemTech, 4, 5, 7, 9, 25–27, 29, 30
Fetal membrane, 166, 185–187, 496
Fibrosis, 23, 76, 81, 83, 86, 88, 91, 93, 96, 100, 102, 108, 182, 234, 243, 283, 288, 289, 292, 334, 336, 343, 435, 437, 440, 441, 444, 448, 449, 468, 498, 499, 501, 534–536, 584
Follicle culture, 259–271

G
Genitourinary syndrome of menopause, 8
Graft revascularization, 279, 281, 283–285, 287, 288, 290–293, 295–298
Granular hydrogels, 295–297
Growth and remodeling, 197
Growth factors, 41, 95, 96, 99, 102, 125, 188–190, 239, 261, 263, 268, 286, 293–295, 306, 316, 324, 331, 333, 338, 341, 343, 346, 350, 373, 374, 379, 380, 382, 383, 444, 495, 496, 500, 502, 504, 566, 589
Gynecology, 46, 62

H
Homeostasis, 41, 45, 129, 150, 166, 366, 373, 376, 412, 414, 434, 436, 437, 447, 449, 499, 607
Hormones, 7, 44, 66, 75, 131, 191, 206, 233, 269, 278, 367, 394, 411, 452, 467, 491, 515, 532, 572, 586, 605
Host response, 73, 79–96, 100–102, 105
Hydrogel scaffolds, 267, 268, 295, 296, 496–503

I
Infertility, 164, 165, 206, 212, 232, 278, 297, 488, 533, 534, 537–540, 543, 545, 583, 592
Inflammation, 7, 13, 81, 83, 91, 93, 96, 97, 103, 105, 107, 220, 221, 233, 234, 285, 287, 333, 334, 350, 374, 398, 419, 420, 435, 437, 440–443, 478, 492, 518, 533, 534, 536, 538, 541, 585, 599, 602, 612
Integrative approaches, 603, 613
Intrauterine devices (IUDs), 14, 488–491, 494, 503, 506
In vitro, 66, 95, 168, 186, 206, 236, 261, 282, 313, 334, 366, 414, 436, 475, 492, 537, 560, 577, 603
In vitro folliculogenesis, 260–263, 267–270
In vitro models, 66, 105, 196, 197, 236, 237, 239, 242, 244, 316–318, 383, 443, 449, 495, 496, 588, 591, 592
In vivo mechanical testing, 9, 10
Ischemia, 197, 283, 285, 295, 476, 478
Isthmus, 121, 122, 127, 130–132, 153

L
Lactation, 395–397, 399, 401, 403, 410, 590, 591

M
Maternal-fetal immunology, 613, 622
Mechanical signaling, 187, 196
Mechanistic modeling, 609, 612–614, 616, 617, 619
Mechanobiology, 181–197, 219–223, 452

Mechanotransduction, 151, 182, 184, 187, 190, 194–197, 216, 217, 398, 449
Menopause, 6–8, 25, 29, 43–45, 48, 62, 65, 66, 96, 129, 130, 163, 232, 379, 395, 397–399, 402, 411, 412, 434, 439, 488, 515, 573, 586, 588, 591, 592, 599, 600, 606
Menstrual cycle, 42, 43, 124, 126, 130–132, 135, 150, 189, 191, 206, 210, 211, 213, 214, 233, 235, 246, 278, 395–397, 412, 414, 416, 536, 537, 561, 572, 583, 586, 591, 599, 606, 616, 620
Mesenchymal stem cells (MSCs), 96, 290, 291, 324, 327, 330, 335, 338–343, 345, 373, 374, 376, 412, 417, 424, 497–500, 521, 534, 536–542, 544, 545, 581–583, 585
Microfluidics, 67, 222, 223, 242, 246, 248, 270, 313, 316–319, 448, 450, 451, 556–558, 562–565, 568–570, 573
Microphysiological systems (MPSs), 316, 560
MicroRNA (miRNA), 472, 493, 498, 517, 532–534, 536, 545
Modeling, 87, 218, 222, 231–248, 313, 318, 319, 342, 374, 421, 447–451, 514, 556, 559, 562, 563, 569–573, 577, 579, 587, 590, 591, 598, 601, 603, 605, 606, 609–619, 621, 622
Myofibroblast activation, 436, 445, 449
Myometrial contractility, 205–224, 579, 585

N
Nanocarriers, 520–523, 526
Nanoformulation, 520, 522, 523, 525–528
Nanomedicine, 467, 519–524
Nanoparticles, 221, 224, 247, 296, 334, 337, 339, 342, 417–420, 462, 465–469, 495, 520–524, 526, 545, 621
Nanotechnology, 520
Natural and synthetic polymers, 60, 242, 265, 266, 314, 329, 330, 380–382, 495–504, 506, 566
New approach methodologies (NAMs), 559, 560, 621
Nucleic acids, 328, 462, 464, 467–469, 472, 532, 545

O
Obstetrics, 23, 72, 121, 127, 150, 163–169, 186, 196, 213, 473, 476, 479–481, 619
Organoids, 218–219, 313–316, 319, 330, 332, 420, 495, 496, 560, 563, 568, 578, 588–591, 621
Organ-on-a-chip (OoC), 67, 448, 451, 555–573, 608, 621
Orthopedic tissues, 409–425
Osteoblast, 367–376, 379, 380, 382, 398, 417–419, 421, 422
Osteoclast, 370, 371, 373–376, 378, 398, 401, 417, 418
Osteogenic differentiation, 332, 340, 342, 345, 368, 376, 418, 420, 441–443
Osteoporosis, 278, 372, 378, 379, 383, 402, 416, 417, 519
Ovarian cancer, 468, 489, 513–528, 542, 543, 546, 570, 572, 580
Ovarian tissue transplantation, 277–298

P
Pelvic floor, 4–7, 10, 12, 13, 15, 16, 20–22, 28–30, 44, 48, 72, 77, 534, 546, 585
Pelvic floor disorders, 4, 16, 20, 21, 541
Pelvic floor dysfunction (PFD), 7, 16, 22, 533, 534, 541–542, 546
Pelvic organ prolapse (POP), 7, 12, 14, 15, 17, 18, 24, 28, 45, 48, 72, 76, 77, 107, 541
Physicochemical properties, 465, 471
Placenta, 126, 160, 185, 215, 306, 324, 367, 396, 412, 462, 498, 533, 562, 605
Placental disc, 324, 325, 327–332, 344, 346, 350, 351
Polycystic ovary syndrome (PCOS), 236, 261, 267, 532–534, 537–538
Polymeric drug delivery, 466
Population heterogeneity, 618, 619
Postpartum, 9, 11, 42–43, 45, 48, 122, 128, 135–137, 151, 168, 185, 191, 195, 196, 206, 207, 211, 213, 217, 396, 397, 400, 401, 599
Postpartum remodeling, 217
Precision maternal care, 622
Precision medicine, 573, 609, 620–621
Preeclampsia, 185, 188, 190, 306, 312, 396, 532–534, 540–543, 584, 590, 591
Pregnancy, 4, 37, 61, 122, 150, 182, 206, 233, 281, 306, 324, 367, 395, 410, 462, 489, 533, 561, 584, 597
Pregnancy and parturition, 42–43, 47, 168, 185, 205, 206
Pregnancy modeling, 471
Progesterone, 42, 127, 192, 193, 195, 196, 206, 210, 211, 215, 216, 233, 261, 306, 367, 370, 373, 395, 399, 412–416, 425, 515, 589, 599–601
Prolactin, 396, 397, 399

R

Receptor-mediated drug delivery, 493
Regenerative medicine, 59–61, 292, 297, 324, 325, 330, 338, 342, 344, 350, 380, 386, 425, 533, 544, 577, 580
Reperfusion, 278, 283, 285, 287, 290–291, 298
Reproductive biology, 600
Reproductive health, 37, 151, 169, 197, 531–546, 562, 566, 572, 573, 580, 585, 586, 600, 601, 619

S

Selective estrogen receptor modulators (SERMs), 413, 414, 419, 420, 425
Sex-based differences, 380–386, 410, 445, 448
Sex differences, 365–386, 394, 403, 410–411, 415, 421, 424, 425, 436, 437, 439, 446, 448, 452, 573
Sex hormone bioavailability, 414
Sex-informed biomaterial design, 411
Sex steroid hormones, 402, 412–416, 499
Smooth muscle cells, 38, 40, 62, 64–66, 131, 134, 150, 151, 165, 185, 191–195, 206–209, 214–219, 223, 327, 341, 422, 569
Stem cells, 60, 95, 124, 219, 237, 269, 295, 313, 324, 367, 411, 496, 542, 558, 583
Stiffness, 17, 40, 64, 80, 136, 152, 182, 217, 241, 261, 296, 315, 327, 383, 400, 424, 439, 496, 561, 566, 585, 622
Strength, 5, 8, 15, 20–22, 25, 29, 39, 45, 62, 64, 65, 73, 74, 77, 81, 83, 93, 97, 100, 102, 103, 106, 152, 155, 156, 158–159, 162, 186, 211, 212, 266, 329, 331, 333, 338, 372, 378, 379, 383, 394, 403, 410, 411, 434, 501, 584, 585
Sustained drug delivery, 524
Synthetic mesh, 24, 73, 76–101, 103–105, 107, 546
Systems biology, 597–622

T

Testosterone, 367, 370, 371, 373, 379, 412–416, 425, 437, 537, 538, 599, 600
Therapeutic devices, 7, 12, 20–25, 30
Therapeutics, 7, 94, 169, 197, 218, 233, 343, 380, 409, 441, 462, 492, 515, 532, 559, 577, 617
Therapy, 7, 76, 245, 278, 324, 370, 413, 465, 491, 515, 533, 577, 599
Three dimensional (3D), 36, 125, 194, 197, 214, 223, 241, 246, 261, 313, 315, 316, 318, 329, 452, 467, 495, 496, 556, 557, 569, 581, 586
Time-dependence, 155, 156, 159–160, 162
Tissue engineering, 48, 59, 103, 137, 219, 244, 270, 292, 313, 324, 366, 403, 421, 446, 501, 520, 557, 577
Tissue models, 439, 578, 580, 587
Tissue regeneration, 102, 329, 333, 411, 421, 494–503, 580, 581, 585
Tissue remodeling, 20, 105, 107, 169, 185, 196, 263, 338, 411, 414, 416, 435, 565
Tissue-specific hormone production, 412
Transplacental antibody transfer, 615
Trophoblast, 127, 186, 188–190, 307, 308, 312–314, 316, 317, 319, 325, 330, 340, 349, 476, 479–480, 498, 533, 539, 540, 569–571, 582, 584, 601, 602, 616, 618

U

Uterine cancer, 489, 494, 503
Uterine fibroids, 129, 164–165, 192, 193, 206, 209, 217–219, 223, 488, 492, 503, 546
Uterine peristalsis, 126, 205–224
Uterus, 6, 42, 64, 72, 121, 149, 185, 205, 235, 270, 282, 312, 397, 415, 476, 487, 534, 578

V

Vagina, 5, 36, 61, 72, 121, 150, 194, 212, 415, 489, 541, 571, 578
Vaginal extracellular matrix, 35–48, 67, 102
Vaginal health, 3–31
Vaginal wall structure, 37

W

Women's health, 4, 9, 29–31, 108, 514, 520, 534, 546, 555–573, 598–601, 603–607, 609, 613, 616, 619–621
Women's health immunoengineering, 619–620
Women's reproductive health, 531–546, 562, 566, 572, 600, 619
Wound repair, 39, 96, 97, 324, 328, 332, 334–336, 338–340, 342, 344, 345, 349

X

Xenograft, 99, 100, 284–292, 297, 366, 480, 527

MIX
Papier aus verantwortungsvollen Quellen
Paper from responsible sources
FSC® C105338

If you have any concerns about our products,
you can contact us on
ProductSafety@springernature.com

In case Publisher is established outside the EU,
the EU authorized representative is:
Springer Nature Customer Service Center GmbH
Europaplatz 3, 69115 Heidelberg, Germany

Printed by Libri Plureos GmbH
in Hamburg, Germany